D1310740

ULTRASTRUCTURAL PATHOLOGY OF THE CELL

A Text and Atlas of Physiological and Pathological Alterations in Cell Fine Structure

FEROZE N. GHADIALLY

M.D., Ph.D., D.Sc.(Lond.), M.R.C.Path.

Professor and Joint Head of Pathology, University of Saskatchewan, Saskatoon, Canada
Formerly Reader in Neoplastic Diseases and Senior Lecturer in Experimental Pathology, University of Sheffield, England

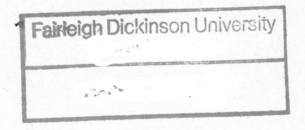
BUTTERWORTHS

London and Boston

THE BUTTERWORTH GROUP

ENGLAND

Butterworth & Co (Publishers) Ltd
London: 88 Kingsway, WC2B 6AB

AUSTRALIA

Butterworth Pty Ltd
Sydney: 586 Pacific Highway, NSW 2067
Melbourne: 343 Little Collins Street, 3000
Brisbane: Commonwealth Bank Building,
  King George Square, 4000

SOUTH AFRICA

Butterworth & Co (South Africa) (Pty) Ltd
Durban: 152–154 Gale Street

NEW ZEALAND

Butterworths of New Zealand Ltd
Wellington: 26–28 Waring Taylor Street, 1

CANADA

Butterworth & Co (Canada) Ltd
Toronto: 2265 Midland Avenue,
  Scarborough, Ontario, M1P 4S1

USA

Butterworths (Publishers) Inc
161 Ash Street,
Reading, Mass. 01867

First published 1975

© Feroze M. Ghadially, 1975

ISBN 0 407 00011 9

Library of Congress Cataloging in Publication Data
Ghadially, Feroze Novroji, 1920–
    Ultrastructural pathology of the cell.

    Bibliography: p.
    Includes index.
    1. Pathology, Cellular. I. Title.
[DNLM: 1. Cells. 2. Cytology-Atlases. 3. Pathology. 4. Pathology-Atlases.
QZ4 G411u]
RB25.G4   599'.08'765   75-14308
ISBN 0-407-00011-9

Printed in England by Page Bros (Norwich) Ltd

Preface

There can hardly be a disease or pathological process where electron microscopy has not added new details and dimensions to existing knowledge. The innumerable published papers and books on the ultrastructure of tissues altered by disease or experimental procedures bear eloquent testimony to the many major contributions made by this technique.

Although the student interested in the pathology of certain systems, organs, and tissues such as liver (David, 1964), muscle (Mair and Tomé, 1972), synovial joints (Ghadially and Roy, 1969), kidney (Dalton and Haguenau, 1967) and peripheral nervous system (Babel *et al.*, 1970) is now catered for and excellent books dealing with the ultrastructure of normal cells and tissues are available (e.g. Fawcett, 1967; Porter and Bonneville, 1973; Lentz, 1971; Rhodin, 1974), there is as yet no book from which one may learn in a systematic fashion about the numerous changes that occur in cellular organelles and inclusions as a result of disease or experimental procedures. On confronting an unfamiliar or unknown morphological alteration in some particular cellular structure the questions that arise are: (1) has this been seen before? (2) if so, in what situations has such a change been seen? (3) what is the significance of the change? and (4) how can one retrieve information on this point from the formidable, scattered literature on the ultrastructure of normal and pathological tissues?

It is my hope that this book will help to answer such questions and serve as a brief textbook and atlas of cellular pathology at the ultrastructural level. Within its covers I have collected, classified, described and illustrated various alterations that are known to occur in cellular organelles and inclusions as a result of changing physiological states, diseases and experimental situations.

In keeping with the traditional practice adopted in many past pathology texts, each chapter commences with a discourse on normal structure and function. This is followed by essays devoted to various morphological alterations that have hitherto been witnessed. The introduction and preliminary essays on well known normal structures (e.g. nucleus and mitochondria) are, of necessity, brief. They do little more than set the scene and outline the classification and nomenclature employed. The advanced electron microscopist may find that some of the passages in these essays are of a rather elementary nature, but this material is included on the assumption that some readers may not be too familiar with current electron microscopic concepts and topics. Less well known normal structures (e.g. rod-shaped tubular bodies and nuclear bodies) are dealt with more fully, for information on such structures is often not easy to find and unfamiliarity with such structures is likely to lead to errors of interpretation.

The sections dealing with morphological alterations and lesions follow a fairly standard pattern in most instances. A brief introduction dealing with matters such as definition, nomenclature, correlations with light microscopy, and historical aspects of the subject is followed by a morphological description supported by accompanying illustrations. After this comes a section where I have listed the sites and situations in which the particular morphological alteration has been seen and the authors who have reported its occurrence. This section often contains numerous references. (Some readers may find these lists irksome, but they are essential for the research worker and student seeking further information.) Then follows a discussion and interpretation of the morphological change under survey. The principle I have followed here is to present as many known theories and ideas as possible even though I may not be in sympathy with some of them. I have also often indicated what I have come to think about the matter as a result of my own studies and reading of the literature. However, I do not feel that an author should judge every issue, and I have, at times, done little more than report as faithfully as I can the views propounded by others. Not all essays follow the above-mentioned pattern for there are instances where the story is told more profitably within a different format. For example, instead of devoting a section to every change in mitochondrial morphology which has been suspected as representing an involuting or degenerating mitochondrion, I have collected these changes into a section entitled 'mitochondrial involution and elimination'.

One of the functions I would like this book to serve is as a gateway to the relevant literature. Since this is not a book primarily devoted to normal structure and function (even though a substantial number of pages are devoted to such matters), the references in sections dealing with well known normal structures are somewhat sparse. When dealing with little known normal structures or with alterations and lesions, I have tried to include virtually every reference on the subject that I am aware of. When such citations are few they are all presented in the text; when too many, I have included review articles and also tried to include the earliest and latest paper on the topic.

Although the format is designed primarily for those who examine pathological tissues with the electron microscope, I hope that this book will also be of interest to the teacher of pathology and the practising pathologist. This book is not for the individual who has no knowledge of cell fine structure at all (there can be few who fall into this category today!) nor is it for the expert ultrastructural pathologist. It is addressed to the much larger intermediate group of workers who may wish to acquire a basic knowledge of general ultrastructural pathology on which they may pursue their own special interests with greater confidence and a wider understanding.

The teacher of pathology attempting to relate classical pathology with the now familiar concepts of cell ultrastructure has had to search through a wide variety of books and journals and at best may only find patchy information. The hospital pathologist, similarly, has up to now had little reason to embark on the exhausting pursuit through the published literature, often in journals which are not on his usual reading list, in search of clues which might lead to a better understanding, or an earlier or more precise diagnosis of human disease. However, in some fields such as the interpretation of the liver, renal and muscle biopsy and the diagnosis of viral and storage diseases and certain tumours the electron microscope is already proving its worth. The scope of electron microscopy will undoubtedly extend into wider areas of diagnostic histopathology. Further, more and more papers in journals of pathology now incorporate the results of ultrastructural studies, and the reader unfamiliar with the range and limitations of electron microscope technology may well be at a loss in attempting to interpret published work.

Today it is not possible to present to the student an up-to-date account of many pathological processes and disease states without discussing ultrastructural changes. Cell injury, cloudy swelling, necrosis, fatty degeneration of the liver, the detoxification of many drugs by the liver, brown atrophy of the heart and lipofuscin, pigmentary disorders of the skin and melanomas, haemorrhage, haemosiderin, erythrophagocytosis and siderosomes, glycogen storage diseases, lipoidosis, Wilson's disease, silicosis, rheumatoid arthritis and melanosis coli are all better understood by virtue of a knowledge of the underlying fine structural changes.

Correlations between light and electron microscopic findings are singularly interesting and satisfying and I have lost no opportunity of dwelling upon such matters. However, the function of electron microscopy is not simply the resolving of old controversies bequeathed by light microscopists. Electron microscopy is a science in its own right with its practitioners, problems and preoccupations. Many structures such as the endoplasmic reticulum and polyribosomes were unheard of in the light microscopic era, while the structural details of others such as the nucleolus, centrioles and cilia were but poorly resolved. The presence of the nuclear envelope and the cell membrane were suspected and the existence of the Golgi complex doubted. Clearly, alterations in such structures belong to the realms of ultrastructural pathology, and correlations with light microscopy are often tenuous and at times non-existent. Such findings may not have a direct appeal to the light microscopist but such matters cannot be ignored for they have materially altered our thinking about cellular physiology and pathology. Indeed, the main preoccupation of this book is with such matters, but I hope that I have presented this material in a manner which will make interesting reading for both light and electron microscopists.

F.N.G.

REFERENCES

Babel, J., Bischoff, A. and Spoendlin, H. (1970). *Ultrastructure of the Peripheral Nervous System and Sense Organs.* Stuttgart: Georg Thieme
Dalton, A. J. and Haguenau, F. (1967). *Ultrastructure of the Kidney.* New York and London: Academic Press
David, H. (1964). *Submicroscopic Ortho- and Patho-Morphology of the Liver.* Oxford: Pergamon Press
Fawcett, D. W. (1967). *The Cell: Its Organelles and Inclusions.* Philadelphia and London: Saunders
Ghadially, F. N. and Roy, S. (1969): *Ultrastructure of Synovial Joints in Health and Disease.* London: Butterworths
Lentz, T. L. (1971). *Cell Fine Structure.* Philadelphia and London: Saunders.
Mair, W. G. P. and Tomé, F. M. S. (1972). *Atlas of the Ultrastructure of Diseased Human Muscle.* Edinburgh and London: Churchill Livingstone
Porter, K. R. and Bonneville, M. A. (1973). *Fine Structure of Cells and Tissues,* 4th Edn. Philadelphia: Lea and Febiger
Rhodin, J. A. G. (1974). *Histology.* New York and London: Oxford University Press

Acknowledgements

Some of the material included in this book stems from research projects executed by my co-workers and myself. This work was supported by the Medical Research Council of Canada and the Canadian Arthritis and Rheumatism Society. I thank these organizations for their support.

It is my pleasant duty also to acknowledge the help given by my friends and colleagues Dr. O. G. Dodge, Dr. E. I. Grodums, Dr. T. E. Larsen, Dr. J. W. Newstead, Dr. E. W. Parry and Dr. L. F. Skinnider who read through whole or part of the typescript and made many useful criticisms and suggestions. Several colleagues have been most helpful in obtaining biopsies of human tissues and also donated material from their experimental animals. These include Dr. B. Bharadwaj (human myocardium), Dr. L. W. Oliphant (tunicate oocyte), Dr. W. E. DeCoteau (lupus kidney), Dr. W. B. Firor (dog myocardium), Dr. W. H. Kirkaldy-Willis, Dr. D. M. Mitchell and Dr. W. A. Silver (articular tissues), Dr. D. McFadden (bronchial mucosa) and Dr. E. W. Parry (Ehrlich ascites tumour).

My thanks are also due to Mrs. C. Dick, Mrs. A. J. LeFebvre, Mrs. E. Williams and Mr. N. Yong for processing tissues, cutting ultrathin sections and preparing the innumerable prints from which the final plates were made. The task of typing and arranging the references has been carried out by Mrs. M. McHaffie and Mrs. B. Taylor. Their patience and skill are gratefully acknowledged.

Worth recording also is the remarkable patience and courtesy of my publishers who waited for five instead of the anticipated two years for the typescript and illustrations of this book. The task of producing this work has been greatly facilitated by the skill and knowledge of the editorial staff of Butterworths.

The electron micrographs published in this work spring mainly from work carried out with various colleagues and co-workers. These include Dr. R. L. Ailsby, Mr. R. Bhatnagar, Dr. J. A. Fuller, Dr. T. E. Larsen, Dr. P. N. Mehta, Dr. A. F. Oryschalk. Dr. E. W. Parry, Dr. S. Roy and Dr. L. F. Skinnider. Their ceaseless efforts in making this material available cannot be over-rated. In the text and/or legends to the illustrations their contributions are duly identified. Of the 520 electron micrographs (on 221 plates) published in this work, 96 come from other sources. For these illustrations I am indebted to the following authors and journals.

P. Barland, A. B. Novikoff and D. Hamerman (1964) *Am. J. Path.* **44**, 853: Plate 128, Fig. 1.

S. Chandra (unpublished): Plate 117, Figs. 1 and 3; (1968) *Lab. Invest.* **18**, 422: Plate 117, Fig. 2.

A. Coimbra and A. Lopez-Vaz (1967) *Arthritis Rheum.* **10**, 337: Plate 128, Figs. 2–5.

M. L. Cook and J. G. Stevens (1970) *J. Ultrastruct. Res.* **32**, 334: Plate 202, Figs. 1, 2 and 3.

H. A. Dahl (1963) *Z. Zellforsch. mikrosk. Anat.* **60**, 369: Plate 218, Fig. 5.

W. C. Davis, S. S. Spicer, W. B. Greene and G. A. Podgett (1971) *Lab. Invest.* **24**, 303: Plate 148, Figs. 1 and 2.

I. R. Duncan and F. K. Ramsey (1965) *Am. J. Path.* **47**, 601: Plate 221, Figs. 1–3.

B. Flaks and A. Flaks (1970) *Cancer Res.* **30**, 1437: Plate 15, Fig. 2; Plate 33, Figs. 1–3.

J. M. Frasca, O. Auerbach, V. Parks and W. Stoeckenius (1965) *Expl Molec. Path.* **4**, 340: Plate 14; (1967) **6**, 261: Plate 125, Figs. 1–4.

C. E. Ganote and J. B. Otis (unpublished): Plate 120.

G. C. Godman and N. Lane (1964) *J. Cell. Biol.* **21**, 353: Plate 86, Figs. 1 and 2.

N. K. Gonatas G. Margolis and L. Kilham (1971) *Lab. Invest.* **24**, 101: Plate 186, Figs. 1 and 2.

E. I. Grodums (unpublished): Plate 31, Figs. 1 and 2; Plate 77, Figs. 1 and 2; Plate 118, Fig. 2; Plate 194.

M. L. Grunnet and P. R. Spilsbury (1973) *Archs Neurol.* **28**, 231: Plate 138.

T. Ishikawa and Y. F. Pei (1965) *J. Cell Biol.* **25**, 402: Plate 75, Figs. 1–5.

R. W. Mahley, M. E. Gray, R. L. Hamilton and V. S. LeQuire (1968) *Lab. Invest.* **19**, 358: Plate 90, Fig. 2.

A. Martinez-Palomo (unpublished): Plate 198, Figs. 1 and 2; (1970) *Lab. Invest.* **22**, 605: Plate 200, Figs. 1 and 2.

H. Matsuda and S. Sugiura (1970) *Invest. Ophthal.* **9**, 919: Plate 171, Figs. 1–5.

T. Nagano and I. Ohtsuki (1971) *J. Cell. Biol.* **51**, 148: Plate 191.

T. Nakai, F. L. Shand and A. F. Howatson (1969) *Virology* **38**, 50: Plate 37, Figs. 1–3.

J. D. Newstead (unpublished): Plate 95, Fig. 2; Plate 178, Fig. 1.

F. T. Oteruelo (unpublished): Plate 173.

E. W. Parry (unpublished): Plate 77, Fig. 6; Plate 78, Fig. 2; Plate 199, Fig. 3; (1969) *J. Path.* **97**, 155: Plate 155, Fig. 1; (1970) *J. Anat.* **107**, 505: Plate 178, Fig. 2.

S. Roy (1967) *Ann. rheum. Dis.* **26**, 517: Plate 89, Fig. 1.

F. T. Sanel and M. J. Lepore (1968) *Expl Molec. Path.* **9**, 110: Plate 110, Fig. 2.

E. E. Schneeberger-Keeley and E. J. Burger (1970) *Lab. Invest.* **22**, 361: Plate 206, Figs. 1 and 2.

F. H. Shipkey, R. A. Erlandson, R. B. Bailey, V. I. Babcock and C. V. Southam (1967) *Expl Molec. Path.* **6**, 39: Plate 12, Figs. 1–4.

E. Stubblefield and B. R. Brinkley (1967) In *Formation and Fate of Cell Organelles*, Vol. 6, p. 175, Ed. by K. B. Warren, Academic Press: Plate 42; Plate 43, Figs. 1 and 2; Plate 44, Figs. 1 and 2.

B. Tandler, R. V. P. Hutter and R. A. Erlandson (1970) *Lab. Invest.* **23**, 567: Plate 76, Figs. 1–3.

L. T. Threadgold and R. Lasker (1967) *J. Ultrastruct. Res.* **19**, 238: Plate 53, Figs. 1–3; (unpublished): Plate 53, Fig. 4.

T. Tillack and V. Marchesi (1970) *J. Cell Biol.* **45**, 649: Plate 196, Figs. 2 and 3.

D. N. Wheatley (unpublished): Plate 216, Fig. 1; Plate 218, Figs. 2–4; (1969) *J. Anat.* **105**, 351: Plate 218, Fig. 1.

Y. C. Wong and R. C. Buck (1971) *Lab. Invest.* **24**, 55: Plate 220, Fig. 4.

T. Yamamoto (1969) *Microbiology* **1**, 371: Plate 36, Fig. 1; (unpublished): Plate 36, Fig. 2.

D. Zucker-Franklin (1969) *J. clin. Invest.* **48**, 165: Plate 185, Figs. 1–4.

I am also grateful to the following journals for permission to use illustrations from past publications of which I am a co-author.

Ann. rheum. Dis.
F. N. Ghadially and P. Mehta: (1971) **30**, 31: Plate 179; Plate 180.
F. N. Ghadially and S. Roy: (1967) **26**, 426: Plate 153, Figs. 1–3; Plate 154.
F. N. Ghadially, G. Meachim and D. H. Collins: (1965) **24**, 136: Plate 136, Figs. 4 and 5.
P. Mehta and F. N. Ghadially: (1973) **32**, 75: Plate 91, Fig. 1; Plate 189, Figs. 1 and 2.
S. Roy and F. N. Ghadially: (1966) **25**, 402: Plate 139, Fig. 1; (1967) **26**, 26: Plate 85, Fig. 2;
    Plate 201, Fig. 1; (1969) **28**, 402: Plate 142, Figs. 1 and 2; Plate 143, Figs. 1 and 2.

Archs Path.
F. N. Ghadially, J. A. Fuller and W. H. Kirkaldy-Willis: (1971) **92**, 356: Plate 10, Fig. 3; Plate 17.
L. E. Skinnider and F. N. Ghadially: (1973) **95**, 139: Plate 159, Fig. 3; Plate 187, Fig. 2.
L. E. Skinnider and F. N. Ghadially: (1974) **98**, 58: Plate 149.

Cancer
F. N. Ghadially and P. Mehta: (1970) **25**, 1457: Plate 2; Plate 108.
F. N. Ghadially and E. W. Parry: (1965) **18**, 485: Plate 155, Fig. 2; (1966) **19**, 1989: Plate 27, Fig.
    2; Plate 68; Plate 77, Fig. 5; Plate 88, Fig. 1; Plate 115, Fig. 1; Plate 135, Fig. 1.
F. N. Ghadially and L. E. Skinnider: (1972) **29**, 444: Plate 210, Figs. 2 and 3; Plate 212, Fig. 3.
E. W. Parry and F. N. Ghadially: (1965) **18**, 1026: Plate 130, Figs. 2 and 3; (1966) **19**, 821: Plate
    60, Figs. 1 and 2.

Experientia
F. N. Ghadially and L. E. Skinnider: (1971) **27**, 1217: Plate 211, Fig. 4.
F. N. Ghadially, A. F. Oryschak and D. M. Mitchell: (1974) **30**, 649: Plate 204, Figs. 1 and 4.

J. Bone Jt Surg.
F. N. Ghadially and S. Roy: (1969) **49**E, 1636: Plate 141, Figs. 3 and 5.
F. N. Ghadially, P. N. Mehta and W. H. Kirkaldy-Willis: (1970) **52**A, 1147: Plate 91, Fig. 2.

J. Path.
R. L. Ailsby and F. N. Ghadially: (1973) **109**, 75: Plate 219; Plate 220, Fig. 3.
T. E. Larsen and F. N. Ghadially: (1974) **114**, 69: Plate 216, Fig. 2.
L. E. Skinnider and F. N. Ghadially: (1973) **109**, 1: Plate 211, Figs. 1 and 2; Plate 212, Figs. 1 and
    2.
F. N. Ghadially and L. E. Skinnider (1974): **114**, 113: Plate 72, Fig. 2.

J. Path. Bact.
F. N. Ghadially and E. W. Parry: (1966) **92**, 313: Plate 151, Figs. 1 and 2; Plate 152, Figs. 1 and
    2.
S. Roy and F. N. Ghadially: (1967) **93**, 555: Plate 87, Figs. 1 and 2.

Ultrastructure of Synovial Joints in Health and Disease, Butterworths
F. N. Ghadially and S. Roy (1969): Plate 8; Plate 25; Plate 84; Plate 85, Fig. 1; Plate 89, Fig. 2;
    Plate 93; Plate 94, Figs. 1 and 2; Plate 98; Plate 114; Plate 135, Fig. 2; Plate 139, Figs. 2–4;
    Plate 140; Plate 141, Figs. 1, 2 and 4; Plate 170, Fig. 2; Plate 215, Fig. 1.

Contents

CHAPTER I

Nucleus

INTRODUCTION

Our knowledge of the fine structure of the interphase nucleus is relatively recent. Early studies were concentrated mainly on the new and intriguing structures revealed by the electron microscope in the cytoplasm and not on the nucleus which revealed only an assortment of granules intermingled with some fibrous and amorphous material. The sentiments of that era are recorded by Moses (1956), who stated 'Most electron-microscopists acknowledge that the nucleus appears to be as remarkable for its lack of obvious ordered detail as the cytoplasm is for the richness in it'. Dissatisfaction with the state of affairs was expressed by many workers and is epitomized by Bernhard and Granboulan (1963), who stated 'In electronmicroscopical cytology the interphase nucleus of the normal somatic cell has been the neglected orphan compared with cytoplasmic organelles'. Such sentiments have been reiterated even in recent times, for example by Kaye (1969), who states 'Research on the nucleus seems remarkably unfruitful compared with that on cytoplasmic organelles when results achieved by similar efforts are considered'.

However, disenchantment with electron microscopic studies on the nucleus stems mainly from failure to elucidate satisfactorily the structure of chromatin and chromosomes· and the variations that might underlie cell differentiation, function and neoplastic transformation. Excluding this, the electron microscope has revealed much that is new and interesting, as evidenced by the fact that this chapter on the nucleus is the largest in this book.

Outstanding among these achievements are the studies on the nuclear envelope, and the nucleolus. There is much here of interest for both the student of normal structure and the pathologist. Similarly, our knowledge of viral and non-viral inclusions has been enhanced, and many an old controversy regarding the nature of these inclusions has been settled. This subject, of course, is of great interest to pathologists; hence I have dealt with it in some detail in this chapter. It is amazing how much more one can discern in these inclusions with the light microscope once their ultrastructural features are recognized.

On the other hand, as already indicated, light microscopic studies of the mitotic nucleus and its chromosomes have proved more rewarding than studies of ultrathin sections through these structures. Since ultrastructural studies on pathologically altered mitoses are few and as yet of very limited interest, only the interphase nucleus is dealt with in this chapter; the mitotic nucleus receives only passing mention in this and later chapters.

In ultrathin sections examined with the electron microscope, many nuclei show a degree of irregularity of form quite beyond that expected from their light microscopic appearance. It need hardly be pointed out that this is no shrinkage artefact, since other organelles such as mitochondria are not crenated or shrunken. This phenomenon, although at first perplexing, can be readily explained when one considers that the thinness of the sections employed in electron microscopy gives a virtually two-dimensional view of the state of affairs at the plane of section, while the much thicker sections employed for light microscopy may be regarded as several superimposed thin sections where projections and indentations which overlie each other cancel out and give a smooth appearance to the nuclear margin. No doubt the higher magnification employed in electron microscopy also contributes to this phenomenon by revealing small irregularities which would appear insignificant or be beyond the resolving power of the light microscope.

Thus the electron microscope shows that many nuclei which one had come to regard as smooth and round or oval, can in fact be quite irregular and at times beset by an unsuspected slender deep invagination (e.g. lymphocyte nucleus). The significance of such irregularity of nuclear shape is obscure and the operative mechanisms poorly understood. However, a few interesting studies and speculations regarding this point are worth recording.

Perhaps the best known example here is the nucleus of smooth and striated muscle which in ultrathin sections often shows a markedly folded or convoluted appearance. This has now been correlated with the state of the cell, the nucleus being unfolded and elongated in the relaxed phase and ovoid and invaginated after contraction of the muscle cell (Lane, 1965; Franke and Schinko, 1969). Similar changes also occur in the nuclei of endothelial cells of blood vessels, and it is reasonable to assume that this, too, may be correlated with the state of the vessel wall (*Plate 1*).

Instances may be cited where complexity of nuclear form is related to maturation and ageing of the cell. The classical example here is the polymorphonuclear neutrophil leucocyte where the nucleus becomes segmented and lobed as the cell increases in age. In mature normal articular

Plate 1

Folded and invaginated nuclei (E) are seen in the endothelial cells of this collapsed blood vessel from the subsynovial tissue of man. × 14,000 (*Ghadially and Roy, unpublished electron micrograph*)

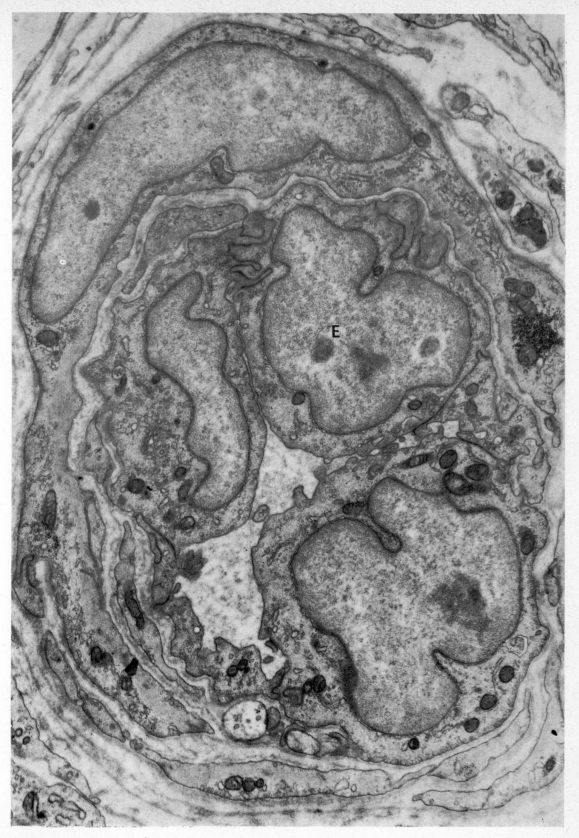

cartilage there is a population of cells which apparently do not divide but suffer *in situ* necrosis, with resultant loss of cells as the animal ages. Barnett *et al.* (1963) have observed an increased complexity of nuclear form in this ageing population of cells. There is also evidence that hepatic and adrenal cell nuclei (Kleinfeld and Koulish, 1957; Sobel *et al.*, 1969a) of man show invaginations of the nuclear envelope and complexity of nuclear form more frequently in older age groups.

Irregularity of nuclear form provides an increased area of contact between the nucleus and the cytoplasm, and in some cases at least this seems to denote increased nucleocytoplasmic exchanges and heightened metabolic activity. In this connection it is interesting to note that some of the most irregular and branched nuclei occur in the cells of silk-spinning glands of certain insects and that such nuclei evolve by a series of steps from unremarkable oval nuclei of the cells of the Malpighian tubule (Lozinski, 1911). Here increasing metabolic activity is clearly associated with an increasing complexity of nuclear form. Support for this hypothesis may also be found in the case of tumours where complex nuclear form is associated with a high metabolic activity. The marked irregularities of shape assumed by neoplastic nuclei are well known to the light microscopist. The electron microscope reveals even more dramatically, the extremes of complex and bizarre forms that the nuclei of tumour cells can assume (*Plate 2*). At times the nucleus is so extensively segmented or invaded by numerous invaginations that it assumes an almost sponge-like character. Remarkable also are the nuclei of leucocytes in Sézary's syndrome (believed to be the leukaemic phase of mycosis fungoides), which show a cerebriform appearance in blood smears, but appear serpentine or drawn out into a mass of overlapping narrow ribbons in ultrathin sections examined with the electron microscope (Lutzner and Jordan, 1968).

Invaginations of the nuclear envelope lead to the formation of pseudoinclusions. These, and further discussion on the mode of formation of such invaginations, are dealt with on page 50.

Plate 2

Giant cell from a well differentiated osteogenic sarcoma of man showing two irregular nuclear profiles with small pedunculated masses of nuclear substance connected by complex filamentous stalks. Also seen are two transversely cut centrioles (C). ×9,500 (*From Ghadially and Mehta, 1970*)

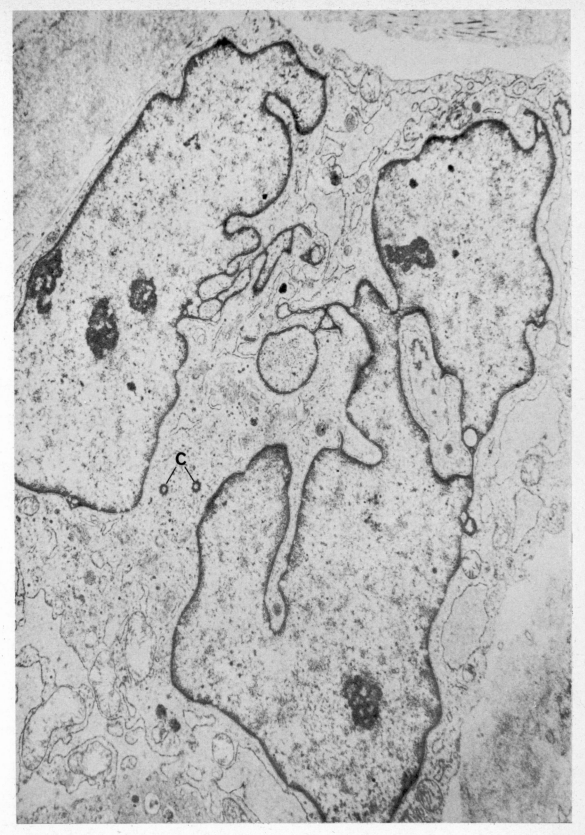

DNA occurs in the nucleus combined with histones and other proteins. This combination constitutes chromatin. Two forms of chromatin are known to occur in the interphase nucleus: (1) a condensed, presumably inactive, form called heterochromatin, which is basophilic with the light microscope and presents as collections of rounded or irregular-shaped electron-dense granules in ultrathin sections (*Plate 3*); and (2) an active form called euchromatin, which is dispersed in the nuclear matrix and stains feebly or not at all with basic dyes. This form cannot be confidently identified in electron micrographs either.

In the mitotic nucleus (*Plate 4*) the chromosomes present as elongated bodies constricted at one or more places, and are seen to be composed of heterochromatin which has a structure similar to the heterochromatin areas of the interphase nucleus, except that it is somewhat more densely packed (particularly at metaphase). Thus the heterochromatin of the interphase nucleus is generally looked upon as the unexpanded segments of chromosomal chromatin, while the euchromatin is regarded as the functional expanded portion of the chromosome engaged in synthetic activity within the interphase nucleus. In the mature spermatozoa the chromatin is highly compacted so that it appears as a homogeneous electron-dense mass in the sperm head (*Plate 5*). Even so it can be shown by treatment with alkaline thioglycolate that the chromatin is still strikingly fibrillar (Lung, 1972).

For some time now the term chromatin, coined on the basis of the tinctorial reaction of this nuclear material to basic dyes, has been restricted to indicate only the DNA-containing Feulgen-positive areas in the nucleus and not the basophilic, but Feulgen-negative, nucleolus. In suitably prepared tissues viewed with the electron microscope, aggregates of electron-dense granules having the characteristic intranuclear chromatin distribution (chromatin pattern) are visualized. Hence, the term chromatin has been retained by electron microscopists even though no tinctorial reaction is involved and the ultrastructural techniques used are not specific for the demonstration of DNA.

In ultrathin sections through interphase nuclei, aggregates of chromatin have a granular appearance. However, it is well established that the structural units of chromatin are fibrillar and at high magnifications images that can be interpreted as fibrils cut in various planes can be discerned. It would appear that ultrathin sections are singularly unsuitable for studying the structure of chromatin and other techniques, such as negative staining, whole mounts of chromosomes and scanning electron microscopy, have been employed to elucidate the structure of chromatin. Even so, despite numerous studies the size and arrangement of chromatin fibres in the interphase and mitotic nucleus has not been unequivocally established. Studies on the tissues

---

Plate 3

Plasma cell from bronchial mucosa of man showing the characteristic cart-wheel or clock-face distribution of heterochromatin aggregates. Centrally placed nucleolus (N), marginated chromatin (A), chromatin centres (B), and nucleolus-associated chromatin (C) can be readily identified in this material, which was fixed in cacodylate-buffered osmium and stained with uranium and lead. × 34,000

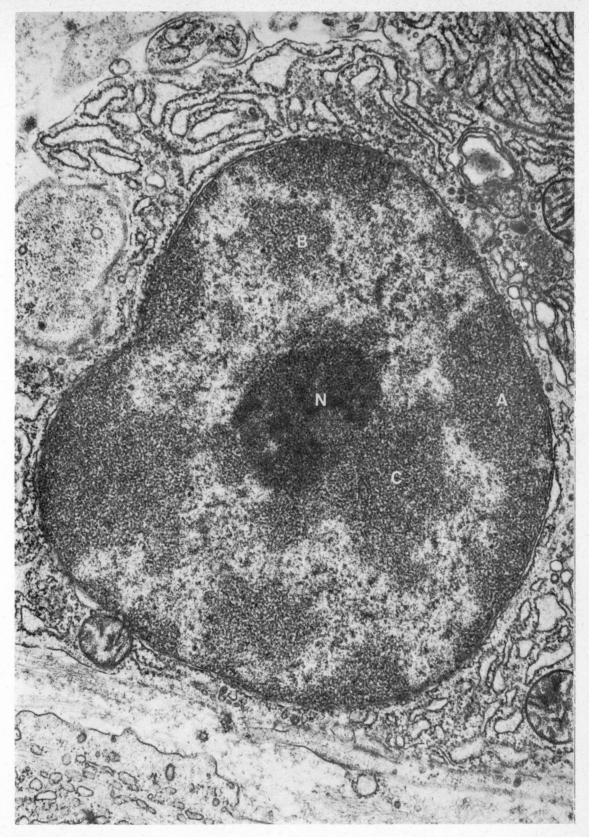

of higher plants, insects and various vertebrates have given figures for the diameter of chromatin fibres which range from 30 to 500 Å (40 to 150 Å in ultrathin sections) (Ris, 1956, 1962; De Robertis, 1956; Moses, 1960; Porter, 1960; Miyai and Steiner, 1965; Abuelo and Moore, 1969; Kaye, 1969; Golomb and Bahr, 1971; Golomb et al., 1971). In suitably treated whole mounts of chromosomes the chromatin fibres are found to have a diameter of 240 ± 50 Å. Most of this material, however, is protein which can be removed by treatment with trypsin. The trypsin-resistant DNA core measures 25–50 Å in diameter (Abuelo and Moore, 1969).

It is generally believed that the granular appearance of chromatin seen in ultrathin sections results from sections through tightly coiled filaments, but some believe that the chromatin fibres form an interlacing, branching network (Yasuzumi, 1960; Hay and Revel, 1963).

In tissues fixed in osmium (collidine- or veronal-acetate-buffered) and stained with lead, nuclei have a somewhat homogeneous appearance and condensations of chromatin with the pattern familiar to light microscopists are either absent or barely discernible (see, for example, Plate 1). The closest approach to the familiar chromatin pattern is seen when tissues are fixed in glutaraldehyde, post-fixed in osmium and stained with uranium and lead.

This difference is attributable to the staining techniques employed (see Plate 188) and also to the fixative and buffer used. It is clear that lead is a poor stain for chromatin, while uranium, particularly alcoholic uranium, stains chromatin intensely. (Uranium can combine with DNA in amounts sufficient to increase the dry weight by a factor of almost 2 (Huxley and Zubay, 1961).) In my experience, tissues fixed in cacodylate-buffered osmium, and stained with uranium and lead, give a good visualization of the familiar chromatin pattern (Plate 3) only a little less compact and dense than that obtained from glutaraldehyde fixation and double staining with uranium and lead.

It has been argued in the past that osmium may be a poor fixative for chromatin and that the difference observed is due to loss of DNA. This idea has to be discarded, for ultraviolet spectrometry has shown that little, if any, DNA is lost by this process, and the work of Moses (1956) has shown that the characteristic chromatin pattern can be demonstrated with the Feulgen technique in osmium-fixed nuclei that do not show this pattern with the electron microscope.

Chromatin aggregates occur in certain preferred sites in the nucleus and it is this phenomenon which produces the familiar chromatin pattern. Such aggregates of chromatin may be designated as follows (Plate 3).

Plate 4

Ultrathin section through chromosomes of a mitotic nucleus. From monkey kidney cells in culture. ×25,000

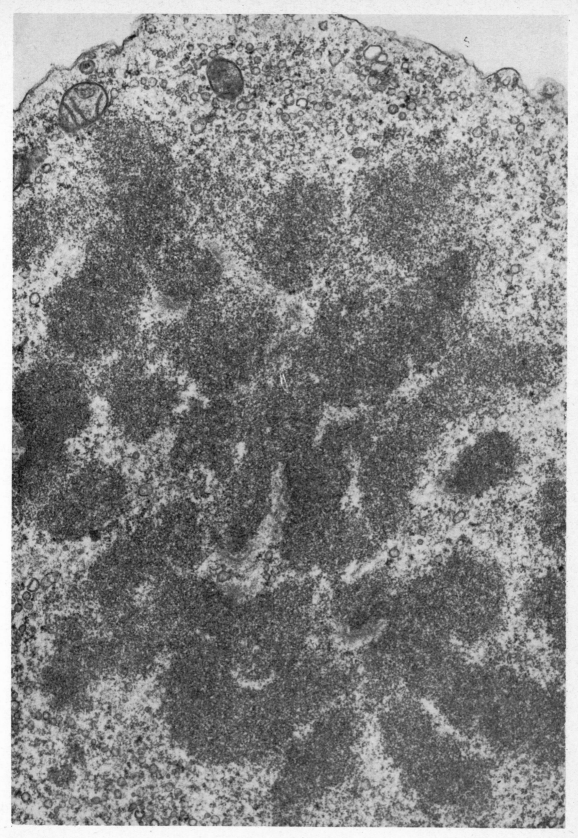

(1) *Peripheral or marginal chromatin*: irregular-shaped masses of chromatin adjacent to the nuclear envelope, between the nuclear pores. There is a clear area devoid of chromatin granules immediately behind the nuclear pores.

(2) *Chromatin centres*: randomly distributed chromatin aggregates within the nuclear matrix.

(3) *Nucleolus-associated chromatin*: focal aggregates of chromatin granules along the periphery of the nucleolus.

(4) *Intranucleolar chromatin*: although the nucleolus contains mainly protein and RNA and is Feulgen negative, numerous studies have shown that it contains a small amount of DNA also (see review by Miller and Beatty, 1969).

It is now clear that not only the distribution but also the proportion of heterochromatin to euchromatin varies from one cell type to another. Since it is well established that the average amount of DNA in the somatic cell nuclei from various tissues of a given species is constant, one can argue that in nuclei poorly endowed with heterochromatin there will be more of the metabolically active euchromatin (Fawcett, 1967). Thus one may expect that metabolically active cells will have a paler-staining nucleus with fewer and smaller heterochromatin masses. This thesis is borne out by the fact that stem cells or blast cells have paler nuclei, and that in a maturing series of cells such as the red blood cells an increasing concentration of heterochromatin masses becomes evident as the cell matures, and becomes metabolically less active.

An apparent exception to the rule is the plasma cell with its familiar chromatin pattern (clock-face or cart-wheel) of large heterochromatin masses. This cell, with its abundant rough endoplasmic reticulum, is known to be actively engaged in the synthesis of antibodies. Fawcett (1967) has put forward two interesting suggestions to explain this anomaly. He states, 'It is conceivable that in a cell so highly specialized in its function only a small proportion of its DNA may be needed in an active form to direct the narrow range of synthetic activities in its cytoplasm. Alternatively one may speculate that all the transcription of information necessary for continuing synthesis of antibody took place at an earlier stage in the differentiation of the plasma cell before its nucleus acquired its definitive coarse chromatin pattern.'

However, when attempting to correlate the metabolic activity of a cell with its degree of nuclear staining by basophilic dyes, or with chromatin aggregates seen with the electron microscope, one must take another factor into consideration. Thus although the total amount of DNA per nucleus is remarkably constant in a given species, the concentration of DNA is very variable, as evidenced by variations in nuclear size, and there is also a striking difference in the nature and amount of total protein of various nuclei.

Plate 5

Mouse spermatozoon, showing extreme condensation of chromatin. In this form the chromatin is metabolically inert and serves only an archival function, transmitting genetic information to the next generation. × 23,000

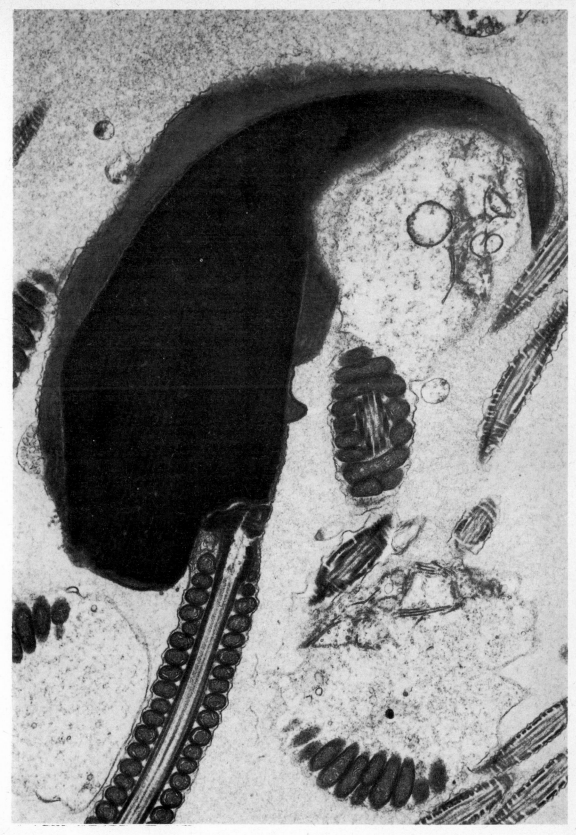

According to Mirsky and Osawa (1961) it is this factor which is largely responsible for the difference in staining characteristics of nuclei, and they point out that there is a significant correlation between the amount of residual protein (non-histone protein) and metabolic activity of the cell. Thus liver and kidney cells with high metabolic activity have relatively large amounts of nuclear residual protein as compared to the nuclei of metabolically sluggish cells such as lymphocytes and nucleated erythrocytes.

Light microscopists have long been familiar with the nuclear changes seen in malignant tumour cells and also with the fact that none of these changes taken singly is specific for the neoplastic state. It had been hoped that the electron microscope would reveal specific morphological alterations which could be regarded as the hallmark of malignancy, but such a hope has not fructified. The chromatin pattern of tumour nuclei is very variable but not characteristic or distinctive (Bernhard and Granboulan, 1963). The electron microscope does little more than tell us what we already know, namely that tumour cell nuclei are highly pleomorphic. Nuclei with large coarse lumps of heterochromatin and pale nuclei poor in heterochromatin content both occur in tumours (see, for example, *Plate 21*). Indeed, one can more confidently identify tumour cells with the light microscope than with the electron microscope.

Students of pathology are well aware of the nuclear changes in necrosis, designated as pyknosis, karyorrhexis and karyolysis. The terms 'necrosis' and 'cell death' are often used interchangeably, but I shall here use the term necrosis, as does Robbins (1969), in a stricter sense to imply morphological changes occurring after cell death. One need hardly point out that cells examined in fixed tissues, though dead, do not show the morphological features of necrosis, and that some time (at least 8 hours for rat liver; Majno *et al.*, 1960) must elapse between the death of the cell in the living organism (or outside it) before the classical changes we call necrosis are detectable in the nucleus by light microscopy. Viewed this way, necrosis may also be looked upon as an early stage prior to frank autolysis.

Plate 6

Cells harvested from a pleural effusion in a case of lymphocytic leukaemia. (*Ghadially and Skinnider, unpublished electron micrographs*)

Fig. 1. Pyknosis. × 20,000
Fig. 2. Karyorrhexis. × 20,000.

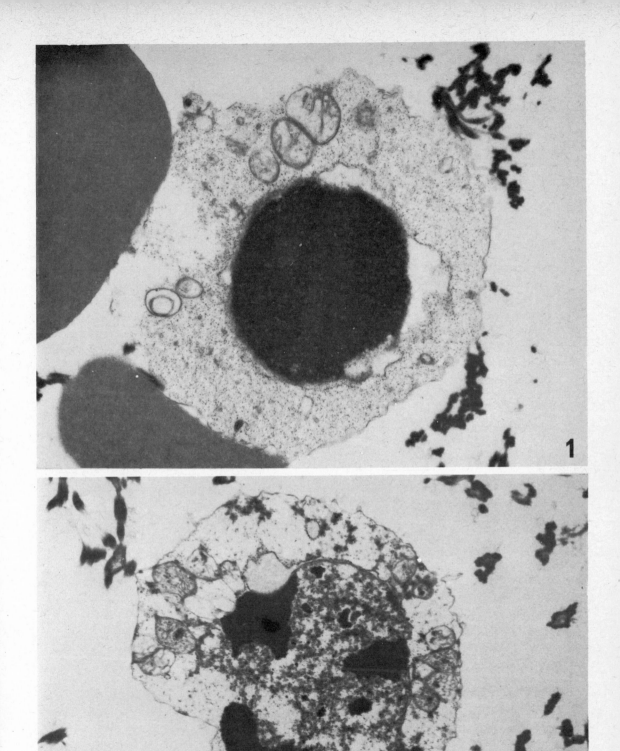

The large literature on cell injury, cell death, necrosis and autolysis can hardly be discussed here. My main purpose is to illustrate the electron microscopic equivalents of the nuclear changes associated with necrosis. Since these changes involve the distribution of chromatin they are considered in this section of the text, but changes also occur in the other nuclear components such as the nucleolus and nuclear envelope.

Pyknosis involves a shrinkage of the nucleus and condensation of the chromatin (*Plate 6, Fig. 1*). In karyorrhexis the nuclear chromatin is aggregated or clumped into numerous masses, and later released by rupture of the nuclear envelope (*Plate 6, Fig. 2*). In karyolysis the nuclear envelope remains reasonably intact but the contents are partially or completely lost (*Plate 7, Fig. 2*). Such ultrastructural appearances amply vindicate what has long been taught about these nuclear changes to students of pathology. But although one can find electron microscopic images that correlate well with our light microscopic concepts of pyknosis, karyorrhexis and karyolysis, there are also other images which cannot confidently be fitted into one of these three well known categories.

Electron microscopic studies have in fact focused attention on a much more common and consistent pattern of nuclear change in the necrotic cell, which is spoken of as chromatin margination. Here a condensation of the chromatin occurs along or adjacent to the inner membrane of the nuclear envelope, while chromatin disappears from other parts of the nucleus. Such a condensation may present in ultrathin sections as a complete ring, a crescent-shaped mass or irregular clumps of condensed chromatin (*Plate 7*) set at the periphery of the nucleus. Such changes are seen in necrosis resulting from the action of various noxious agents, such as viral infection, x-rays or ischaemia.

Margination of chromatin appears to be a fairly early change that occurs in the nucleus after irreversible injury leading to cell death (*Plate 7*). Trump *et al.* (1963, 1965a, b) studied this phenomenon in slices of mouse liver incubated in aseptic conditions for various periods of time prior to

---

Plate 7

Fig. 1. Rabbit liver fixed 1 hour after death of the animal. Chromatin margination is evident in this necrotic hepatocyte nucleus, as also are woolly focal densities in the mitochondria (arrow) which are considered to be evidence of irreversible cell injury. Endoplasmic reticulum and mitochondria are, however, not swollen in this instance. × 20,000

Fig. 2. Two nuclei from an ovarian carcinoma are seen in this electron micrograph. The one on the left shows karyolysis, while the one on the right may be interpreted as an intermediate stage between margination and lysis. × 11,000

14

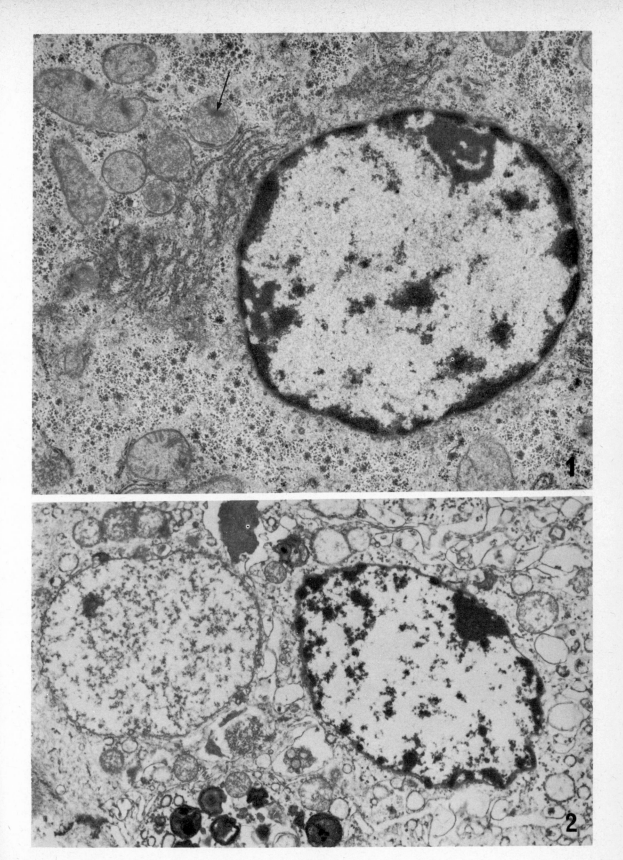

fixation. They report that the earliest nuclear change seen is chromatin margination and that this is detectable after 30 minutes but is not well developed until 2 hours after excision of liver tissue. (It should, however, be noted that mild degrees of chromatin margination are probably reversible and that this is not inevitably followed by cell death.)

Chromatin margination is also seen in so-called physiological necrosis (necrobiosis); that is to say, in cells that die normally in the body. An excellent site for studying this phenomenon is articular cartilage where *in situ* necrosis of chondrocytes normally occurs. We have occasionally noted chromatin margination in such cells. Another interesting alteration of nuclear morphology seen in a chondrocyte which has suffered *in situ* necrosis is illustrated in *Plate 8, Fig. 1*. Here the nucleus is crenated and the nuclear contents have a homogeneous appearance. No chromatin masses or nucleoli are discernible. Such a change may be designated homogenization of the nucleus, and it is worth noting that this type of change is at times seen also in other cells besides chondrocytes. Necrosis of chondrocytes is followed by disintegration and dispersal of cell fragments (*Plate 8, Fig. 2*) and lipidic debris derived from them into the matrix (Ghadially *et al.*, 1965; Ghadially and Roy, 1969a).

This section began by noting that necrosis follows cell death. However, the precise point at which a cell may be pronounced dead is debatable. In analogy with somatic death, one may argue that just as all the tissues do not die or cease functioning simultaneously, so also not all the organelles. Electron microscopic studies tend to support such an idea. The earliest signs of cell injury seen after a large variety of insults lie in the cytoplasm. These consist of loss of intramitochondrial dense granules, swelling of mitochondria (page 140) and dilation and vesiculation of the cisternae of the endoplasmic reticulum (page 222). This is the equivalent of cloudy swelling, a change that is reversible. Trump *et al.* (1965a, b), from their study of necrosis in isolated liver slices, concluded that when (1 hour after excision of liver tissue) mitochondria came to contain flocculent electron-dense masses (*Plate 7*), the point of no return had been reached. Thus it would appear that the changes that occur in the nucleus may be secondary to derangements of mitochondrial morphology and energy production.

Plate 8

Necrotic chondrocytes from the articular cartilage of a 6-month-old rabbit. (*From Ghadially and Roy, 1969a*)

Fig. 1. The nucleus (N) is crenated and its contents are homogeneous. The distended cisternae (C) of the rough endoplasmic reticulum and disintegrating mitochondria (M) can be easily recognized. ×23,000

Fig. 2. Another pattern of chondrocyte necrosis and disintegration is seen in this electron micrograph. In this shrunken cell lying in a lacuna (L) organelles can no longer be identified. The dark masses (M) probably represent fragmented nuclear remnants. Cell processes (P) and lipidic debris (D) derived from them are seen among the radially oriented collagen fibres (C) in the matrix. ×21,000

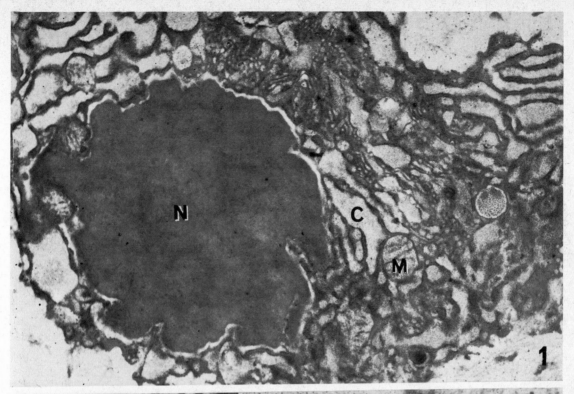

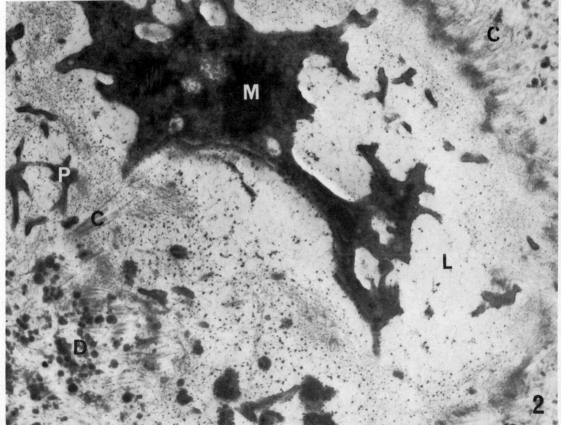

INTERCHROMATIN AND PERICHROMATIN GRANULES

The nuclear sap (karyoplasm, nucleoplasm, nuclear matrix) of living cells has a clear lipid appearance, but much fibrillar and granular material can be discerned in this region by electron microscopy. Hence this region of the nucleus is sometimes referred to by electron microscopists as the interchromatin area or substance (that is to say, the material lying between the chromatin) and the two types of granules seen in this region as the interchromatin and perichromatin granules. Besides these granules the nuclear matrix also contains euchromatin and fibrillary material of low density, believed to be protein.

Perichromatin granules, as their name implies, usually lie on the borders of chromatin areas. These electron-dense, solitary, spherical granules are separated from the adjacent chromatin by an electron-lucent halo. The granule itself measures 300–350 Å in diameter; the over-all diameter including the halo is about 750 Å (Watson, 1962; Bernhard and Granboulan, 1963). It has been estimated that the hepatocyte nucleus contains 500–2,000 such granules.

Interchromatin granules are highly electron dense. They vary in diameter from 150 to 500 Å (Granboulan and Bernhard, 1961; Bernhard and Granboulan, 1963; Jezequel and Marinozzi, 1963; Swift, 1963) and frequently have an angular shape. They often occur as clusters in the nuclear matrix, but single granules or short linear arrays of granules are also quite common.

The function and chemical composition of interchromatin and perichromatin granules have not been clearly established. It has been suggested (Watson, 1962; Bernhard and Granboulan, 1963) that both RNA and DNA may be present in the perichromatin granules. Currently, both types of granules are regarded as nuclear ribosomes. It seems likely that these granules are involved in the synthesis of nuclear proteins.

Little is known about the frequency and distribution of these granules in various cell types, but they can be easily demonstrated in hepatocytes and pancreatic acinar cells. An abundance of interchromatin granules is seen in various tumours (*Plate 9*). According to Bernhard and Granboulan (1963), interchromatin granules are seen more frequently in tumour cells, and Reddy and Svoboda (1968) have observed that, 'In chronic studies of carcinogenesis in rat liver the most consistent ultrastructural alteration is an apparent increase in interchromatinic granules'. An abundance of perichromatin granules has also been noted in some tumours; for example, scirrhous carcinoma of the breast (Murad and Scarpelli, 1967). I, too, have at times been impressed by the abundance of either interchromatin or perichromatin granules in tumour nuclei. My experience is that in a given tumour one or the other type of granule is prominent, but not both. Prominent or enlarged perichromatin granules in tumours and other pathological tissues have at times been mistaken for virus particles.

Plate 9

Fig. 1. Osteogenic sarcoma of man. The tumour cell nucleus contains clusters of markedly electron-dense interchromatin granules (IC), and a few perichromatin granules (arrows) separated from the adjacent chromatin by a halo. × 27,000

Fig. 2. High power view of perichromatin granules from the nucleus of a rat hepatocyte (arrows). × 84,000

18

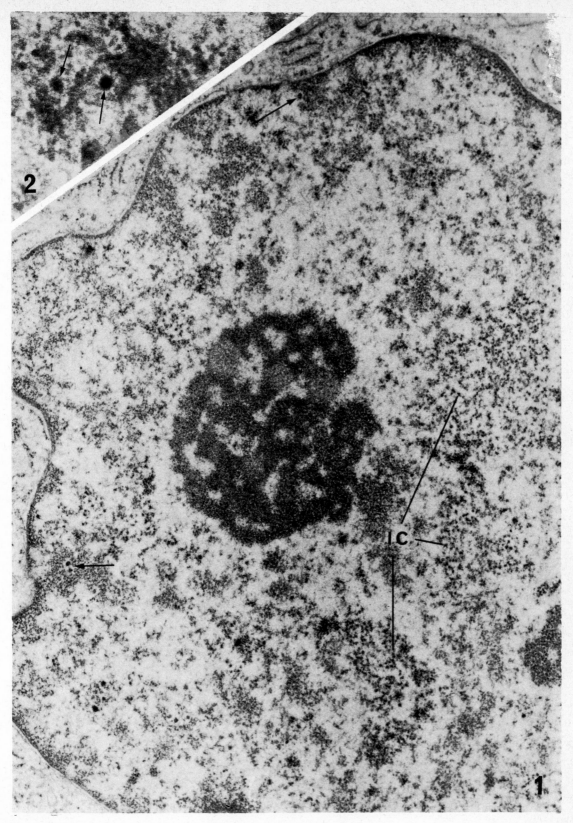

In electron micrographs the nuclear envelope is seen to consist of two membranes separated by a perinuclear cistern, generally about 200–300 Å wide (Watson, 1955, 1959). The outer membrane of the nuclear envelope is often studded with a few or many ribosomes, and in favourable sections continuities between it and the rough endoplasmic reticulum are demonstrable, as is also a continuity between the cisternae of the rough endoplasmic reticulum and the perinuclear cistern (*Plate 10*)

At intervals along the surface of the envelope the two membranes fuse, producing 'fenestrations' 300–1,000 Å in diameter, called nuclear pores (Watson, 1959; Oberling and Bernhard, 1961). In tangential sections through the nucleus the pores are seen as circular annuli, often with a dense granule or knob in the centre (Rhodin, 1963).

Often a diaphragm is seen guarding the pore but at times no such structure is visualized. Sometimes a thin membrane is seen extending across the pore, but, as Barnes and Davis (1959) point out, such an image can be produced by non-equatorial sections through an annular opening. Whether a true diaphragm exists or whether such images are the product of sectioning geometry and thickness of section employed, have been extensively debated (see critique by Stevens and Andre, 1969). Our view is that pores both with and without diaphragms occur in nuclei of various cell types. In any case, the pores cannot be regarded as simple holes or fenestrations in the nuclear envelope through which material small enough can pass unimpeded. This is attested to by many experimental studies (see below), including studies on the electrical properties of the nuclear envelope (Loewenstein and Kanno, 1963). The pores in fact delimit channels extending from the nucleoplasm to the cytoplasm, and at high magnifications are seen to contain oriented fibrillar material (Watson, 1959). The channel material and pores are referred to as the 'pore complexes' by Watson (1959) and as the 'annular complexes' by Wischnitzer (1958).

Numerous studies on the passage of substances across the nuclear membrane show that small molecules such as sugars, amino acids and polypeptides readily pass from the cytoplasm into the nucleus, but various proteins such as ovalbumin, serum albumin and globulin do not behave in this fashion even though the molecular size of these proteins is smaller than the diameter of nuclear pores (Mirsky and Osawa, 1961; Feldherr, 1962; Baud, 1963).

Since nuclear pores are potential pathways of nucleocytoplasmic exchanges, one may postulate that there might be a correlation between the metabolic activity of the cell and the number and size of nuclear pores. Such a correlation has been elegantly demonstrated by Merriam (1962) in the nuclear envelope dissected off frog oöcyte nuclei. In this study, envelopes from immature oöcytes at the onset of yolk deposition were compared with those from mature oöcytes, and it

Plate 10

Fig. 1. Nuclear envelope of rat hepatocyte, showing transversely cut nuclear pores (P) and continuity of the outer membrane of the nuclear envelope with the rough endoplasmic reticulum (arrows). × 58,000

Fig. 2. Tangentially sectioned rat hepatocyte nucleus showing an *en face* view of nuclear pores which present as annuli. × 34,000

Fig. 3. Profile of a pore with a diaphragm. From repair tissue in articular cartilage. Same nucleus as in *Plate 17.* × 82,000 (*From Ghadially, Fuller and Kirkaldy-Willis, 1971*)

Fig. 4. Nucleus of a polymorphonuclear neutrophil leucocyte showing profiles of two pores without diaphragms and one (arrow) where a thin membrane is seen across the pore opening. × 52,000

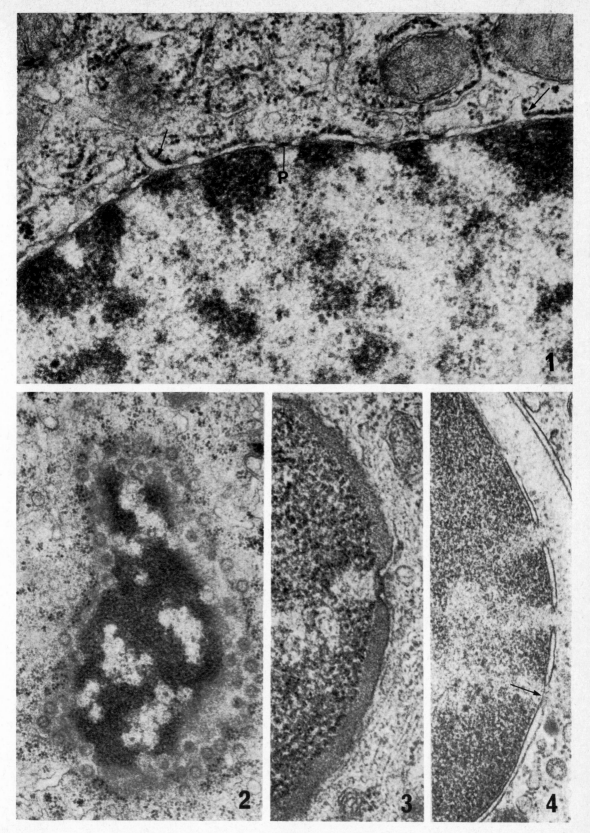

was found that envelopes from the metabolically more active, immature form had: (1) 40 per cent more pores per unit area; (2) larger annuli; and (3) the central dot or knob seen more frequently than in the envelopes from mature oöcytes.

A reduction in the number of pores with diminished metabolic activity is indicated by the studies of: (1) Yasuzumi *et al.* (1967), who found very few nuclear pores in the testicular Leydig cells of old men (over 70 years) as compared to young men (20 to 25 years); (2) Blackburn and Vinijchaikul (1969), who found that in kwashiorkor, where there is a severe amino-acid deficiency, there is a reduction in the number of nuclear pores per nuclear section (11 per nuclear section as compared to the normal 18·7 per nuclear section), in the nuclei of pancreatic acinar cells; and (3) Zucker-Franklin (1968), who found fewer nuclear pores in circulating polymorphonuclear neutrophil leucocytes than in their marrow precursors.

Besides the numerical variations in pores already discussed, an interesting situation regarding nuclear pores in the liver of ethionine intoxicated rats (Miyai and Steiner, 1965) is worth mentioning. In this example, *en face* projections or pores appearing as annuli were frequently seen—often in sections well away from the nuclear pole or even near the equator, a site where one would normally expect to see pore profiles and not annuli. These authors suggest that this phenomenon may be due to the stretching of the nuclear envelope and a consequent rotation of the pore complexes. However, as these authors themselves point out, it is difficult to see why, if this were the case, the pores retain their circular form and do not suffer distortion from stretching.

A phenomenon similar to the above was observed by us in non-neoplastic liver tissue adjacent to a human hepatoma (Ghadially and Parry, 1966) and in the livers of rats bearing subcutaneous carcinogen-induced or transplanted tumours (Parry and Ghadially, 1967). In these livers we found a high incidence of sections of nuclei showing numerous prominent pore annuli (*Plate 11*), but in normal rat liver such sections were very rare and the pores appeared fewer, smaller and less distinct. The mechanism of production of this phenomenon and its significance is obscure.

It is, however, worth noting that while in ethionine intoxication there is a suppression of protein synthesis, the liver of the tumour-bearing host is markedly enlarged and there is evidence of increased protein synthesis in all but the terminal stages of the life of the tumour-bearing host (Greenstein, 1954; Wiseman and Ghadially, 1958).

Plate 11

Hepatocyte nucleus (N) from the liver of a rat bearing a transplanted tumour in its flank. Numerous prominent pore annuli, some with a central dot (arrow), are seen in this section which cuts the nucleus at a little distance from the pole. Numerous polyribosomes (P) are abundant in the cytoplasm. × 48,000 (*Parry and Ghadially, unpublished electron micrograph*)

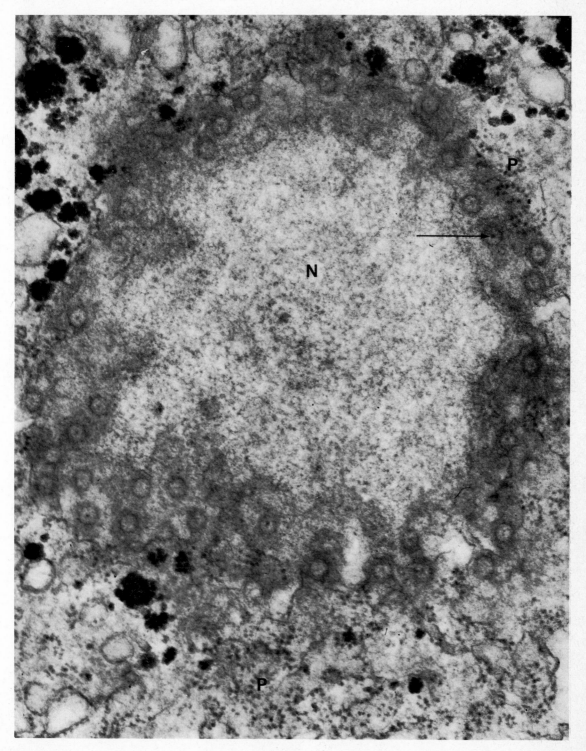

THICKENING, PROLIFERATION AND REDUPLICATION OF NUCLEAR ENVELOPE

Complex morphological changes occur in the nuclear envelope in cells infected with the herpes group of viruses (for references, see third paragraph), certain types of adenoviruses (Gregg and Morgan, 1959) and cytomegalovirus (Patrizi *et al.*, 1967). Details of the morphological picture vary, apparently depending upon the type of virus and variety of infected cell. These changes have been found in infected tissues of man, experimentally produced disease in laboratory animals and numerous infected tissue culture cell lines grown *in vitro*. We shall illustrate and discuss the changes that occur in the nuclear membrane using herpesvirus as an example.

A sequence of events that occurs in the nuclear envelope is clearly related to the passage of nucleocapsids from the nucleus to the cytoplasm (*Plate 12, Figs. 1–4*). The viral core and the surrounding shell, called the capsid (made of units called capsomeres), are assembled in the nucleus. The viral particle (core and capsid) then migrates to the nuclear envelope and, with the approach of the virus, the inner membrane of the nuclear envelope develops a focal thickening and becomes evaginated and encloses the virus. It is now clear from many studies (Shipkey *et al.*, 1967; Darlington and Moss, 1968; Leestma *et al.*, 1969) that, as the viral particle escapes from the nucleus, it acquires one or two membranous coats from the nuclear envelope. It may also derive further membranous coats from other membranous structures in the cell, and thus single virions or groups of virions may come to lie in vacuoles within the cytoplasm. Most workers believe that the primary membranous coat arises from the nuclear envelope but some contend that it can also be derived from cytoplasmic membranes and the Golgi (Epstein, 1962; Siminoff and Menefee, 1966; Leestma *et al.*, 1969).

Besides the changes in the nuclear envelope noted above, there also occur a variety of complex alterations which defy detailed description in the limited space available. These multitudinous morphological alterations stem from a combination of various changes designated as thickening, proliferation, reduplication and fusion of the membranes of the nuclear envelope. These patterns of change have been extensively studied and described in the literature. They may be briefly catalogued as follows: (1) electron-opaque macular thickening of the inner membrane of the nuclear envelope and the associated portion of a round or flattened vesicle which is believed to develop by a process of reduplication of the inner membrane of the nuclear envelope (Swanson *et al.*, 1966; Moore and Pickren, 1967; Roy and Wolman, 1969); (2) proliferation of inner

---

Plate 12

Figs. 1–4. Electron micrographs arranged in a sequence to depict the probable manner in which a virus particle migrates from the nucleus (N) to the cytoplasm. Thickening of the inner membrane of the nuclear envelope in proximity to the virus is clearly seen in *Figs. 1–3*, as is also an increasing evagination of the nuclear envelope. *Fig. 4* depicts the virus about to be detached from the nuclear envelope. From centre outwards one can discern the dense viral core, the capsid and two ensheathing membranous coats continuous with the inner and outer membranes of the nuclear envelope. All figs. × 100,000 (*From Shipkey, Erlandson, Bailey, Babcock and Southam, 1967*)

Figs. 5 and 6. Nuclei of herpesvirus-infected monkey kidney cells in culture. These two electron micrographs show that the vesicular profiles (arrow) seen in *Fig. 5* could be sections through shelf-like elongations (arrow) of the inner membrane of the nuclear envelope as seen in *Fig. 6*. × 45,000; × 40,000

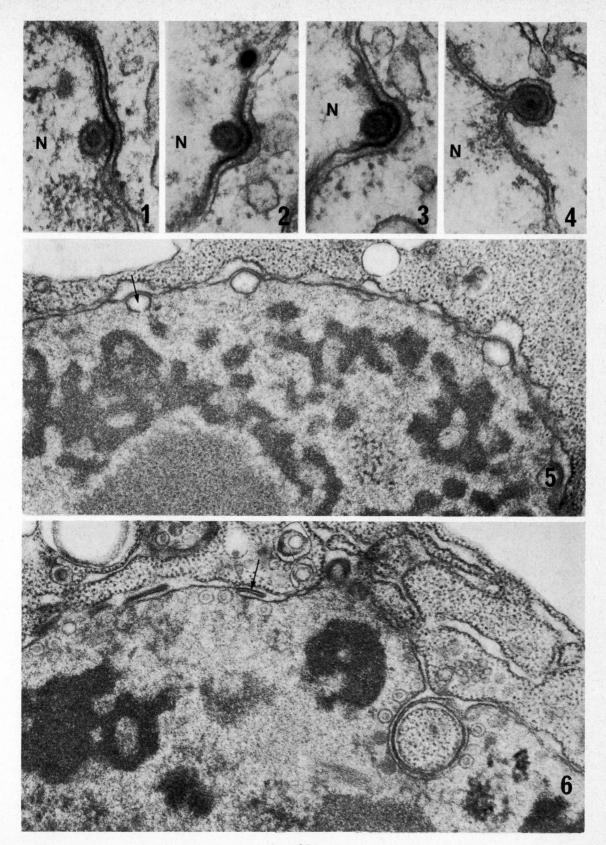

membrane of the nuclear envelope, forming vesicles within the nucleus containing virus particles (Darlington and Moss, 1968); (3) extensive proliferation of the nuclear membranes, producing pod-like or finger-like extensions into the nucleus and/or cytoplasm (Shipkey *et al.*, 1967; Nii *et al.*, 1966, 1968); (4) thickening of long lengths of nuclear membrane, even in areas where no contact with virus particles is observed (Swanson *et al.*, 1966; Shipkey *et al.*, 1967); (5) reduplication of inner nuclear membrane (Epstein, 1962); (6) extensive proliferation and reduplication of the inner membrane of the nuclear envelope, with complex folds and macular densities along its length (Leestma *et al.*, 1969); and (7) proliferation, thickening and fusion, leading to the formation of concentric lamellar membranous arrays within and outside the nucleus (Nii *et al.*, 1968).

Some of these morphological alterations are shown in the accompanying illustrations (*Plates 12* and *13*). In *Plate 12, Fig. 5*, are depicted the 'vesicles' that have frequently been described in the literature and are believed to arise by a process of reduplication of the inner membrane of the nuclear envelope. However, as demonstrated in *Plate 12, Fig. 6*, at least some of these so-called vesicles may be sections through shelf-like extensions of the inner membrane of the nuclear envelope extending along the perinuclear cistern. *Plate 13, Fig. 1*, is a good example of how elaborate and extensive the membranous proliferations can be in herpesvirus-infected cells. Here the proliferated nuclear membranes have grown mainly outwards into the cytoplasm but in *Plate 13, Fig. 2*, the membranes have grown inwards into the nucleus to form membranous whorls. The dense 'lines' within these whorls have been interpreted as evidence of membrane thickening and/or fusion of adjacent membranes.

The precise significance of the many alterations seen in the nuclear envelope have not been elucidated. Leestma *et al.* (1969) have proposed that 'the redundant foldings of the nuclear membranes may represent a proliferative reaction, to proteins or lipid–protein components of the nearby virus'. Watson and Wildy (1963) have shown that the capsid contains virus-specific antigens while the membranous coat contains host cell antigens. Fluorescent antibody studies by Shipkey *et al.* (1967) have shown that the thickened inner membrane of the nuclear envelope and the coat derived from this contain viral antigens also. Thus it would appear that thickening of the nuclear membrane denotes the accumulation of viral antigens at this site.

Plate 13

Herpesvirus-infected monkey kidney cells in culture.

Fig. 1. The proliferated nuclear envelope is seen extending as complex folds into the cytoplasm. Note the marginated clumps of chromatin (C) and numerous viral particles in the nucleus and cytoplasm and also a few on the cell membrane (arrow). × 22,000

Fig. 2. Proliferation of the nuclear envelope extending into the nucleus, giving rise to whorled membranous structures. Note also the collection of virus particles in the nucleus (arrow). × 27,000

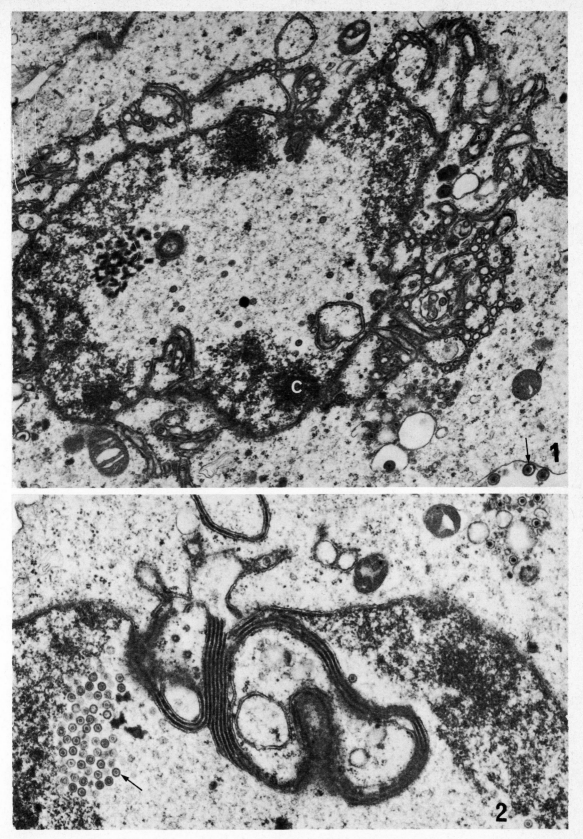

Many reports suggest that extrusion of nuclear material into the cytoplasm can occur via the formation of blebs, evaginations or pouches from the surface of the nucleus. Particularly interesting is the time-lapse cinematographic study by Hsu and Lou (1959) with Cloudman melanoma cells in culture where, upon adding fresh culture medium, a burst of nuclear activity and bleb formation was precipitated.

Bleb formation as a mechanism for nucleocytoplasmic exchanges has also been claimed to occur in (1) oöcytes and adenocarcinoma of frog kidney in culture (Duryee and Doherty, 1954; Duryee, 1956); (2) cultures of human tonsillar epithelium (Pomerat *et al.*, 1954); (3) salivary gland cells of third larval instar of *Drosophila melanogaster* (Gay, 1956); (4) dissociated cells of rat myocardium (Kyte, 1964) and (5) ultraviolet-irradiated cells of *Tetrahymena pyriformis* (Shepard, 1964).

In most of the above-mentioned examples one can be reasonably certain that both membranes of the nuclear envelope were involved in the formation of the bleb and that material was probably being conveyed from the nucleus, but in many other reports this is doubtful. Conversely there are other examples where presumably only the outer membrane of the nuclear envelope suffered evagination (Watson, 1955; Moses, 1956; Wischnitzer, 1958; Swift, 1959; Hadek and Swift, 1962). Such evaginations of the outer membrane lead to the formation of quite small vesicles which are also implicated in nucleocytoplasmic exchanges (Baud, 1963).

Convincing electron microscopic evidence of bleb formation involving both layers of the nuclear envelope comes from the work of Clark (1960), on the exocrine cells of the rat pancreas, and Frasca *et al.* (1965), who have elegantly demonstrated this phenomenon in the ciliated columnar cells from the bronchial epithelium of four patients (*Plate 14*). Often a series of vacuoles derived from the nucleus were seen lying in the cytoplasm. Disintegration of the more distally placed vacuoles was noted, and it is suggested that this may provide a means of transfer of nuclear material to the cytoplasm.

The question raised by these studies on nuclear bleb formation is whether this is a normal phenomenon, or the sign of a damaged or a sick cell. Arguments supporting both these contentions can be given, but on the available data one cannot reach any definite conclusion. Certainly there is nothing overtly abnormal that one can detect from electron micrographs of cells showing this phenomenon. It is worth recalling that Clark (1960) found nuclear evagination in the pancreas of normal rats, and, although the patients studied by Frasca *et al.* (1965) had grave pathological changes in their lungs, the mucosa used for study was collected well away from the site of disease.

If, for the sake of argument, one concedes that nuclear bleb formation is a normal phenomenon, then it becomes difficult to explain why it has not been reported more frequently in the electron microscopy literature. Tissue culture studies indicate that this is an intermittent phenomenon which proceeds with some rapidity. It is conceivable, therefore, that the failure to visualize nuclear blebs more frequently may be related to the transient nature of this phenomenon and the ever-annoying problem of the smallness of the sample that can be examined with the electron microscope.

Plate 14

Multiple double-membrane-bound 'vacuoles', derived by a process of evagination of the nuclear envelope, are seen in this cell from the bronchial mucosa of man. The bleb (B) nearest to the nucleus (N) is seen to be an evagination with the limiting membranes of the bleb continuous with the two membranes of the nuclear envelope. Besides amorphous and electron-lucent material, this bleb also contains electron-dense granules resembling the chromatin in the nucleus. × 23,000 (*From Frasca, Auerbach, Parks and Stockenius, 1965*)

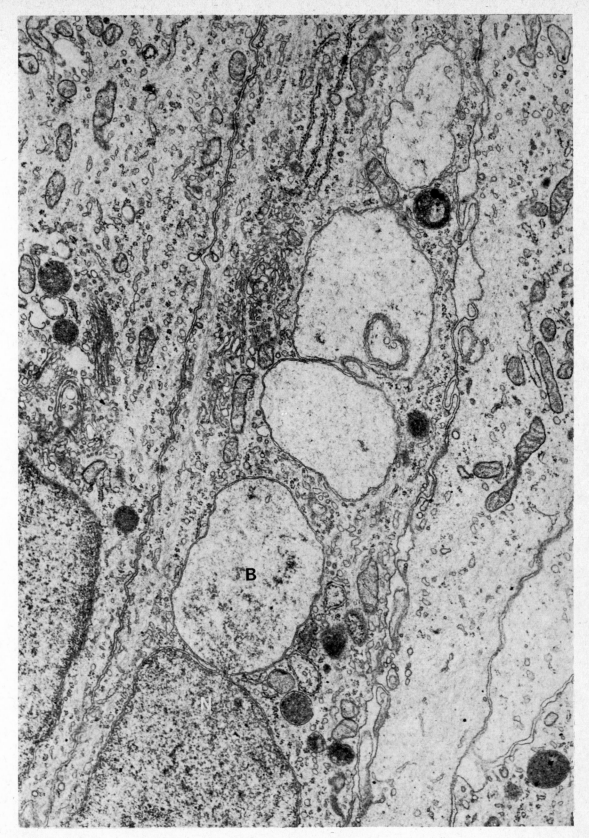

INTRANUCLEAR AND INTRANUCLEOLAR LAMELLAE, TUBULES AND VESICLES

Membrane-bound structures such as lamellae, tubules and vesicles have at times been found in nuclei; in many instances their origin from the inner membrane of the nuclear envelope has been convincingly demonstrated, as has continuity between the interior of such tubules and lamellae and the perinuclear cistern. The distinction between tubules and lamellae can be made in favourable ultrathin sections on the basis that when tubules are present some of these are likely to be cut transversely and give the characteristic circular profile but lamellae, being large flattened sac-like structures, will appear like longitudinally sectioned tubules and circular profiles will be absent.

One of the most highly organized lamellar systems is that of the annulate lamellae, which usually occur in the cytoplasm but are sometimes seen also in the nucleus (see Chapter 6). Intranuclear annulate lamellae are derived from the inner membrane of the nuclear envelope, and indeed both intranuclear annulate lamellae and membranous formations of the type discussed in this section of the text can coexist in the same nucleus.

Lamellar and tubular systems arising from the inner membrane of the nuclear envelope may come into close association with the nucleolus, or penetrate and ramify in this structure. Examples of this have been seen in: (1) normal human endometrial cells during the early secretory phase of the menstrual cycle (Clyman, 1963; Moricard and Moricard, 1964; Ancla and De Brux, 1965; Terzakis, 1965); (2) salamander and crayfish oöcytes (Miller, 1966; Kessel and Beams, 1968); and (3) a strain of Novikoff hepatoma cells (Babai et al., 1969; Karasaki, 1970).

Intranuclear tubules, lamellae and vesicles (*Plate 15*) have been seen in: (1) a Rous sarcoma (Bucciarelli, 1966); (2) a variety of transplantable ascites tumours of rats and mice (Hoshino, 1961; Yasuzumi and Sugihara, 1965; Levine et al., 1968; Locker et al., 1968); (3) pulmonary adenomas and adenocarcinomas of mice (Flaks and Flaks, 1970); (4) a cell from human acute leukaemia (*Plate 15, Fig. 1*); (5) rat and mouse hepatocytes after exposure to sodium tetraphenyl boron (Parry, 1971); and (6) herpesvirus-infected cells (*Plate 15, Fig. 3*). It has already been noted that in certain virus infections (page 22) proliferation of the membranes of the nuclear envelope occurs. While often quite complex structures are produced, sometimes the nucleus contains simpler lamellar formations (*Plate 15, Fig. 3*).

The significance of the intranuclear membrane-bound structures described above is not well understood. However, virtually all authors note that cells in which these changes occur are not dying cells, but cells with a normal or increased metabolic activity. Thus it has been suggested, particularly where such formations touch the nucleolus, that these membrane-bound structures probably facilitate nucleocytoplasmic exchanges.

Plate 15

Fig. 1. Nucleus of a leukaemic leucocyte showing intranuclear vesicles and/or tubules. The nuclear envelope is not clearly visualized because of tangential sectioning. However, infoldings of the inner membrane (arrow), depicting the probable manner in which these structures arise, can be discerned. × 44,000

Fig. 2. A group of intranuclear tubules, most cut longitudinally and some transversely (arrow), are seen in this electron micrograph. From murine pulmonary tumour. × 33,000 (*From Flaks and Flaks, 1970*)

Fig. 3. Membrane-bound intranuclear structures in this nucleus represent sections through lamellae rather than tubules, as no circular profile of a transversely cut tubule is seen. Whether these lamellae are annulate or not is difficult to say. There are occasional interruptions along their length which could be interpreted as profiles of annuli. From monkey kidney cell culture infected with herpesvirus. × 24,000

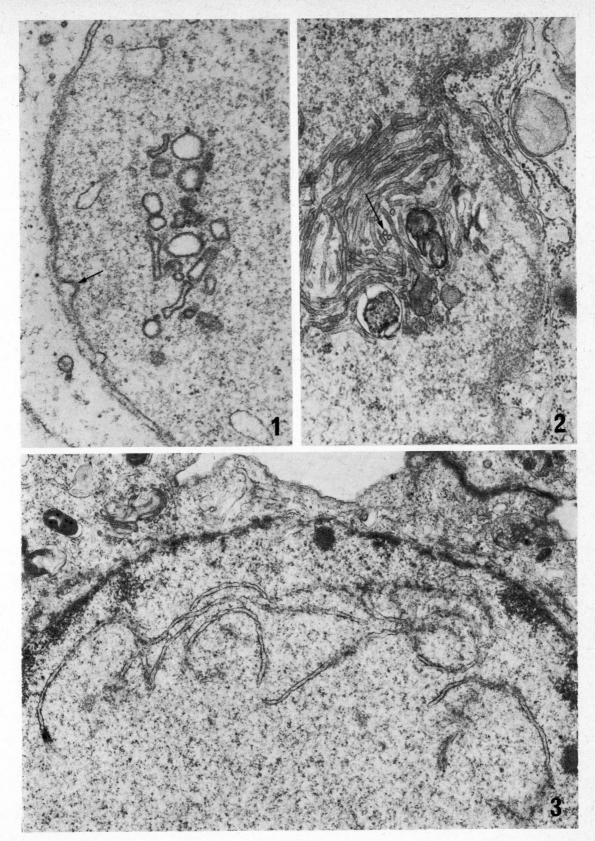

In electron micrographs the fibrous lamina presents as a fine-textured medium-density zone adjacent to the inner membrane of the nuclear envelope. In *Amoeba proteus* (Pappas, 1956; Mercer, 1959), *Gregarina melanopli* (Beams *et al.*, 1957) and neurons of the ventral nerve cord of *Hirudo medicinalis* (Gray and Guillery, 1963; Coggeshall and Fawcett, 1964), the fibrous lamina is a complex prominent structure measuring 900–2,000 Å thick. Filaments 30–50 Å thick have been demonstrated in the fibrous lamina of *Hirudo* (Coggeshall and Fawcett, 1964). In sections perpendicular to the nuclear envelope, the fibrous lamina of *Amoeba proteus* (*Plate 16, Fig. 1*) is seen to delineate a system of cylindrical compartments. In tangential cuts through this region the lamina has a honeycombed appearance (*Plate 16, Figs. 2* and *3*). In the region of the nuclear pores this layer is either very thin or absent.

A fibrous lamina has now been demonstrated in some vertebrate cells also. However, the lamina in these instances is thinner (usually less than 300 Å) and presents as a band of medium to moderately high density lying between the inner surface of the nuclear envelope and the marginal condensates of heterochromatin. Fawcett (1966) has found that, in contrast to the situation in the leech where the fibrous lamina is absent over the pores, in the vertebrate cells studied by him the fibrous lamina continues either unaltered or as an attenuated band across the pores. Patrizi and Poger (1967), however, have failed to find such continuity in their material. Further they found that the lamina was thicker and more marked in glutaraldehyde-fixed material, but we (Ghadially *et al.*, 1974) found no difference in thickness between the lamina of tissues fixed in cacodylate-buffered osmium or glutaraldehyde.

Filaments have been convincingly demonstrated in the lamina of *Hirudo* but not in the lamina of vertebrate cell nuclei. If they do exist, they are likely to be very thin and therefore difficult to demonstrate in this slender compact structure. However, the texture of the lamina is in keeping with the idea that it contains filaments, and in analogy with the lamina in invertebrates it is best to retain the term fibrous lamina. The situation here is analogous to that of chromatin where the fibrillary nature is also difficult to demonstrate in ultrathin sections.

Plate 16

Fibrous lamina in *Amoeba proteus* (*Ghadially and Bhatnagar, unpublished electron micrographs*)

Fig. 1. Section through the nucleus, showing fibrous lamina delineating the cylindrical compartments. × 42,000
Fig. 2. Tangential section, showing the honeycomb pattern of fibrous lamina. × 40,000
Fig. 3. Tangential cut through tip of nucleus, showing nuclear pores lying over the cylindrical openings in the lamina (arrow). × 44,000

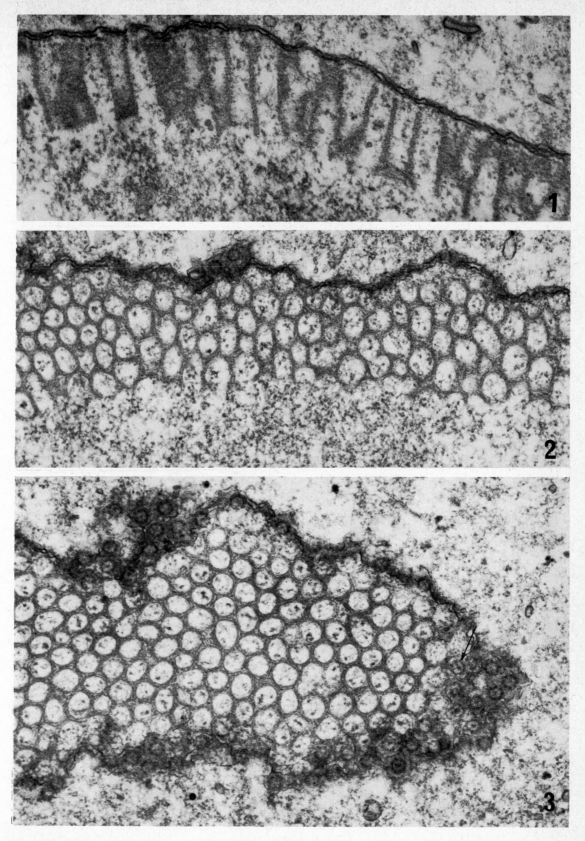

The fibrous lamina is now known to occur in various normal vertebrate cells such as Schwann cells, endothelial cells, fibroblasts, smooth muscle cells, interstitial cells of the testis, intestinal epithelial cells, cells of Brünner's glands and amniotic cells in cultures (Fawcett, 1966; Patrizi and Poger, 1967; Kalifat *et al.*, 1967; Leeson and Leeson, 1968). We (Oryschak *et al.*, 1974) have noted a fibrous lamina in chondrocytes of normal articular cartilage of man, rabbit, cow, horse and dog. However in 2-month-old rabbits the lamina was absent or under 45 Å thick but in older rabbits and other animals mentioned, the mean thickness of the lamina lay between 200 and 300 Å.

Nuclei with fibrous lamina have also been found in experimental and pathological states such as: (1) cells of a mixed tumour of salivary gland (Kumegawa *et al.*, 1969); (2) reticular cells and immature plasma cells from a case of Hodgkin's disease (Sanel and Lepore, 1968); (3) repair tissue filling surgically produced deep defects in articular cartilage (Ghadially *et al.*, 1971, 1972); (*Plate 17*) and (4) synovial intimal cells in cases of rheumatoid arthritis and a patient with multiple sclerosis, psoriasis and arthritis (Ghadially *et al.*, 1974).

During studies on the healing of surgically produced deep defects in articular cartilage of the knee joint of rabbits we found fibrous laminae up to 950 Å in thickness (Ghadially *et al.*, 1972). A hole passing through the articular cartilage and violating subchondral bone soon becomes filled with repair tissue arising from the marrow spaces. Later, metaplastic transformation to cartilage occurs. During the early stages (two weeks) the nuclei in the repair tissue show only a thin (353 ± 9 Å) fibrous lamina, but at three months the lamina is remarkably well developed (725 ± 15 Å). At six months the lamina is reduced in size (370 ± 10 Å).

Little is known about the structure and function of the fibrous lamina. Its distribution among various cell types, and possible variations in physiological and pathological states still remain to be determined. Its occurrence in large nuclei, such as those of the leech neurons, suggested that it might have a skeletal or supportive function, that is to say it may act as a fibrous reinforcement to the nuclear envelope. However, the discovery that cells with not particularly large nuclei also have a fibrous lamina has now cast doubt on this theory. The waxing and waning of the lamina in repair tissue in articular cartilage shows that this is not a static structure of fixed dimensions for a given cell type, but that it is a dynamic component of the nucleus, capable of undergoing hypertrophy and involution in physiologically or pathologically altered states. Fawcett (1966) has suggested that, since in vertebrates the fibrous lamina extends across the pores, it may function as a selective barrier in nucleocytoplasmic exchanges.

Plate 17

Nucleus of a cell from repair tissue filling a surgically produced deep defect in articular cartilage showing a prominent fibrous lamina (F). Also seen is a nuclear pore with a well developed diaphragm (arrow), and others where no such diaphragm is evident in the plane of sectioning. Fixed in cacodylate-buffered osmium and stained with uranium and lead. × 58,000 (*From Ghadially, Fuller and Kirkaldy-Willis, 1971*)

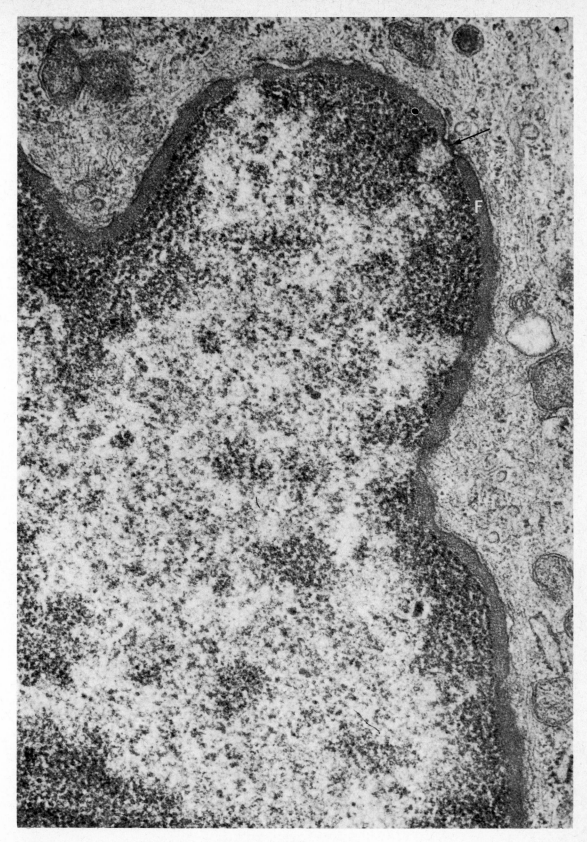

35

Nucleoli are readily visualized by a variety of light microscope techniques. The study of living cells shows them as refractile bodies that can move about in the nucleus and also fuse and divide. In fixed material the RNA-rich nucleolus stains intensely with a variety of basic dyes but is Feulgen negative, except for the rim of Feulgen-reactive nucleolus-associated chromatin. In suitable specimens, after silver impregnation the nucleolus shows two components: a branching anastomosing coarse thread-like structure called the nucleolonema, in the meshes of which are entrapped one or more rounded structures called the pars amorpha or fibrillar centres (see below). Both the light microscope and the electron microscope show that not all nucleoli have an open or reticular nucleolonema. In many the nucleolonema is compacted to varying degrees so that the thread-like appearance is partially or completely lost (*Plate 18*).

With the electron microscope the nucleolus is seen to contain granular (150–200 Å diameter) and fibrillary (50 Å diameter and 300–400 Å long) elements but these are not dispersed homogeneously throughout the nucleolus (Swift, 1963; Granboulan and Granboulan, 1964; Marinozzi, 1964; Smetana and Busch, 1964; Brinkley, 1965; Hyde *et al.*, 1965; Terzakis, 1965; Bernhard, 1966; Bernhard and Granboulan, 1968; Hay, 1968). Besides these granules and fibrils, which are susceptible to ribonuclease digestion and are hence believed to contain RNA, there is also said to be some pepsin-digestible amorphous protein and DNA in the nucleolus (Hay and Revel, 1962; Granboulan and Granboulan, 1964; Marinozzi and Bernhard, 1964; Schoefl, 1964; Lord and Lafontaine, 1969; Recher *et al.*, 1970).

With the electron microscope the nucleolonema is seen to be composed of granules set in a fibrillary matrix, but the proportion of granules and fibrillary material varies in different zones of the nucleolonema. This produces light and dark areas at times referred to as the light and dense components of the nucleolus (*Plates 18* and *19*). The dense areas comprise compacted filaments (this is difficult to demonstrate except at high magnifications in suitable preparations) in which granules are scanty or absent. The light areas are rich in granules set in a sparse filamentous matrix. Such zones are also discernible in compact nucleoli where a thread-like nucleolonema is not seen.

Much confusion exists regarding the electron-microscope equivalent of the light microscopist's pars amorpha. This is largely a continuation of the confusion which has reigned in the light microscope literature where at times the pars amorpha is described as lying within the nucleolus and in other instances the nucleolus is described as embedded in a structureless mass called the pars amorpha. The interstices of the nucleolonema are permeated by the nuclear matrix (*Plate 18, Fig. 1*) and at times such regions have erroneously been called pars amorpha by electron microscopists.

Plate 18

Fig. 1. Nucleolus from dog myocardium with a reticular nucleolonema. Light granular (G) and dense fibrillar (F) components can be discerned, as can rounded areas which might be called pars amorpha or fibrillar centres (C). Note how the nuclear matrix extends into the interstices of the nucleolus (arrows). × 46,000

Fig. 2. Nucleolus from hypertrophic myocardium of man obtained at open heart surgery. A compact nucleolus is seen in which no obvious nucleolonema can be discerned. Dense fibrillary zones (F), light granular zones (G) and fibrillary centres (C) are easily discerned. × 35,000

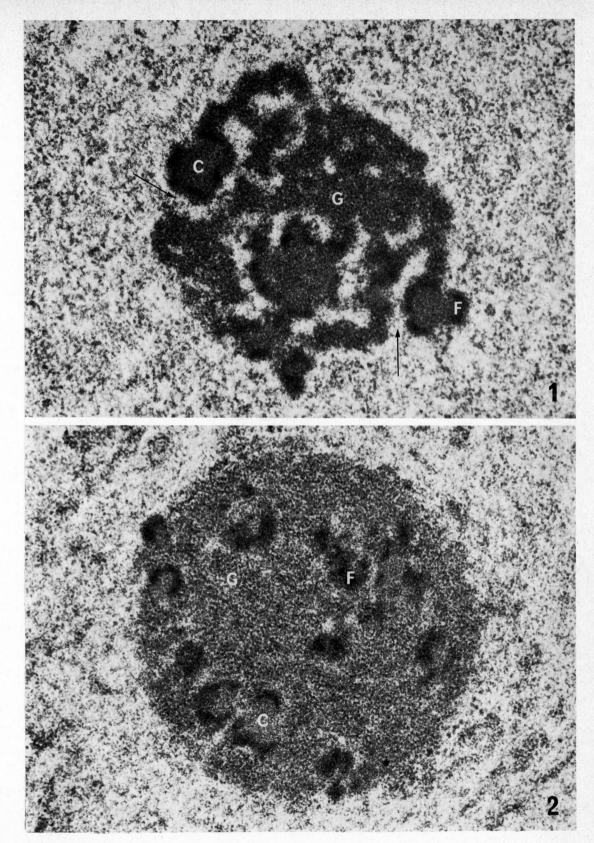

If this term is to be retained at all by electron microscopists, it should be used, as by Fawcett (1967) and many others, to describe the rounded zones of light density and texture that are encountered in nucleoli. However, such regions also appear to contain 50 Å diameter filaments, similar to those in the rest of the nucleolus except that they are not compacted as in the dense zones of the nucleolonema. These rounded structures have now been described by various names, two common ones being 'fibrillar centres' and 'nucleolini'. Since the nucleolonema is visualized as a thread-like structure in only some nucleoli, and as the status of the term pars amorpha is debatable, there is a growing tendency to ignore these terms and speak only of light and dark components or granular and fibrillary parts of the nucleolus. Therefore, in the text which follows and the illustrations accompanying this section, I have indicated the 'pars amorpha' as fibrillar centres.

The prominence of the nucleolus in proliferating cells such as embryonic cells, stem cells, cells in tissue culture, tumour cells and cells producing a protein-rich secretory product such as pancreatic acinar cells has long suggested that the nucleolus plays a key role in protein synthesis (Caspersson and Schultz, 1940; Caspersson and Santesson, 1942; Caspersson, 1950). Since then evidence has accumulated which shows that this is because the nucleolus is involved in the production and distribution of RNA and is the site of synthesis of the precursors of ribosomal RNA (Perry, 1964, 1966, 1969). Such evidence includes the demonstration of a similarity of base composition between nucleolar and ribosomal RNA (Edstrom et al., 1961), the inhibition of ribosomal RNA synthesis after destruction of the nucleolus by ultraviolet microbeam irradiation (Perry, 1964) and work on the anucleolate mutant of *Xenopus laevis* which is unable to produce ribosomal RNA (Brown and Gurdon, 1964). The steps involved in the synthesis and maturation of ribosomal RNA and its combination with protein to form ribosomal subunits and ultimately ribosomes and polyribosomes in the cytoplasm have also been described (see review by Perry, 1969).

Enlargement of the nucleolus is a well known feature of tumour cells (*Plate 19*). This pheno-menon, first observed by Pianese (1896), has been demonstrated by McCarty (1937) and by many others since to be true for a large number and variety of tumours. Although this enlargement can be quite impressive, and is a fairly constant feature of the neoplastic state, it is by no means the hallmark of malignancy. Thus Stowell (1949) showed that nucleoli larger than those occurring in malignant hepatoma can be found in regenerating rat liver after partial hepatectomy. Early nucleolar enlargement has been observed in the skin of mice painted with carcinogens, but here

---

Plate 19

Figs. 1 and 2. Nucleolar pleomorphism in malignant tumours. *Fig. 1* shows a compact but enlarged nucleolus from an adenocarcinoma (primary site probably the stomach or colon). *Fig. 2* shows an enlarged irregular nucleolus with a reticular nucleolonema (N), from an anaplastic bronchial carcinoma. Nucleolus-associated heterochromatin (H) is well demonstrated in *Fig. 1* while numerous small fibrillar centres (F) are seen in *Fig. 2*. Nuclear matrix (M) extending into the nucleolus is also seen. × 32,000; × 28,000

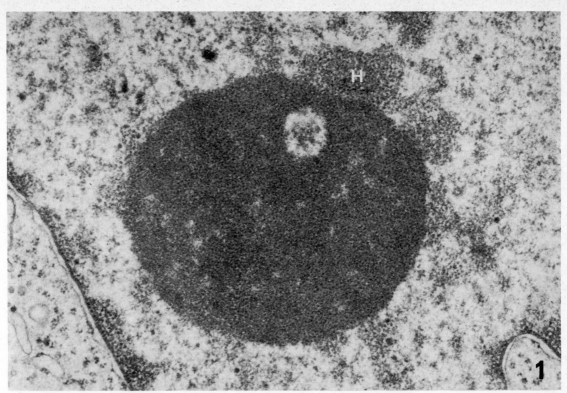

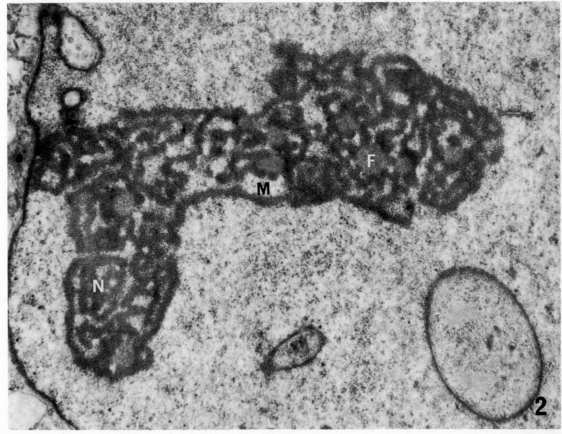

also it is largely related to the hyperplastic rather than the neoplastic state engendered by such treatment (Cowdry and Paletta, 1941; Cooper, 1956). Other similar non-specific nucleolar changes in malignancy include margination of nucleolus (page 42), irregularity of shape, and an increase in numbers of nucleoli. The latter is said to be related to the aneuploidy of cancer cells, but splitting of pre-existing nucleoli also seems to be involved.

We have noted that nucleolar hypertrophy is associated with heightened protein synthesis. It is therefore conceivable that regressive changes might be evident in the nucleolus when cells, once engaged in such active synthesis, have ceased to do so.

It is interesting to note that light microscopists have for long described 'vacuoles' in nucleoli and noted that the number of vacuoles increase with the age of the cell, after irradiation, after treatment with acridine derivatives, or when growing cell cultures at low temperatures (for references, see Busch *et al.*, 1963)—situations where one would suspect that protein synthesis had been depressed. A pattern seen in ultrathin sections which probably reflects regressive changes is called the ring-shaped nucleolus. Here the nucleolonema forms a thin shell surrounding one or two pale fibrillary centres (*Plate 20, Fig. 1*).

In a series of papers, Smetana and his colleagues (for references, see Smetana *et al.*, 1970a, b) have described ring-shaped nucleoli in various cells such as human lymphocytes, plasmacytes, monocytes, differentiated lymphosarcoma cells, myeloblasts and promyelocytes of acute myeloblastic leukaemia, and in mature (but not in immature) smooth muscle cells. They conclude from these studies that 'The finding of ring-shaped nucleoli in these different cell types apparently indicates that the presence and formation of such nucleoli represents a general phenomenon that reflects a reduced but continuing synthesis of ribosome precursors in the nucleolus.' Similarly, tissue culture studies (for references, see Love and Soriano, 1971) also show that when nucleolar RNA synthesis is inhibited by thymidine, or when the cells are in a quiescent state, the fibrillar centres are few, large and prominent, while during active growth the nucleolonema is prominent and the fibrillary centres form numerous small discrete spherules. Our observations are in keeping with these findings, and in *Plate 20, Figs. 2 and 3*, are illustrated some extreme examples of nucleolar atrophy which we have encountered. One of these was found in a smooth muscle cell of the involuting rat uterus, two days after delivery. Here the nucleolus is reduced to a very thin shell-like structure and shows large spaces occupied by some fibrillary material and nuclear matrix.

Plate 20

Fig. 1. Ring-shaped nucleolus from a plasmacytoid cell found in human bronchial mucosa. The nucleus of this cell showed the characteristic cart-wheel pattern but little rough endoplasmic reticulum was evident in the cytoplasm. × 45,000

Fig. 2. Nucleolus from a rat kidney tubule cell. This animal had been on an Atromid S-containing diet for a long period. The cytoplasm of this cell appeared oedematous and contained few organelles. × 50,000

Fig. 3. Nucleolus from involuting rat uterus. The nucleolonema (N) is reduced to a thin shell-like structure, surrounding pools of nuclear matrix (M) and fibrillary material (F). × 56,000

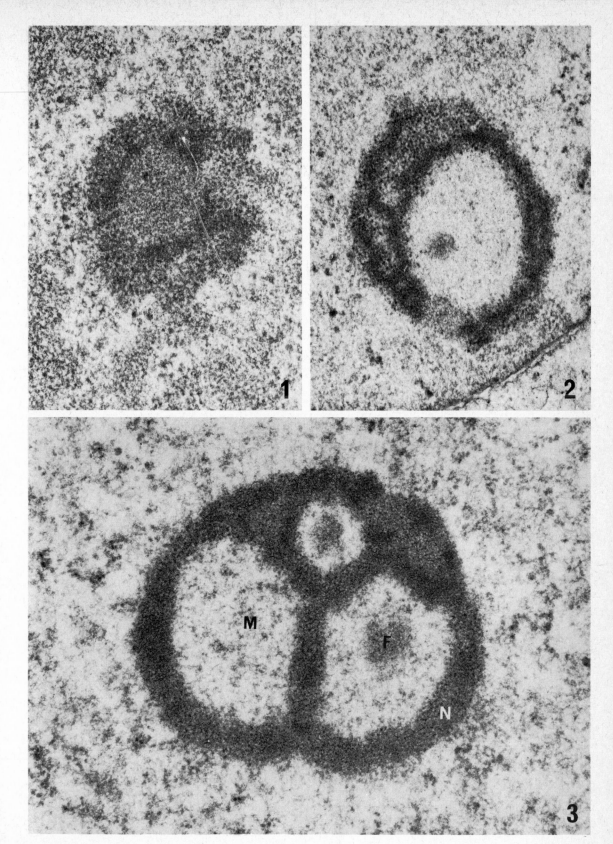

The nucleolus can move within the nucleus and examples may be cited to show that, in states of active protein synthesis, it may come to lie against the nuclear membrane. This phenomenon is referred to as nucleolar margination.

Thus in the growing oöcyte of amphibia most of the numerous nucleoli that occur in this cell type are located at the inner membrane of the nuclear envelope. When the oöcyte matures they shrink and lie in the central region of the nucleus, and after fertilization and during early cleavage, when protein synthetic activity is very low, the nucleoli are not visible (Mirsky and Osawa, 1961). Particularly interesting is the situation seen in the neurons of the fish, *Lophius*, for the direction of movement of the nucleolus which occurs with change in synthetic activity is toward the segment of nuclear membrane proximal to the axon base, and it is in the cytoplasm in this region where most of the synthetic activity is carried on (Hydén, 1943). Intense protein synthetic activity occurs in the regenerating liver of the rat after partial hepatectomy, and Swift (1959) has noted that some 50 per cent of the nucleoli move to the nuclear margin.

Evidence of the type presented above indicates that nucleolar margination is a sign of increased protein synthesis. It is therefore not surprising to find that nucleolar margination is frequently seen in a variety of tumours, and that in some instances, such as the adenocarcinoma illustrated in *Plate 21*, many marginated nucleoli can be seen in a single field of view.

Although as a general rule there is a positive correlation between the degree of malignancy and the rate of growth of a tumour, this is not invariably so, and even some benign tumours are known to have a rapid growth phase. An example of this is the keratoacanthoma, a benign usually self-regressing tumour which mimics a carcinoma both in its histological appearance and in its rapid growth rate (Ghadially, 1961, 1971; Ghadially *et al.*, 1963). Such tumours can be produced experimentally (Ghadially, 1958) and we (Ghadially and Parry, unpublished observation) have observed frequent nucleolar margination during the growth phase of this benign tumour (*Plate 22, Fig. 1*).

Plate 21

A fragment of human adenocarcinoma (same case as *Plate 19, Fig. 1*) found in ascitic fluid. Most of the nucleoli seen in this electron micrograph are marginated (arrows). Note also the irregularity of nuclear shape and the variability of heterochromatin content. The two nuclei at the top corner of the electron micrograph contain abundant heterochromatin aggregates, and would thus appear hyperchromatic at light microscopy, while the remainder are poor in heterochromatin content and would present a paler appearance. × 7,000

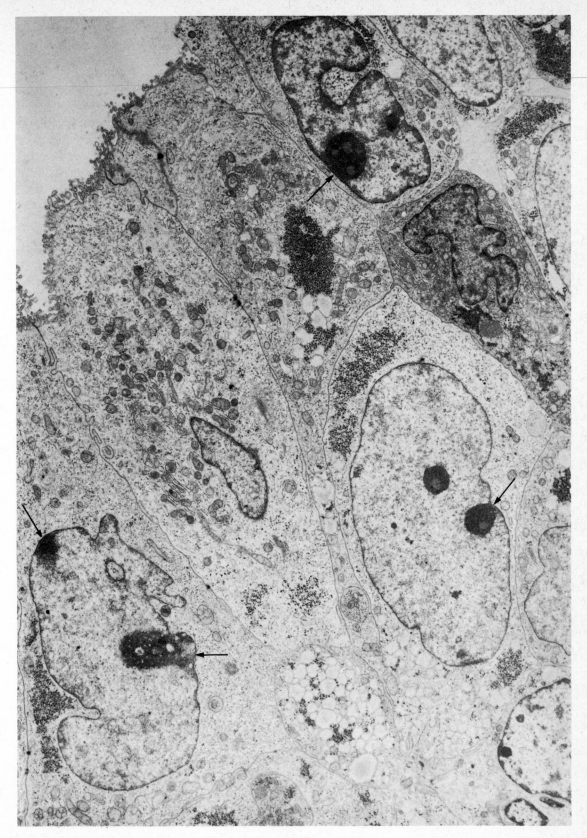

43

Irregularities of nuclear shape (page 4), invaginations of the nuclear envelope and pseudo-inclusions (page 50) are common features of the neoplastic nucleus, and in some tumours such deep invaginations are seen to make contact with or penetrate the nucleolus (*Plate 22, Figs. 2 and 3*). This phenomenon has been recorded in the Ehrlich ascites tumour (Oberling and Bernhard, 1961) and has been observed by us (Ghadially and Oryschak, unpublished observation) in bronchial carcinoma cells found in a pleural effusion (*Plate 22*). In this example, innumerable tumour cells showed this close association between nucleolus and invaginations of the nuclear envelope. Examples were seen where multiple invaginations were present, in a single nucleus, each contacting one or more nucleoli.

The phenomenon of nucleolar margination has led many observers to speculate that such an arrangement facilitates nucleocytoplasmic exchanges. For although an occasional marginated nucleolus may be found in the cells of any tissue, it is seen much more frequently in rapidly growing cells and in cells engaged in the production of a protein-rich secretory product (e.g. pancreatic cells). Thus regarding nucleolar margination, Oberling and Bernhard (1961) state, 'One can assume that transportation of nucleolar products towards the cytoplasm is highly facilitated by this arrangement'. Clear morphological evidence on this point is, however, lacking. If exchanges do occur at such sites of contact, they are probably at a molecular level undetectable by current techniques. One may at times find ribosomes in the cytoplasm adjacent to a marginated nucleolus, and even a nuclear pore may be detected in the area, but this cannot be accepted as proof of transfer from nucleolus to cytoplasm, as has sometimes been suggested.

Plate 22

Fig. 1. Cells from keratoacanthoma of rabbit skin, produced by repeated applications of 9:10-dimethyl-1:2-benzanthracene. Enlarged and marginated nucleoli are seen in the nuclei of this tumour. × 5,500

Fig. 2. Carcinoma of the bronchus. A deep invagination of the nuclear envelope (E) containing cytoplasmic material (C) is seen in contact with the nucleolus (NU). Nucleus (N), intratcyopasmic lipid droplet (L). × 17,500

Fig. 3. (From the same specimen as *Fig. 2.*) A pseudo-inclusion containing cytoplasmic structures (C) is seen in close association with a nucleolus (NU). × 18,500

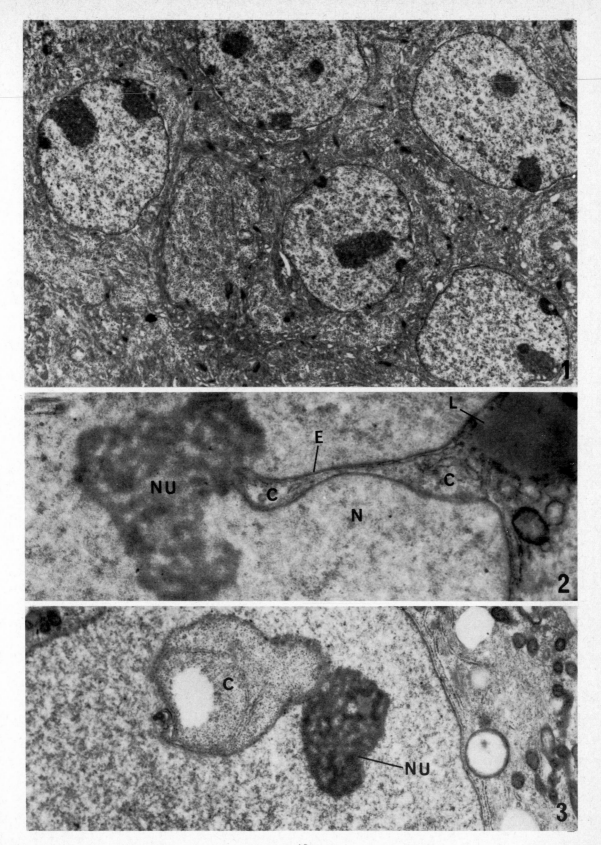

It has already been noted (page 36) that the normal nucleolus is largely made up of granules and fibrillary material and that focal variations in the proportion of fibrils and granules produce the light and dark zones of the nucleolus. The dark areas comprise compacted fibrils, while the light areas are mainly granular. In the phenomenon referred to as nucleolar segregation there is separation and migration of the fibrillary from the granular component (*Plates 23 and 24*). This change is to some extent reversible but the process may lead to wide separation and dispersal of the components, and ultimately to a total disintegration of the nucleolus.

In assessing nucleolar segregation, two main points must be borne in mind: one is the degree of separation, that is to say how far the segregated components have moved apart, and the second is the purity of segregation. Thus in some instances the segregation may be quite pure and one can distinguish the dense fibrillary component quite clearly from the much lighter granular component, but in other instances (impure segregation) there is only a marginal difference in densities, for both granules and fibrils are present in each component, there being only a relative difference in the amount of granules and fibrils in the segregated parts. Yet another not too common factor may affect the final image that is seen in electron micrographs; the density of the fibrillary component is due to close packing of the fibrils; if these are not well packed, this component may also present as a light area.

It is worth recalling that the fibrils of the nucleolus are extremely fine and, in the dense areas, form a closely packed meshwork. Thus the fibrillary nature of the dense component is difficult to demonstrate in sectioned material where only short lengths of the cut fibrils are present. Examination of the margins of the dense areas at high magnifications usually demonstrates the fibrils for here they are not so tightly packed.

Various patterns of nucleolar segregation are recognized, perhaps the best known being the nucleolar cap. Here, the dense filamentous component forms a crescentic, hemispherical, cone-shaped or cap-like mass over the granular component of the nucleolus (*Plate 23*). Sometimes two caps are formed and wider separation of segregated components may also occur.

In other instances the filamentous component departs from the granular component as numerous small dense masses, from one pole of the nucleolus or in a radiate fashion (*Plate 24, Figs. 1, 2 and 4*). The significance and mechanisms involved in the production of these different patterns is not known. A correlation between aetiological agent and pattern of nucleolar segregation does not seem to exist.

Plate 23

Nucleolar segregation produced in rat hepatocyte nucleoli by actinomycin D (*Ghadially and Ailsby, unpublished electron micrographs*)

Figs. 1–3. Nuclear caps are shown. The denser fibrillary component forming the cap is indicated by arrows. Note also the nucleolus associated heterochromatin (H). $\times 29,000$; $\times 35,000$; $\times 56,000$
Fig. 4. Further separation of segregated components is illustrated here. The segregation is quite impure; the component richer in fibrils (arrow) can barely be identified $\times 56,000$

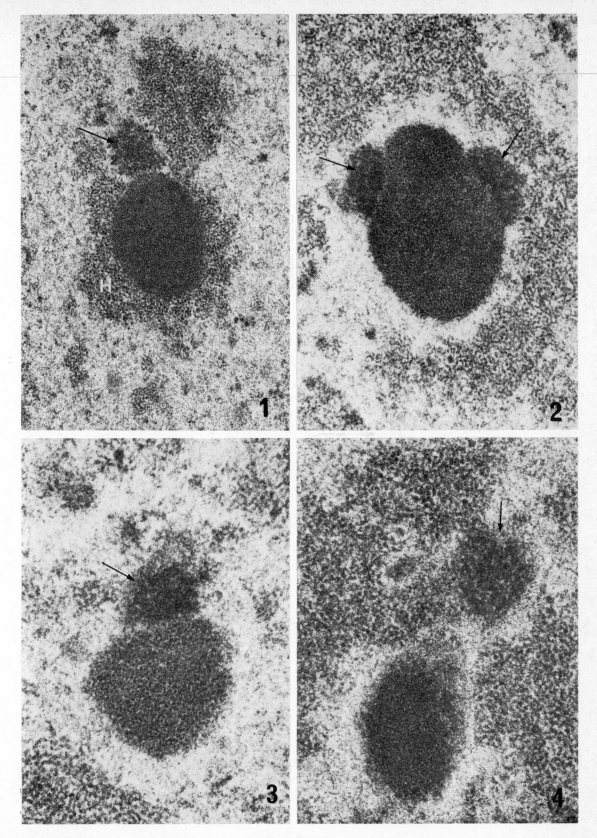

47

Thus nucleolar cap formation, which is the characteristic form of segregation seen after actinomycin D administration, has also been seen in herpesvirus-infected cells (Sirtori and Bosisio, 1966).

Nucleolar segregation has been produced in a variety of cells (most studies are on rat hepatocytes) by numerous agents such as: (1) actinomycin D (Schoefl, 1964; Oda and Chiga, 1965; Chiga *et al.*, 1966; De Man and Noorduyn, 1967); (2) mitomycin C (Lapis and Bernhard, 1965; Kume *et al.*, 1967; Goldblatt *et al.*, 1969); (3) 4-nitroquinoline-*N*-oxide (Reynolds *et al.*, 1963; Lazarus *et al.*, 1966); (4) proflavine, acridine orange (Simard, 1966; Reynolds and Montgomery, 1967); (5) ethionine (Miyai and Steiner, 1967; Shinozuka *et al.*, 1968); (6) dimethylnitrosoamine, 3'methyl-4-dimethyl-aminoazobenzene, aflatoxin B, lasiocarpine, tannic acid (Svoboda *et al.*, 1966, 1967; Reddy and Svoboda, 1968); (7) cycloheximide (Harris *et al.*, 1968); (8) herpesvirus (Sirtori and Bosisio, 1966; Swanson *et al.*, 1966; Leestma *et al.*, 1969); (9) Coxsackie virus (Weiss and Meyer, 1972); (10) myoplasma (Jezequel *et al.*, 1967); and (11) flying spot ultraviolet nuclear irradiation (Montgomery *et al.*, 1966). It will be observed that the list of agents which can produce nucleolar segregation contains many carcinogens and antimetabolites.

Simard and Bernhard (1966) postulated that nucleolar segregation probably reflects DNA binding and inhibition of DNA-dependent RNA synthesis because of the loss of template activity of DNA, and this view has found favour with many students of this subject. Reddy and Svoboda (1968) have pointed out that many hepatocarcinogens and also some other agents which produce nucleolar segregation produce a decrease in the activity of RNA polymerase, an enzyme known to catalyse the synthesis of RNA, and that two carcinogens, 3-methylcholanthrene and thioacetamide, which do not produce nucleolar segregation show an increase in RNA polymerase activity and RNA synthesis. Further, it can be observed that the list of agents which produce nucleolar segregation also contains many compounds not known to be carcinogenic. Hence one may conclude that this phenomenon is not a prerequisite for the production of a tumour.

Plate 24

Fig. 1. Small dense masses comprising the fibrillary component (F) are seen sequestrated from the main nucleolar mass containing numerous granules (G). From herpesvirus-infected monkey kidney cells in culture. ×41,000

Fig. 2. A more advanced form of segregation is seen in this electron micrograph. The fibrillary component (F) is represented by small dense bodies radiating from the centrally placed granular component (G). Virus particles (V). From the same material as *Fig. 1.* ×33,000

Fig. 3. Another pattern of nucleolar segregation, where the granular (G) and fibrillar components (F) have each formed a hemispherical mass. From the same material as *Fig. 1.* ×49,000

Fig. 4. An unusual pattern of nucleolar segregation is depicted here. In the centre of the nucleolus is an enlarged fibrillar centre (C). Adjacent to this is the granular component (G) and, surrounding this, the dense fibrillary component (F) which is broken up into discrete small masses. From an early tumour nodule (fibrosarcoma) produced in the subcutaneous tissue of the rat by an injection of 9:10-dimethyl 1:2-benzanthracene. ×40,000 (*Ghadially and Bhatnagar, unpublished electron micrograph*)

48

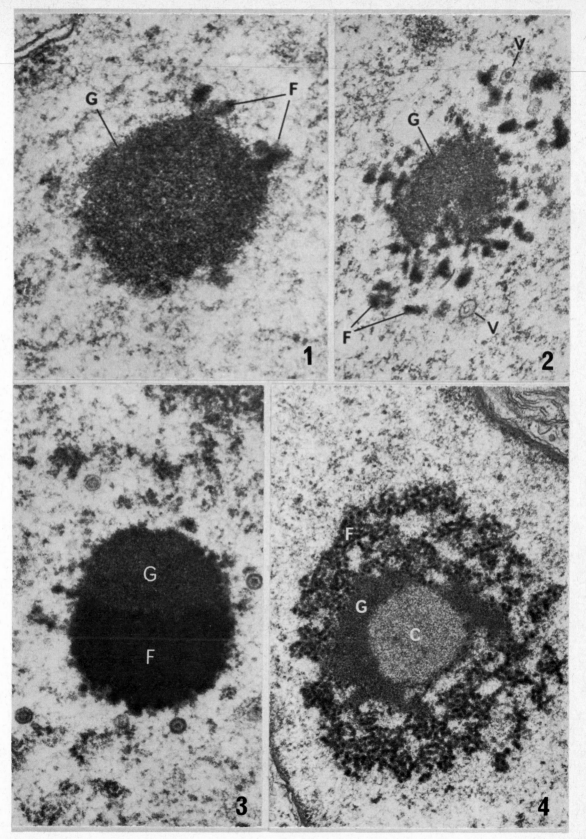

c

49

PSEUDOINCLUSIONS AND TRUE INCLUSIONS

Nuclear inclusions occurring in a variety of tissues of man and other animals have been studied extensively by light microscopy for over 60 years. (For references see Sobel *et al.*, 1969a). Distinction between viral and non-viral inclusions could not be made with confidence and many non-viral inclusions were assumed to be viral ones.

Electron microscopic studies have now made it amply clear that most nuclear inclusions contain cytoplasmic structures and are non-viral. It is also evident that a large majority of these inclusions are, in fact, pseudoinclusions (*Plate 25*), for the apparently included material does not lie free in the nuclear matrix but is separated from it by an invagination of the nuclear envelope. Virtually every cytoplasmic organelle and inclusion has, at one time or another, been found within such pseudoinclusions. True inclusions, where the included material lies free in the nuclear matrix, are somewhat rarer.

The morphology of pseudoinclusions is illustrated by two examples in *Plate 25*, *Fig. 1*, and it can be seen that an invagination in longitudinal section will appear as a pseudoinclusion in transverse section. Serial sections show that fusion of membranes in narrow-necked invagination can occur (Leduc and Wilson, 1959a), sequestrating the double-membrane-bound inclusion within the nucleus. At this stage one can argue that the included material is still not truly within the nucleus and hence such inclusions should be regarded as pseudoinclusions. However, dissolution of the covering membranes may occur and ultimately convert a pseudoinclusion into a true inclusion where the included material mingles with the nuclear matrix. Characteristically, pseudoinclusions are lined by the two membranes of the nuclear envelope and, as one would expect, the inner membrane is studded with ribosomes just like the outer membrane of the nuclear envelope, while condensed chromatin may be seen lying round the outer membrane of the inclusion as it does along the inner membrane of the nuclear envelope.

Pseudoinclusions show marked variations in size. Very large inclusions, as large as normal nuclei, were noted in the enlarged hepatocytes of mice fed a methionine-rich diet to which bentonite was added (Leduc and Wilson, 1959a, b). An extreme example of this has been reported by Bloom (1967), where virtually the entire cytoplasmic mass with its organelles and inclusions formed an inclusion within the nucleus, which was reduced to a thin shell lying just under the cell membrane. The number of inclusions seen in a single nucleus is also variable. Occasionally, the entire nucleus is studded with multiple inclusions (*Plate 26*, *Fig. 1*).

Plate 25

Fig. 1. Human synovial intimal cell showing an irregular nucleus (nucleus, N; cytoplasm, C). An invagination such as that seen at A will appear as a pseudoinclusion (B) in transverse section. The characteristic double membrane lining such inclusions can barely be discerned at this low magnification. × 33,000 (*From Ghadially and Roy, 1969*)

Fig. 2. Acute leukaemic cell from peripheral blood, showing an invagination (I) and a pseudoinclusion containing a mitochondrion (M) with longitudinally orientated cristae. A few ribosomes can be seen along the inner membrane of the inclusion (arrow). × 42,000 (*Ghadially and Skinnider, unpublished electron micrograph*)

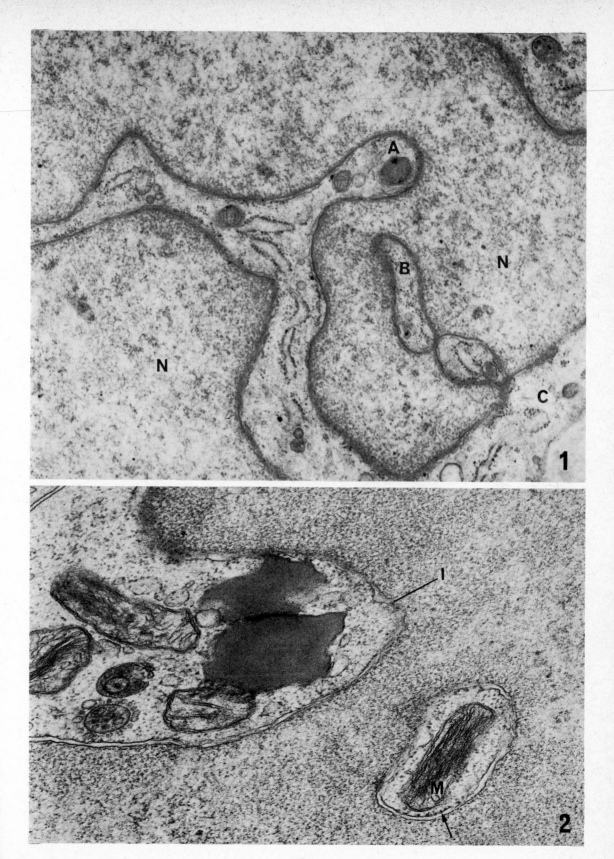

Changes often occur in the structures trapped in an inclusion (*Plate 26*, *Fig. 2*). Organelles such as rough endoplasmic reticulum and mitochondria frequently show degenerative changes which lead to the formation of membranous whorls and myelin figures. It would appear that such changes are more likely to occur when the invagination has a narrow opening or when the opening is occluded, and it has been suggested that normal structures promptly degenerate in such an unfavourable environment (Kleinfeld *et al.*, 1956; Leduc and Wilson, 1959a).

A variety of drugs which cause toxic injury to cells can produce nuclear invaginations and inclusions, and Sobel *et al.* (1969a) have postulated that in most of these instances there is an increased cytoplasmic volume (swelling) which probably leads to the extrusion of cytoplasmic material into the nucleus. In this respect the observations of Wessel (1958) are interesting, for they suggest that pseudoinclusions can be transient. In colchicine-injected mice he noted a swelling of hepatocytes and formation of nuclear inclusions which regressed when the effect of the drug had worn off and the swelling had subsided.

A study of published data indicates that nuclear inclusions are seen infrequently in young animals, including man, but with advancing years there is an increase in the number of both hyperploid nuclei and inclusions. This is suggested by the work of: (1) Sobel *et al.* (1969a) on human material; (2) Olitsky and Casals (1945) who observed invaginations of the nuclear envelope in the liver of two strains of mice and found that they were more frequent in older animals; and (3) Andrew *et al.* (1943) who observed nuclear inclusions more frequently in the liver of older mice and men.

A variety of true inclusions occurs in the nucleus, besides those containing cytoplasmic components; for example, inclusions produced by viruses and lead. These and other true inclusions are dealt with in later sections of this chapter. However, it is worth making a few brief comments here about the manner in which cytoplasmic components may come to lie in the nuclear matrix. It has already been pointed out that dissolution of the membranes enclosing a pseudoinclusion can produce a true inclusion. Other theories have also been offered to explain how true inclusions may occur. It has thus been suggested that organelles as large as mitochondria can gain access to the interior of the nucleus via enlarged nuclear pores, or that organelles may become accidentally incorporated within the nucleus during mitosis (Brandes *et al.*, 1965; Bucciarelli, 1966; Bloom, 1967). The latter event is particularly liable to occur with frequent or abnormal mitoses. Such a view is in keeping with the observation that nuclear inclusions are commonly encountered in many tumours, but it should be noted that even in this example most of the inclusions are pseudoinclusions dependent upon irregularity of nuclear shape. (See pages 2–4 for further discussion on this topic.)

Inclusions have been seen in such a large variety of tumours that it would be impossible to list all instances. Perhaps of special interest are the human and experimentally produced melanomas, for true inclusions of pigment granules may be found in the nucleus. However, such inclusions have also been observed in naevi and in the choroid of human and animal eyes (Ludford, 1924; Apitz, 1937; Sobel *et al.*, 1969a).

Plate 26

Fig. 1. Nucleus of synovial intimal cell from a rabbit with experimentally produced haemarthrosis showing numerous pseudoinclusions. In one of the inclusions the included cytoplasmic vesicles and other structures are well preserved (A); in others there is evidence of structural disorganization, while in the inclusion marked 'B' a myelin figure has evolved by this process. × 37,000 (*Ghadially and Roy, unpublished electron micrograph*)

Fig. 2. Hepatocyte from liver tissue adjacent to a hepatoma in man. The nucleus contains many small inclusions and large myelin figures, probably derived by degenerative changes in the contents of a pseudoinclusion. × 20,000. (*Ghadially and Parry, unpublished electron micrograph*)

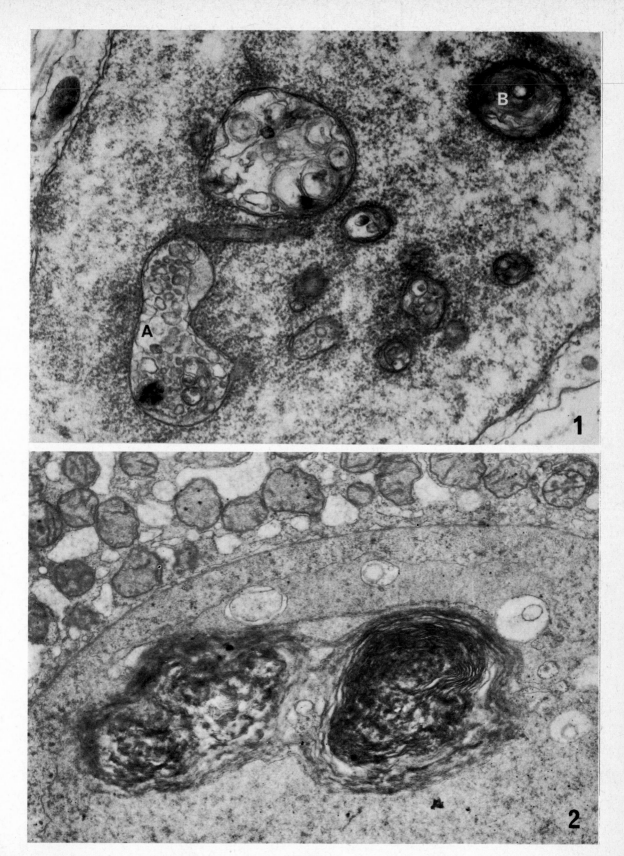

Intranuclear glycogen deposits were first described by Ehrlich (1883) in the hepatocytes of patients suffering from diabetes mellitus. In routine histological sections such deposits present as clear vacuolar inclusions. With the electron microscope, characteristic plumbophilic dense particles are seen. In most instances only monoparticulate glycogen is observed but in rare instances rosettes or rosette-like formations have also been found.

Glycogen deposits may present as large irregular-shaped masses within the nucleus, or they may form a compact rounded mass surrounded by fibrillary material (*Plate 27*). Solitary glycogen particles or small groups of particles may also be seen lying free in the nuclear matrix. Invaginations of the nuclear envelope are not seen around these inclusions, so these deposits are regarded as true inclusions.

Glycogen deposits have been seen in hepatocyte nuclei in: (1) diabetes mellitus (Ehrlich, 1883; Chipps and Duff, 1942; Tanikawa and Igarashi, 1963; Caramia *et al.*, 1967, 1968; Schulz and Hahnel, 1969; Sobel *et al.*, 1969b); (2) Graves's disease and Hodgkin's disease (Cazal and Mirouze, 1951); (3) infective hepatitis (Biava, 1963; Wills, 1968); (4) Wilson's disease and Gilbert's disease (Sobel *et al.*, 1969b); (5) glycogen storage disease type I, but not type II (Sheldon *et al.*, 1962; Baudhuin *et al.*, 1964); (6) lupus erythematosus (Sparrow and Ashworth, 1965); and (7) normal well-fed tadpoles (Himes and Pollister, 1962).

Intranuclear glycogen has been seen in a biopsy of human myocardium obtained at open heart surgery but the reason for this occurrence could not be ascertained (*Plate 28*). Intranuclear glycogen has also been seen in tumour cell nuclei, such as: (1) hepatomas of mouse (Shelton, 1955) and man (Ghadially and Parry, 1966); (2) a chicken sarcoma (Binggeli, 1959); (3) Ehrlich ascites tumours (Novikoff, 1957; Scholz and Pawletz, 1969); and (4) Novikoff ascites rat hepatoma cells incubated with tritium-labelled D-glucose (Karasaki, 1971).

Plate 27

From human liver adjacent to a hepatoma.

Fig. 1. Part of a large glycogen (G) deposit lying in the nucleus (N) is seen in this electron micrograph (*Ghadially and Parry, unpublished electron micrograph*) ×72,000

Fig. 2. A focal deposit of glycogen (A) surrounded by some fibrillary material is seen in this electron micrograph. Such a deposit is sometimes referred to as an intranuclear glycogen body. Smaller deposits of glycogen (B) are scattered in the nuclear matrix. (*From Ghadially and Parry, 1966*). ×80,000

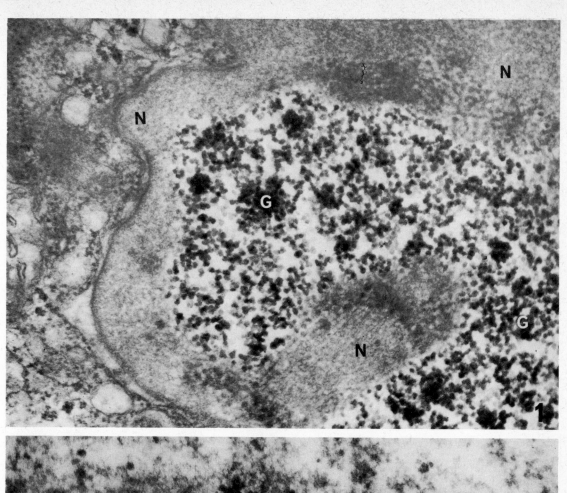

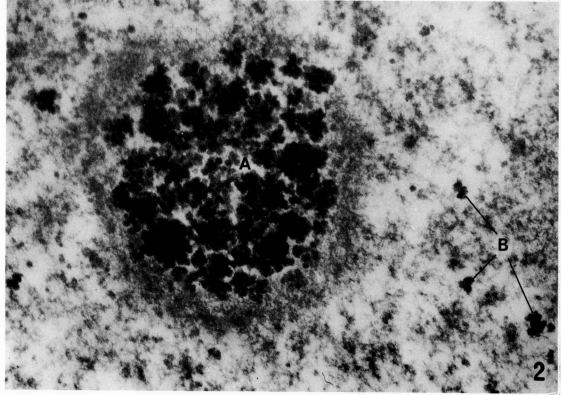

The idea that glycogen arrives in the nucleus via pseudoinclusions or that it enters the nucleus via the nuclear pores finds little support from recent studies. Himes and Pollister (1962) suggested that glycogen in the nucleus may be synthesized *in situ* and this hypothesis is supported by the recent work of Karasaki (1971), who incubated hepatoma cells with tritium-labelled D-glucose and found that massive accumulations of glycogen can occur rapidly in nuclei without similar deposits in the cytoplasm at a period of active DNA synthesis when the nuclear envelope is intact. He noted an inverse relationship between deposits in the cytoplasm and nucleus, a point that has often also been made by those studying such deposits in human liver.

It is worth noting that focal glycogen deposits of the type illustrated in *Plate 27, Fig. 2*, can at times be confused with the fibrillogranular type of nuclear body as illustrated in *Plate 41, Fig. 6*. In this example distinction between the two is not too difficult because the glycogen forms pseudo-rosettes, but this is not always the case. Nuclear bodies that bear a remarkable resemblance to some examples of focal glycogen deposits (e.g. those observed by Caramia *et al.*, 1967, 1968) are illustrated by Murad and Murthy (1970) in a chordoma, and by Wyatt *et al.* (1970) in a rhabdomyoma. In the latter example the bodies were PAS-positive but diastase-resistant. The focal deposits of glycogen, called glycogen bodies by Caramia *et al.* (1967, 1968), were also PAS-positive but susceptible to diastase digestion. Thus it would appear that we are dealing here with two distinct entities which may at times be difficult to distinguish on morphological grounds alone. Finally, it is worth noting that the term 'glycogen body' has also been used to describe glycogen membrane arrays in the cytoplasm (Chapter V and *Plate 120*), so this term should be avoided or the focal deposits of glycogen described more fully as the intranuclear glycogen body.

Plate 28

From human myocardium obtained at open heart surgery. The nucleus of this myocardial cell contains accumulations of monoparticulate glycogen (G) similar to such deposits in the cytoplasm (g). × 35,000

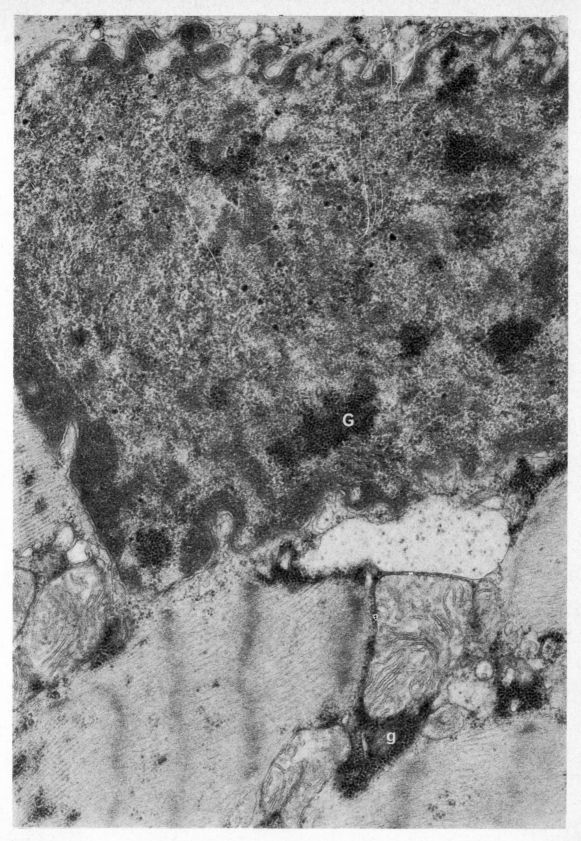

Both false and true lipid inclusions occur in the nucleus. In the former instance lipid forms but a part of a pseudoinclusion which also contains a variable amount of cytoplasm and often also some organelles. The true inclusion is seen as one or more lipid droplets lying free in the nuclear matrix (*Plate 29*). As a rule no membrane surrounds such droplets but at times a membrane or membrane-like structure (characteristic trilaminar structure has not been demonstrated) can be discerned closely applied to the lipid droplet (*Plate 29, Fig. 1*). However, it is unlikely that this is derived from the nuclear envelope, for a double membrane is not seen and at times cytoplasmic lipid also has such a 'membranous' structure around it. It is my experience that such 'membrane-bound' lipid droplets occur in the nucleus only when similar 'membrane-bound' lipid occurs in the cytoplasm.

The morphology of lipid droplets depends upon several factors such as the amount and degree of saturation of the fatty acids present, and the manner in which the tissue is processed. (For fuller discussion, see page 448.) Thus in electron micrographs lipids show varying degrees of electron density ranging from very low to very high, or it may be totally removed during processing and appear as a hole. The contours of the lipid droplet may be smooth and round, ruffled or crenated. These are but a few of the many variations of lipid droplet morphology that one observes in electron micrographs. However, all such variations of morphology seen in cytoplasmic lipid are also seen in intranuclear lipid inclusions, and there is usually a close similarity between the two in any given specimen.

It would be futile to attempt to list all instances in which intranuclear lipid inclusions have been sighted, for lipid inclusions are perhaps the commonest form of true nuclear inclusions. An occasional such inclusion may be encountered in a variety of normal tissues, particularly where lipid droplets normally occur in the cytoplasm. Thus an occasional intranuclear lipid inclusion is found in normal liver but they occur more frequently in situations where there is an increase in cytoplasmic lipid droplets. In normal synovial intimal cells lipid has not been seen in the nucleus, but in lipohaemarthrosis the synovial cells are loaded with lipid droplets and intranuclear lipid inclusions also occur (Ghadially and Roy, 1969b). Intranuclear lipid inclusions have often been noted in a variety of tumours. Passing mention of the occurrence of intranuclear lipid inclusions abounds in the literature, but detailed description or comment about the mechanism by which such inclusions arise is made in only a few instances. Such studies deal mainly

---

Plate 29

Fig. 1. A nucleus from an adenocarcinoma of the stomach of man showing 'membrane-bound' crenated lipid inclusions (L). × 31,000

Fig. 2. Leukaemic lymphocyte from peripheral blood of man. An electron-dense crenated lipid droplet (L) is seen in the nucleus. × 32,000

Fig. 3. Nucleus from small intestinal epithelial cell of a rat bearing a subcutaneous sarcoma showing a medium density lipid droplet (L) in the nucleus. × 48,000

Fig. 4. Human hepatoma cell nucleus showing a vacuolar electron-lucent area (L) which could be interpreted as lipid removed during tissue processing. × 49,000

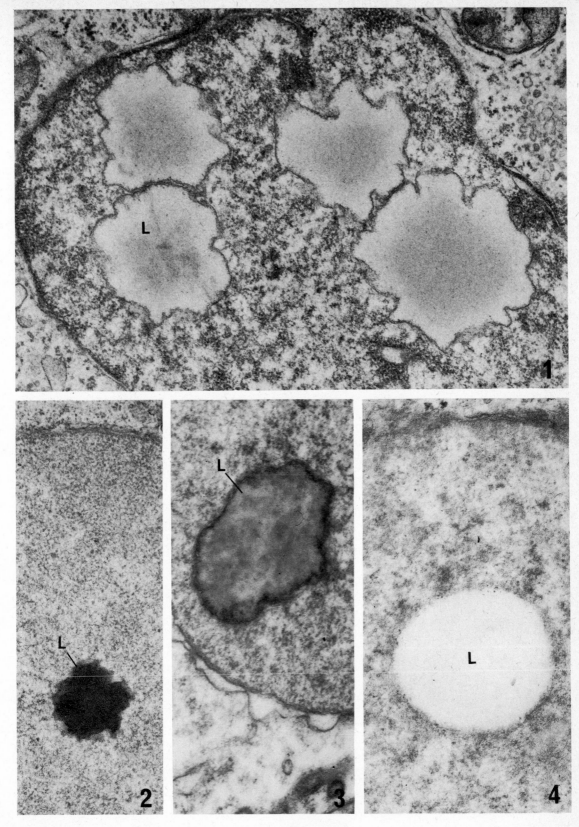

with hepatomas, and liver cells, after various treatments such as partial hepatectomy and thio-acetamide treatment (Kleinfeld and Von Haam, 1959; Leduc and Wilson, 1959a, b; Rouiller and Simon, 1962; Hruban *et al.*, 1965; Toker and Trevino, 1966; Smith *et al.*, 1968).

Regarding the mechanism of production of intranuclear lipid inclusions, the findings of Leduc and Wilson (1959a) are of interest. They found numerous pseudoinclusions containing lipid and variable amounts of cytoplasmic material. As long as there was cytoplasmic material present separating the lipid droplet from the invaginated nuclear envelope the characteristic double membrane lining of such inclusions could be easily identified, but when lipid alone was present no surrounding membrane could be seen. About such lipidic inclusions studied in serial sections they comment: 'although double membranes could not be resolved around the inclusions that were entirely occupied by a lipid droplet, one such inclusion well within the nucleus was found to which the double membrane extended, then disappeared as if obscured by or dissolved in the lipid'. In this connection it is worth noting that when close association of lipid and mitochondria occurs (page 126) the outer mitochondrial membrane also seems to disappear as if obscured by or dissolved in the lipid.

My observations on intranuclear lipid inclusions seen in many situations support the idea that lipid droplets enter the nucleus at least in some instances in a manner similar to pseudo-inclusions, but alterations and dissolution of the membranes of the invaginating nuclear envelope occur during this process, thus liberating the lipid into the nuclear matrix. This point is made in *Plate 30*, which depicts the probable sequence of events.

Plate 30

Fig. 1. Cell from ascitic effusion in a case of ovarian carcinoma. Intranuclear lipid inclusions and cytoplasmic lipid droplets were of frequent occurrence in many cells. Appearances seen in this electron micrograph may be interpreted as an early stage of formation of intranuclear lipid inclusions. Three lipid droplets are seen, two of which have indented the nucleus. Probable dissolution of nuclear envelope is seen at one point (arrow), while at other points (arrowheads) the envelope appears altered and dense. × 31,500

Fig. 2. Acute leukaemic cell from peripheral blood. Lipid droplets were plentiful in both cytoplasm and nucleus and could be detected also in smears examined with the light microscope. Appearances seen here may be interpreted as a lipid droplet in the process of entering the nucleus. The expected double membrane is not seen around the lipid droplet but electron-dense material probably derived from it is seen on the surface of the lipid. Invaginated inner membrane of the nuclear envelope can just be discerned at the neck of the inclusion (arrow). × 40,000

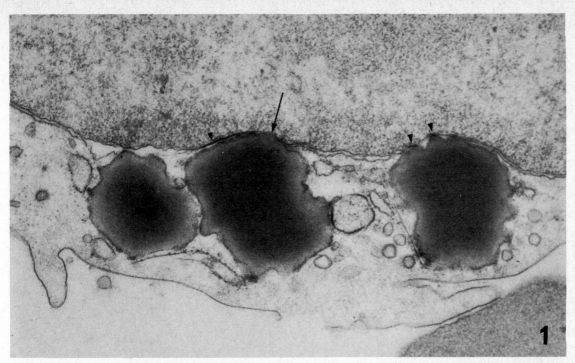

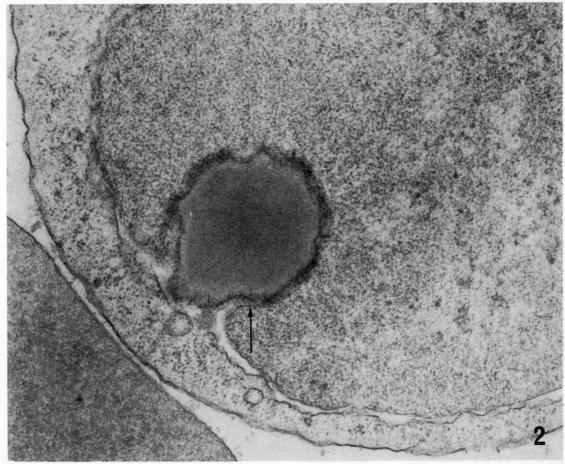

61

Crystalline, paracrystalline or crystalloid inclusions (see page 170 for definitions of these terms) have now been observed in virtually every cell compartment, including the nucleus, and are generally assumed to be protein, but only in some instances has the protein been characterized. The morphology of crystals and the appearances they present in ultrathin sections will be dealt with when crystals in mitochondria (page 170) and cytoplasm (page 452) are considered.

Perhaps the best known and most extensively studied is the crystal of Reinke found in the cytoplasm of the interstitial cells (Leydig cells) of the human testis after puberty. Occasionally, this crystal is also seen in the nucleus of the interstitial cell and, since it is not surrounded by membranes but lies free in the nuclear matrix, it is considered to be a true inclusion. The idea that this inclusion is produced in the nucleus is supported by the demonstration of tubular inclusions in the nucleus similar to those in the cytoplasm from which such crystals are believed to arise (Yasuzumi *et al.*, 1967; De Kretser, 1967, 1968).

Rarer than the Reinke crystal and not too well known is the crystalloid of Lubarsch found in the cytoplasm of spermatogonia of the human testis. It is said to be composed of filaments 80–130 Å wide with a 130–450 Å spacing between them. Dense granules resembling ribosomes are intermingled with the filaments. Such a crystalloid inclusion has also once been noted lying free in the nuclear matrix, but ribosome-like particles were absent (Sohval *et al.*, 1971). Intranuclear crystals have also been found in the phagocytic cells of ovarian tissues in echinoderms. Thus in *Arbacia punctulata* the crystal is said to be composed of spherical units 100 Å in diameter, and cytochemical studies show that it is rich in iron (Karasaki, 1963).

Perhaps the most important group of intranuclear crystals are those associated with virus infection, and this possibility must always be considered when an intranuclear crystal is sighted in an unexpected situation. It should be noted that at times the term 'virus crystal' is used to describe virus particles deployed in crystalline arrays within the nucleus, as in the case of adenovirus illustrated in *Plate 36, Fig. 1*. These are not relevant here. It is the protein crystals (which also occur in some virus-infected cells) that form the subject under discussion in this section.

Thus intranuclear crystals, which in some instances were histochemically characterized as protein, have been seen in the nuclei of cells infected with (1) certain types of adenovirus (Morgan *et al.*, 1957; Givan and Jézéquel, 1969), (2) Coxsackie virus (Jézéquel and Steiner, 1966), (3) measles virus (Kallman *et al.*, 1959), and (4) herpesvirus (a single small crystalloid inclusion seen is illustrated in *Plate 35, Fig. 2*). There is now much evidence linking measles virus infection and subacute sclerosing panencephalitis in man (for references, see Koestner and Long, 1970), and Grodums (unpublished) has found crystals in the cerebral neurons of a case of this disease (*Plate 31*), but proof of measles infection was not obtained in this case. Crystals have also been reported to occur in the hepatocyte nuclei of foxes, jackals and apparently normal dogs, but it has been suggested that they, too, may indicate a latent viral infection (for references, see Jézéquel and Steiner, 1966; Givan and Jézéquel, 1969).

Thus it would appear that crystal formation is seen in quite a variety of virus infections in various cells, both *in vitro* and *in vivo*. It is not clear whether the crystalline protein is host or viral protein, but it has been suggested that excessive protein production probably occurs in the nucleus, and that when a critical concentration is reached crystallization ensues.

Plate 31

Figs. 1 and 2. Intranuclear crystalline or paracrystalline inclusions found in cerebral neurons in a case of subacute sclerosing panencephalitis. ×78,000 and 97,000. (*Grodums, unpublished electron micrograph*)

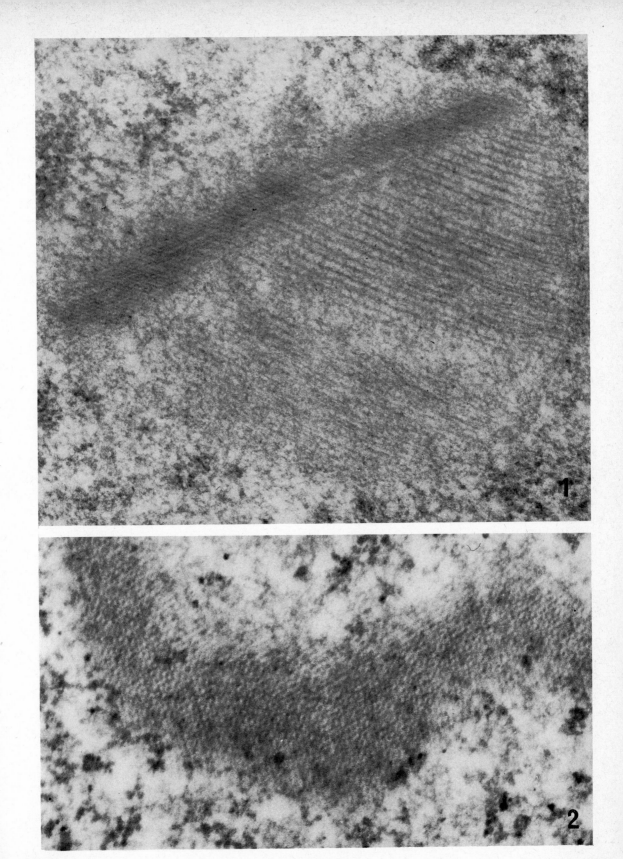

INTRANUCLEAR HAEMOGLOBIN INCLUSIONS

Haemoglobin is usually thought to be localized in the cytoplasm of erythroid cells. Its occurrence in the nucleus has in the past been doubted or denied (e.g. Maximow and Bloom, 1948). Perhaps the first convincing evidence of the presence of intranuclear haemoglobin stems from the analysis of isolated avian erythrocyte nuclei by Stern *et al.* (1951).

Intranuclear deposits of haemoglobin present as areas of moderate electron density with an appearance similar to the haemoglobin-containing cytoplasm of the erythroid cells. In suitable specimens an uninterrupted continuity of intracytoplasmic and intranuclear haemoglobin is seen via the nuclear pores (*Plate 32*). Usually the deposits are lighter than the condensed chromatin masses, but if the chromatin is not well condensed or stained and the cell is well haemoglobinized the densities are reversed (see, for example, Figs. 16 and 17 in Fawcett and Witebsky, 1964).

Intranuclear haemoglobin has been reported to occur in: (1) the erythrocytes of lower vertebrates such as fish, amphibians, reptiles and birds (Stern *et al.*, 1951; O'Brien, 1960; Davies, 1961; Tooze and Davies, 1963; Fawcett and Witebsky, 1964); and (2) erythroblasts (normoblasts) of mammals such as rabbit, dog and man (Jones, 1959; Davies, 1961; Grasso *et al.*, 1962; Simpson and Kling, 1967) in hepatic and adult medullary phases of erythopoiesis (Firkin, 1969).

However, evidence for the presence of intranuclear haemoglobin in human material and also other mammals is somewhat scanty, and rests solely on the occasional demonstration of areas within the nucleus of a density and texture similar to that of the haemoglobinized cytoplasm.

It is generally thought that haemoglobin probably migrates from the cytoplasm into the nucleus via the nuclear pores in the later stages of erythropoiesis as the nucleus becomes pyknotic. The converse possibility, however, is not denied. At least in the case of the chick embryo, histochemical studies suggest that during erythropoiesis haemoglobin first appears in the nucleus (O'Brien, 1960), and immunological and electrophoretic studies (Wilt, 1967) on haemoglobin from isolated nuclei have shown that it consists of only one of the three haemoglobins of the embryonic chicken. Whether intranuclear haemoglobin synthesis occurs in man and other mammals, and whether such synthesis contributes a particular type of haemoglobin, remains to be determined.

Plate 32

Erythrocyte from peripheral blood of a canary, showing intranuclear haemoglobin (∗). The similarity of texture and density between the haemoglobinized cytoplasm and the included material is evident, as is continuity between the two (arrow). ×37,000

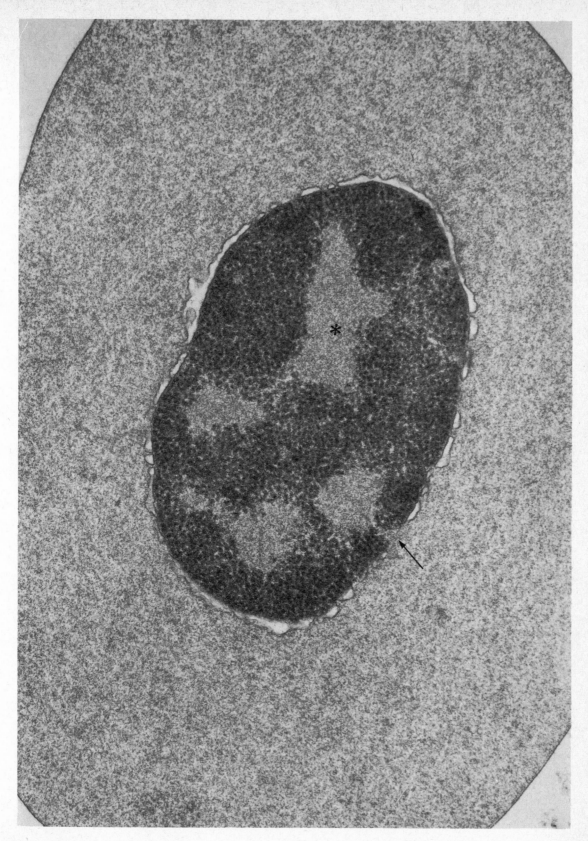

INTRANUCLEAR CONCENTRIC LAMINATED INCLUSIONS

The concentric laminated inclusion is a rare variety of intranuclear inclusion about which little is known. It is composed of alternating concentric shells of electron-dense and electron-lucent material. A single, smooth-surfaced, loose-fitting crenated membrane usually separates the inclusion from the nuclear matrix (*Plate 33*). Connections with the nuclear envelope have not been observed.

Intranuclear laminated inclusions of this type have been observed in: (1) oviduct epithelium of hens (Johnston, 1962); (2) mucus-secreting cells of human labial salivary glands (Tandler and Denning, 1969); (3) adenocarcinoma of paratid gland (Erlandson and Tandler, 1972); (4) murine pulmonary adenomas and adenocarcinomas (Flaks and Flaks, 1970); and (5) a synovial cell from an apparently healthy rabbit (*Plate 33, Fig. 4*).

It will be observed from the above-mentioned list that these inclusions occur in cells capable of elaborating a mucoid secretory product. Tandler *et al.* (1969) noted that such inclusions in labial glands occurred in immature mucous cells, but not in cells containing abundant secretory products. Thus these inclusions may be related to the secretory cycle of the mucus-producing cells. In the hen's oviduct epithelium, Johnston (1962) found similar laminated inclusions both in the cytoplasm and nucleus and suggested that this might be a type of nuclear secretion. However, the laminated bodies portrayed in the cytoplasm are reminiscent of cytolysosomes.

The manner in which these inclusions arise is not clear. In the labial glands they may have arisen from inclusions containing multiple electron-dense lipid droplets, which were also often seen. The inclusions found by Flaks and Flaks (1970) in the murine tumours also at times contain material which could be lipid. Intranuclear tubular inclusions were also frequently seen in these tumours and it was suggested that they participate in the formation of these inclusions.

The inclusions in the labial salivary gland are reported to be eosinophilic but difficult to detect in H and E stained sections. Some stained with Nile blue sulphate (neutral phospholipids) while others were PAS-positive but diastase-resistant. They were also Feulgen-negative.

Plate 33

Figs. 1–3. Electron micrographs showing a variety of intranuclear concentric laminated inclusions found in pulmonary adenomas and adenocarcinomas of mice. ×16,000; ×25,000; ×21,000 (*From Flaks and Flaks, 1970*)

Fig. 4. An intranuclear concentric laminated inclusion found in an apparently normal human synovial cell. This is the only example of a laminated inclusion we have seen. ×46,000 (*Ghadially and Roy, unpublished electron micrograph*)

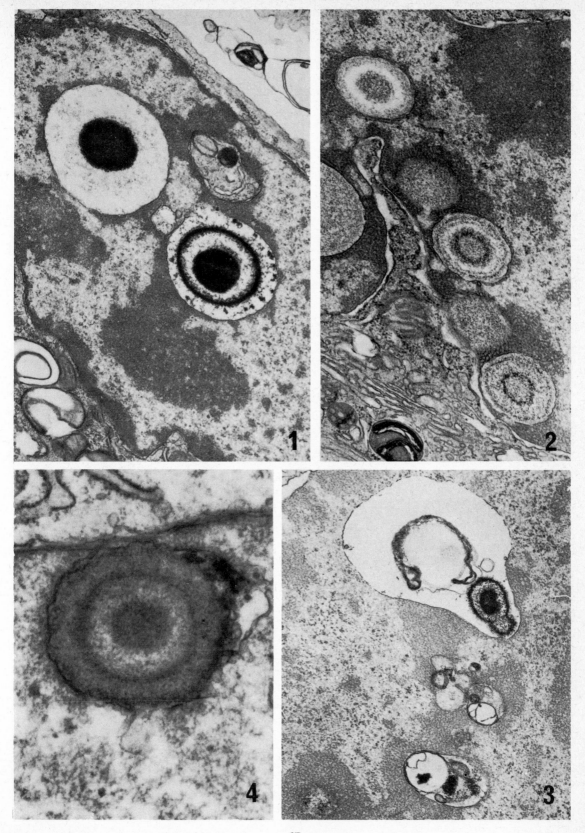

INTRANUCLEAR LEAD INCLUSIONS

The toxicity of lead has been recognized since the time of Hippocrates, but the characteristic intranuclear inclusions that occur were first described in 1936 by Blackman. In the rat such inclusions occur in the proximal tubular epithelial cells of the kidney (*Plate 34*), but in other animals such as the pig, rabbit and man, both kidney and liver contain such inclusions. The extensive early literature on lead poisoning has been reviewed by Calvery (1938). Many papers dealing with the morphology and chemistry of intranuclear lead inclusions have also been published (Blackman, 1936; Finner and Calvery, 1939; Wachstein, 1949; Bracken *et al.*, 1958; Landing and Nakai, 1959; Beaver, 1961; Gueft and Molnar, 1961; Angevine *et al.*, 1962; Watrach and Vatter, 1962; Dallenbach, 1964; Goyer, 1968; Richter *et al.*, 1968; Goyer *et al.*, 1970).

The typical lead inclusion presents as a body with a dense central core enveloped in a cortex of matted and radiating filaments. The early lesion starts in a zone between the nucleolus and nuclear envelope and is clearly not derived from these structures. As the lesion increases in size it displaces the nucleolus and assumes a central position, and at light microscopy it could be mistaken for a viral inclusion. Numerous conflicting reports on the histochemistry of these lesions have been published, but it seems reasonably certain now that these inclusions are acid-fast to carbol fuschin (indicating presence of proteins rich in sulphydryl groups), contain little or no lipid or carbohydrate, and probably no DNA or RNA either. About the latter (DNA, RNA), however, there is much uncertainty in the literature. Nevertheless, the presence of protein has been confirmed by enzyme digestion studies on epon-embedded material (Richter *et al.*, 1968) and on inclusions isolated from tissue homogenates. The fibrillary cortex soon disappears after such treatment (Goyer *et al.*, 1970).

Although the presence of lead in these inclusions has long been suspected, unequivocal demonstration of this was not achieved until recently. The first convincing evidence on this point came from the work of Dallenbach (1965) who, by autoradiography, demonstrated the presence of lead in the inclusions of animals that had received radioactive lead. Goyer *et al.* (1970) have now isolated and analysed these inclusions and they report that the lead is bound to protein, in a relatively constant ratio. They found that about 80–90 per cent of the renal lead resides in the nucleus and that at least 50 per cent can be recovered with the inclusions. They postulate that 'the inclusion body may therefore function as a store or a depot for intracellular lead'.

Plate 34

Three nuclei containing highly electron-dense lead inclusions are seen in this section of rat kidney tubule. The animal had received 0·5 per cent lead acetate in drinking water for two months. × 19,500 (*Ghadially and Bhatnagar, unpublished electron micrograph*)

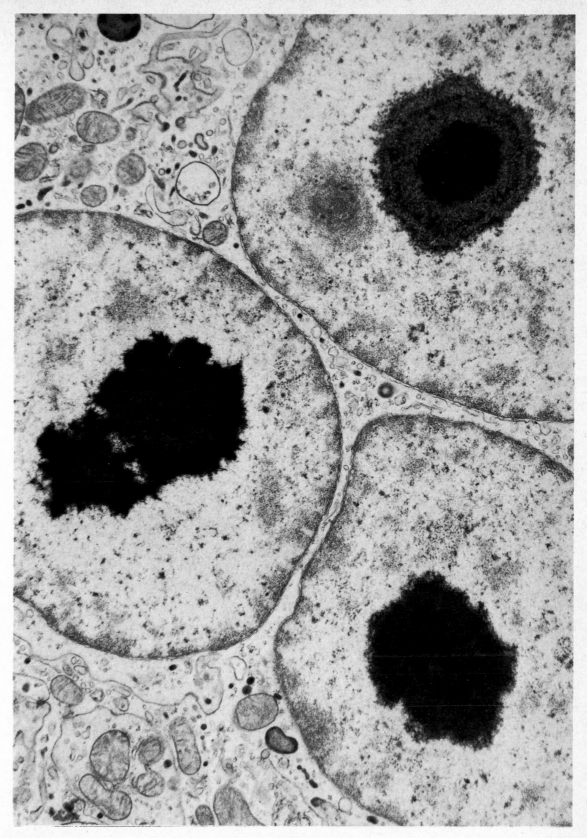

Viruses may be synthesized in the nucleus and/or cytoplasm. Most DNA viruses such as adeno, papova and herpes are synthesized in the nucleus but some, such as pox viruses, are produced in the cytoplasm. Almost all RNA viruses are assembled in the cytoplasm, but some (e.g. myxoviruses) involve both nucleus and cytoplasm. It is beyond the scope of this work to illustrate and discuss the morphological changes produced in the nucleus by the large number of known viruses. Here we shall deal briefly with the nuclear inclusions produced by two DNA viruses (adeno and herpes simplex) and one RNA virus (measles).

Various types of inclusions are seen in the nuclei of virus-infected cells. These include viral particles, precursors of such particles, malformed viral components and also structures derived by alterations of nuclear components. In herpesvirus and adenovirus infections such viral particles may be found scattered randomly in the nucleus or aligned close to the nuclear envelope. The particles may be solitary, in clusters, in linear arrays or in crystalline formations. Herpesvirus rarely forms crystalline structures but large viral crystals are quite common with adenovirus (*Plates 35 and 36*).

Intranuclear herpesvirus particles usually present as a DNA-containing core and a protein envelope called the capsid. The two are separated by a less dense interval. The core measures 350–500 Å in diameter and is usually rounded, but it may be bar-shaped and appear solid or hollow. To a large extent the appearance depends upon type of fixation. Thus bar-shaped and solid cores are frequent after permanganate fixation, while hollow cores are said to be characteristic of osmium fixation. Some capsids appear empty. This is because cores are absent; it is not a sectioning artefact (Swanson *et al.*, 1966). The capsids often appear spherical. However, the

---

Plate 35

From monkey kidney cells in culture infected with herpes simplex virus. Fixed briefly (30 minutes) in glutaraldehyde, post-fixed in osmium and stained with uranium and lead.

Fig. 1. A group of virus particles are seen lying in the nucleus adjacent to the marginated chromatin (M). Various morphological variations are depicted here. Thus we can see dense or solid cores (S), hollow cores (H), and capsids (C) without cores. × 58,000

Fig. 2. Beside a chromatin aggregate (C) lie numerous malformed capsids (M), occasional virus particles and a para-crystalline inclusion (P). × 45,000

Fig. 3. Vermicellar bodies (V) are seen in the nucleus of this herpesvirus-infected cell. × 28,000

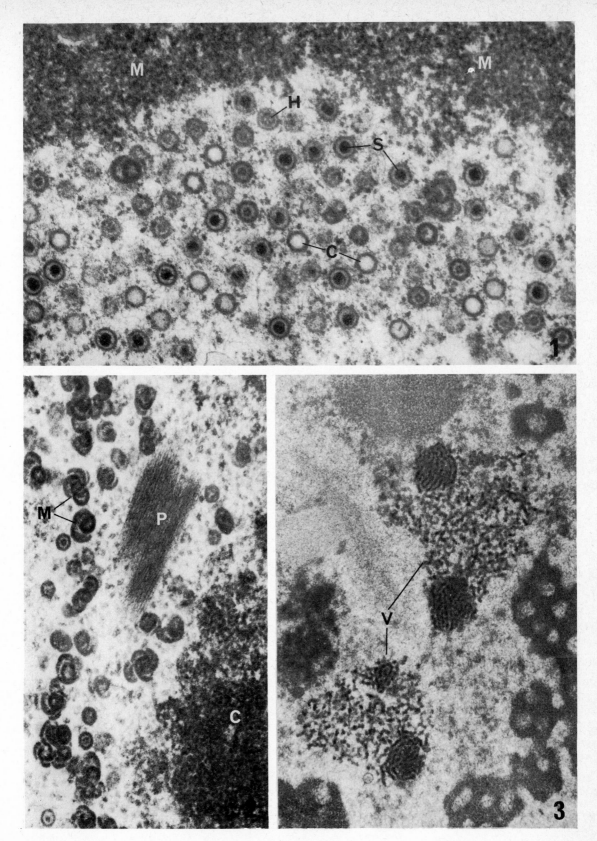

pentagonal or hexagonal shape expected from sections through these virus particles which are known to have an icosahedral symmetry can at times be discerned in ultrathin sections. Herpes-virus particles are singularly resistant to a variety of treatments that cause gross disruption of cellular architecture. Thus such particles have been demonstrated in autopsy material, paraffin-embedded material and in tissues kept in formaldehyde fixatives for up to four years (Roy and Wolman, 1969).

In measles-infected cells the situation is quite different, for the virus presents as an aggregate of tubules believed to be composed of viral nucleoprotein (*Plate 37*). Such aggregates may be focal and rounded or quite large and almost entirely fill the nucleus, leaving little besides occasional clumps of marginated chromatin. Such aggregates of tubules occur also in the cyto-plasm and, while budding from the cell surface, become enveloped in cell membrane to form measles virions. The intranuclear tubules, however, appear to be trapped in the nucleus. Few or none succeed in maturing into measles virions (Nakai *et al.*, 1969).

As mentioned earlier, the nucleus of the virus-infected cell contains other inclusions besides virus particles. Thus crystals or paracrystalline inclusions are at times seen in a variety of virus-infected cells but it is not clear whether this is host or viral protein (page 62). In herpes-infected cells collections of malformed capsids are at times encountered (*Plate 35, Fig. 2*), or a character-istic but rather rare inclusion called the vermicellar body (*Plate 35, Fig. 3*) may be found. This body is made up of intertwining filamentous or rod-like elements. The morphology of this plexiform inclusion is better appreciated in relatively thick sections, for in very thin sections it presents as dense granules, which may be confused with disintegrating and clumped nuclear and

---

Plate 36

From a culture of canine kidney cell line infected with canine adenovirus.

Fig. 1. Nucleus showing crystalline arrays of adenovirus. × 40,000 (*From Yamamoto, 1969*)
Fig. 2. Nucleus containing ring-shaped inclusions. × 24,000 (*Yamamoto, unpublished electron micrograph*)

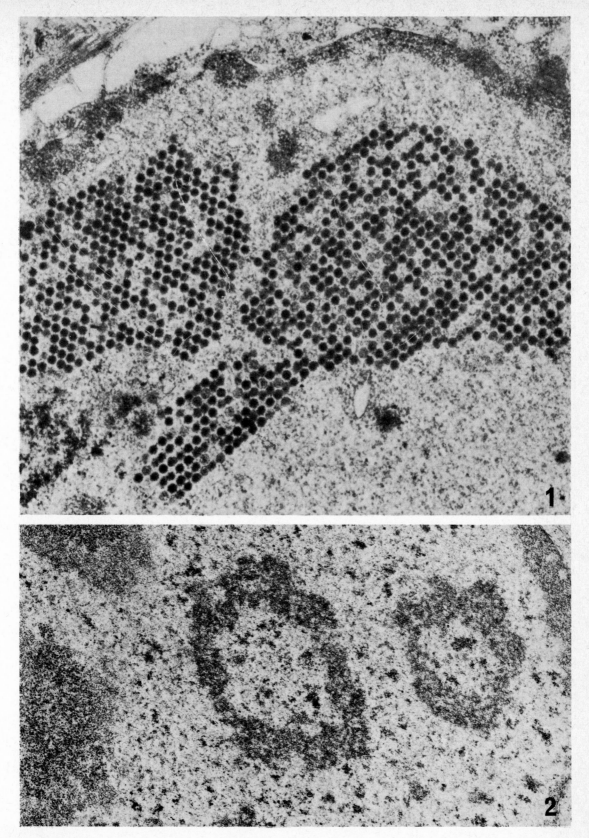

nucleolar material. The diameter of the vermicellar rods is of the same order as the diameter of viral cores and the staining reaction is also similar. Therefore, the vermicellar body might be looked upon as the site of core production, but one would argue that, since this structure is so rarely seen, this is not the way cores are normally produced, and that the vermicellar body probably represents deranged or frustrated core production.

In adenovirus-infected cells, Yamamoto and Shahrabadi (1971) have shown that viral DNA is synthesized in ring-shaped inclusions which develop within a few hours after infection (*Plate 36, Fig. 2*). Such inclusions readily incorporate tritiated thymidine into DNA and later the labelled DNA is found incorporated in viral particles.

Many of the changes that occur in the nucleus of virus-infected cells, particularly herpesvirus-infected cells, have already been described (pages 24–27). Such changes include thickening and reduplication of the nuclear envelope, margination of chromatin, increase in interchromatin and perichromatin granules, and segregation and scattering of nucleolar components. Other, mostly later, changes include rupture of nuclear membranes, chromatin dispersion and degeneration, disappearance of interchromatin and perichromatin granules, absence of a recognizable nucleolus, but presence of granular or fibrillar structures reminiscent of nucleolar material. Such alterations produce a variety of intranuclear bodies, the precise origin and nature of which it is at times difficult to be certain.

Plate 37

Intranuclear inclusions produced by measles virus (*From Nakai, Shand and Howatson, 1969*)

Fig. 1. A focal aggregate of viral tubules in the nucleus of a BSC-1 cell (a cell line derived from green monkey kidney). × 110,000

Fig. 2. Extensive formation of viral tubules has replaced the normal nuclear contents. From a primary culture of Rhesus monkey kidney. × 47,000

Fig. 3. Part of an intranuclear aggregate of viral tubules is shown here at a higher magnification. × 140,000

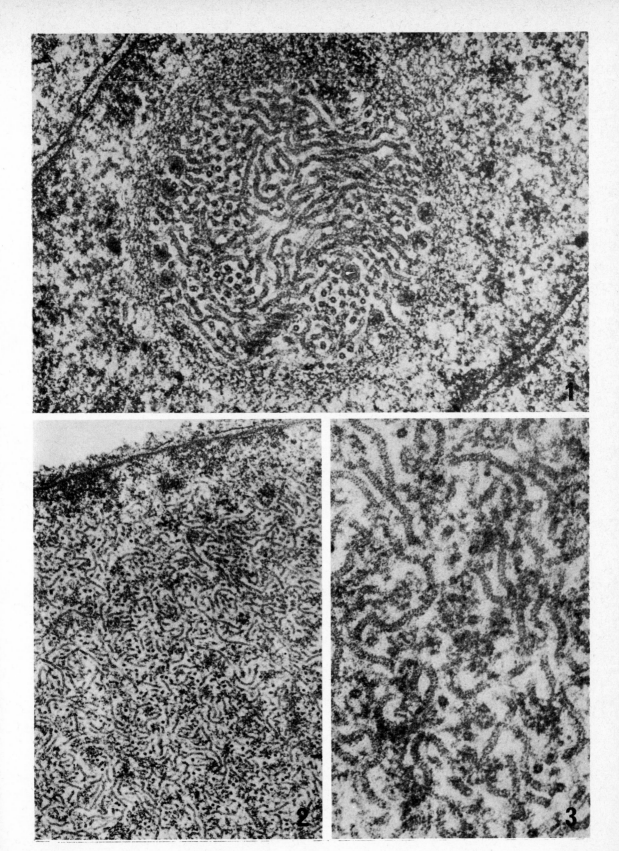

Nuclear projections may present as a sessile or pedunculated nodule, tag, filament, club or drumstick arising from the surface of the nucleus. Such projections are best noted in whole cells examined with the light microscope. They have been seen more frequently in neutrophil poly-morphonuclear leucocytes than in other cell types. In an ultrathin section the chance of encountering, say, a solitary filament or drumstick (e.g. the well known drumstick containing chromatin of the XX chromosome pair in the human female) is small, and even more remote is the possibility of cutting such structures along their entire length so that their shape can be recognized. Thus when an object resembling a drumstick is seen in an ultrathin section (*Plate 38*), it is much more likely to be a section through a sheet-like or membranous formation with a thickened margin.

Ultrastructural studies have drawn attention to a structure, which at first sight appears like a pseudoinclusion placed adjacent to the nuclear envelope. This hood or cowl-like formation presents as a 'drumstick' in one plane of sectioning, but in a plane at right angles to this it presents as a band or bridge of nuclear material approximately 400 Å thick, arising from the surface of the nucleus to form a pocket in which lies a rounded mass of cytoplasmic material (*Plate 33*) or nuclear material (*Plate 39*). Such structures have been variously referred to as blisters, blebs, projections and pockets. The last term is preferable to others which have already been used to designate various other alterations of nuclear morphology.

In rare instances one may encounter a pocket which shows two 'chromatin bands' (*Plate 39, Fig. 3*) and somewhat more frequently one may also encounter circular or oval loops of chromatin lying free in the cytoplasm (*Plate 38, Fig. 1*). In some instances no doubt such loops may be connected to the main nuclear mass in another plane, but serial sectioning has shown (Clausen and Von Hamm, 1969) that at times such loops are completely detached from the nucleus.

As hinted earlier, some confusion exists regarding the nomenclature of nuclear pockets, and at times appearances such as those seen in *Plate 38, Fig. 1* have been called projections by electron microscopists. Bearing this in mind one can state that nuclear pockets and 'projections' have been observed in: (1) Burkitt's lymphoma (lymphoid cells and cultures derived from them) and other lymphomas including lymphocytic leukaemia of man (Achong and Epstein, 1966;

Plate 38

Polymorphonuclear neutrophil leucocytes from an ascitic effusion in a patient with adenocarcinoma of the ovary. Both the figures in this plate show sections through nuclear pockets cut in different planes.

Fig. 1. Section showing a side view or profile of a nuclear pocket (P) with extension of cytoplasmic material (∗) into the pocket. Such an appearance has at times been called a nuclear projection. Also seen is a loop of nuclear material enclosing cytoplasmic structures (C). × 32,000

Fig. 2. Section showing an *en face* view of a nuclear pocket. The inner (I) and outer (0) membranes of the nuclear envelope are continued over the surface of the pocket. The inner surface of the pocket under the chromatin band (B) is similarly lined and contains cytoplasmic material (C). Note that the perinuclear cistern (P) is continued on both sides of the band of chromatin (B) forming the nuclear pocket. × 60,000

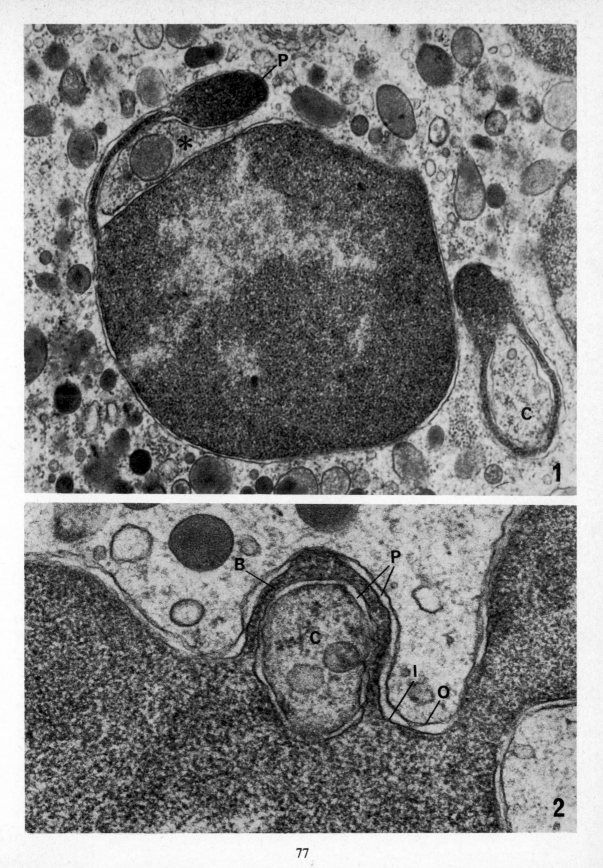

Dorfman, 1968; Ghadially and Skinnider, unpublished observation) (*Plate 39*); (2) avian lymphomatosis (Marek's disease) (Fujimoto *et al.*, 1970); (3) thymocytes of fetal guinea-pig and man (Sebuwufu, 1966; Toro and Olah, 1966); (4) granulocytes of patients treated with cystosine arabinoside (Ahearn *et al.*, 1967) and fluorouracil (Stalzer *et al.*, 1965); (5) granulocytes of pernicious anaemia patients (Stalzer *et al.*, 1965); (6) neutrophils and eosinophils of children with D_1 (13–15) trisomy and partial C trisomy (Huehns *et al.*, 1964; Lutzner and Hecht, 1966); (7) myeloblastic and monoblastic leukaemic cells of man (Anderson, 1966; McDuffie, 1967); (8) circulating neutrophils of four persons with bronchial cancer (Clausen and Von Hamm, 1969) (6–16 per cent of neutrophils showed nuclear pockets in the cancer patients, but only one nuclear pocket was seen from the blood of five normal individuals); (9) neutrophils and monocytes in malignant ascites resulting from an ovarian carcinoma (*Plate 38*); and (10) on rare occasions, neutrophils, lymphocytes and monocytes of apparently healthy individuals (Huhn, 1967; Smith and O'Hara, 1967).

Apparently about 1 per cent of circulating neutrophils in normal individuals may show nuclear pockets (Bessis, personal communication quoted by Clausen and Von Haam, 1969) but this number is considerably increased in leukaemic individuals and persons exposed to irradiation.

A review of my electron micrographs and those published by others shows that there are at least two morphological varieties of nuclear pockets: those that contain cytoplasmic material and those that contain nuclear material. Whether they are related, and whether one form evolves into another, is, however, not apparent. A process of pseudoinclusion production could explain how cytoplasm-containing nuclear pockets arise, but this can hardly explain the manner in which pockets containing sequestrated nuclear material are formed. In this respect the illustrations in the paper by Lutzner and Hecht (1966) are interesting, for they suggest that such pockets may be formed within the nucleus by sequestration of a rounded mass of chromatin. These authors state that 'these findings suggest a sequence of events whereby peripheral chromatin is separated by clefts into coiled pedunculated processes within the nucleus, which uncoil and project into the cytoplasm and which may then separate completely from the nucleus'.

Another reason why the idea that the cytoplasm-containing nuclear pockets are no more than marginally placed pseudoinclusions is not too appealing is that it does not explain why a chromatin band of fairly constant width forms the wall of the pocket. Attention is drawn by Clausen and Von Haam to the thickness of chromatin loops and bands or bridges around pockets which, in their material, measured 400 Å, a figure similar to that which I find in my material.

On the basis of these observations and a review of the literature on the incidence of nuclear pockets (which they call blebs) in various states Clausen and Von Haam (1969) point out that, 'There is a strong correlation between the reported occurrence of nuclear blebs and chromosomal abnormalities, either unusual numbers, breakage or a defect in nucleoprotein synthesis,' and that blebs may be the morphologic expression of chromatin dislocation resulting from such chromosomal abnormalities.

Plate 39

Figs. 1 and 2. Acute lymphocytic leukaemia cells from peripheral blood of man showing nuclear pockets which contain sequestrated nuclear material. × 54,000; × 44,000 (*Ghadially and Skinnider, unpublished electron micrographs*)

Fig. 3. A monocyte from the same source as in *Plate 36*, showing an unusual pocket with two chromatin bands. × 70,000 (*Ghadially and Skinnider, unpublished electron micrograph*)

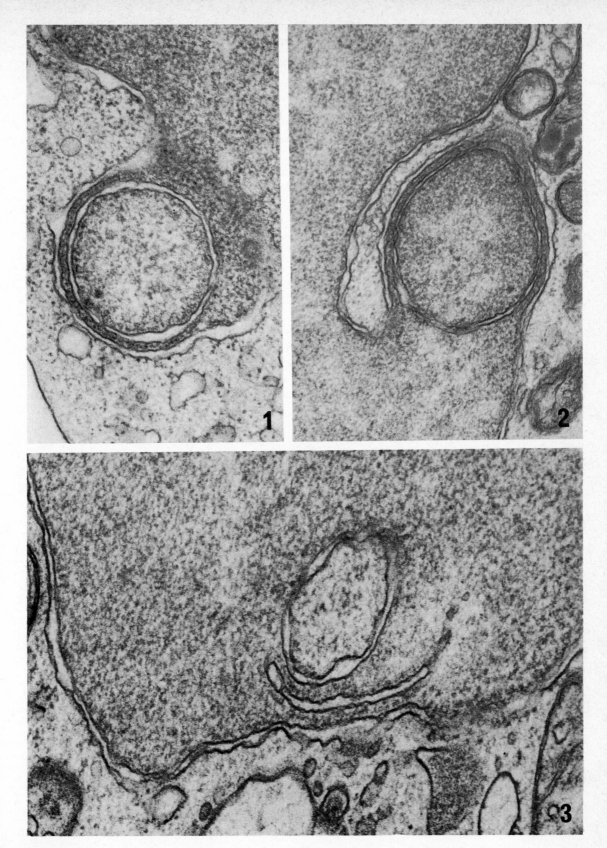

The term 'nuclear bodies' is used to describe a group of intranuclear structures of diverse morphology (*Plates 40 and 41*). Several attempts have been made to classify nuclear bodies on the basis of their ultrastructural appearance. For example, Bouteille *et al.* (1967) divided them into types I to V, Vazquez *et al.* (1970) into types I to IV, Popoff and Stewart (1968) into types I to III, and Krishan *et al.* (1967) into groups a, b and c. Little is gained by this exercise, and therefore in this text will be used the descriptive terms which, although cumbersome at times, convey the meaning more clearly.

The simplest type of nuclear body is composed of fibrils (approximately 50–70 Å diameter) which may be randomly orientated or arranged in concentric or annular formations. More than one such body may occur in a nucleus and they are easily spotted because there is usually a clear halo around them (*Plate 40*). Another variety of nuclear body is composed of fibrils and granules. Such fibrillogranular bodies may contain only a few granules set in a fibrillary matrix or there may be many granules surrounded by a fibrillary cortex (*Plate 41*). Some examples of these are likely to be confused with focal glycogen deposits in the nucleus (see page 56). Occasionally, one encounters nuclear bodies which contain fine tubules or vesicles surrounded by a fibrillary cortex. Finally, there is a complex group of large nuclear bodies, which besides the usual fibrils and perhaps some small granules, may also contain one or more structures such as vesicles, tubules, large electron-dense masses and lipid. Such bodies are of rarer occurrence. Only the simpler varieties of nuclear bodies, that is to say the fibrillar and smaller varieties of fibrillogranular bodies with sparse granules, are commonly encountered in normal tissues of plants and animals.

Nuclear bodies have been reported to occur in the following situations: (1) normal plants (Lafontaine, 1965; Sankaranarayanan and Hyde, 1965; Büttner, 1968); (2) normal animal tissues (Farquhar and Palade, 1962; Horstmann, 1962, 1965; Horstmann *et al.*, 1966; Latta and Maunsbach, 1962a, b; Weber and Frommes, 1963; Ishikawa, 1964; Nicander, 1964; Brooks and Siegel, 1967; Henry and Petts, 1969; Misrabi, 1969; Dixon, 1970; Masurovsky *et al.*, 1970; Van Noord *et al.*, 1972); (3) a variety of tumours, such as Shope papilloma, bronchial carcinoid and carcinoma, ependymomas, gliomas, meningiomas, leukaemias, Hodgkin's disease, Waldenström's macroglobulinaemia, squamous cell carcinoma, melanoma, rhabdomyoma, and tumours of salivary gland (De The *et al.*, 1960; Hinglais-Guillard *et al.*, 1961; Bessis and Thiery, 1962; Ogawa, 1962; Bernhard and Granboulan, 1963; Bessis *et al.*, 1963; Robertson, 1964; Robertson and Maclean, 1965; Brooks and Siegel, 1967; Bouteille *et al.*, 1967; Krishan *et al.*, 1967; Kuhn, 1967; Kierszenbaum, 1968; Vazquez *et al.*, 1970; Wyatt *et al.*, 1970); (4) in tissues or cultures infected with adenovirus, herpes zoster and herpes simplex, human cytomegalovirus, polyoma, SV40, Shope papilloma, varicella, vaccinia and wart virus (for references, see Granboulan *et al.*, 1963; Patrizi and Middlekamp, 1969); (5) drug action (Torack, 1961; Swanbeck and Thyresson, 1964; Simard, 1966; Ulrich and Kidd, 1966); (6) immunological stimulation (Simar, 1969; Dumont and Roberts, 1971); and (7) hormonal stimulation (Lemaire, 1963; Weber *et al.*, 1964; Horstmann, 1965; Simar and Lemaire, 1966; Dahl, 1970).

Plate 40

Nucleus of cell from human bronchial mucosa, showing fibrillary nuclear bodies surrounded by a clear halo (arrows). × 32,000

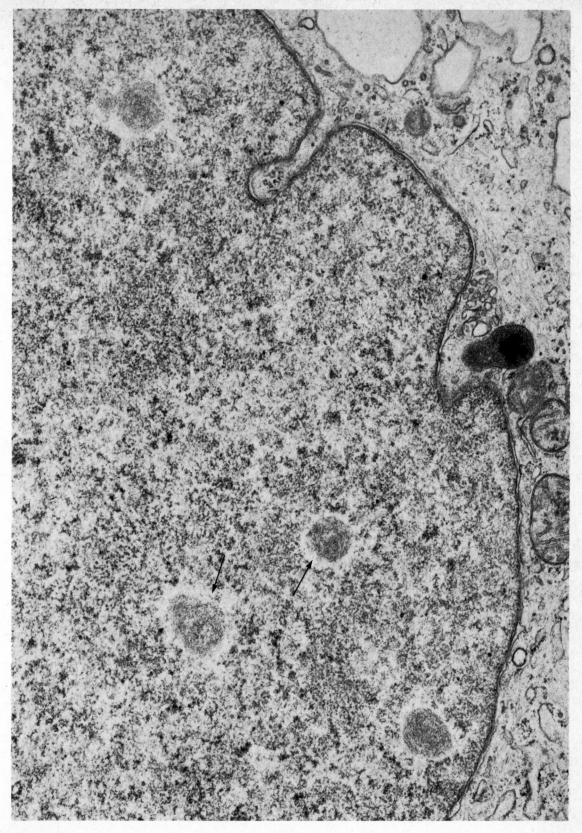

D

Nuclear bodies have been observed in such a wide variety of tissues that many authors now consider them to be a normal constituent of the nucleus, and probably of universal occurrence. A review of the literature also indicates that when cells are stimulated to activity by a variety of means an increase in numbers, size and complexity of the nuclear bodies is observed. Thus in the zona fasciculata of the calf adrenal after ACTH stimulation the fibrillogranular nuclear body transforms into a large multiloculated vesicular structure (Weber *et al.*, 1964). Numerous nuclear bodies occur in the epithelium of the dog epididymis, but these are absent or less frequent in the young, castrated or oestrogen-treated animal (Lemaire, 1963; Simar and Lemaire, 1966). Horstmann (1962) has noted a close relationship between the differentiation of nuclear bodies and maturation of the epididymis in man. An increase in the number and size of nuclear bodies is reported by Dahl (1970) in ovarian tissue after clomiphene or gonadotropin treatment.

Similarly, there are experiments which indicate that nuclear bodies increase in size, number and complexity in inflammation and after immunological stimulation. For example, it has been found that after intravenous injection of various micro-organisms in hamsters the peritoneal macrophages contain large complex nuclear bodies (Dumont and Roberts, 1971). When to this is added the fact that most of the larger nuclear bodies are seen in tumours, and that cells in culture and virus-infected cells show abundant nuclear bodies, one has to concede that these bodies are a sign of stimulated or metabolically active cells.

Despite numerous studies the nature and function of these bodies remain obscure. There is also much doubt about their chemical composition, for conflicting reports abound in the literature. For example, the fibrillogranular body which can at times be large enough to locate with the light microscope, has been reported to be basophilic by some authors and eosinophilic by others (Wyatt *et al.*, 1970). Cytochemical studies have not revealed DNA or RNA in the simpler nuclear bodies, and the fibrillary nuclear body is said to contain only protein (Krishan *et al.*, 1967). However, in larger complex bodies enzyme digestion studies suggest that the fibrillary component contains RNA while the dense granular component contains DNA (Sankaranarayanan and Hyde, 1965; Simar, 1969). This is in keeping with the observation of Vazquez *et al.* (1970), that the granules of the large fibrillogranular bodies in gliomas are Feulgen-positive.

Plate 41

Fig. 1. A nuclear body with a concentric arrangement of its components. From full-term human placenta. ×77,000

Fig. 2. A nuclear body with a fibrillary cortex and some microtubules. From bronchial mucosa of heavy smoker. ×40,000

Fig. 3. A fibrillary nuclear body with an annular configuration. From liver of phenobarbitone-treated hamster. ×48,000

Fig. 4. From the same nucleus as *Fig. 3.* More annular fibrillary nuclear bodies and also one that could be a compact spherical body as in *Plate 40*, or a tangential cut through an annular one. ×42,000

Fig. 5. A nuclear body containing vesicles. From human chronic lymphocytic leukaemia. ×66,000

Fig. 6. Fibrillogranular nuclear body from the same case as *Fig. 2.* ×55,000

Fig. 7. A nuclear body containing a lipid droplet, numerous dense structures with paler centres and a fibrillary cortex. From liver of phenobarbitone-treated hamster. ×65,000

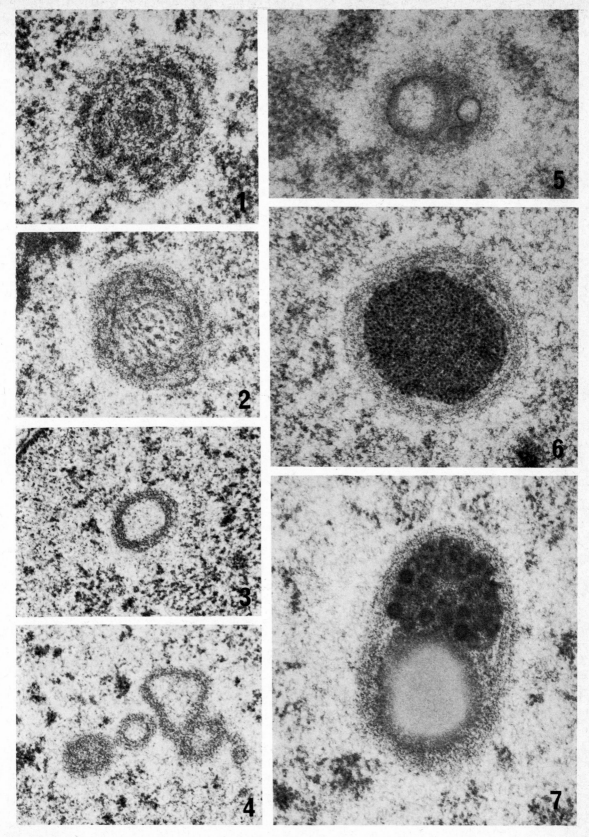

Abuelo, J. G. and Moore, D. E. (1969). 'The human chromosome. Electron microscopic observations on chromatin fiber organization.' *J. Cell Biol.* **41**, 73

Achong, B. G. and Epstein, M. A. (1966). 'Fine structure of the Burkitt tumour.' *J. natn. Cancer Inst.* **36**, 877

Ahearn, M. J., Lewis, C. W. and Campbell, L. A. (1967). 'Nuclear bleb formation in human bone marrow cells during cytosine arabinoside therapy.' *Nature, Lond.* **215**, 196

Ancla, M. and De Brux, J. (1965). 'Occurrence of intranuclear tubular structures in the human endometrium during the secretory phase, and of annulate lamellae in hyperestrogenic states.' *Obstet. Gynec.* **26**, 23

Anderson, D. R. (1966). 'Ultrastructure of normal and leukemic leukocytes in human peripheral blood.' *J. Ultrastruct. Res.* (Suppl. 9), 26

Andrew, W., Brown, H. M. and Johnson, J. (1943). 'Senile changes in the liver of mouse and man, with special reference to the similarity of the nuclear alterations.' *Am. J. Anat.* **72**, 199

Angevine, J. M., Kappas, A., DeGowin, R. L. and Spargo, B. H. (1962). 'Renal tubular nuclear inclusions in lead poisoning. A clinical and experimental study.' *Archs. Path.* **73**, 486.

Apitz, K. (1937). 'Uber die pigmentbildung in den zellkernen melanotischer geschwulste: I. Beitrag zur pathologie des zellkernes.' *Virchows Arch. path. Anat. Physiol.* **300**, 89

Babai, F., Tremblay, G. and Dumont, A. (1969). 'Intranuclear and intranucleolar tubular structures in Novikoff hepatoma cells.' *J. Ultrastruct. Res.* **28**, 125

Barnes, B. G. and Davis, J. M. (1959). 'The structure of nuclear pores in mammalian tissue.' *J. Ultrastruct. Res.* **3**, 131

Barnett, C. H., Cochrane, W. and Palfrey, A. J. (1963). 'Age changes in articular cartilage of rabbits.' *Ann. rheum. Dis.* **22**, 389

Baud, C. A. (1963). 'Nuclear membrane and permeability.' In *Intracellular Membrane Structure*, p. 323. Ed. by S. Seno and E. V. Cowdry. Okayama: Okayama Press

Baudhuin, P., Hers, H. G. and Loeb, H. (1964). 'An Electron microscopic and biochemical study of type II glycogenosis.' *Lab. Invest.* **13**, 1139.

Beams, H. W., Tahmisian, T. N., Devine, R. and Anderson, E. (1957). 'Ultrastructure of the nuclear membrane of a Gregarine parasitic in grasshoppers.' *Expl Cell Res.* **13**. 200

Beaver, D. L. (1961). 'The ultrastructure of the kidney in lead intoxication with particular reference to intranuclear inclusions.' *Am. J. Path.*, **39**, 195

Bernhard, W. (1966). 'Ultrastructural aspects of the normal and pathological nucleolus in mammalian cells.' *Natn. Cancer Inst. Monogr.* **23**, 13

— and Granboulan, N. (1963). 'The fine structure of the cancer cell nucleus.' *Expl Cell Res.* (Suppl. 9), 19

—— (1968). 'Electron microscopy of the nucleolus in vertebrate cells.' In *The Nucleus.* Ed. by A. Dalton and F. Haguenau. New York: Academic Press

— Febure, H. L. and Cramer, R. (1959). 'Electron microscopic demonstration of a virus in cells infected *in vitro* by the polyma agent'. *C.r. Acad. Sci.* **249**, 483

Bessis, M. J. and Thiery, J. P. (1962). 'Etude au microscope electronique sur les leucemies humanes. II. Les leuccemies lymphocytaines. Comparison avec la leucemie de la souris de souche A. K.' *Nouv. Rev. franc. Hematol.* **2**, 387

— Breton-Gorius, J. and Binet, J. L. (1963). 'Etude comparee du plasmocytome et du syndrome de Waldenstrom. Examen au microscope electronique.' *Nouv. Rev. franc. Hematol.* **3**, 159

Biava, C. (1963). 'Identification and structural forms of human particulate glycogen.' *Lab. Invest.* **12**, 1179

Binggeli, M. F. (1959). 'Abnormal intranuclear and cytoplasmic formations associated with a chemically induced transplantable chicken sarcoma.' *J. biophys. biochem. Cytol.* **5**, 143

Blackburn, W. R. and Vinijchaikul, K. (1969). 'The pancreas in kwashiorkor. An electron microscopic study.' *Lab. Invest.* **20**, 305

Blackman, S. S., Jr. (1936). 'Intranuclear inclusion bodies in kidney and liver caused by lead poisoning.' *Bull. Johns Hopkins Hosp.* **58**, 384

Bloom, G. D. (1967). 'A nucleus with cytoplasmic features.' *J. Cell. Biol.* **35**, 266

Bouteille, M., Kalifat, S. R. and Delarue, J. (1967). 'Ultrastructural variations of nuclear bodies in human diseases.' *J. Ultrastruct. Res.* **19**, 474

Bracken, E. C., Beaver, D. L. and Randall, C. C. (1958). 'Histochemical studies of viral and lead-induced intranuclear bodies.' *J. Path. Bact.* **75**, 253

Brandes, D., Schofield, B. H. and Anton, E. (1965). 'Nuclear mitochondria?' *Science*, **149**, 1373

Brinkley, B. R. (1965). 'The fine structure of the nucleolus in mitotic division of Chinese hamster cell in vitro.' *J. Cell. Biol.* **27**, 411

Brooks, R. E. and Siegel, B. V. (1967). 'Nuclear bodies of normal and pathological human lymph node cells. An electron microscopic study.' *Blood*, **29**, 269

Brown, D. D. and Gurdon, J. B. (1964). 'Absence of ribosomal R.N.A. synthesis in the anucleolate mutant of Xenopus laevis.' *Proc. natn. Acad. Sci., U.S.A.* **51**, 139

Bucciarelli, E. (1966). 'Intracellular cisternae resembling structures of the Golgi complex.' *J. Cell. Biol.* **30**, 664

Busch, H., Byvoet, P. and Smetana, K. (1963). 'The nucleolus of the cancer cell: a review.' *Cancer Res.* **23**, 313

Büttner, D. W. (1968). 'Elektronenmikroskopische beobachtung von sphaeridien in karyoplasma der pauropsidenzelle.' *Z. Zellforsch. mikrosk. Anat.* **85**, 527

Calvery, H. O. (1938). 'Chronic effects of ingested lead and arsenic; a review and correlation.' *J. Am. med. Ass.* **111**, 1722

Caputo, R. and Bellone, A. G. (1966). 'On a new type of intranuclear microbodies observed in bullous mucosynechial and atrophic dermatitis (occular pemphigus).' *J. invest. Derm.* **47**, 141

Caramia, F., Ghergo, F. G. and Menghini, C. (1967). 'A glycogen body in liver nuclei.' *J. Ultrastruct. Res.* **19**, 573

—— Branciari, C. and Menghini, G. (1968). 'New aspect of hepatic nuclear glycogenosis in diabetes.' *J. clin. Path.* **21**, 19

Caspersson, T. O. (1950). *Cell Growth and Cell Function: a cytochemical study.* New York: W. W. Norton

— and Santesson, L. (1942). 'Studies on protein metabolism in the cells of epithelial tumors.' *Acta Radiol.* (Suppl.), **46**, 1

— and Schultz, J. (1940). 'Ribonucleic acids in both nucleus and cytoplasm and the function of the nucleolus.' *Proc. natn. Acad. Sci., U.S.A.* **26**, 507

Cazal, P. and Mirouze, J. (1951). 'Une anomalie mal connue des cellules hépatiques: les noyaux vacuolaires et leur signification physiopathologique probable dans le syndrome d'adaptation.' *Presse méd.* **59**, 571

Chiga, M., Kume, F. and Millar, R. C. (1966). 'Nucleolar alteration produced by actinomycin D and the delayed onset of hepatic regeneration in rats.' *Lab. Invest.* **15**, 1403

Chipps, H. D. and Duff, G. L. (1942). 'Glycogen infiltration of liver cell nuclei.' *Am. J. Path.* **18**, 645

Clark, W. H. (1960). 'Electron microscope studies of nuclear extrusions in pancreatic acinar cells of the rat.' *J. biophys. biochem. Cytol.* **7**, 345

Clausen, K. P. and Von Haam, E. (1969). 'Fine structure of malignancy-associated changes (MAC) in peripheral human leukocytes.' *Acta cytol.* **13**, 435

Clyman, M. J. (1963). 'A new structure observed in the nucleolus of the human endometrial epithelial cell.' *Am. J. Obstet. Gynec.* **86**, 430

Coggeshall, R. E. and Fawcett, D. W. (1964). 'The fine structure of the central nervous system of the leech *Hirudo medicinalis.*' *J. Neurophysiol.* **27**, 229

Cooper, N. C. (1956). 'Early cytological changes produced by carcinogens.' *Bull. N.Y. med. Soc.* **32**, 79

Cowdry, E. V. and Paletta, F. X. (1941). 'Changes in cellular, nuclear and nucleolar sizes during methylcholanthrene epidermal carcinogenesis.' *J. Natn. Cancer. Inst.* **1**, 745

Dahl, E. (1970). 'Studies on the fine structure of ovarian interstitial tissue. 6. Effects of clomiphene on the thecal gland of the domestic fowl.' *Z. Zellforsch. mikrosk. Anat.* **109**, 227

Dallenbach, F. D. (1964). 'Phenolrotausscheidung and trypanblauspeicherung bei der blei-nephropathie der ratte.' *Virchows Arch. path. Anat. Physiol.* **338**, 91

— (1965). 'Uptake of radioactive lead by tubular epithelium of the kidney.' *Verh. deutsch. Ges. Path.* **49**, 179

Darlington, R. W. and Moss, L. H. (1968). 'Herpes virus envelopment.' *J. Virol.* **2**, 48

Davies, H. G. (1961). 'Structure in nucleated erythrocytes.' *J. biophys. biochem. Cytol.* **9**, 671

De Kretser, D. M. (1967). 'Changes in the fine structure of the human testicular interstitial cells after treatment with human gonadotrophins.' *Z. Zellforsch. mikrosk. Anat.* **83**, 344

— (1968). 'Crystals of Reinke in the nuclei of human testicular interstitial cells.' *Experientia* **24**, 587

De Man, J. C. H. and Noorduyn, N. J. (1967). 'Light and electron microscopic radioautography of hepatic cell nucleoli in mice treated with actinomycin D.' *J. Cell. Biol.* **33**, 489

De Robertis, E. (1956). 'Electron microscopic observations on the submicroscopic morphology of the meiotic nucleus and chromosomes.' *J. biophys. biochem. Cytol.* **2**, 785

De The, G., Riviere, M. and Bernhard, W. (1960). 'Examen au microscope electronique de la tumeur VX 2 du lapin domestique derivee du papillome de shape.' *Bull. Cancer* **47**, 569

Dixon, J. S. (1970). 'Nuclear bodies in normal and chromatolytic sympathetic neurons.' *Anat. Rec.* **168**, 179

Dorfman, R. F. (1968). 'Diagnosis of Burkitt's tumor in the United States.' *Cancer* **21**, 563

Dumont, A. and Roberts, A. (1971). 'Ultrastructure of complex nuclear bodies produced experimentally in hamster peritoneal macrophages.' *J. Ultrastruct. Res.* **36**, 483

Duryee, W. R. (1956). 'Precancer cells in amphibian adenocarcinoma.' *Ann. N.Y. Acad. Sci.* **63**, 1280

— and Doherty, J. R. (1954). 'Nuclear and cytoplasmic organoids in the living cell.' *Ann. N.Y. Acad. Sci.* **58**, 1210

Edstrom, J. E., Grampp, W. and Schor, N. (1961). 'The intracellular distribution and heterogeneity of ribonucleic acid in starfish oocytes.' *J. biophys. biochem. Cytol.* **11**, 549

Ehrlich, P. (1883). 'Ueber das Vorkommen Von Glykogen im Diabetischen und in Normalen organismus.' *Z. klin. Med.* **6**, 33

Epstein, M. A. (1962). 'Observations on the mode of release of herpes virus from infected HeLa cells.' *J. Cell Biol.* **12**, 589

Erlandson, R. A. and Tandler, B. (1972). 'Ultrastructure of acinic cell carcinoma of the parotid gland.' *Archs Path.* **93**, 130

Farquhar, M. G. and Palade, G. E. (1962). 'Functional evidence for the existence of a third cell type in the renal glomerulus. Phagocytosis of filtration residues by a distinctive "third" cell.' *J. Cell Biol.* **13**, 55

Fawcett, D. W. (1966). 'On the occurrence of a fibrous lamina on the inner aspect of the nuclear envelope in certain cells of vertebrates.' *Am. J. Anat.* **119**, 129

— (1967). *The Cell: Its Organelles and Inclusions.* Philadelphia and London: Saunders

— and Witebsky, F. (1964). 'Observations on the Ultrastructure of nucleated erythrocytes and thrombocytes, with particular reference to the structural basis of their discoidal shape.' *Z. Zellforsch. mikrosk. Anat.* **62**, 785

Feldherr, C. M. (1962). 'The nuclear annuli as pathways for nucleocytoplasmic exchanges.' *J. Cell Biol.* **14**, 65

Finner, L. L. and Calvery, H. O. (1939). 'Pathologic changes in rats and in dogs fed diets containing lead and arsenic compounds.' *Archs. Path.* **27**, 433

Firkin, B. G. (1969). 'The fine structure and chemistry of haemopoietic tissue.' In *The Biological Basis of Medicine,* Vol. 3. Ed. by E. E. Bittar and N. Bittar. New York and London: Academic Press

Flaks, B. and Flaks, A. (1970). 'Fine structure of nuclear inclusions in murine pulmonary tumour cells.' *Cancer Res.* **30**, 1437

Franke, W. W. and Schinko, W. (1969). 'Nuclear shape in muscle cells.' *J. Cell Biol.* **42**, 326

Frasca, J. M., Auerbach, O., Parks, V. and Stoeckenius, W. (1965). 'Electron microscope observations of nuclear evaginations in bronchial epithelium.' *Expl Molec. Path.* **4**, 340

Fujimoto, Y., Okada, M. and Okada, K. (1970). 'Electron microscopic studies on Marek's disease. V. Light and electron microscopic observations on skeletal muscle lesions.' Proc. 70th Meet. of Jap. Soc. Vet. Sci. *Jap. J. vet. Sci.* **32**, 221

Gay, H. (1956). 'Chromosome-nuclear membrane-cytoplasmic interrelations in Drosophila.' *J. biophys. biochem. Cytol.* **2**, No. 4 Suppl., 407

Ghadially, F. N. (1958). 'Comparative morphological study of keratoacanthoma of man and similar experimentally produced lesions in rabbit.' *J. Path. Bact.* **75**, 441

—(1961). 'The role of hair follicle in origin and evolution of some cutaneous neoplasms of man and experimental animals.' *Cancer* **14**, 801

—(1971). 'Keratoacanthoma.' In *Dermatology in General Medicine*, pp. 425. Ed. by T. B. Fitzpatrick and D. P. Johnson. New York and Maidenhead: McGraw-Hill

— and Mehta, P. N. (1970). 'Ultrastructure of osteogenic sarcoma.' *Cancer* **25**, 1457

— and Parry, E. W. (1966). 'Ultrastructure of a human hepatocellular carcinoma and surrounding non-neoplastic liver.' *Cancer* **19**, 1989

— and Roy, S. (1969a). *Ultrastructure of Synovial Joints in Health and Disease*. London: Butterworths.
(1969b). 'Ultrastructural changes in the synovial membrane in lipohaemarthrosis.' *Ann. Rheum. Dis.* **28**, 529

— Barton, B. W. and Kerridge, D. F. (1963). 'The etiology of keratoacanthoma.' *Cancer* **16**, 603

— Meachim, G. and Collins, D. H. (1965). 'Extracellular lipid in matrix of human articular cartilage.' *Ann. rheum. Dis.* **24**, 136

— Fuller, J. A. and Kirkaldy-Willis, W. H. (1971). 'Ultrastructure of full-thickness defects in articular cartilage.' *Archs Path.* **92**, 356

— — and Bhatnagar, R. (1972). 'Waxing and waning of nuclear fibrous lamina.' *Archs Path.* **94**, 303

— Oryschak, A. F. and Mitchell, D. M. (1974). 'Nuclear fibrous lamina in pathological human synovial membrane.' *Virchows Arch. Abt. B Zellpath.* **15**, 223

Givan, K. F. and Jézéquel, A. (1969). 'Infectious canine hepatitis: a virologic and ultrastructural study.' *Lab. Invest.* **20**, 36

Goldblatt, P. J., Sullivan, R. J. and Farber, E., (1969). 'Induction of partial nucleolar segregation in hepatic parenchymal cells by actinomycin D, following inhibition of ribonucleic acid synthesis by ethionine'. *Lab Invest.* **20**, 283

Golomb, H. M. and Bahr, G. F. (1971). 'Scanning electron microscopic observations of surface structures of isolated human chromosomes.' *Science* **171**, 1024

— — and Borgaonkar, D. S. (1971). 'Analysis of human chromosomal variants by quantitative electron microscopy. I. Group D chromosome with giant satellites.' *Genetics* **69**, 123

Goyer, R. A. (1968). 'The renal tubule in lead poisoning. 1. Mitochondrial swelling and aminoaciduria.' *Lab. Invest.* **19**, 71

— May, P., Cates, M. M. and Krigman, M. R. (1970). 'Lead and protein content of isolated intranuclear inclusion bodies from kidneys of lead-poisoned rats.' *Lab. Invest.* **22**, 245

Granboulan, N. and Bernhard, W. (1961). 'Cytochimie ultrastructurale. Exploration des structures nucleaires par digestion enzymatique.' *C. r. Soc. Biol.* **155**, 1767

— Tournier, P., Wicker, R. and Bernhard, W. (1963). 'An electron microscopic study of the development of SV40 virus.' *J. Cell. Biol.* **17**, 423

— and Granboulan, P. (1964). 'Cytochimie ultrastructurale du nucleole. I. Mise en evidence de chromatine a l'interieur du nucleole.' *Expl Cell. Res.* **34**, 71

Grasso, J. A., Swift, H. and Ackerman, G. A. (1962). 'Observations on the development of erythrocytes in mammalian fetal liver.' *J. Cell. Biol.* **14**, 235

Gray, E. G. and Guillery, R. W. (1963). 'On nuclear structure in the ventral nerve cord of the leech *Hirudo medicinalis*.' *Z. Zellforsch. mikrosk. Anat.* **59**, 738

Greenstein, J. P. (1954). 'Chemistry of the tumour-bearing host.' In *Biochemistry of Cancer*, p. 507. New York: Academic Press

Gregg, M. B. and Morgan, C. (1959). 'Reduplication of nuclear membranes in HeLa cells infected with adenoviruses.' *J. biophys. biochem. Cytol.* **6**, 539

Gueft, B. and Molnar, J. J. (1961). 'The lead poisoned liver cell under the electron microscope.' In *Abstracts of the 58th Annual Meeting of the American Association of Pathologists and Bacteriologists,* Chicago, Ill, p. 45.

Hadek, R. and Swift, H. (1962). 'Nuclear extrusion and intracisternal inclusions in the rabbit blastocyst.' *J. Cell Biol.* **13**, 445

Harris, C., Grady, H. and Svoboda, D. (1968). 'Alterations in pancreatic and hepatic ultrastructure following acute cyclohexemide intoxication.' *J. Ultrastruct. Res.* **22**, 240

Hay, E. D. (1968). 'Structure and function of the nucleolus in developing cells.' In *The Nucleus*, pp 2–79. Ed. by A. Dalton and F. Haguenau. New York: Academic Press

— and Revel, J. P. (1962). 'The D.N.A. component of the nucleolus studied in autoradiographs viewed with the electron microscope.' In *Fifth Int. Congr. Electron Microscopy, Philadelphia.* Vol. 2, pp 1–7. New York: Academic Press

— — (1963). 'The fine structure of the DNP-component of the nucleus. An electron microscopic study utilizing autoradiography to locate DNA syntheses.' *J. Cell. Biol.* **16**, 29

Henry, K. and Petts, V. (1969). 'Nuclear bodies in human thymus.' *J. Ultrastruct. Res.* **27**, 330

Himes, M. M. and Pollister, A. W. (1962). 'Glycogen accumulation in the nucleus.' *J. Histochem. Cytochem.* **10**, 175

Hinglais-Guillard, N., Moricard, R. and Bernhard, W. (1961). 'Ultrastructure des cancers pavimentex invasip du col uterin chez la femme.' *Bull. Cancer* **49**, 283

Horstmann, E. (1962). 'Elektronenmikroskopie des menschlichen nebenhodenepithels.' *Z. Zellforsch. mikrosk. Anat.* **57**, 692

— (1965). 'Die kerneinschlüsse im nebenhodenepithel des hundes.' *Z. Zellforsch. mikrosk. Anat.* **65**, 770

— Richter, R. and Roosen-Runge, E. (1966). 'Zur elektronenmikroskopie der kerneinschlüsse im menschlichen neben-hodenepithel.' *Z. Zellforsch. mikrosk. Anat.* **69**, 69

Hoshino, M. (1961). 'The deep invagination of the inner nuclear membrane into the nucleoplasm in the ascites hepatoma cells.' *Expl Cell Res.* **24**, 606

Hruban, Z., Swift, H. and Rechcigl, M., Jr. (1965). 'Fine structure of transplantable hepatomas of the rat.' *J. natn. Cancer Inst.* **35**, 459

Hsu, T. C. and Lou, T. Y. (1959). 'Nuclear extrusions in cells of Cloudman melanoma *in vitro*.' In *Pigment Cell Biology*. pp. 315–325. Ed. by M. Gordon. New York: Academic Press

Huehns, E. R., Lutzner, M. and Hecht, F. (1964). 'Nuclear abnormalities of the neutrophils in the D_1 (13–15) trisomy syndrome.' *Lancet* **1**, 589

Huhn, D. (1967). 'Nuclear pockets in normal monocytes.' *Nature, Lond.* **216**, 1240

Huxley, H. E. and Zubay, G. (1961). 'Preferential staining of nucleic acid-containing structures for electron microscopy.' *J. biophys. biochem. Cytol.* **11**, 273

Hyde, B. B., Sankaranarayanan, K. and Birnstiel, M. L. (1965). 'Observations on fine structure in pea nucleoli *in situ* and isolated.' *J. Ultrastruct. Res.* **12**, 652

Hyden, H. (1943). 'Die funktion des kernkörperchens bei der Eiweibbildung in Nervenzellen.' *Z. mikrosk.-anat. Forsch.* **54**, 96

Ishikawa, H. (1964). 'Peculiar intranuclear structures in sympathetic ganglion cells of a dog.' *Z. Zellforsch. mikrosk. Anat.* **62**, 822

Jézéquel, A. M. and Marinozzi, V. (1963). 'A Propos de certains composants granulaires du noyau reveles par la fixation aux aldehydes,' *J. Microscopie* **2**, 34 (abstract)

— and Steiner, J. W. (1966). 'Some ultrastructural and histochemical aspects of coxsackie virus-cell interactions.' *Lab. Invest.* **15**, 1055

— Shreeve, M. M. and Steiner, J. W. (1967). 'Segregation of nucleolar components in mycoplasma-infected cells.' *Lab. Invest.* **16**, 287

Johnston, H. S. (1962). 'Nuclear inclusions in the epithelium of the hen's oviduct.' *Z. Zellforsch. mikrosk. Anat.* **57**, 385

Jones, O. P. (1959). 'Formation of erythroblasts in the fetal liver and their destruction by macrophages and hepatic cells.' *Anat. Rec.* **133**, 294

Kalifat, S. R., Bouteille, M. and Delarue, J. (1967). 'Etude ultrastructurale de la lamelle dense observée au contact de la membrane nucleaire interne.' *J. Microscopie* **6**, 1019

Kallman, F., Adams, J. M., Williams, R. C. and Imagawa, D. T. (1959). 'Fine structure of cellular inclusions in measles virus infections.' *J. biophys. biochem. Cytol.* **6**, 379

Karasaki, S. (1963). 'Studies on amphibian yolk. I. The ultrastructure of the yolk platelet.' *J. Cell. Biol.* **18**, 135

— (1970). 'An electron microscope study of intranuclear canaliculi in Novikoff hepatoma cells.' *Cancer Res.* **30**, 1736

— (1971). 'Cytoplasmic and nuclear glycogen synthesis in Novikoff ascites hepatoma cells.' *J. Ultrastruct. Res.* **35**, 181

Kaye, J. S. (1969). 'The ultrastructure of chromatin in nuclei of interphase cells and in spermatids.' In *Handbook of Molecular Cytology*, p. 362. Ed. by A. Lima-de-Faria. Amsterdam and London: North Holland Publ.

Kessel, R. G. and Beams, H. W. (1968). 'Intranucleolar membranes and nuclear-cytoplasmic exchange in young cray-fish oocytes.' *J. Cell Biol.* **39**, 735

Kierszenbaum, A. L. (1968). 'The ultrastructure of human mixed salivary tumors.' *Lab. Invest.* **18**, 391

Kleinfeld, R. and Koulish, S. (1957). 'Cytological aspects of mouse and rat liver containing nuclear inclusions.' *Anat. Rec.* **128**, 433

— and Von Haam, E. (1959). 'Effect of thioacetamide on rat liver regeneration. II. Nuclear RNA in mitosis.' *J. biophys. biochem. Cytol.* **6**, 393

— Greider, M. H. and Frajola, W. J. (1956). 'Electron microscopy of intranuclear inclusions found in human and rat liver parenchymal cells.' *J. biophys. biochem. Cytol.* (Suppl. 4) **2**, 435

Koestner, A. and Long, J. F. (1970). 'Ultrastructure of canine distemper virus in explant tissue cultures of canine cerebellum.' *Lab. Invest.* **23**, 196

Krishan, A., Uzman, B. G. and Hedley-Whyte, E. T. (1967). 'Nuclear bodies, a component of cell nuclei in hamster tissues and human tumors.' *J. Ultrastruct. Res.* **19**, 563

Kuhn, C. H. (1967). 'Nuclear bodies and intranuclear globulin inclusions in Waldenstrom's macroglobulinemia.' *Lab. Invest.* **17**, 404

Kume, F., Maruyama, S., D'Agostino, A. N. and Chiga, M. (1967). 'Nucleolus change produced by mithramycin in rat hepatic cell.' *Expl Molec. Path.* **6**, 254

Kumegawa, M., Cattoni, M. and Stimson, P. G. (1969). 'Electron microscopy of intranuclear inclusions in a mixed tumor.' *Am. Acad. Oral. Path.* **28**, 89

Kyte, J. (1964). 'Nuclear extrusion in dissociated rat heart cells.' *Z. Zellforsch. mikrosk. Anat.* **62**, 495

LaFontaine, J. G. (1965). 'A light and electron microscope study of small, spherical nuclear bodies in meristematic cells of *Allium cepa, Vicia faba* and *Raphanus sativus*.' *J. Cell. Biol.* **26**, 1

Landing, B. H. and Nakai, H. (1959). 'Histochemical properties of renal lead-inclusions and their demonstration in urinary sediment.' *Am. J. clin. Path.* **31**, 499

Lane, B. P. (1965). 'Alterations in the cytologic detail of intestinal smooth muscle cells in various stages of contraction.' *J. Cell Biol.* **27**, 199

Lapis, K. and Bernhard, W. (1965). 'The effect of mitomycin C on the nucleolar fine structure of KB cells in culture.' *Cancer Res.* **25**, 628

Latta, H. and Maunsbach, A. B. (1962a). 'The juxtaglomerular apparatus as studied electron microscopically.' *J. Ultra-struct. Res.* **6**, 547

—— (1962b). 'Relations of the centrolobular region of the glomerulus to the juxtaglomerular apparatus.' *J. Ultrastruct. Res.* **6**, 562

Lazarus, S. S., Vethamany, V. G., Shapiro, S. H. and Amsterdam, D. (1966). 'Histochemistry and fine structure of 4-nitroquinoline-N-oxide-induced nuclear inclusions.' *Cancer Res.* **26**, 2229

LeBuis, J. J. (1966). 'Alterations ultrastructurales nucleaire et nucleolaires de cellules Kb infectées par l'adenovirus type 12.' *J. Microscopie* **5**, 59a

Leduc, E. H. and Wilson, J. W. (1959a). 'An electron microscope study of intranuclear inclusions in mouse liver and hepatoma.' *J. biophys. biochem. Cytol.* **6**, 427

—— (1959b). 'A histochemical study of intranuclear inclusions in mouse liver and hepatoma.' *J. Histochem. Cytochem.* **7**, 8

Leeson, T. S. and Leeson, C. R. (1968). 'The fine structure of Brunner's glands in man.' *J. Anat.* **103**, 263

Leestma, J. E., Bornstein, M. B., Sheppard, R. D. and Feldman, L. A. (1969). 'Ultrastructural aspects of *Herpes simplex* virus infection in organized cultures of mammalian nervous tissue.' *Lab. Invest.* **20**, 70

Lemaire, R. (1963). 'Recherches morphologiques, cytochimiques et experimentales sur les inclusions nucleaires dans l'epididyme du chien.' *Arch. Biol.* **3**, 342

Levine, A. S., Nesbit, N. E., White, J. G. and Yarbro, J. W. (1968). 'Effects of fractionated histones on nucleic acid synthesis in 6C3HED mouse ascites tumor cells and in normal spleen cells.' *Cancer Res.* **28**, 831

Locker, J., Goldblatt, P. J. and Leighton, J. (1968). 'Some ultrastructural features of Yoshida ascites hepatoma.' *Cancer Res.* **28**, 2039

Loewenstein, W. R. and Kanno, Y. (1963). 'Some electrical properties of a nuclear membrane examined with a micro-electrode.' *J. gen. Physiol.* **46**, 1123

Lord, A. and LaFontaine, J. G. (1969). 'The organization of the nucleolus in meristematic plant cells. A cytochemical study.' *J. Cell Biol.* **40**, 633

Love, R. and Soriano, R. Z. (1971). 'Correlation of nucleolini with fine structural nucleolar constituents of cultured normal and neoplastic cells.' *Cancer Res.* **31**, 1030

Lozinski, P. (1911). 'I. Wissenschaftliche mitteilungen. 1. Uber die Malpighischen gefabe der Myrmeleonidenlarven als Spinndrusen.' *Zool. Anz.* **38**, 401

Ludford, R. J. (1924). 'Nuclear activity during melanosis.' *J. Roy Micro. Soc.* **13**, 28

Lung, B. (1972). 'Ultrastructure and chromatin disaggregation of human sperm head with thioglycolate treatment.' *J. Cell Biol.* **52**, 179

Lutzner, M. A. and Hecht, F. (1966). 'Nuclear anomalies of the neutrophil in a chromosomal triplication. The D_1 (13–15) trisomy syndrome.' *Lab. Invest.* **15**, 597

—— and Jordan, H. W. (1968). 'The ultrastructure of an abnormal cell in Sezary's syndrome.' *Blood* **31**, 719

McCarty, W. C. (1937). 'Further observations on the macronucleolus of cancer.' *Am. J. Cancer* **31**, 104

McDuffie, N. G. (1967). 'Nuclear blebs in human leukaemic cells.' *Nature, Lond.* **214**, 1341

Majno, G., La Gattuta, M. and Thompson, T. E. (1960). 'Cellular death and necrosis. Chemical, physical and morphologic changes in rat liver.' *Virchows Arch. path. Anat. Physiol.* **333**, 421

Marinozzi, V. (1964). 'Cytochimie ultrastructurale du nucleole-RNA et proteines intranucleolaires.' *J. Ultrastruct. Res.* **10**, 433

—— and Bernhard, W. (1964). 'Presence dans le nucleole de deux types de ribonucleoproteins morphologiquement distincts.' *Expl Cell Res.* **32**, 595

Masurovsky, E. B., Benitez, H. H., Kim, S. U. and Murray, M. R. (1970). 'Origin, development and nature of intra-nuclear rodlets and associated bodies in chicken sympathetic neurons.' *J. Cell Biol.* **44**, 172

Maximow, A. and Bloom, W. (1948). *Textbook of Histology*. Philadelphia and London: Saunders

Mercer, E. H. (1959). 'An electron microscopic study of *Amoeba proteus*.' *Proc. R. Soc. B.* **150**, 216

Merriam, R. W. (1962). 'Some dynamic aspects of the nuclear envelope.' *J. Cell Biol.* **12**, 79

Miller, O. L., Jr. (1966). 'Structure and composition of peripheral nucleoli of salamander oocytes.' *Natn Cancer Inst. Monogr.* **23**, 53

—— and Beatty, Barbara R. (1969). 'Nucleolar structure and function.' In *Handbook of Molecular Cytology*. Ed. by A. Lima-de-Faria. Amsterdam and London: North Holland Publ. Company

Mirsky, A. E. and Osawa, S. (1961). 'The interphase nucleus.' In *The Cell*, Vol. 2, p. 677. Ed. by J. Brachet and A. E. Mirsky. New York: Academic Press

Misrabi, M. (1969). 'Intranuclear inclusions in neurons and glial cells in the spiral cord of foetal, neonatal and adult rats.' *J. Anat.* **104**, 588

Miyai, K. and Steiner, J. W. (1965). 'Fine structure of interphase liver cell nuclei in subacute ethionine intoxication.' *Expl Molec. Path.* **4**, 525

—— (1967). 'Fine structure of interphase liver cell nuclei in acute ethionine intoxication.' *Lab. Invest.* **16**, 677

Montgomery, P. O'B., Jr., Reynolds, R. C. and Cook, J. E. (1966). 'Nucleolar "caps" induced by flying spot ultraviolet nuclear irradiation.' *Am. J. Path.* **49**, 555

Moore, G. E. and Pickren, J. W. (1967). 'Study of a virus-containing hematopoietic cell line and a melanoma cell line derived from a patient with a leukemoid reaction.' *Lab. Invest.* **16**, 882

Morgan, C., Goldman, G. C., Rose, H. M., Howe, C. and Huang, J. S. (1957). 'Electron microscopic and histochemical studies of an unusual crystalline protein occurring in cells infected by type 5 adenovirus. Preliminary observations.' *J. biophys. biochem. Cytol.* **3**, 505

Moricard, R. and Moricard, F. (1964). 'Modifications cytoplasmiques et nucleaires ultrastructurales uterines au cours de l'état follicoluteinique à glycogene massif.' *Gynec. Obstet.* **63**, 203

Moses, M. J. (1956). 'Studies on nuclei using correlated cytochemical, light and electron microscope techniques.' *J. biophys. biochem. Cytol.* **2**, No. 4 Suppl., 397

— (1960). 'Patterns of organization in the fine structure of chromosomes. In *4th Int. Congr. Electron Microscopy*, p. 199. Berlin: Springer

Murad, T. M. and Murthy, M. S. N. (1970). 'Ultrastructure of a chordoma.' *Cancer* **25**, 1204

— and Scarpelli, D. G. (1967). 'The ultrastructure of medullary and scirrhous mammary duct carcinoma.' *Am. J. Path.* **50**, 335

Nakai, T., Shand, F. L. and Howatson, A. F. (1969). 'Development of measles virus *in vitro*.' *Virology* **38**, 50

Nicander, L. (1964). 'Fine structure and cytochemistry of nuclear inclusions in the dog epididymis.' *Expl Cell Res.* **34**, 533

Nii, S., Morgan, C., Rose, H. M. and Rosenkranz, H. S. (1966). 'Analytical studies of the development of *Herpes simplex* virus.' In *Proceedings of the 6th international congress of electron microscopy*, Vol. 2, p. 201. Ed. by R. Uyeda. Tokyo: Maruzen

——— (1968). 'Electron microscopy of *Herpes simplex* virus. II. Sequence of development.' *J. Virol.* **2**, 517

Novikoff, A. B. (1957). 'A transplantable rat liver tumor induced by 4-dimethylaminoazobenzene.' *Cancer Res.* **17**, 1010

Oberling, Ch. and Bernhard, W. (1961). 'The morphology of the cancer cells.' In *The Cell.* Vol. 5, p. 405. Ed. by J. Brachet and A. E. Mirsky. New York: Academic Press

O'Brien, B. R. A. (1960). 'The presence of hemoglobin within the nucleus of the embryonic chick erythroblast.' *Expl Cell Res.* **21**, 226

Oda, A. and Chiga, M. (1965). 'Effect of actinomycin D on the hepatic cells of partially hepatectomised rats: an electron microscopic study.' *Lab. Invest.* **14**, 1419

Ogawa, K. (1962). 'Elektronenoptische untersuchungen bei eunem fall von sogenannten Hodgkensarkom.' *Frankfurt Z. Path.* **71**, 677

Olitsky, P. K. and Casals, J. (1945). 'Certain affections of the liver that arise spontaneously in so-called normal stock albino mice.' *Proc. Soc. exp. Biol. Med.* **60**, 48

Oryschak, A. F., Ghadially, F. N. and Bhatnagar (1974). 'Nuclear fibrous lamina in chondrocytes of articular cartilage.' *J. Anat.* **118**, 3

Pappas, G. D. (1956). 'The fine structure of the nuclear envelope of *Amoeba proteus*.' *J. biophys. biochem. Cytol.* **2**, Suppl. 4, 431

Parry, E. W. (1971). 'Membrane-bounded intranuclear structures in hepatocytes after exposure to sodium tetraphenyl boron.' *J. Path.* **104**, 210

— and Ghadially, F. N. (1967). 'Ultrastructure of the livers of rats bearing transplanted tumours.' *J. Path. Bact.* **93**, 295

Patrizi, G. and Middelkamp, J. N. (1969). '*In vivo* and *in vitro* demonstration of nuclear bodies in vaccinia infected cells.' *J. Ultrastruct. Res.* **28**, 275

— and Poger, M. (1967). 'The ultrastructure of the nuclear periphery. The zonula nucleum limitans.' *J. Ultrastruct. Res.* **17**, 127

— Middelkamp, J. N. and Reed, C. A. (1967). 'Reduplication of nuclear membranes in tissue culture cells infected with guinea pig cytomegalovirus.' *Am. J. Path.* **50**, 779

Perry, R. P. (1964). 'Role of the nucleolus in ribonucleic acid metabolism and other cellular processes.' *Natn. Cancer Inst. Monogr.* **14**, 73

— (1966). 'On ribosomal biogenesis.' *Natn. Cancer Inst. Monogr.* **23**, 527

—(1969). 'Nucleoli: the cellular sites of ribosome production.' In *Handbook of Molecular Cytology*. Ed. by A. Lima-de-Faria. Amsterdam and London: North Holland Publ.

Pianese, G. (1896). 'Beitrag zur histologie und aetiologie des carcinoms. Histologische und experimentelle untersuchungen. Aus dem Italieneschen ubersetzt von R. Teuscher. I–II. Histologische untersuchungen. *Ziegler's Beitr.* **142**, Suppl. 1, 1

Pomerat, C. M., Lefeber, C. G. and Smith, McD. (1954). 'Quantitative cine analysis of cell organoid activity.' *Ann. N.Y. Acad. Sci.* **58**, 1311

Popoff, N. and Stewart, S. E. (1968). 'The fine structure of nuclear inclusions in the brain of experimental golden hamsters.' *J. Ultrastruct. Res.* **23**, 347

Porter, K. R. (1960). 'Problems in the study of nuclear fine structure.' In *4th Int. Congr. Electron Microscopy*, Vol. 2, p. 186. Berlin: Springer

Recher, L., Whitescarver, J. and Briggs, L. (1970). 'A cytochemical and radioautographic study of human tissue culture cell nucleoli.' *J. Cell Biol.* **45**, 479

Reddy, J. and Svoboda, D. J. (1968). 'The relationship of nucleolar segregation to ribonucleic acid synthesis following the administration of selected hepatocarcinogens.' *Lab. Invest.* **19**, 132

Reynolds, R. C. and Montgomery, P. O'B., Jr. (1967). 'Nucleolar pathology produced by acridine orange and pro-flavine.' *Am. J. Path.* **51**, 323

— and Karney, D. H. (1963). 'Nucleolar "caps" a morphologic entity produced by the carcinogen 4-nitroquinoline-N-oxide.' *Cancer Res.* **23**, 535

Rhodin, J. A. G. (1963). *An Atlas of Ultrastructure*. Philadelphia, Pa: Saunders

Richter, G. W., Kress, Y. and Cornwall, C. C. (1968). 'Another look at lead inclusion bodies.' *Am. J. Path.* **53**, 189

Ris, H. (1956). 'A study of chromosomes with the electron microscope.' *J. biophys. biochem. Cytol.* **2**, Supp. 4, 385

— (1962). 'Interpretation of ultrastructure in the cell nucleus.' In *The Interpretation of Ultrastructure*, Vol. 1, p. 69. Ed. by R. J. Harris. New York: Academic Press.

Robbins, S. L. (1969). *Pathology*, 3rd ed. Philadelphia and London: Saunders

Robertson, D. M. (1964). 'Electron microscopic studies of nuclear inclusions in meningiomas.' *Am. J. Path.* **45**, 835

— and Maclean, J. D. (1965). 'Nuclear inclusions in malignant gliomas.' *Archs Neurol., Chicago* **13**, 287

Rouiller, C. and Simon, G. (1962). 'Contribution de la microscopie electronique au progres de nos connaissances en cytologie et en histo-pathologie hepatique.' *Revue int. Hépat.* **12**, 167

Roy, S. and Wolman, L. (1969). 'Electron microscopic observations on the virus particles in *Herpes simplex* encephalitis.' *J. clin. Path.* **22**, 51

Sanel, F. T. and Lepore, M. J. (1968). 'Granular and crystalline deposits in perinuclear and ergastoplasmic cisternae of human lamina propria cells.' *Expl Molec. Path.* **9**, 110

Sankaranarayanan, K. and Hyde, B. B. (1965). 'Ultrastructural studies of a nuclear body in peas with characteristics of both chromatin and nucleoli.' *J. Ultrastruct. Res.* **12**, 748

Schoefl, G. J. (1964). 'The effect of actinomycin D on the fine structure of the nucleolus.' *J. Ultrastructure Res.* **10**, 224

Scholz, W. and Paweletz, N. (1969). 'Glykogenablagerung in zellkernan des Ehrlich-ascites-tumors.' *Z. Krebsforsch.* **72**, 211

Schulz, H. and Hahnel, E. (1969). 'Die ultrastruktur des Glykogen in Lochkernen der menschlichen Leberepithelzellen bei Diabetes mellitus.' *Virchows Arch. Abt. B. Zellpath.* **3**, 282

Sebuwufu, P. H. (1966). 'Nuclear blebs in the human foetal thymus.' *Nature, Lond.* **213**, 1382

Sheldon, H., Silverberg, M. and Kerner, I. (1962). 'On the differing appearance of intranuclear and cytoplasmic glycogen in liver cells in glycogen storage disease.' *J. Cell. Biol.* **13**, 468

Shelton, E. (1955). 'Hepatomas in mice: factors affecting rapid induction of high incidence of hepatomas by *o*-amino-azotoluene.' *J. Natn. Cancer Inst.* **16**, 107

Shepard, D. C. (1964). 'Production and elimination of excess DNA in ultraviolet-irradiated Tetrahymena.' *J. Cell. Biol.* **23**, Abstr. No. 178, 86A

Shinozuka, H., Goldblatt, P. J. and Farber, E. (1968). 'The disorganization of hepatic cell nucleoli induced by ethionine and its reversal by adenine.' *J. Cell Biol.* **36**, 313

Shipkey, F. H., Erlandson, R. A., Bailey, R. B., Babcock, V. I. and Southam, C. M. (1967). 'Virus biographies. II. Growth of *Herpes simplex* virus in tissue culture.' *Expl Molec. Path.* **6**, 39

Simar, L. J. (1969). 'Ultrastructure et constitution des corps nucleaires dans les plasmocytes.' *Z. Zellforsch. mikrosk. Anat.* **99**, 235

— and Lemaire, R. (1966). 'Etude ultrastructurale des inclusions nucleaires de l'epididyme du chien.' *C.r. Acad. Sci., Paris* **262**, 1455

Simard, R. (1966). 'Specific nuclear and nucleolar ultrastructural lesions induced by proflavin and similarly acting antimetabolites in tissue culture.' *Cancer Res.* **26**, 2316

— and Bernhard, W. (1966). 'Le phenomène de la segregation nucleolaire specificité d'action de certains antimetabolites.' *Int. J. Cancer* **1**, 463

Siminoff, P. and Menefee, M. G. (1966). 'Normal and 5-bromo-deoxyuridine inhibited development of *Herpes simplex* virus.' *Expl Cell Res.* **44**, 241

Simpson, C. F. and Kling, J. M. (1967). 'The mechanism of denucleation in circulating erythroblasts.' *J. Cell Biol.* **35**, 237

Sirtori, C. and Bosisio, M. (1966). 'Oncolysis by *Herpes simplex*.' *Lancet* **1**, 96

Smetana, K. and Busch, H. (1964). 'Studies on the ultrastructure of the nucleoli of the Walker tumor and rat liver.' *Cancer Res.* **24**, 537

— Gyorkey, F., Gyorkey, P. and Busch, H. (1970a). 'Studies on the ultrastructure of nucleoli in human smooth muscle cells.' *Expl Cell Res.* **60**, 175

— — — — (1970b). 'Comparative studies on the ultrastructure of nucleoli in human lymphosarcoma cells and leukemic lymphocytes.' *Cancer Res.* **30**, 1149

Smith, G. F. and O'Hara, P. T. (1967). 'Nuclear pockets in normal leukocytes.' *Nature, Lond.* **215**, 773

Smith, E. B., Nosanchuk, J. S., Schnitzer, B. and Swarm, R. (1968). 'Fatty inclusions and microcysts. Thioacetamide-induced fatty inclusions in nuclei of mouse liver cells and hepatoma cells.' *Archs Path.* **85**, 175

Sobel, H. J., Schwarz, R. and Marquet, E. (1969a). 'Non-viral nuclear inclusions. 1. Cytoplasmic invaginations.' *Archs Path.* **87**, 179

— — — (1969b). 'Non-viral inclusions. 2. Glycogen and lipid.' *Lab. Invest.* **20**, 604 (abstract)

Sohval, A. R., Suzuki, Y., Gabrilove, J. L. and Churg, J. (1971). 'Ultrastructure of crystalloids in spermatogonia and Sertoli cells of normal human testis.' *J. Ultrastruct. Res.* **34**, 83

Sparrow, W. T. and Ashworth, C. T. (1965). 'Electron microscopy of nuclear glycogenesis.' *Archs Path.* **80**, 84

Stalzer, R. C., Kiely, J. M., Pease, G. L. and Brown, A. L. (1965). 'Effect of 5-fluorouracil on human hematopoiesis.' *Cancer* **18**, 1071

Stern, H., Allfrey, V., Mirsky, A. E. and Saetren, H. (1951). 'Some enzymes of isolated nuclei.' *J. gen. Physiol.* **35**, 559

Stevens, B. J. and Andre, J. (1969). 'The nuclear envelope.' In *Handbook of Molecular Cytology*, p. 837. Ed. by A. Lima-de-Faria. Amsterdam and London: North-Holland Publ.

Stowell, R. E. (1949). 'Alterations in nucleic acids during hepatoma formation in rats fed *p*-dimethylaminoazobenzene.' *Cancer* **2**, 121

Svoboda, D., Grady, H. J. and Higginson, J. (1966). 'Aflatoxin B$_1$ injury in rat and monkey liver.' *Am. J. Path.* **49**, 1023

— Racela, A. and Higginson, J. (1967). 'Variations in ultrastructural nuclear changes in hepatocarcinogenesis.' *Biochem. Pharmac.* **16**, 651

Swanbeck, G. and Thyresson, N. (1964). 'Electron microscopy in intranuclear particles in lichen ruber planus.' *Acta derm-vener.* **44**, 105

Swanson, J. L., Craighead, J. E. and Reynolds, E. S. (1966). 'Electron microscopic observations on *Herpes virus hominis* (*Herpes simplex* virus) encephalitis in man.' *Lab. Invest.* **15**

Swift, H. (1959). 'Studies on nucleolar function.' In *Symposium on Molecular Biology*, p. 266. Ed. by R. E. Zirkle. Chicago, Ill: University of Chicago Press

— (1963). 'Cytochemical studies on nuclear fine structure.' *Expl Cell. Res.* Suppl. **9**, 54

Tandler, B., Denning, C. R., Mandel, I. D. and Kutscher, A. H. (1969) 'Ultrastructure of human labial salivary glands. II. Intranuclear inclusions in the acinar secretory cell.' *Z. Zellforsch. mikrosk. Anat.* **94**, 555

Tanikawa, K. and Igarashi, M. (1963). 'Electron microscopic observations of the liver in diabetes mellitus with special attention to the intranuclear glycogen of the liver cell.' *J. Electron Micro.* **12**, 117

Terzakis, J. A. (1965). 'The nucleolar channel system of human endometrium.' *J.Cell. Biol.* **27**, 293

Toker, C. and Trevino, N. (1966). 'Ultrastructure of human primary hepatic carcinoma.' *Cancer* **19**, 1594

Tooze, J. and Davies, H. G. (1963). 'The occurrence and possible significance of hemoglobin in the chromosomal regions of mature erythrocyte nuclei of the newt, *Triturus cristatus cristatus.*' *J. Cell Biol.* **16**, 501

Torack, R. M. (1961). 'Ultrastructure of capillary reaction to brain tumors.' *Archs Neurol., Chicago* **5**, 416

Toro, I. and Olah, I. (1966). 'Nuclear blebs in the cells of the guinea-pig thymus.' *Nature, Lond.* **212**, 315

Trump, B. F., Goldblatt, P. J. and Stowell, R. E. (1963). 'Nuclear and cytoplasmic changes during necrosis *in vitro* (autolysis); an electron microscopic study.' *Am. J. Path.* **43**, 23a

— — — (1965a). 'Studies on necrosis of mouse liver *in vitro*. Ultrastructural alterations in the mitochondria of hepatic parenchymal cells.' *Lab. Invest.* **14**, 343

— — — (1965b). 'Studies of necrosis *in vitro* of mouse hepatic parenchymal cells. Ultrastructural alterations in endoplasmic reticulum, Golgi's apparatus, plasma membrane and lipid droplets.' *Lab. Invest.* **14**, 2000

Ulrich, J. and Kidd, M. (1966). 'Subacute inclusion body encephalitis. A histological and electron microscopical study.' *Acta neuropath.* **6**, 359

Van Noord, M. J., Van Pelt, Frida, G., Hollander C. F. and Daems, W. T. (1972). 'The development of ultrastructural glomerular alterations in *Praomys (mastomys) natalensis*. An electron microscopic study.' *Lab. Invest.* **26**, 364

Vazquez, J. J., Ortuno, G. and Cervos-Navarro, J. (1970). 'An ultrastructural study of spheroidal nuclear bodies found in gliomas.' *Virchows Arch. Abt. B. Zellpath.* **5**, 288

Wachstein, M. (1949). 'Studies on inclusion bodies. 1. Acid fastness of nuclear inclusion bodies that are induced by ingestion of lead and bismuth.' *Am. J. clin. Path.* **19**, 608

Watrach, A. M. and Vatter, A. E., Jr. (1962). 'The nature of inclusion bodies in lead poisoning.' In *Proc. Fifth Int. Congr. for Electron Microscopy*, p. VV–II. Ed. by S. S. Breese. New York: Academic Press

Watson, M. L. (1955). 'The nuclear envelope. Its structure and relation to cytoplasmic membranes.' *J. biophys. biochem. Cytol.* **1**, 257

— (1959). 'Further observations on the nuclear envelope of the animal cell.' *J. biophys. biochem. Cytol.* **6**, 147

— (1962). 'Observations on a granule associated with chromatin in the nuclei of cells of rat and mouse.' *J. Cell Biol.* **13**, 162

Watson, D. H. and Wildy, P. (1963). 'Some serological properties of *herpes virus* particles studied with the electron microscope.' *Virology* **21**, 100

Weber, A. F. and Frommes, S. P. (1963). 'Nuclear bodies: their prevalence, location and ultrastructure in the calf.' *Science* **141**, 912

— Whipp, S., Usenik, E. and Frommes, S. P. (1964). 'Structural changes in the nuclear body in the adrenal zona fasciculata of the calf following the administration of ACTH.' *J. Ultrastruct. Res.* **11**, 564

Weiss, M. and Meyer, J. (1972). 'Comparison of the effects of Coxsackie virus A9 and of actinomycin D on the nucleolar ultrastructure of monkey kidney cells.' *J. Ultrastructure Research* **38**, 411

Wessel, W. (1958). 'Electronenmikroskopische untersuchungen von intranuclearen einschlusskorpern.' *Virchows Arch. path. Anat. Physiol.* **331**, 314

Wills, E. J. (1968). 'Acute infective hepatitis.' *Archs Path.* **86**, 184

Wilt, F. H. (1967). 'The control of embryonic hemoglobin synthesis.' In *Advances in Morphogenesis,* vol. 6, p. 89. Ed. by M. Abercrombie and T. Brachet. New York: Academic Press

Wischnitzer, S. (1958). 'An electron microscope study of the nuclear envelope of amphibian oocytes.' *J. Ultrastruct. Res.* **1**, 201

Wiseman, G. and Ghadially, F. N. (1958). 'A biochemical concept of tumour growth, infiltration and cachexia.' *Br. med. J.* **2**, 18

Wyatt, R. B., Schochet, S. S. and McCormick, W. F. (1970). 'Rhabdomyoma light and electron microscopic study of a case with intranucuclear inclusions.' *Archs Otolar.* **92**, 32

Yamamoto, T. (1969). 'Correlation of electron and light microscopy on the replication of a canine adenovirus.' *Microbiology* **1**, 371

— and Shahrabadi, M. S. (1971). 'Enzyme cytochemistry and autoradiography of adenovirus-infected cells as determined with the electron microscope.' *Can. J. Microbiol.* **17**, 249

Yasuzumi, G. (1960). Licht und electronenmikroskopische studien an kernhaltigen erythrocyten. *Z. Zellforsch mikrosk. anat.* **51**, 325

— and Sugihara, R. (1965). 'The fine structure of nuclei as revealed by electron microscopy. The fine structure of Ehrlich ascites tumor cell nuclei in preprophase.' *Expl Cell Res.* **37**, 207

— Nakai, Y., Tsubo, I., Yasuda, M. and Sugioka, T. (1967). 'IV. The intranuclear inclusion formation in Leydig cells of aging human testis.' *Expl Cell Res.* **45**, 261

Zucker-Franklin, D. (1968). 'Electron microscopic studies of human granulocytes: structural variations related to function.' *Semin. Hemat.* **5**, 109

CHAPTER II

Centrioles

INTRODUCTION

The existence of centrioles and their association with the process of mitosis has been recognized by light microscopists for many years (Van Beneden, 1876). In the historic work *The Cell in Development and Heredity*, Wilson (1925) described them as 'granules of extreme minuteness, staining intensely with iron haematoxylin, crystal violet, and some other dyes, and often hardly to be distinguished from a microsome save that it lies at the focus of astral rays'.

Another intracellular structure, the basal body of cilia and flagella, has also long been observed by light microscopists and believed to be related to centrioles (Henneguy, 1897; Lenhossek, 1898). The ultrastructure of centrioles and basal bodies has been studied by several workers (DeHarven and Bernhard, 1956; Sorokin, 1962; Renaud and Swift, 1964; Forer, 1965; Stubblefield and Brinkley, 1967) and it is now clear that the two structures are morphologically identical (Stubblefield and Brinkley, 1967) and that the basal body is no more than a centriole in another type of activity.

In suitably stained light microscopic preparations, a pair of centrioles is usually seen in a cell. These present in electron micrographs as short cylindrical bodies, usually lying at right angles to one another. Collectively they comprise the diplosome which usually lies in the juxtanuclear region partially surrounded by the Golgi complex. The region in which the centrioles lie is called the centrosome, and the line joining the centrosome to the centre of the nucleus is referred to as the cell axis. In some cells, such as those of certain epithelia, the diplosomal centrioles lie not in the juxtanuclear position but under the apical portion of the cell membrane.

Although in most instances only a single pair of centrioles is seen, it should be remembered that well before the cell enters mitosis the centrioles replicate (Mazia, 1961). At this stage four centrioles (i.e. two pairs) are seen. Each pair then migrates to the poles of the mitotic apparatus. The megakaryocyte, with its peculiar nucleus derived through cycles of division and fusion of daughter nuclei without cell division (cytokinesis), may contain as many as 40 centrioles. Neoplastic and other varieties of giant cells formed either by repeated division of the nucleus without cytokinesis or a fusion of cells also contain multiple centrioles.

Ultrastructural studies have demonstrated that centrioles are hollow cylindrical bodies about 0·1–0·25 μ in diameter and 0·3–0·7 μ in length (*Plates 42 and 43*). The cylindrical wall of the centriole is composed of nine longitudinally orientated, evenly spaced triplets of tubules or fibres set in a dense matrix. The tubules or subfibres of each triplet are designated A, B and C as indicated in *Plate 44, Fig. 1*. It is not established unequivocally whether these structures are tubules or fibres. Fawcett (1967) points out, 'all three have a dense rim and a less dense center giving them a hollow appearance but it has not been established whether they are actually tubules or solid fibers with a dense cortex and a light interior'. He prefers to call them fibres or subfibres. Despite such quite valid contentions, most workers have adopted the term 'tubules'. Certainly the structures look like tubules and one could argue that, unless proven to the contrary, the benefit of the doubt should rest with the term 'tubules' or 'microtubules'. In keeping with current practice, I shall continue to call these and other similar structures in the mitotic apparatus and cilia and flagella as tubules or microtubules rather than filaments.

When viewed in transverse section the triplets appear like the arms of a pyrotechnic pin-wheel, for the line joining the centres of the three microtubules forms an angle of approximately 30 degrees to the tangent of the cylindrical wall (Fawcett, 1967).

The detailed anatomy of the centriole is quite complex and difficult to discern. Rarely is a centriole cut exactly transversely or longitudinally. More frequent are oblique sections (*Plate 43, Fig. 3*), where the features mentioned above cannot be appreciated. Even in sections close to the transverse plane, all the tubules are often not clearly visualized, because they follow a low-pitched helical course and not a course parallel to the long axis of the organelle. Excellent illustrations and a detailed account of the anatomy of the centriole as seen in cultured fibroblasts of the Chinese hamster may be found in Stubblefield and Brinkley's (1967) paper. Here only a brief description of some of these features will be presented, derived mainly from that work.

The 'cavity' within the hollow cylindrical centrioles contains many interesting structures besides material resembling the cytoplasm. In sections (transverse, oblique or longitudinal) through the centriole a small vesicle 600 Å in diameter is sometimes seen (*Plate 43*). The significance and function of this structure are entirely unknown, but it has been seen in the centrioles of a wide variety of cells and is probably of universal occurrence. Another component which is singularly difficult to demonstrate is the internal helix which spirals the entire length of the cylinder just under the triplets (*Plate 42*).

Plate 42

Two parent centrioles cut transversely are seen in company with immature daughter centrioles sectioned longitudinally. One of the lower parent centrioles is slightly obliquely sectioned so that a fairly large segment of the internal helix is revealed (arrow). Note also the numerous microtubules radiating from the centrioles. ×40,000 (*From Stubblefield and Brinkley, 1967*)

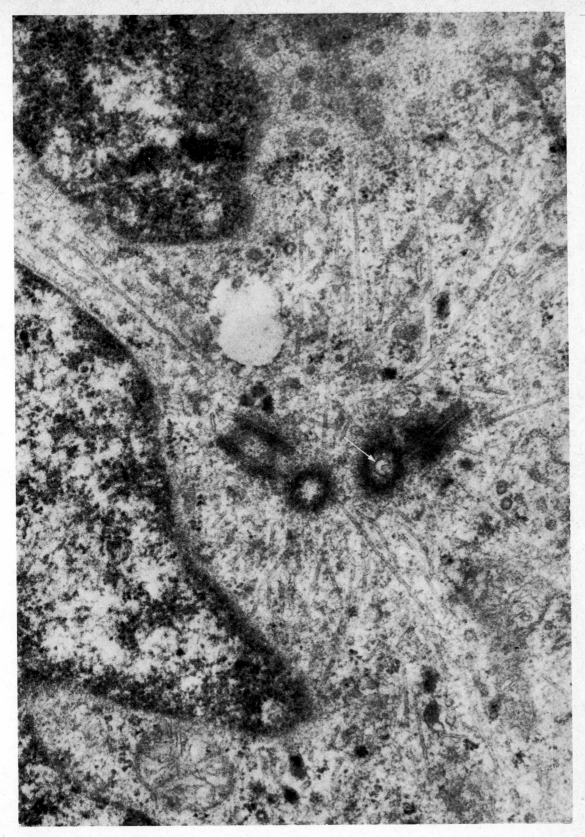

95

Since the centriole has a rotational symmetry (ninefold), it is possible to perform a Markham analysis on this structure (Markham *et al.*, 1963). Briefly, this involves making a multiple exposure photograph from an electron micrograph of a transverse section of a centriole, rotated through a 40-degree angle between each of nine exposures. Such treatment enhances structures that repeat at 40 degrees and tends to obliterate the randomly distributed structures and 'noise' in the electron micrograph. Using this technique, Stubblefield and Brinkley (1967) have shown a faint double structure, called the triplet base, on which the triplet blade rests. The innermost dense part of this structure forms a foot-like appendage continuous with the microtubule A (*Plate 44, Fig. 1*). On Markham analysis performed on thicker sections where a substantial part of the arc of the internal helix is included, it can be shown that this helical structure contacts the 'feet' mentioned above.

Markham analysis of transverse sections at one end of the centriole reveals another structure which has been called the cart-wheel. This has been seen in the centrioles and basal bodies of several species (Gibbons and Grimstone, 1960; Gall, 1961). (In some protozoon centrioles more than one cart-wheel is present.) The cart-wheel has a ninefold symmetry and presents as nine radial spokes arising from a hub at the centre of the centriole and extending to the triplet base. A structure with eightfold symmetry, called the octagonal end structure, is seen in the end opposite to the cart-wheel (Stubblefield and Brinkley, 1967). It is probably homologous to the basal plate of basal bodies.

Adjacent to, and at times continuous with, the centriole are seen various pericentriolar structures or satellites whose function and significance is obscure. They show numerous diverse forms, such as knob-like dense bodies, radial arms extending from one end of the centriole, or electron-dense granular and fibrillary masses quite separate from the centriole.

Plate 43

Fig. 1. Cross-section of a centriole from a Chinese hamster fibroblast cultivated *in vitro*. × 120,000 (*From Stubblefield and Brinkley, 1967*)

Fig. 2. Longitudinal section of a centriole from a mitotic cell. Note the central vesicle (V) and adjacent cytoplasmic microtubules (arrows). × 140,000 (*From Stubblefield and Brinkley, 1967*)

Fig. 3. Obliquely sectioned centrioles from a rat sarcoma. The section has passed through the central vesicle (V) in one of the centrioles. × 102,000

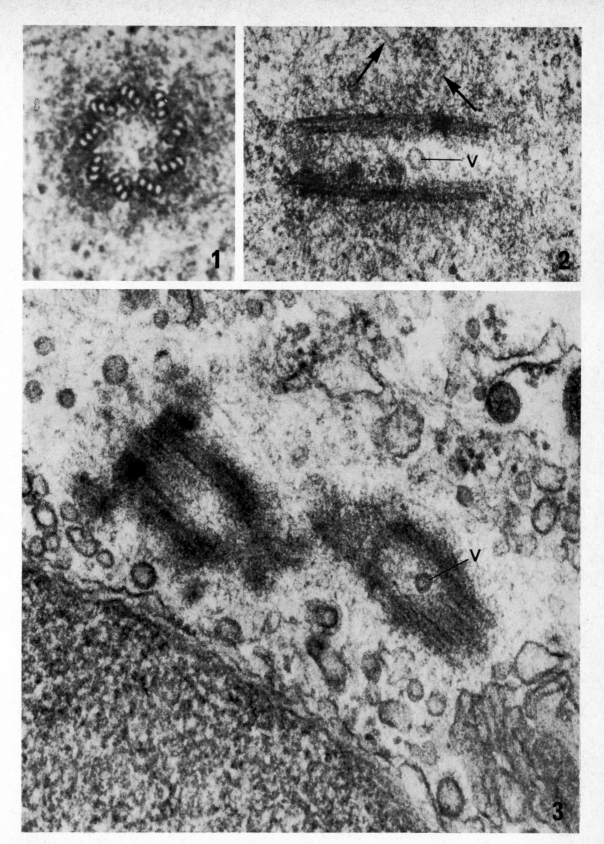

Microtubules are at times seen radiating from the centrioles (*Plates 42 and 43*), particularly in rapidly growing cells where parts of the mitotic spindle persist during interphase. Many more microtubules are seen when the cell is preparing to enter the mitotic phase. A basic function of the centriole is the production of microtubules.* Thus it produces the pole-to-pole microtubules of the mitotic apparatus, the elongation of which is involved in chromosome separation during mitosis, and also the astral rays, some of which are said to attach to the cell membrane and probably play a part in cytokinesis (see review by Mazia, 1961).

Centrioles or basal bodies also produce the microtubules of cilia and flagella. It is interesting to note that some of the microtubules of the mitotic spindle tend to occur in pairs as do the peripheral doublets in cilia. However, the microtubules of the mitotic apparatus arise at right angles to the wall of the centriole, while the nine peripheral doublets of the axial microtubule complex of cilia arise as a continuation of the inner two microtubules (A and B) of the centriolar triplets (Gibbons and Grimstone, 1960).

Centrioles are self-replicating organelles but the process involved is not one of fission whereby a structure divides to produce two equivalent daughter units, but a generative mechanism which involves the production of a procentriole from or near the end of the parent. The procentriole is a short cylindrical body with a structure similar to the parent centriole. Growth and lengthening of the procentriole at right angles to the parent produces a mature centriole (*Plate 44, Fig. 2*). According to some observers, basal bodies are also produced in a similar fashion from pre-existing centrioles (Gall, 1961; Mizukami and Gall, 1966; Steinman, 1968; Kalnius and Porter, 1969), but others claim that basal bodies arise also from the granular and filamentous bodies found in the neighbourhood of centrioles and elsewhere in the cell (Dirksen and Crocker, 1966; Sorokin, 1968; Dirksen, 1971) (see also page 518).

* The word 'produces' is used here and later on this page in a broad sense, to cover two suggestions found in the literature: (1) that microtubular proteins are synthesized by the centriole, or (2) that they are assembled or organized by the centriole from pre-existing subunits in the cytoplasm.

Plate 44

Fig. 1. High-resolution photograph obtained by the Markham technique using the centriole image shown in *Plate 43, Fig. 1.* The microtubules A, B and C are clearly visualized, as are the triplet base and dense foot (circle). × 460,000 (*From Stubblefield and Brinkley, 1967*)

Fig. 2. A procentriole (arrow) is seen arising as a short cylindrical structure at right angles to a parent centriole. Numerous centriolar satellites are also present. × 48,000 (*From Stubblefield and Brinkley, 1967*)

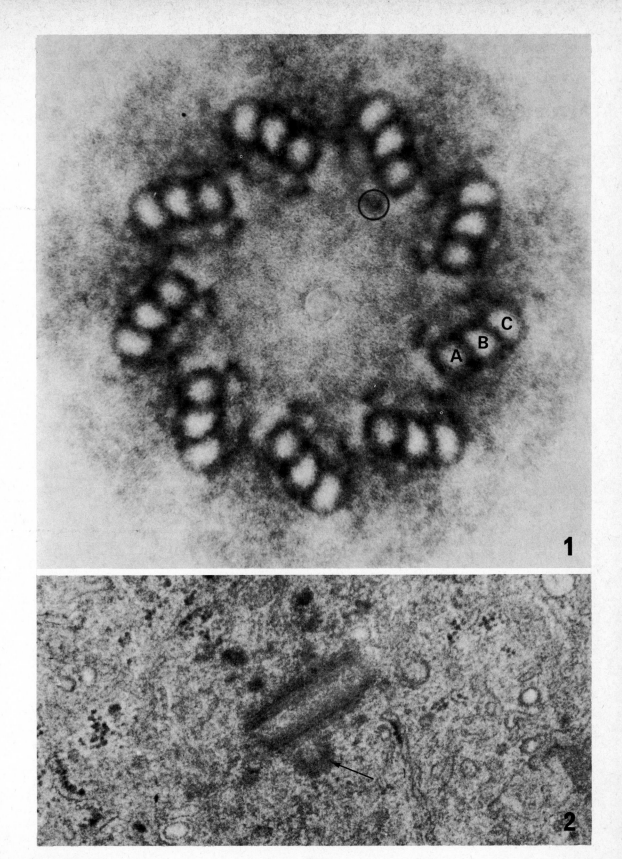

REFERENCES

De Harven, E. and Bernhard, W. (1956). 'Etude au microscope electronique de l'ultrastructure du centriole chez les vertebres.' *Z. Zellforsch. mikrosk. Anat.* **45**, 378

Dirksen, E. R. (1971). 'Centriole morphogenesis in developing ciliated epithelium of the mouse oviduct.' *J. Cell Biol.* **51**, 286

— and Crocker, T. T. (1966). 'Centriole replication in differentiating ciliated cells of mammalian respiratory epithelium. An electron microscope study.' *J. Microscopie* **5**, 629

Fawcett, D. W. (1967). *The Cell: Its Organelles and Inclusions.* Philadelphia and London: Saunders

Forer, A. (1965). 'Local reduction of spindle fiber birefringence in living nephrotoma suturalis (Loew) spermatocytes induced by ultraviolet microbeam irradiation.' *J. Cell Biol.* **25**, 95

Gall, J. G. (1961). 'Centriole replication. A study of spermatogenesis in the snail viviparus.' *J. biophys. biochem. Cytol.* **10**, 163

Gibbons, I. R. and Grimstone, A. V. (1960). 'On flagellar structure in certain flagellates.' *J. biophys. biochem. Cytol.* **7**, 697

Henneguy, L. F. (1897). 'Les rapports des cils vibratiles avec les centrosomes.' *Arch. anat. microscop.* **1**, 481

Kalnins, V. I. and Porter, K. R. (1969). 'Centriole replication during ciliogenesis in the chick tracheal epithelium.' *Z. Zellforsch. mikrosk. Anat.* **100**, 1

Lenhossek, M. von (1898). *Verhandl. dent. Anat. Ges. Jena* **12**, 106

Markham, R., Frey, S. and Hills G. J. (1963). 'Methods for the enhancement of image detail and accentuation of structure in electron microscopy.' *Virology* **20**, 88

Mazia, D. (1961). 'Mitosis and the physiology of cell division.' In *The Cell,* Vol. III, p. 77. Ed. by J. Brachet and A. E. Mirsky. New York: Academic Press

Mizukami, I. and Gall, J. (1966). 'Centriole replication. II. Sperm formation in the fern Marsilea and the cycad Zamia.' *J. Cell Biol.* **29**, 97

Renaud, F. L. and Swift, H. (1964). 'The development of basal bodies and flagella in *Allomyces arbusculus.' J. Cell Biol.* **23**, 339

Sorokin, S. P. (1962). 'Centrioles and the formation of rudimentary cilia by fibroblasts and smooth muscle cells.' *J. Cell Biol.* **15**, 363

— (1968). 'Reconstructions of centriole formation and ciliogenesis in mammalian lungs.' *J. Cell Sci.* **3**, 207

Steinman, R. M. (1968). 'An electron microscopic study of ciliogenesis in developing epidermis and trachea in the embryo of *Xenopus laevis.' Am. J. Anat.* **122**, 19

Stubblefield, E. and Brinkley, B. R. (1967). 'Architecture and function of the mammalian centriole.' In *Formation and Fate of Cell Organelles,* vol. 6, p. 175. Ed. by K. B. Warren. New York and London: Academic Press

Van Beneden, E. (1876). *Bull. acad. roy. med. Belg.* **42**, Ser. II, 35

Wilson, E. B. (1925). *The Cell in Development and Heredity,* 3rd ed. New York: Macmillan

CHAPTER III

Mitochondria

INTRODUCTION

The term 'mitochondrion' was introduced by Benda (1902) to describe certain thread-like or granular components seen in cells. In living cells these organelles are seen to make slow sinuous movements accompanied by changes in size and shape. They also appear to divide and recombine. Mitochondria show many variations in size, shape and fine structure, yet they are sufficiently characteristic to be distinguishable from other cell organelles in electron micrographs. Mitochondria are now known to occur in the cytoplasm of all aerobic eucaryotic cells.

The main morphological features can be summarized by defining a mitochondrion as a double-membrane-bounded body containing matrix, a system of cristae and, frequently, some dense granules (Palade, 1952, 1953; Sjostrand, 1956; Dalton and Felix, 1957; Howatson and Ham, 1957; Rouiller, 1960; Lehninger, 1965). This highly characteristic pattern of organization is found to hold true for the mitochondria of vertebrates, invertebrates, protozoa and plants.

Although the basic morphology of the mitochondrion is so characteristic, innumerable variations on this central theme occur. Such variations can be considered in terms of species differences, tissue or organ differences, physiological and functional activity, and pathological states.

It is now well established that the mitochondrion is the major source of cellular ATP. Since it supplies the cell with most of its usable energy it is considered to be the power-house or power-plant of the cell (Siekevitz, 1957; Lehninger, 1960, 1961, 1965; Racker, 1968). In cell fractions prepared by homogenization of eucaryotic cells, enzymes of the Krebs cycle, oxidative phosphorylation and respiratory chain are found to be largely confined to the mitochondrial fraction while the enzymes of anaerobic glycolysis occur in the unsedimented supernatant (cytoplasmic matrix or hyaloplasm).

Fractionation of disrupted mitochondria has shown that most of the Krebs cycle enzymes are located in the matrix and the electron transport and oxidative phosphorylation enzymes form molecular assemblies in or on the inner mitochondrial membrane covering the wall and cristae (see also page 102). Stalked spheres about 85 Å in diameter, covering the surface of the inner mitochondrial membrane facing the matrix, have been found in negatively stained preparations of ruptured mitochondria. The inner membrane and its spheres are thought to be the site of oxidative phosphorylation. The stalks of the inner membrane spheres are probably a preparation artefact. The idea that each sphere may be a complete 'respiratory assembly' has been abandoned because the spheres are too small to hold all the enzymes responsible for electron transport and associated phosphorylation. They are thought to represent the F_1 coupling factor for oxidative phosphorylation, a protein with a diameter of approximately 80 Å and molecular weight 280,000 (Kagawa *et al.*, 1966; Racker, 1968, 1969; Lehninger, 1970).

MITOCHONDRIAL MORPHOLOGY AND ENZYME CONTENT

To demonstrate the ultrastructural anatomy of the mitochondrion and its component parts I shall here employ a mitochondrion with lamellar or plate-like cristae (*Plate 45*) as this type of mitochondrion is the one most commonly encountered in a majority of the cells of higher animals.

This organelle is bounded by two membranes, an external limiting membrane (about 70 Å thick) and an inner membrane (about 50 Å thick) from which arise the cristae. These membranes enclose two chambers, which are not connected with each other. The outer chamber is the space between the two membranes. The inner or matrix chamber is bounded by the internal membrane, and contains the matrix which is usually more electron dense than the contents of the outer chamber.

The cristae mitochondriales are seen as a system of membranous laminae or plate-like structures lying within the mitochondrion. They arise from the inner membrane and traverse a variable distance across the width of the organelle. The cristae are infoldings of the inner membrane, enclosing a cleft-like space which is continuous with the outer chamber. In favourable sections the membranous layers of the cristae are seen to be continuous with the inner membrane of the mitochondrial envelope.

In ultrathin sections not all the cristae within a mitochondrion are visualized, for some of them are cut obliquely or tangentially. This is particularly so in long, thin mitochondria which are often slightly bent and sometimes quite tortuous. Here an appearance is created as if some parts of the mitochondrion are lacking in cristae. Since sectioning geometry can produce this kind of effect, it is extremely difficult to decide in a given example whether the cristae are truly missing or not in a particular segment of a mitochondrion.

In the mitochondria of most cells the matrix contains some electron-dense granules 300–500 Å in diameter. These are referred to by various terms such as 'dense granules', 'intramitochondrial granules' or 'matricial granules', or 'matrical granules'.

It is now well established that the inner and outer mitochondrial membranes have different permeabilities and chemical compositions. For example, the outer membrane is permeable to sucrose but the inner membrane is not. The evolution of techniques which permit the separation of the outer membrane, inner membrane and matrix have made possible the direct chemical analysis of these components and indicated the locations of various mitochondrial enzymes. The results of these studies have been summarized most lucidly by Lehninger (1970). The localization of some mitochondrial enzymes according to this author is as follows: *Outer membrane*: monoamine oxidase, fatty acid thiokinases, kynurenine hydroxylase, rotenone-insensitive cytochrome *c* reductase. *Space between the membranes*: adenylate kinase, nucleoside diphosphokinase. *Inner membrane*: respiratory chain enzymes, ATP-synthesizing enzymes, α-keto acid dehydrogenases, succinate dehydrogenase, D-β-hydroxybutyrate dehydrogenase, carnitine fatty acyl transferase. *Matrix*: citrate synthase, isocitrate dehydrogenase, fumarase, malate dehydrogenase, aconitase, glutamate dehydrogenase, fatty acid oxidation enzymes.

Plate 45

Mitochondria from kidney tubule of mouse, showing the double-membraned envelope (E), lamellar cristae (C), matrix (M) and dense granules (circle). At the base of a crista (arrow) continuity between the inner membrane of the mitochondrion and the membranes of the crista can be discerned. In some zones (∗) the cristae are presumably tangentially cut and hence not visualized in the electron micrograph. × 54,000

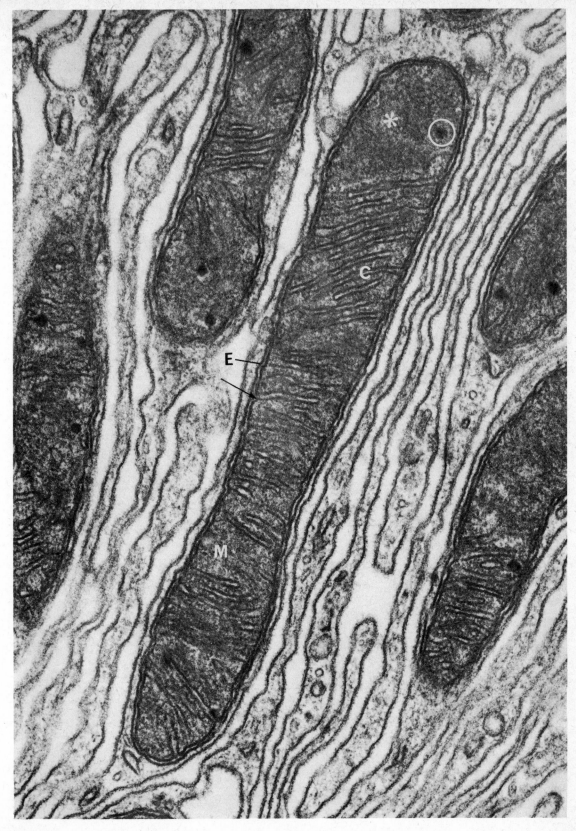

103

Mitochondria show many diverse variations of form and internal structure. Some of the patterns produced are dependent on the type and orientation of the cristae. Examples of such variations are described in later pages, but it is worth noting that there are two main types of cristae—lamellar and tubular—and that many of the other variations could be regarded as stemming from these two basic forms.

As already noted (page 102), lamellar cristae are believed to arise from the inner mitochondrial membrane as thin plate-like or shelf-like infoldings extending a variable distance into the mitochondrial matrix. Continuity between the inner membrane of the mitochondrion and the membranes of the crista is occasionally demonstrable but since such images are rare it has been suggested that the failure to demonstrate such continuity more frequently may be due to the vagaries of sectioning geometry and also because the base of attachment of the cristae to the inner membrane may be quite narrow. Other alternatives have also been debated; namely, that not all cristae are attached to the inner membrane, or that they are detached during tissue preparation.

The length of the cristae and the extent to which they penetrate the mitochondrial matrix is quite variable. For example, in hepatocyte mitochondria many of the cristae barely reach the centre of the mitochondrion. In the mitochondria of muscle tissue and kidney tubules, they penetrate far deeper, often extending across almost the entire width of the organelle and at times are seen to be continuous with the inner mitochondrial membrane on the opposite side. The number of cristae per mitochondrion also varies greatly, and as a rule this is related to the metabolic activity of the tissue (see page 106).

Tubular cristae also show many variations of morphological detail (*Plate 47*). In transverse section they show the circular profile expected of a tubular structure, but in longitudinal sections they may present as (1) short blind-ending tubules (villous cristae), (2) irregular meandering or tortuous tubules, or (3) long tubules extending right across the width of the organelle, sometimes continuous with the inner mitochondrial membrane on the opposite side.

In higher animals, mitochondria with tubular cristae are comparatively rare and occur only in certain sites. However, in certain protozoans and other lower forms, mitochondria with tubular cristae are of common occurrence (*Plate 46, Fig. 1*). In man and in laboratory animals mitochondria containing tubular cristae occur in cells which are involved in cholesterol metabolism and the production of steroids, such as the cells of the adrenal cortex, ovary and interstitial cells of the testis. It is interesting to note that all these cells are also well endowed with smooth endoplasmic reticulum.

In some mitochondria both lamellar and tubular cristae occur. Hepatocyte mitochondria may contain an occasional tubular crista while the adrenal cortex mitochondria may at times contain a few lamellar cristae also.

Plate 46

Fig. 1. A group of mitochondria from Amoeba proteus, showing tubular cristae. × 42,000

Fig. 2. Suprarenal cortex from a case of Cushing's syndrome. Note the mitochondria with tubular cristae and abundant vesicular smooth endoplasmic reticulum. × 35,000

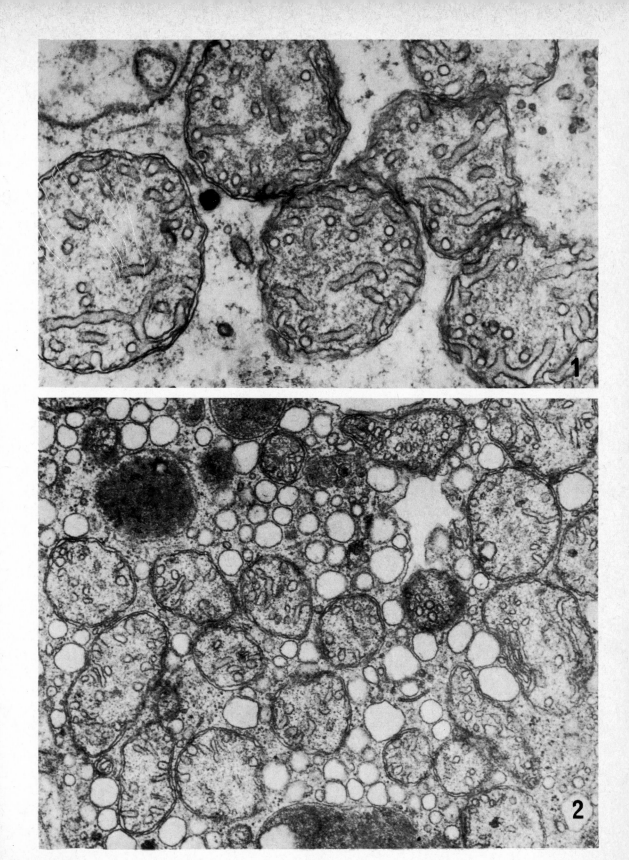

It is widely held that there is a positive correlation between the metabolic activity of a tissue and the number and size of mitochondria and also the number, size, surface area and concentration of cristae. This point may be illustrated by comparing the mitochondria from two extreme examples (*Plate 47*), the high energy transforming (chemical to mechanical) flight muscle of the dragon-fly, and the metabolically depressed liver of a frog collected in the winter.

The general validity of the thesis stated above is attested by many examples. Thus large mitochondria with abundant cristae occur in: (1) brown adipose tissue, where energy is required for the synthesis of lipid prior to storage, and later for the breakdown of lipid to yield heat and raise the body temperature during arousal from hibernation; (2) various epithelia where energy is needed for active transport of ions across membranes (e.g. kidney tubules); and (3) continuously active muscle tissue with a high energy demand, like that of the heart and diaphragm. Comparatively speaking, most examples of skeletal muscle and smooth muscle have fewer mitochondria with less abundant cristae. (For references, more details and further examples, see reviews by Rouiller, 1960; Novikoff, 1961; Lehninger, 1965.)

In the myocardium of birds, Slautterback (1965) has noted a relationship between heart rate and mitochondrial size and complexity of cristae structure. Similarly cardiac, uterine or skeletal muscle hypertrophy is accompanied or preceded by an increase in mitochondrial mass and also an increase in the concentration of cristae (see page 146).

Exceptions or apparent exceptions to the thesis stated above have also been recorded. Leeson and Leeson (1969) found complex mitochondrial forms with abundant cristae in rat palatine muscle, and they note that 'mitochondrial concentrations in muscle fibers of the palate are much more extensive than those in the diaphragmatic (red) fibers'. The reason for this is not clear, for one would not expect palatine muscle to be more demanding in energy requirement than the diaphragm. However, as these authors suggest, it is conceivable that palatine muscle may possess hitherto unknown, peculiar or unusual physiological properties. In malignant tumours, the mitochondria are pleomorphic and examples of mitochondria with sparse or numerous cristae may be found in the same tumour and even in an individual tumour cell. The mitochondrial population is also quite variable but often the mitochondria appear to be too few and the cristae too sparse to support the obviously heightened metabolic activity and rapid growth rate. The historical work of Warberg (1956, 1962) showed the predominance of glycolysis over respiration in the energy metabolism of many tumours, and this may well explain the apparent paradox of this fast-growing tissue which as a rule is not particularly well endowed with mitochondria.

Plate 47

Fig. 1. Liver of a winter-starved frog, showing abundant glycogen deposits (G) and mitochondria (M) with sparse cristae. × 28,000

Fig. 2. Dragon-fly flight muscle, showing voluminous mitochondria (M) with abundant complex cristae. Note also the close association between the smooth endoplasmic reticulum (arrow) and the mitochondria (page 130). × 34,000

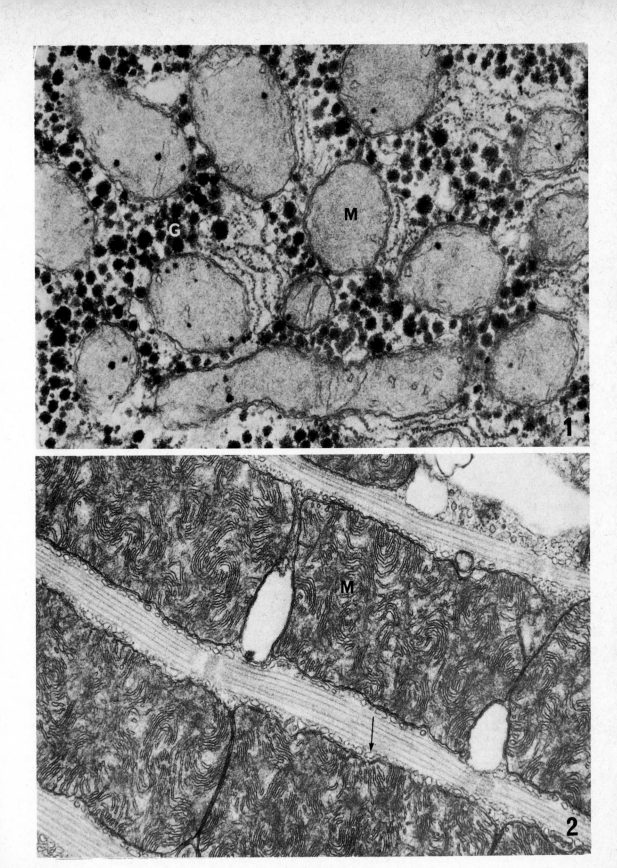

Mitochondria containing cristae which in ultrathin sections present as crescentric, annular, spiral or concentric formations have been noted to occur in certain normal and pathological tissues (*Plate 48*). Examples of both lamellar and tubular cristae showing this kind of orientation have been observed.

In ultrathin sections, mitochondria with concentric cristae are often found in company with mitochondria with stacked parallel cristae, and it is thought that in such instances the stacked cristae appearance may represent a longitudinal section through cristae which on transverse section would appear concentric (Leeson and Leeson, 1969; Hug and Schubert, 1970).

Mitochondria with concentric cristae have been reported to occur in: (1) axons of lobsters (Geren and Schmitt, 1954); (2) spermatids of snails (Beams and Tahmisian, 1954; Grasse *et al.*, 1956); (3) normal mammalian myocardium (on rare occasions) (Moore and Ruska, 1957; Stenger and Spiro, 1961); (4) hearts of birds such as the quail (quite frequently) (Slautterback, 1965); (5) soft palate of the normal rat (Leeson and Leeson, 1969); (6) a case of idiopathic cardiomyopathy (Hug and Schubert, 1970; this was associated with an increased mycocardial glycogen phosphorylase activity, suggesting hypermetabolism); (7) a case of severe hypermetabolism of non-thyroid origin (Luft *et al.*, 1962); (8) cases of myopathy (Hulsmann *et al.*, 1967; D'Agostino *et al.*, 1968); (9) rhabdomyosarcoma (Polack *et al.*, 1971); and (10) Warthin's tumour (adeno-lymphoma of salivary gland) (Tandler and Shipkey, 1964).

Mitochondria with crescentic or concentrically arranged tubular cristae have been seen in the ovarian theca lutein cells of mouse (Rhodin, 1963) and in the rat adrenals after spironolactone administration (Fisher and Horvat, 1971). This transformation of adrenal mitochondrial morphology was regarded as an expression of increased or altered aldosterone production or secretion or both. Mitochondria with a few annular or concentric cristae may also be found in the adrenal cortex of the cow (see *Plates 74 and 77*).

An analysis of the above-mentioned examples indicates that mitochondria with concentric cristae occur in tissues with a naturally high metabolic activity or when metabolic activity is increased in disease or by experimental procedures. It is debatable, however, whether such mitochondria are in fact metabolically more active than others, or represent a sequence of change in the life-span of the mitochondrion, heralding degenerative changes leading ultimately to lysosomal degradation and myelin figure formation. The latter idea finds some support at least in the case of some pathologically altered tissues. For example, such a sequence is suggested by Hug and Schubert's (1970) observations in the mitochrondria in cardiomyopathy and by the illustrations of mitochondria in rat adrenals after spironolactone administration (Fisher and Horvat, 1971). Furthermore, there is evidence that mitochondria in adenolymphoma (Tandler and Shipkey, 1964) may be biochemically defective, and in the patient studied by Luft *et al.* (1962) there was uncoupling of oxidative phosphorylation. In any case the two ideas are not mutually exclusive or incompatible, for it is conceivable that at some stage these mitochondria may be metabolically quite active, and later suffer degenerative changes.

Plate 48

Normal rat myocardium, showing mitochondria with concentric cristae. ×41,000

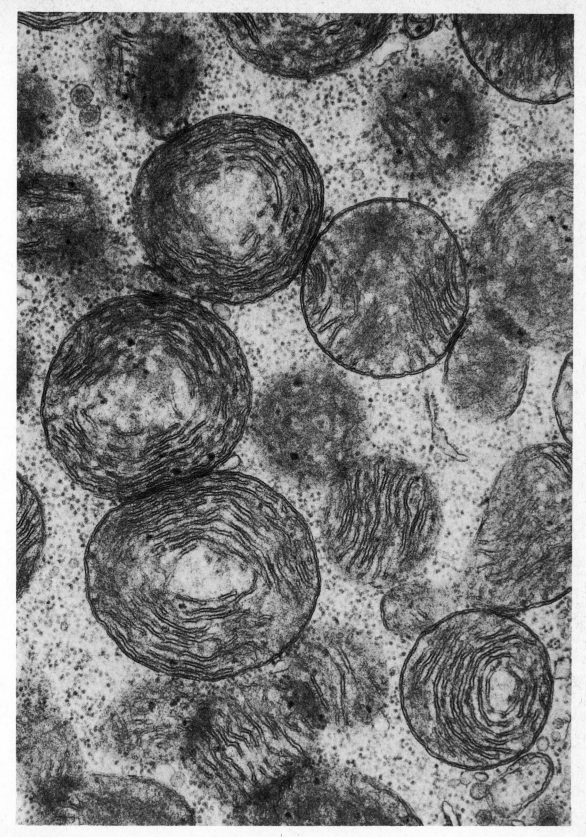

The term 'zig-zag' is applied to cristae which exhibit sharp angulations of their membranes, and pursue a zig-zag rather than the usual, more or less straight, course across the mitochondrion (*Plate 49*). Mitochondria with zig-zag cristae show many different patterns, depending upon the plane of sectioning and on whether the zig-zag courses of neighbouring cristae are in register or out of register. In the former instance they are easily recognized as zig-zag cristae, but in the latter instance when angulations of adjacent cristae make contact and probably fuse, a complex honeycombed pattern enclosing irregular or cylindrical compartments of matrix is produced (for illustrations depicting this phenomenon, see Fawcett, 1967). Frequently all the cristae in a mitochondrion show a zig-zag conformation, but at times only a few are so affected, the rest following a straight course.

Mitochondria with zig-zag or angulated cristae have been noted in various cells, such as: (1) giant amoeba, *Pelomyxa carolinensis, wilson,* (*Chaos chaos* L.) (Pappas and Brandt, 1959); (2) chloride cells from the gills of *Fundulus heteroclitus* and glandular cells from gastric mucosa of the frog (Revel *et al.*, 1963; Fawcett, 1967); (3) myocardium of the canary, and occasionally of sparrow hearts, but rarely in hearts of the zebra-finch, quail or goose (Slautterback, 1965); (4) ventricle and atrium of cats (Fawcett and McNutt. 1969; McNutt and Fawcett, 1969); (5) myocardium of epinephrine-treated rats and, on rare occasions, normal animals (Ferrans *et al.*, 1970); (6) dog heart preserved for 18 hours with plasma–dextran perfusate (Ferrans *et al.*, 1971); (7) hypertrophied human myocardium (*Plate 49*); (8) skeletal muscle from a man with severe hypermetabolism of non-thyroid origin (Luft *et al.*, 1962; Ernster and Luft, 1963); (9) skeletal muscle of rats treated with thyroxine (Gustafsson *et al.*, 1965); and (10) palatine muscle of the rat (Leeson and Leeson, 1969).

Mitochondria with zig-zag cristae have mostly been observed in metabolically active tissues. Since this type of configuration obviously results in an increase in membrane surface per unit volume of mitochondrion, it has been suggested (Pappas and Brandt, 1959) that this is a more efficient mitochondrion better suited to meet high metabolic needs.

Plate 49

Mitochondrion with zig-zag cristae. From a biopsy of hypertrophied human myocardium obtained during open-heart surgery. ×90,000

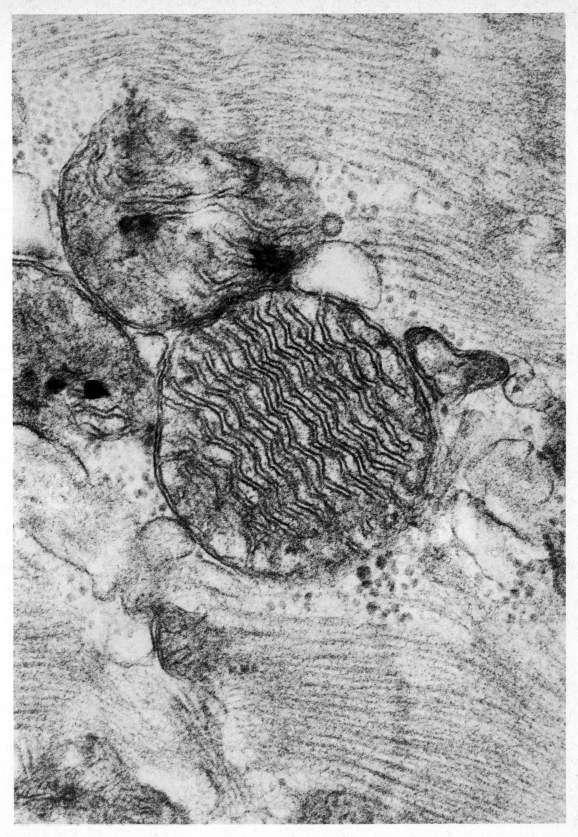

Mitochondria with fenestrated cristae seem to be of rare occurrence. Frequently such cristae occur in close-packed parallel arrays, and when sectioned transversely numerous discontinuities (fenestrations) may be noted along the course of such cristae (*Plate 50*). It is, however, in sections parallel to the surface of the cristae that the circular or nearly circular fenestrae are readily identified. This is particularly so when the fenestrae in adjacent cristae are in register, for in such instances clear matrix-filled channels traversing the mitochondrion at right angles to the cristae are formed.

The finest example of mitochondria with fenestrated cristae so far recorded (Smith, 1963) is that found in the flight muscle of the blowfly (*Calliphora erythrocephala*). Here the fenestrae are in perfect register and are evenly spaced over the cristae. Mitochondria with fenestrated cristae have also been seen: (1) in the myocardium of the shrew (Slautterback, 1961); (2) in birds such as canaries and sparrows (Slautterback, 1965); and (3) in the palatine muscle of the rat (Leeson and Leeson, 1969). In these instances, however, accurate juxtaposition of fenestrae in adjacent cristae is not evident as in the case of the blowfly.

Mitochondria with fenestrated cristae occur in metabolically active tissues and one may suggest that, in these mitochondria packed with cristae, continuity of the matrix chamber and short diffusion paths are achieved by the fenestrae in the cristae.

Plate 50

Mitochondria with fenestrated cristae from the myocardium of a canary.

Fig. 1. In two of the mitochondria where the cristae are sectioned transversely the fenestrae are seen as interruptions along the course of the cristae (arrow). Note that the fenestrae in adjacent cristae are out of register in most instances. × 42,000

Fig. 2. The section has passed parallel to the surface of the cristae in most of the mitochondria shown in this illustration. Mitochondrial matrix and dense granules are clearly seen lying within the fenestrae (circle) of the cristae. × 41,000

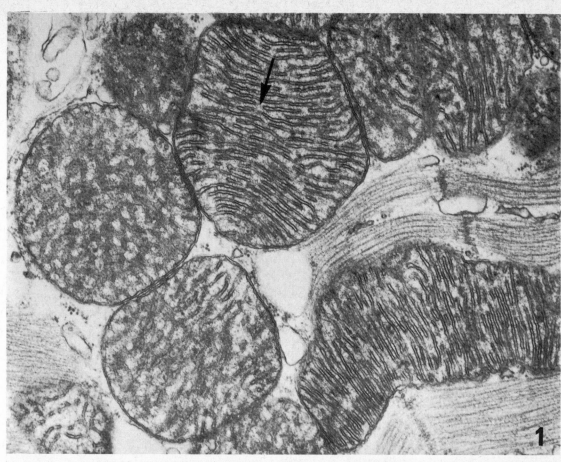

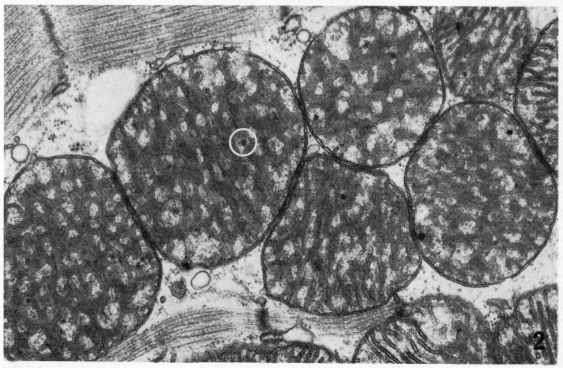

E

Mitochondrial cristae usually pursue a transverse course, lying at right angles to the long axis of the mitochondrion, but in this interesting variation of mitochondrial inner structure, longitudinally orientated cristae lie parallel to the long axis of the mitochondrion (*Plate 51*). This transformation may be complete or incomplete. In the latter instance one or both poles of the mitochondrion contain transversely orientated cristae while in the remainder of the organelle the cristae are arranged longitudinally.

Some interesting correlations between this morphological transformation and altered mitochondrial enzyme content have been recorded. For example: (1) the cytochrome oxidase activity of the proximal kidney tubules of frogs (*Rana pipiens*) collected in the winter is greatly reduced as compared to freshly caught summer frogs, and in these animals (winter frogs) many of the mitochondria in this region (*Plate 51, Fig. 1*) show partial or complete transformation of the cristae to a longitudinal orientation (Karnovsky, 1962, 1963); (2) Luft *et al.* (1962) have reported a case of non-thyroid hypermetabolism where a partial uncoupling of oxidative phosphorylation was associated with complex alterations of mitochondrial morphology (some of the cristae could be regarded as longitudinally orientated); and (3) in rats exposed to high concentrations of oxygen, mitochondria with longitudinally orientated cristae develop in the great alveolar cells of the lung (Rosenbaum *et al.*, 1969) and it is known from biochemical studies that high oxygen concentrations can act as an inhibitor of several kinds of enzymatic activity, including such exclusively mitochondrial enzymes as succinic dehydrogenase and cytochrome oxidase.

Plate 51

Fig. 1. Mitochondria with longitudinally orientated cristae from a kidney tubule of a winter-starved frog. ×56,000

Fig. 2. Acute leukaemic cell of man. Three mitochondria with longitudinally arranged cristae are seen. One shows complete transformation (C), the other two partial transformation (P). ×45,000 (*Ghadially and Skinnider, unpublished electron micrograph*)

Fig. 3. Acute leukaemic cell of man, showing partially transformed mitochondria, one of which is C-shaped. ×41,000 (*Ghadially and Skinnider, unpublished electron micrograph*)

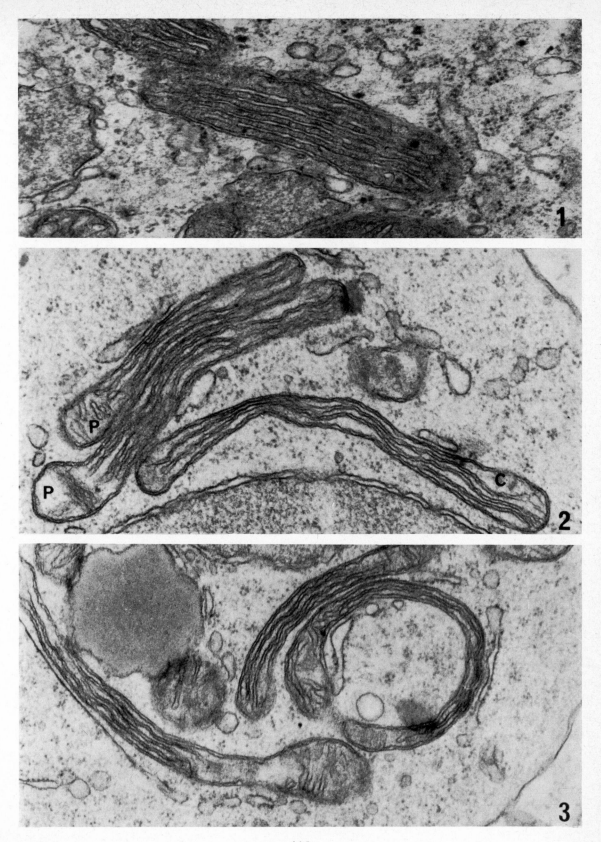

115

However, as Karnovsky has already pointed out, low cytochrome oxidase activity is not invariably associated with horizontally orientated cristae. Thus 'petite mutants' of yeast lack cytochrome oxidase (Ephrussi, 1953) but have unchanged mitochondria with transverse cristae (Yotsuyanagi, 1959), and in the urodele, *Necturus maculosus*, the proximal tubular cells lack cytochrome oxidase but have mitochondria with sparse transverse cristae (Himmelhoch and Karnovsky, 1961). There is a lack of both mitochondria and cytochrome oxidase activity in yeast (*Torulopsis utilis*) grown anaerobically (Linnane *et al.*, 1962).

Besides the examples mentioned earlier, mitochondria with longitudinally orientated cristae have been seen in: (1) the liver of thyrotoxic rats (Greenawalt *et al.*, 1962) and the liver of rats poisoned by ammonium carbonate (David and Kettler, 1961) or copper (Barka *et al.*, 1964); (2) the adrenal cortex (Lever, 1956; De Robertis and Sabatini, 1958; Zelander, 1959); (3) rat skeletal muscle after thyroid hormone treatment (Gustafsson *et al.*, 1965); (4) reactive and regenerating axons in the spinal cord and medulla of rats (Lampert, 1967); (5) renal cell carcinoma (Seljelid and Ericsson, 1965); (6) human ovarian carcinoma (Ghadially, unpublished observation); and (7) acute leukaemic cells in peripheral blood of man (*Plate 51, Figs. 2 and 3*).

In the leukaemic cells studied by us (Ghadially and Skinnider, unpublished observations) and also in some of the examples mentioned above, mitochondria with longitudinally orientated cristae, showed C-shaped or ring-shaped configuration in ultrathin sections. It has been suggested that the ring form may be produced either by the approximation and fusion of the tips of a C-shaped mitochondrion, or that C-shaped and ring-shaped mitochondria represent sections through cup-shaped mitochondria. (For further comments on ring-shaped mitochondria, see pages 158–160.) Transitions from 'ring' forms to electron-dense membranous whorls have also been noted by us and others (*Plate 52, Figs. 2 and 3*). It is worth noting that the ring-shaped mitochondrial form is not invariably associated with longitudinally orientated cristae, and that ring-shaped mitochondria with transversely orientated cristae are probably of more common occurrence (*Plates 73 and 74*).

Plate 52

From acute leukaemic cells of man. (*Ghadially and Skinnider, unpublished electron micrographs*)
Fig. 1. Ring-shaped mitochondrion with partial transformation of cristae. × 74,000
Fig. 2 and 3. Early stages of membranous whorl formation from ring mitochondria where structural details (e.g. paired membranes of cristae) of the partially altered mitochondria can still be discerned. × 58,000; × 66,000

116

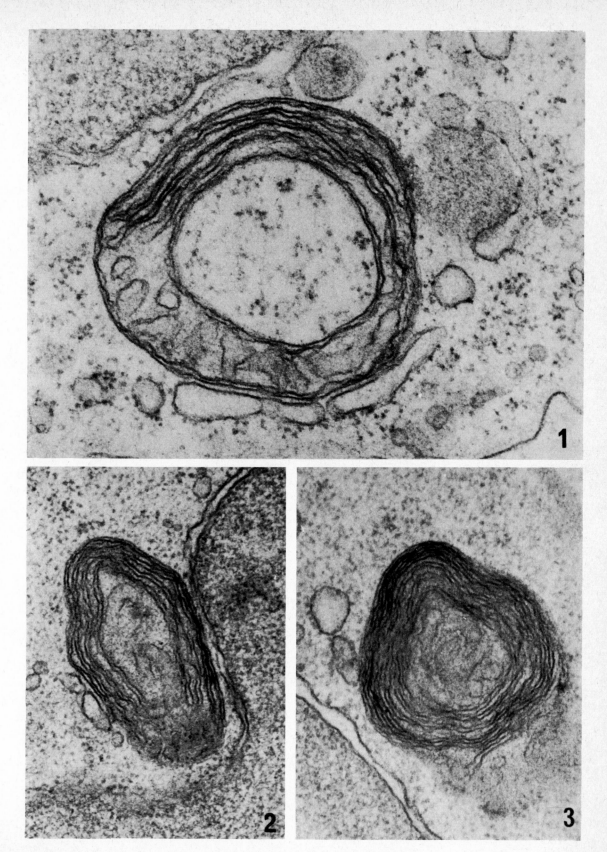

MITOCHONDROGENESIS

Theories regarding the genesis of mitochondria may be divided into three not mutually exclusive groups: (1) *de novo* synthesis; (2) origin from non-mitochondrial structures such as nuclear envelope (Hoffman and Grigg, 1958; Brandt and Pappas, 1959), intracytoplasmic vacuoles or membranes (Linnane *et al.*, 1962; Berger, 1964; Threadgold and Lasker, 1967), cell membrane (Geren and Schmitt, 1954; De Robertis and Bleichmar, 1962), pinocytotic vesicles (Gey, 1956), and microbodies (Rouiller and Bernhard, 1956; Engfeldt *et al.*, 1958); (3) origin from pre-existing mitochondria with or without the prior formation of a partition (Fawcett, 1955; Campiche, 1960; Andre, 1962; Laguens and Bianchi, 1963; Svoboda and Higginson, 1963; Lafontaine and Allard, 1964; Arhelger *et al.*, 1965; Hübner, 1965; Schaffner and Felig, 1965; Glinsmann and Ericsson, 1966; Coupland and MacDougall, 1968; Flaks, 1968; Tandler *et al.*, 1969, 1970; Rifkin and Gahagan-Chase, 1970; Rohr *et al.*, 1970, 1971).

The term '*de novo* synthesis' was used in earlier times to indicate a non-mitochondrial origin of mitochondria from structures not resolvable by light microscopy. Since the disclosure of numerous organelles by the electron microscope, this term is now restricted to mean origin from the cytoplasmic matrix. There is, however, little evidence that this in fact happens. Similarly, most of the claims regarding the origin of mitochondria from other organelles are also singularly tenuous. (See reviews by Novikoff, 1961 and Lehninger, 1965.) For instance, the once-popular theory regarding the origin of mitochondria from microbodies (and vice versa) has lost favour as these structures have come to be recognized as organelles in their own right.

However, the idea that mitochondria may arise from some membrane systems, particularly the cell membrane, is at least theoretically admissible (Lehninger, 1965). Although unequivocal proof of origin of mitochondria from various cytomembranes is still lacking, some very persuasive electron micrographs depicting the possible sequence of events leading to the production of mitochondria in this fashion have been published. For instance, from the morphological standpoint, there are quite convincing reports of origin of mitochondria from (1) the axolemma of the nerve fibres of the infrared receptors in pit vipers (*Crotalus duvissus*) (De Robertis and Bleichmar, 1962), (2) reticular membranes of yeast (*Torulopsis utilis*) grown anaerobically and subsequently aerated (Linnane *et al.*, 1962), and (3) cytoplasmic vacuoles in certain cells in the skin of the larval sardine (*Sardinops carulae*) (Threadgold and Lasker, 1967) (*Plate 353*).

Plate 53

From the integumentary cells of the larval sardine. A possible mode of mitochondrogenesis from cytoplasmic vacuoles is depicted in these electron micrographs. (*Figs. 1–3, From Threadgold and Lasker, 1967; Fig. 4, Threadgold and Lasker, unpublished electron micrograph*)

Fig. 1. This electron micrograph shows a large vacuole into which has invaginated a short cytoplasmic process (arrow) containing some vesicles or tubules. × 30,000

Fig. 2. A further stage of evolution is depicted here. The invaginating cytoplasmic process (P) is now quite large, but still probably continuous with surrounding cytoplasm (arrow). The presumptive parts of the future mitochondrion can now be envisaged as follows: matrix chamber (M), outer chamber or intermembranous space (S) and cristae (C). × 36,000

Fig. 3. The invaginating process has almost completely filled the vacuole and nearly formed a normal mitochondrion. Only in one zone the intermembranous space (S) is still quite large. × 32,000

Fig. 4. A transversely cut normal mitochondrion (A) is seen here, as also is part of another (B) which is in a formative stage similar to that in *Fig. 2*. × 48,000

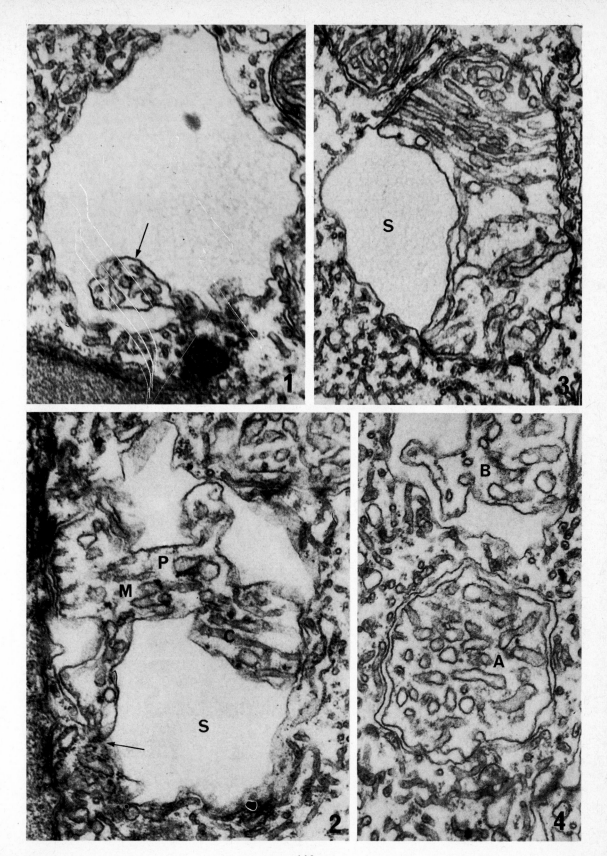

The view that mitochondria arise by a process of division from pre-existing mitochondria is well substantiated by light microscopic studies of living and fixed cells (for references, see De Robertis and Bleichmar, 1962) and by recent studies which show that mitochondria are capable of synthesizing protein and lipoprotein and that they contain DNA and RNA (for references, see Nass and Nass, 1963; Nass and Afzelius, 1965; Leduc *et al.*, 1966; Anderson, 1969; Bergeron and Droz, 1969). In ultrathin sections, mitochondrial profiles with deep indentations or constrictions suggesting fission or budding are sometimes seen (*Plate 54*), but this could be the result of sectioning through an irregular or Y-shaped organelle. Even when a narrow connecting piece is demonstrated by serial sectioning, one cannot be certain whether one is witnessing fusion or fission.

There is, however, one image which can confidently be interpreted as a dividing mitochondrion, and this process may be called partition and division (*Plate 54*, *Fig. 1 and 2*; see also *Plate 76*, *Fig. 3, and Plate 77, Fig. 6*). This observation, first made by Fawcett (1955), has now been confirmed by many studies. It would appear that in this process a partition forms from the inner mitochondrial membrane which divides the matrix chamber into two distinct compartments. A process of pinching off at the level of the partition then separates the two daughter mitochondria. Here again one may contend that this could be either fusion or fission, for a series of static pictures cannot on their own indicate the direction in which a process is moving. However, such arguments are silenced by the fact that partitioned mitochondria are seen in situations where we know an increase in mitochondrial population is occurring. For example, Tandler *et al.* (1968, 1969) have shown that in riboflavin-deficient mice the mitochondria are greatly enlarged but reduced in numbers. If riboflavin is administered to such mice the normal mitochondrial size and number are restored, and during this stage many partitioned mitochondria are seen. Similarly, morphometric analysis of perinatal rat livers has shown (Rohr *et al.*, 1971) that the newly formed post-mitotic hepatocyte has only half the normal number of mitochondria. This is followed by a stage of mitochondrial enlargement (volume doubled) and, later, partition and division so that the hepatocyte eventually contains a mitochondrial population of normal size and number. We (Ghadially, Parry and Bhatnager, unpublished observations) have observed partitioned mitochondria quite frequently in the regenerating post-hepatectomy liver of the rat but they are rarely seen in normal rat liver. Thus it would appear that one of the ways in which a mitochondrion divides is by first laying down a partition.

Finally, it is worth stressing that the three basic theories of mitochondrogenesis are not mutually exclusive, and just because there is now ample evidence that mitochondria do arise from other mitochondria it does not necessarily follow that this is the only way in which mitochondria are born.

Plate 54

Figs. 1 and 2. Partitioned mitochondria found in regenerating rat liver. × 50,000; × 43,000

Figs. 3–6. These electron micrographs show various mitochondrial profiles suggesting impending division, but such appearances could be due to sections through irregularly shaped mitochondria. From rat liver (*Figs. 3–5*) and human bone marrow (*Fig. 6*). × 43,000; × 50,000; × 42,000; × 45,000

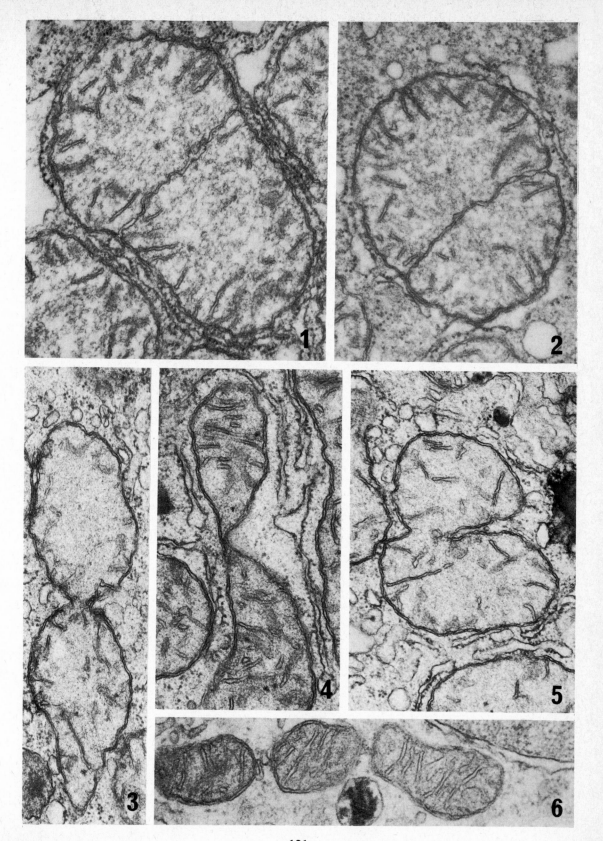

121

It would appear that old effete or damaged organelles can suffer regressive changes and be removed in various ways in the cell. Images which may be interpreted as mitochondrial involution or dissolution are occasionally encountered in normal tissues, but many more are seen in pathological situations. The greater frequency of such changes in pathological states may be looked upon as an activation of normal mechanisms geared to the removal of organelles damaged by noxious influences. The various ways in which it is alleged that mitochondria are got rid of by the cell include: (1) mitochondrial pyknosis; (2) mitochondrial swelling (balloon degeneration); (3) cytolysosome formation; and (4) intracisternal sequestration.

Mitochondrial swelling which is part and parcel of cloudy swelling is a widely recognized and much studied phenomenon (see page 140). The converse change, mitochondrial pyknosis, is not too well recognized and only occasionally mentioned in the literature. Here a striking increase in the density of the matrix and a reduction of mitochondrial size occurs (*Plate 155*). The term 'mitochondrial pyknosis', which so succinctly describes this change was first employed by Wachestein and Besen (1964). These authors demonstrated mitochondrial pyknosis in coagulative necrosis produced in renal tissue with DL-serine. Both mitochondrial swelling and mitochondrial pyknosis were witnessed in adjacent cells and the contrast between these is beautifully illustrated in their paper.

Similar changes which can be interpreted as mitochondrial pyknosis have been observed: (1) in the liver of rats after (*a*) starvation (Rouiller, 1957), (*b*) carcinogenic diets (Rouiller and Simon, 1962), (*c*) necrogenic diets (Svoboda and Higginson, 1963); and (2) in human liver from cases of viral hepatitis (Pavel *et al.*, 1971); pyknotic mitochondria have also been seen in tumours such as (3) hepatomas (Gansler and Rouiller, 1956), (4) experimentally induced renal tumours in hamsters (Mannweiler and Bernhard, 1957), and (5) human ovarian adenocarcinoma (*Plate 55*).

Pyknotic mitochondrial forms bear some resemblance to microbodies and indeed it has been suggested (e.g. Pavel *et al.*, 1971) that such dense mitochondria may represent an intermediate step leading to the formation of microbodies. In view of what is now known about microbodies, this does not seem a likely possibility.

Plate 55

Fig. 1. A cell from human adenocarcinoma of the ovary showing mitochondrial pyknosis. In some instances where the matrix is not too dense, disorientated and fused cristae are discernible. × 7,000

Fig. 2. High power view of two mitochondria from *Fig. 1*, showing altered cristae and a dense matrix containing some intramatricial granules. × 13,500

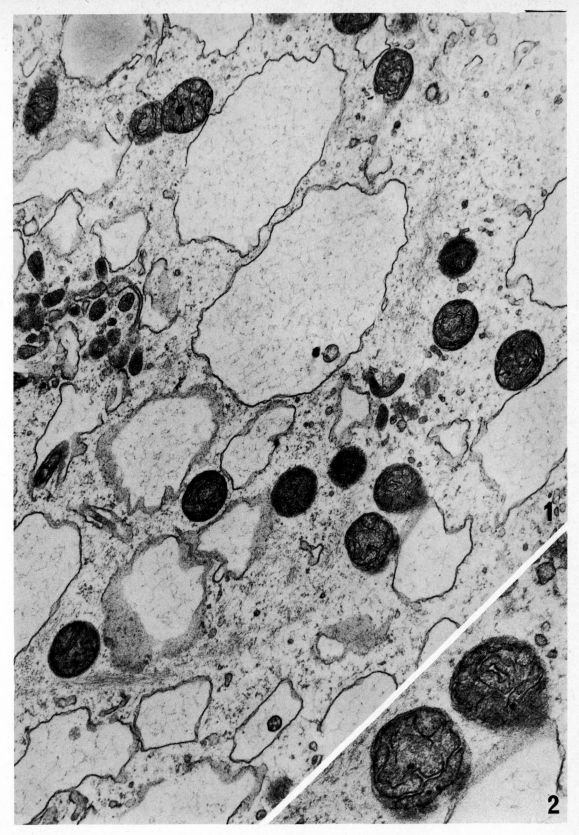

Mitochondrial swelling has at times been regarded as another possible fate that might befall effete mitochondria (Gansler and Rouiller, 1956; Rouiller, 1960). This must be distinguished from the well known variety of mitochondrial swelling which affects virtually every mitochondrion in the cell and is the equivalent of the cloudy swelling and post-mortem change known to light microscopists (see page 140). This is not relevant here. What I wish to demonstrate (*Plate 56, Fig. 1*) is that one may occasionally find one or two grossly swollen mitochondria in company with other perfectly normal-looking mitochondria in a variety of experimental and other situations. Here there is clearly no general derangement of osmotic forces within the cell. The primary defect obviously lies in the swollen mitochondrion itself, and this could well be regarded as an effete or damaged organelle about to suffer dissolution.

The transformation or incorporation of mitochondria into cytolysosomes is perhaps the most common method by which these organelles are eliminated. Such methods of mitochondrial elimination include: (1) development of dense osmiophilic laminated or whorled membranes in mitochondria and conversion of such organelles into lysosomal bodies containing myelin figures; (2) incorporation of mitochondria into pre-existing lysosomes; and (3) sequestration of mitochondria with or without other organelles to form cytolysosomes (*Plate 56, Figs. 2–5*).

Yet another ingenious method of involution is suggested by Pavel *et al.* (1971), which they describe as 'dissolution of mitochondria into the distended cisternae or vesicles of granular or agranular endoplasmic reticulum'. According to this concept the mitochondrion either fuses with the wall of a rough endoplasmic reticulum cistern and discharges its contents, or herniates and falls into it and suffers subsequent dissolution.

This concept is reminiscent of the concept of intracisternal sequestration evoked by Blackburn and Vinijchaikul (1969) to explain the involution of the rough endoplasmic reticulum. Here it is postulated that invaginations of the rough endoplasmic reticulum into the cisternae occur, and portions of the papillary processes thus formed are detached and suffer dissolution (see page 256). One could also look upon intracisternal sequestration as one of the ways in which an autophagic vacuole or cytolysosome commences (see page 300).

Plate 56

Fig. 1. A solitary grossly swollen mitochondrion (M) with lucent matrix and disorganized cristae is seen among numerous normal-looking mitochondria. From the liver of a rat that had been treated with Atromid S. (See also *Plate 66, Fig. 2*, which shows a similar phenomenon in anoxic dog myocardium.) × 33,000

Fig. 2. Whorled membranous bodies (B), probably derived from involuting mitochondria. From monkey kidney cells in tissue culture. × 28,000

Fig. 3. A cytolysosome containing two mitochondria. From the same specimen as *Fig. 1.* × 40,000

Fig. 4. A cytolysosome containing disintegrating mitochondrial remnants and other structures. From the liver of a tumour-bearing rat. × 40,000. (*Ghadially and Parry, unpublished electron micrograph*)

Fig. 5. Cytolysosome containing mitochondrial remnants. From the kidney of a rat poisoned with lead acetate. × 42,000

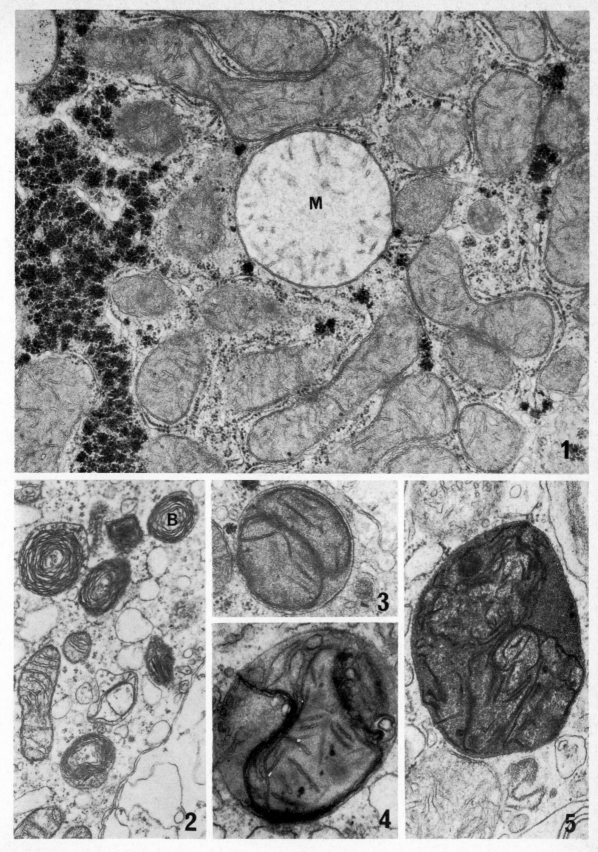

Although in most cells mitochondria appear to be randomly scattered in the cytoplasm, there are many instances where a close association occurs between mitochondria and other organelles and inclusions. Such associations seem to be quite meaningful and provide satisfying examples of correlation between structure and function. Various observations indicate that mitochondria are often located near a supply of substrate, or at sites in the cell known to require the ATP generated by the mitochondrion (Lehninger, 1965).

One of the frequently observed associations is between mitochondria and lipid droplets. Occasional examples of this may be found in a variety of tissues, but this association is of common occurrence in the myocardium, liver, pancreas and brown adipose tissue. A variety of appearances is seen. A single mitochondrion may appear close to, spread out over, or fused to the surface of a small lipid droplet, or numerous mitochondria may be seen surrounding a larger lipid droplet. In other instances the lipid droplet may lie in a deep invagination of the mitochondrial envelope and it is clear that in another plane of sectioning such a droplet could easily be mistaken for a lipid inclusion in the mitochondrion (*Plate 57*, *Figs. 1 and 2*), particularly if the invaginating membranes are not visualized (see below).

Often, when such close contact has occurred, it is impossible to resolve the mitochondrial membranes adjacent to the lipid droplet. Such an appearance could be explained on the basis of oblique sectioning through this area, and it has been debated whether a true continuity between the lipid and the mitochondrial matrix ever occurs (see the discussion in Napolitano and Fawcett, 1958, and in Novikoff, 1961). Some workers have adopted an intermediate view that only the outer membrane of the mitochondrion suffers dissolution but the inner membrane remains intact.

Since mitochondria are known to contain many of the enzymes (see also page 102) necessary for the metabolism of triglycerides (fatty acid oxidases), it has been suggested (Palade and Schidlowsky, 1958; Palade, 1959) that this is a meaningful juxtaposition which brings the mitochondrial enzymes into close association with the lipidic substrate. Close association between mitochondria and lipid is much more frequent and obvious in the liver and pancreas of fasted, rather than fully fed animals. This is in keeping with the idea that in the fasted animal the cells, having depleted much of the glycogen reserves, have shifted to the utilization of lipid to a greater extent than before for their metabolic needs.

However, when mitochondria have been seen in close association with lipid droplets in situations where lipid is accumulating as in brown adipose tissue, it has been suggested that the

---

Plate 57

Fig. 1. Rat hepatocyte mitochondria, showing close association with a lipid droplet (L). × 21,000

Fig. 2. A human myocardial mitochondrion, showing a deep invagination occupied by a lipid droplet (L). × 51,000

Fig. 3. Liver of day-old rat, showing close association of mitochondria with loops of rough endoplasmic reticulum. × 32,000

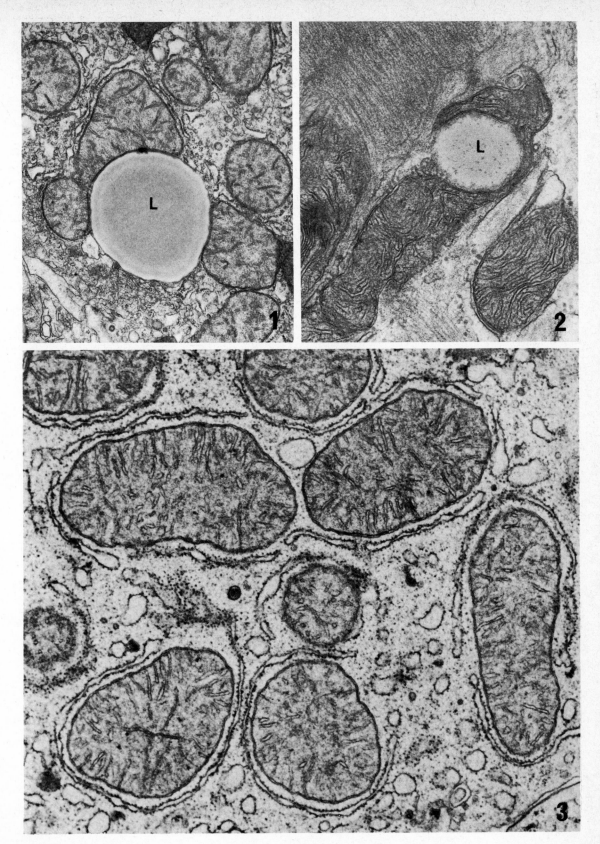

127

organelle may be involved in active synthesis of lipid (Napolitano and Fawcett, 1958). Apparently, most, but perhaps not all, of the enzymes necessary for this are present in the mitochondrion (see page 102). For instance, beef heart mitochondria and also mitochondria from some other sites are capable of quite rapid long-chain fatty acid synthesis (Hulsmann, 1962).

Another example of close association is that seen between the rough endoplasmic reticulum and the mitochondrion. The common pattern seen in such instances consists of curved profiles of rough endoplasmic reticulum, partially or almost completely encircling mitochondria but with a narrow zone of cytoplasm persisting between them (*Plate 57, Fig. 3*). Instances of continuity or apparent continuity have, however, been reported to occur between the mitochondrial membranes and the rough endoplasmic reticulum in the irradiated Rhesus hepatocyte (Ghidoni and Thomas, 1969) and between the mitochondrion and sarcoplasmic reticulum in skeletal and cardiac myocytes (Walker *et al.*, 1965; Walker and Schrodt, 1966; Bowman, 1967).

Even if the vagaries of sectioning geometry are accounted for and one concedes that true contact or continuity has in fact been demonstrated beyond reasonable doubt, one still wonders whether such rare examples of contact are fortuitous or artefactual rather than meaningful. On the other hand, one cannot exclude the possibility that the rarity of such images may indicate a transient but meaningful episode, which does occur in the living cell.

Profiles of rough endoplasmic reticulum wrapping around mitochondria are not so rare, however, particularly in cells engaged in active protein synthesis (e.g. the pancreas), and here is one of many examples where juxtaposition of this organelle to a site of energy utilization occurs. Bernhard and Rouiller (1956) reported that in fasted rats the rough endoplasmic reticulum regresses, but some is still seen around mitochondria. On re-feeding, the reticulum is re-formed

Plate 58

An oblique section through a portion of the distal tubule of mouse kidney. Note the close association of mitochondria with the highly folded basal part of the plasma membrane of the tubular epithelial cells. Basement membrane lining the circumference of the tubule is indicated by arrows. × 21,000

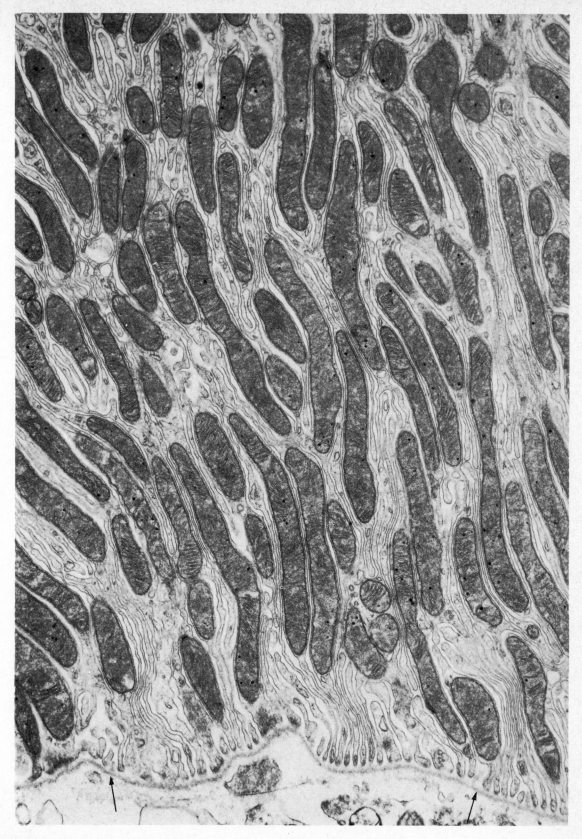

and, according to these authors, the mitochondria provide energy for its regrowth. Similarly in the liver of the newborn rat, where an active growth and proliferation of cells and organelles is in progress, a close association between mitochondria and developing rough endoplasmic reticulum is clearly evident (*Plate 57, Fig. 3*). A close association has also been noted between smooth endoplasmic reticulum and mitochondria (*Plate 47, Fig. 2*), as for example in dragon-fly flight muscle (Smith, 1961) and in the pseudobranch gland of *Fundulus heteroclitus*. In the latter instance this is considered to be related to the high rate of carbonic anhydrase synthesis (Copeland and Dalton, 1959).

One of the most striking associations is that seen between mitochondria and myofilaments. In longitudinal sections of cardiac and skeletal muscle, rows of mitochondria are seen lying closely apposed to such filaments, while in traverse sections through the I-band region, rings or girdles of mitochondria may be seen surrounding groups of myofilaments. It would appear that such an arrangement ensures that the ATP produced by the mitochondria is readily available via short diffusion paths to the myofilaments which need ATP for contraction. (Excellent illustrations supporting this point may be found in Fawcett, 1967.)

Another frequently noted example of mitochondrial associations is the juxtaposition of mitochondria to cell membranes engaged in active transport of ions or other tasks involving high expenditure of energy. Thus in the distal convoluted tubule of the kidney the basal plasma membrane is deeply infolded, and in the cleft-like spaces thus created lodge long slender mitochondria. A similar but not quite so elaborate arrangement is seen in the cells of the proximal tubule of the kidney, striated duct cells of the salivary gland, vestibular cells of cristae ampullaris, and marginal cells of the stria vascularis (for details, see Lentz, 1971). In all these instances a close association occurs over an extensive area between the mitochondrion and the cell membrane, and a topographical situation is created whereby the energy producer is brought into close apposition to the site of energy utilization.

Other examples of proximity of mitochondria to sites of energy utilization may be summarized briefly as follows: (1) in the Schwann cell for energy needed in the synthesis of large expanses of cell membrane to form the myelin sheath (Geren and Schmitt, 1954): (2) in synaptic junctions of axons for energy exchanges during impulse transmission (Palay, 1956); (3) in rat and guinea-pig spermatids for energy needed for the synthesis of the acrosome (Palade, 1952; Watson, 1952; Fawcett, 1959); and (4) in ciliated cells (*Plate 59*) for energy needed for ciliary motion (Lehninger, 1965).

Plate 59
Human bronchial mucosa, showing mitochondrial aggregates in the apical cytoplasm adjacent to ciliary border. × 8,000

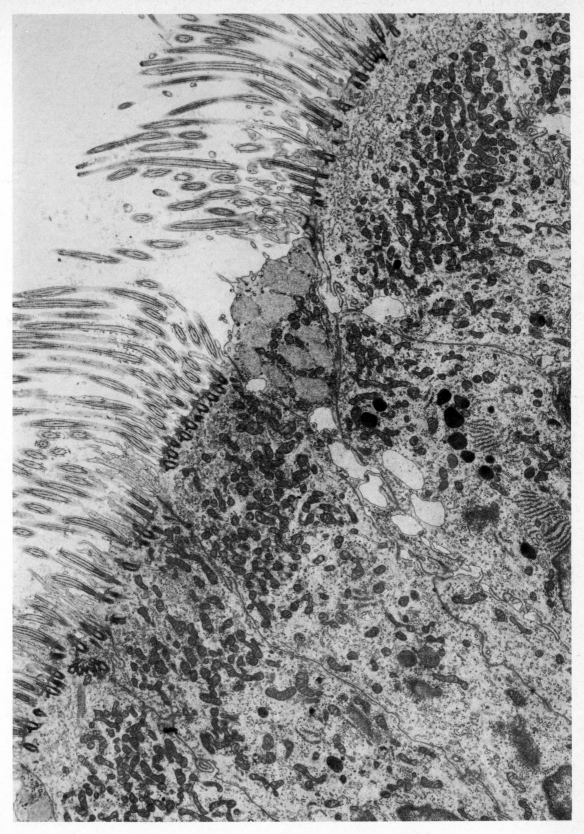

131

The principal alteration here appears to be the protrusion of a knob or finger-like projection (evagination) from one mitochondrion into an invagination in a neighbouring mitochondrion (*Plate 60*). The term' herniation' has been used to describe this phenomenon although it is not strictly correct to do so. The term 'bridge' is also not a very appropriate description of the changes seen. Yet the lack of a better term forces us to continue their use. If membranous structures such as rough endoplasmic reticulum lie between the mitochondria they are dragged into these herniations. Depending upon the plane of section, and further structural modifications, such herniations present as intermitochondrial membranous whorls or bridges or as myelin figures apparently lying free in the mitochondrial matrix.

Such alterations of mitochondrial morphology have been noted in the hepatocytes of experimental animals after: (1) vitamin E deficiency (Sulkin and Sulkin, 1962); (2) necrogenic diet (Svoboda and Higginson, 1963); (3) triparanol and diethanolamine administration (Hruban *et al.*, 1965); (4) riboflavine deficiency (Tandler *et al.*, 1968); (5) *E. coli* endotoxin administration (Boler and Bibighaus, 1967). It has also been seen in (6) the liver of rats bearing carcinogen-induced sarcomas in their flanks during the terminal stages of their life (Parry and Ghadially, 1966); (7) a human hepatoma (Ghadially and Parry, 1966); (8) autonomic ganglion cells of scorbutic guinea-pigs (Sulkin and Sulkin, 1967); and (9) adrenal cortex following hypophysectomy (Volk and Scarpelli, 1966).

The notion that this phenomenon may be dependent on close packing and crenation of mitochondria, due perhaps to the use of hypertonic fixatives or to fluid loss due to other reasons, does not stand up to critical examination, for mitochondrial herniations may affect grossly hydropic mitochondria and can be seen even when only a few mitochondria are present. Sulkin and Sulkin (1962) found that the most striking alteration after prolonged vitamin E deficiency was the occurrence of mitochondrial protrusions projecting into adjacent mitochondria, and this occurs in mitochondria which are markedly swollen. Since during the later phases of the experiment such herniations disappeared and enlarged mitochondria occurred, they suggest that coalescence of mitochondria may have been achieved in this fashion. Similarly, mitochondrial hernias have been implicated in the formation of enlarged or giant mitochondria by other workers (Svoboda and Higginson, 1963; Volk and Scarpelli, 1966; Tandler *et al.*, 1968). In our material such a correlation was not noted, for markedly enlarged or giant mitochondria were not evident, either in the tumour-bearing rat liver or the human hepatoma.

It is also worth noting that, although the union between the mitochondria resembles a joint of the peg-and-socket type rather than a dovetail joint, it is nevertheless quite firm, for such coupled mitochondria can be found also in pellets of isolated mitochondria (Tandler *et al.*, 1968). In view of this, and the subsequent development of myelin figures at this site, it would appear that these junctions represent sites of focal damage and rearrangement of the membrane of the mitochondrial envelope.

Plate 60

Liver to tumour-bearing rat, collected during terminal stage of life. (*From Parry and Ghadially, 1966*)

Fig. 1. Herniation of one mitochondrion into another (arrow). The rough endoplasmic reticulum is dragged into the herniation. × 35,000

Fig. 2. Intermitochondrial bridges (A) of electron-dense whorled membranes or myelin figures are seen connecting adjacent mitochondria. Some (B) appear to lie free in the mitochondrial matrix but they could be continuous with a mitochondrial envelope in another plane. Most of the appearances seen here can be interpreted as transverse or oblique sections through herniations of the type shown in *Fig. 1.* × 48,000

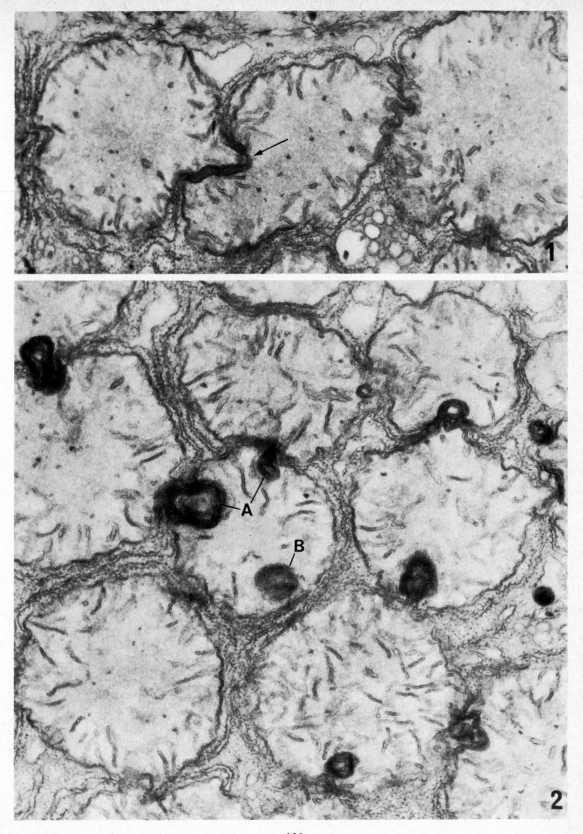

133

It has already been noted (page 102) that the matrices of mitochondria contain electron-dense granules, and that they are more prominent and encountered more frequently in the mitochondria of tissues which transport large quantities of water and ions. Such dense granules measure 200–500 Å in diameter and at times it can be demonstrated that they are composed of subunits measuring 50–70 Å in diameter. There is now ample evidence which indicates that these dense granules represent sites of accumulation of divalent cations. Studies on isolated dense granules indicate that they contain calcium, magnesium, phosphorus and inorganic material. According to Matthews *et al.* (1971), 'Analysis of inorganic constituents indicates a high lipid content, protein and RNA measured by the presence of ribose and traces of lysozyme'.

It has long been known from studies on isolated cell fractions that mitochondria contain relatively large amounts of calcium and magnesium, and it has also been shown that they can accumulate these and other ions, such as strontium and manganese, *in vitro*. Further *in vivo* experimental studies and histochemical studies also implicate mitochondria as sites of divalent cation localization (for references, see Peachey, 1964).

The elegant studies of Peachey (1964), carried out with the excised toad bladder and isolated kidney mitochondria of the rat, show that when the incubating medium contains calcium, strontium or barium, these ions are concentrated in the pre-existing dense granules of the mitochondrial matrix, as evidenced by their increased size and density. This is particularly well demonstrated with barium because of its high atomic number (Ba 56, Sr 38, Ca 20) and, hence, marked electron density as visualized in electron micrographs. Often such deposits assumed the shape of hollow spheres, suggesting that barium had been deposited around a pre-existing matrical granule probably in exchange for other ions at that site. Similarly, in cultures from the heart tissue of day-old rats, Porter and Hogeboom (1964) observed an increase in the size but not the number of matrical-dense granules in the mitochondria of cells exposed to an excess of calcium, strontium or barium ions.

Large electron-opaque granules, often attaining a diameter of 1,000 Å, were observed by Lehninger *et al.* (1963) in the matrix of rat liver mitochondria incubated in a medium containing both calcium and inorganic phosphate, and it has been debated whether such large deposits represent enlarged dense granules or fresh deposits in the matrix.

Peachey (1964) has proposed that divalent cations may be retained in the mitochondrion in two possible forms: (1) bound to organic phosphate in the form of granules pre-existing in the matrix; and (2) as an inorganic precipitate. The concept here is that if modest amounts of calcium ions are presented to the mitochondrion, they will be deposited on the dense granules, but if large amounts of calcium ions, preferably with inorganic phosphate, are offered, they are likely to form *de novo* precipitates of calcium phosphate in the mitochondrial matrix.

Plate 61

Fig. 1. A modest increase in size and perhaps also the number of matrical-dense granules is seen in this group of mitochondria from the kidney tubule of a mouse treated with parathyroid hormone. × 26,000 (*Ghadially and Ailsby, unpublished electron micrograph*)

Fig. 2. Small calcareous deposits (C) are seen in the thickened basement membrane of a kidney tubule. From mouse treated with calcium gluconate. × 27,000 (*Ghadially and Ailsby, unpublished electron micrograph*)

Fig. 3. Numerous laminated bodies (B) are seen at the periphery of the kidney tubules of a mouse treated with calcium gluconate. The membranes which form the laminated bodies are probably derived from the tubular epithelium near or at the plasma membrane. With prolonged treatment such bodies are obliterated by calcium deposits. The dense granules in the mitochondria appear normal in size and number. × 26,000 (*Ghadially and Ailsby, unpublished electron micrograph*)

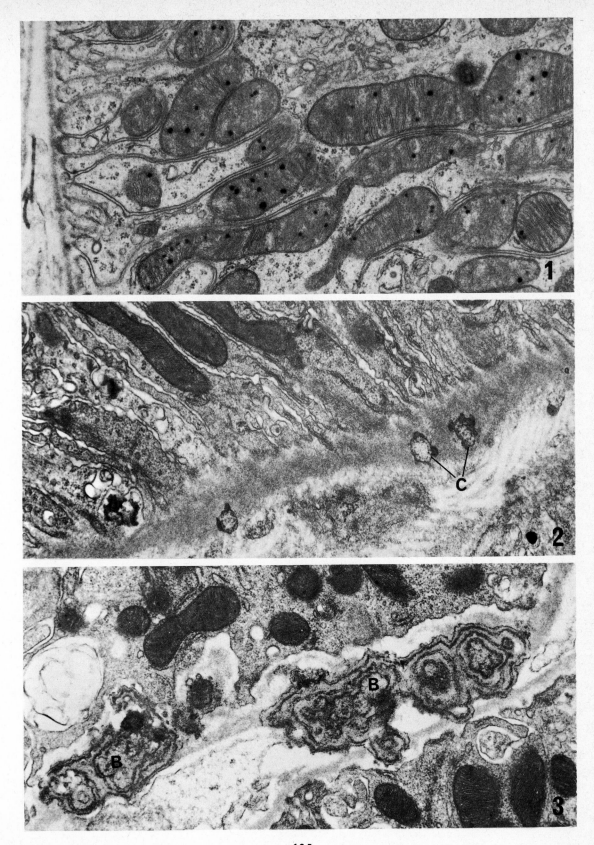

135

An increase in density, size and number of dense granules has been reported to occur in diverse pathological and experimental states. In extreme examples the mitochondrion may be filled with calcium deposits, and fusion of such calcified mitochondria may result in irregular calcified masses within and/or outside the cell.

The more dramatic examples of this kind have been observed following some procedures which produce focal necrosis. It is worth noting that one is not witnessing calcification of necrotic tissue, for intramitochondrial calcification precedes the necrosis and indeed appears to be a factor in its production. Such examples of intramitochondrial calcification include (1) the rat myocardium in magnesium deficiency (Heggtveit et al., 1964) and (2) the kidney tubules of mice after the administration of parathyroid extract (Caulfield and Schrag, 1964).

The effect of experimentally produced hypercalcemia on renal tissues has been the subject of many studies, quite a few at the ultrastructural level (for references, see Duffy et al., 1971). Such studies have revealed essentially three types of lesions in the proximal tubules: (1) changes in dense granules and intramitochondrial calcification; (2) amorphous or crystalline calcium deposits in the cytoplasm; and (3) calcium deposits and calcified laminated bodies in the basement membrane (Plates 61–63).

A clear relationship between the lesion produced and the agent used to produce the hypercalcemia does not seem to exist, but there are probably species differences. Our observations (Ghadially and Ailsby, unpublished) and those of Caulfield and Schrag (1964) show that in mice, parathyroid extract leads to mitochondrial calcification while calcium gluconate does not produce such mitochondrial changes but leads to calcium deposits in the basement membrane (Plate 61, Fig. 2) and in numerous small laminated bodies which develop in this region shortly after (3 days) treatment with calcium gluconate (Plate 61, Fig. 3). In the rat, however, calcium gluconate produces both calcified mitochondria and basement membrane deposits (Duffy et al., 1971).

The sequence of events occurring in the proximal tubule of the mouse after parathyroid hormone treatment is depicted in Plate 61, Fig. 1 and Plates 62 and 63. The earliest change is a modest increase in size and perhaps also the number of intramitochondrial dense granules (Plate 61, Fig. 1). Not all proximal tubules nor all the cells in a proximal tubule show this alteration. Later, cells containing mitochondria with huge dense granules are seen. They may present either as solid or hollow electron-dense spheres (Plate 62).

Plate 62

From the proximal tubule of the kidney of mouse treated with parathyroid hormone. (*Ghadially and Ailsby, unpublished electron micrographs*)

Fig. 1. Large electron-opaque spherules, presumed to be enlarged matrical granules (G), are seen within the mitochondria. One mitochondrion, however, contains normal-sized matrical granules (arrow). ×46,000

Fig. 2. In contrast to *Fig. 1*, most of the calcareous deposits here present as hollow spheres. Note also the tendency of fragmented and disorientated cristae (arrow) to wrap around these highly electron-opaque deposits. ×40,000

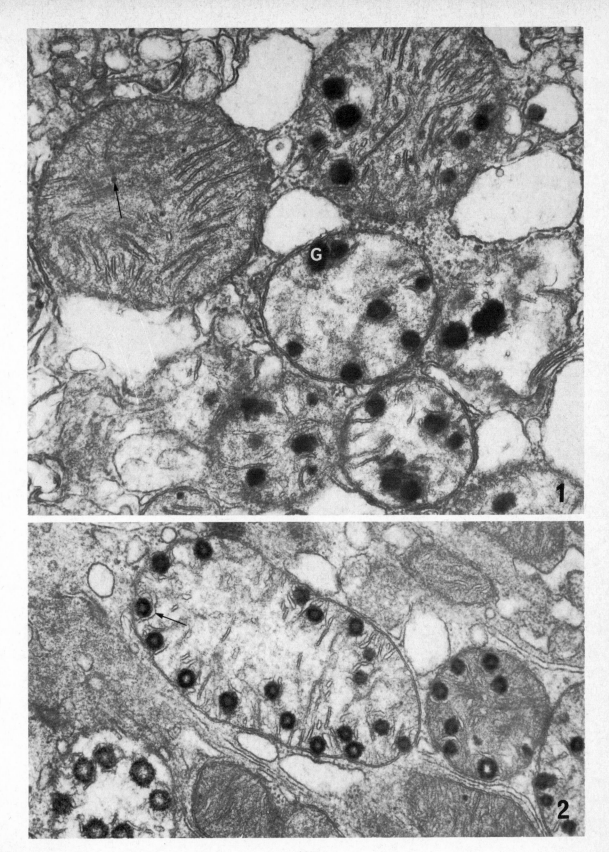

137

In some instances such granules appear to be enveloped in a membrane, probably derived from disintegrating cristae (*Plate 63*). There is no evidence that calcium deposits occur in the intra-cristal space. It is interesting to note that not all mitochondria within a given cell show such changes, and that normal-looking mitochondria with normal-sized dense granules may occur in the same cell. Finally, fusion of calcified mitochondria and/or enlarged dense granules liberated from ruptured mitochondria produce calcareous masses in the cytoplasm and lumen of the kidney tubule.

Numerous other instances of increase in number and size of intramitochondrial dense granules have been reported in the literature. They vary from quite modest changes to changes almost, but not quite, as severe as those discussed earlier. Such examples include: (1) ischaemic dog myocardium (Herdson *et al.*, 1965); (2) rat myocardium after administration of steroids and sodium phosphate (D'Agostino, 1964; Horvath *et al.*, 1970); (3) rat heart poisoned with plasmocid (D'Agostino, 1963); (4) cardiomyopathy associated with a phaeochromocytoma (Alpert *et al.*, 1972); (5) a variety of megamitochondria (see page 148); (6) liver of tumour-bearing rats (Ghadially and Parry, 1965); (7) liver of rats poisoned with carbon tetrachloride (Reynolds, 1963); (8) liver cell necrosis due to heliotrine (Kerr, 1969); (9) chilled dog kidneys used for transplantation (Fisher *et al.*, 1967); (10) muscles of tetanus-intoxicated mouse and man (Zacks and Sheff, 1964; Zacks *et al.*, 1966); and (11) osteoclasts, osteoblasts and gut epithelial cells following the administration of parathormone (Matthews *et al.*, 1971).

A decrease or disappearance of matrical dense granules has also at times been noted to occur. Particularly interesting is the observation by Trump *et al.* (1965a) that the earliest change (15 minutes) which occurs in mouse liver after excision is a disappearance of intramitochondrial dense granules. Similarly, within 10 minutes after occluding the superior mesenteric artery, Brown *et al.* (1970) found a loss of intramitochondrial dense granules in ileal mucosal cells of the dog, and under similar experimental conditions Aho *et al.* (1970) reported a loss of matrical granules in the jejunal mucosal cells. In excised rat and dog kidneys an early disappearance of intramitochondrial dense granules has been noted (MacKay *et al.*, 1968). A decrease in dense granules has also been reported to occur after histamine stimulation of gastric parietal cells and pancreozymin stimulation of pancreas (Fawcett, 1967). Dense granules in hepatocyte mitochondria disappear in normal and tumour-bearing rats 2 hours after partial hepatectomy, but return in both cases 6 hours after the operation (Parry, personal communication).

Plate 63

From kidney of mouse treated with parathyroid hormone. Necrotic cells containing numerous mitochondria with calcareous deposits are seen in the top half of this electron micrograph. Many of the intramitochondrial dense deposits seem to be surrounded by a membrane (arrow). In the lower half of the picture a portion of a kidney tubule containing much necrotic debris, calcified mitochondria (M), and a large calcareous deposit (D) is seen. × 28,000 (*Ghadially and Ailsby, unpublished electron micrograph*)

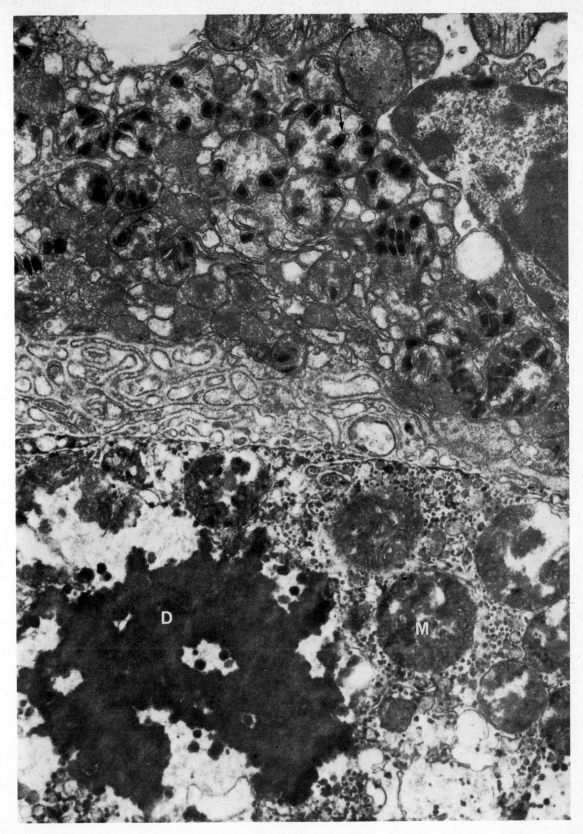

A common and easily recognized variety of mitochondrial enlargement, a swollen or hydropic mitochondrion is due to the entry of water (and solutes) into the organelle, and can be engendered by numerous agents which produce cell damage. Mitochondrial swelling, together with swelling and vesiculation of the rough endoplasmic reticulum, constitutes the change called cloudy swelling by pathologists (see also pages 222–228).

Various alterations of mitochondrial morphology are seen, depending upon the stage reached by the process and also upon which of the two mitochondrial chambers is primarily involved. As pointed out earlier (page 102), there are two compartments in a mitochondrion: (1) the outer or intermembranous chamber lying between the two membranes of the mitochondrial envelope and extending either as a potential space or a cleft-like or tubular space within the cristae, and (2) the inner chamber which contains the mitochondrial matrix. Since the permeability of the inner and outer mitochondrial membranes is known to be different (page 102), it follows that flooding of one or other, or both, chambers may occur.

By far the commonest variety of swelling seen is that due to the involvement of the matrix or inner chamber (*Plate 64*). In the early stages or in mild degrees of swelling there is only a modest increase in the size of the mitochodrion, and dilution of the matrix, as evidenced by a decreased density, is barely discernible. The cristae, however, appear displaced to the periphery and may show varying degrees of disorientation, shortening and reduction in numbers.

In this early stage, the matrix, although somewhat paler, retains its homogeneous character; but with advancing hydration it shows a patchy appearance due to development of multiple electron-lucent foci, and in time frank cavitation of the mitochondrial matrix occurs. Loss of matrix density is due at first to dilution but later there is also loss of matrix substance. Breaks in the mitochondrial-limiting membranes are also encountered, particularly in grossly swollen mitochondria. The intramitochondrial dense granules tend to disappear at an early stage of swelling, but this is not invariably the case.

Plate 64

Mitochondria from the liver of a rat bearing a carcinogen-induced subcutaneous sarcoma, showing varying degrees (increasing from *Figs. 1 to 3*) of swelling of the matrical chamber. (*Ghadially and Parry, unpublished electron micrographs*)

Fig. 1. A slightly swollen mitochondrion (M) showing peripherally placed cristae and a fairly homogeneous, medium-density matrix. Intramitochondrial dense granules are absent. × 32,000

Fig. 2. Markedly swollen mitochondria with peripherally placed, disorientated, and disintegrating cristae. The matrix has a patchy appearance and a break (arrow) is evident in the wall of a mitochondrion. Dense granules are abundant. Note also the vesiculation (V) of the rough endoplasmic reticulum. In pathological terms, this cell is showing cloudy swelling. × 46,000

Fig. 3. This grossly swollen mitochondrion shows frank cavitation of the mitochondrial matrix (M) and loss of cristae. The lower half of the mitochondrial wall is attenuated and probably ruptured (arrow). × 46,000

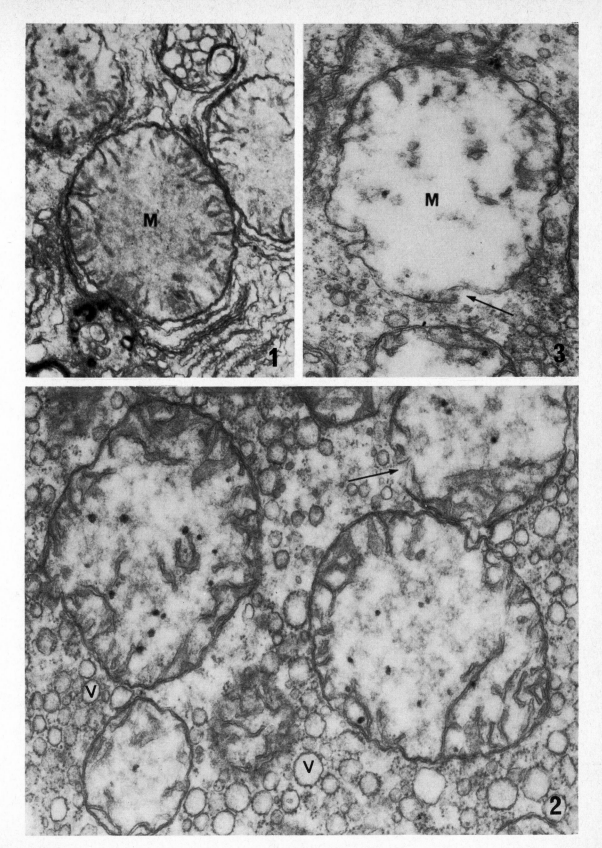

141

Mitochondrial swelling due to influx of water into the outer chamber is usually of a modest degree and is frequently limited to a ballooning of the cristae (intracristal swelling). It is only occasionally accompanied by separation of the inner and outer membrane of the envelope, and even then often only a segment of the wall is affected, forming a 'blister' on the wall of the mitochondrion. In instances where only intracristal swelling is present, there may be no obvious increase in the over-all size of the mitochondrion, and the matrix may appear quite dense. However, with advanced swelling of the intermembranous space, an over-all increase in size of the mitochondrion becomes evident. These remarks apply to mitochondria seen in ultrathin sections of tissues.

Studies with isolated mitochondria and cells or tissues *in vitro* show that similar changes can be produced in mitochondria by various experimental procedures (Trump and Ginn, 1968; Butler and Judha, 1970; Gordon and Bernstein, 1970; Laiho *et al.*, 1971). In such *in vitro* studies normal mitochondria are often referred to as showing an orthodox configuration, and those with dense matrix and swollen cristae as showing a condensed configuration. In Ehrlich ascites tumour cells taken directly from the animal, the mitochondria display a normal configuration, but when such cells are repeatedly washed, transformation of mitochondria to condensed configuration occurs (Gordon and Bernstein, 1970). The mechanism by which this change is produced is not understood. It is thought that such changes are accompanied by conformational changes of the inner membrane protein (Wrigglesworth and Packer, 1968) and that the condensed configuration indicates a 'low energy state' and the orthodox form a 'high energy state' (Hackenbrock, 1968a, b).

Mitochondria with expanded matrical chambers have been produced by the addition of valinomycin to the medium, which produces a rapid potassium ion influx. This has been demonstrated with isolated rat liver mitochondria (Butler and Judha, 1970) and also with the washed Ehrlich ascites cells mentioned earlier. The addition of calcium chloride or phosphate ions also induces swelling of the matrix chamber but there is also much loss of matrix material.

Trump and Bulger (1967, 1968) and Trump and Ginn (1968) have noted, in isolated flounder kidney tubules injured in various ways, that there is first an expansion of the intercristal space and only later is this followed by a swelling of the matrix compartment. Similar sequential swelling of the two chambers has often been observed by us in cultures of herpesvirus-infected cells harvested at different time intervals (*Plates 65 and 66*). Indeed, on occasions, both varieties of swollen mitochondria may be seen in the same cell, and, as Trump and Ginn (1968) point out, at times one portion of the mitochondrion may show intracristal swelling and dense matrix, while the remainder may show marked swelling of the matrix chamber.

Plate 65

Fig. 1. A monkey kidney cell from a culture infected with herpesvirus. Mitochondria cut in various planes clearly show markedly ballooned cristae (C) and a moderately dense matrix (M), but there is no separation of the outer and inner mitochondrial membranes. This (and also *Fig. 2*) is the appearance which is sometimes referred to as a 'condensed configuration'. Numerous dense granules are present. × 41,000

Fig. 2. Two mitochondria, which no doubt escaped while the tissue (frog kidney) was being minced in osmium, are now seen lying free in the embedding medium. Both show markedly ballooned cristae (C), a dense matrix and some intramitochondrial dense granules. There is focal separation of inner and outer membranes (arrow) in one mitochondrion, while in the other the separation is much more extensive. These mitochondria are grossly swollen compared to the mitochondria (M) within the kidney tubule. × 32,000

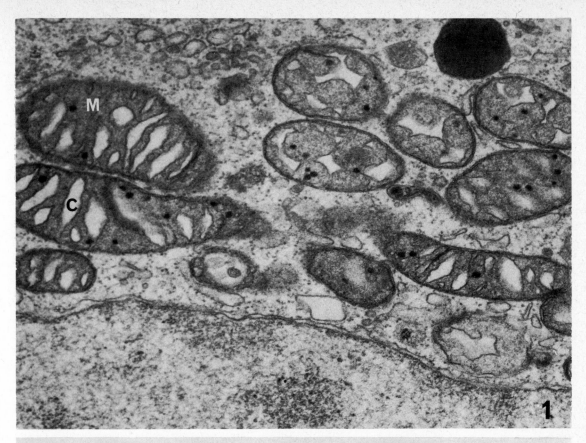

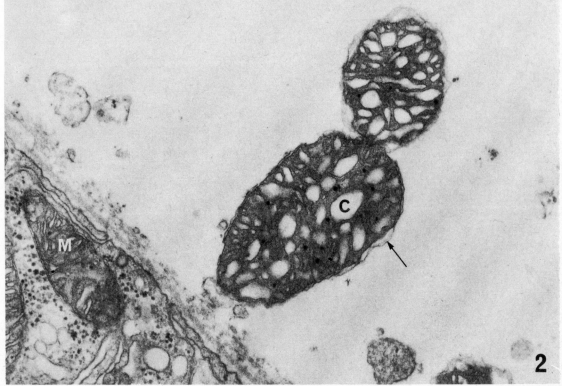

A few of the more recent studies on volume changes in isolated mitochondria have been mentioned above, but a voluminous literature on this subject exists (see reviews by Lehninger, 1962, 1965). These studies, although of great interest, do not directly concern us here, because correlated ultrastructural studies were performed only occasionally, and often artefacts due to the separation procedure and different methods of fixation employed make correlations between these results and what one finds in ultrathin tissue sections difficult. However, these early studies have demonstrated that mitochondria can show two types of swelling: (1) a passive swelling, which can be produced by altering the osmolarity of the medium; and (2) an active swelling, which is dependent on electron transport, and can be brought about in isotonic solutions by adding minute amounts of various swelling-inducer agents, such as phosphorus, calcium and mercury ions, fatty acids, thyroxine, oxytocin, vasopressin, insulin and hydrocortisone. It would appear that in many pathological situations the initial mitochondrial swelling is of the active type, but that later, when the cell becomes flooded with water, a passive enlargement also occurs.

The equivalent of passive swelling is also clearly seen as an artefact in tissues which are fixed in hypotonic solutions (Ogura and Furuta, 1957). Other procedures where mitochondrial swelling might be artefactually introduced in the specimen include hypoxia due to the use of a tourniquet prior to surgical biopsy, delay in collecting tissues, and using blocks of tissues too large to permit rapid penetration of fixative solution (David, 1964; Trump *et al.*, 1965a, b; Ericsson and Biberfeld, 1967). Distinction between this kind of artefactual swelling and that produced by pathological processes which one might be investigating can be difficult or impossible.

Multiple factors appear to be involved in the production of mitochondrial hydrops. Osmotic changes in the external environment of mitochondria are clearly a factor in some cases but, since hydropic and normal mitochondria can at times be found in the same cell (*Plate 66, Fig. 2*; *Plate 56, Fig. 1*), it has been suggested (Rouiller, 1960; David 1964) that the primary chemical derangement can also occur in the organelle itself, and that alterations in membrane permeability may be involved.

Swollen mitochondria (like cloudy swelling) have been observed in almost every type of tissue subjected to a variety of pathological influences. It is so protean a manifestation of cell injury that it would be impossible to list every situation in which this change has been noted. David (1964) lists the following conditions in which mitochondrial swelling has been seen in the liver: starvation, kwashiorkor, choline deficiency, vitamin B_1 deficiency, enteromelia of mouse, hepatitis, yellow fever, x-rays, ethionine intoxication, dimethylaminoazobenzene-feeding, hepatoma, diphtheria toxin, cirrhosis, bile duct obstruction, phosphorus poisoning, hormone action and shock.

The term 'cloudy swelling' was coined by Virchow to describe intracellular water accumulation in cells subject to toxic stress. He believed it to be a primary cause of cell death. (A detailed historical review of this subject has been presented by Cameron, 1952.) The pathogenesis of cloudy swelling is still not fully understood, but it is now believed that it involves a failure of cellular osmotic control mechanisms. It would appear that damage and swelling of mitochondria leads to a suppression of ATP production, which in turn leads to a failure of the ATP-dependent sodium pump at the cell membrane, resulting in the cellular compartments becoming flooded with water.

Plate 66

Fig. 1. Monkey kidney cell from a culture infected with herpesvirus. During the early stages mitochondria with ballooned cristae, as shown in *Plate 65, Fig. 1*, are found. At a later stage such mitochondria suffer swelling of the inner chamber also, producing the appearance shown in this electron micrograph. Note the swollen cristae (C), focal separation of the outer and inner mitochondrial membranes (F), cavitation of the matrix (M), and breaks in the wall of the mitochondrion (arrow). ×49,000

Fig. 2. Dog myocardium subjected to anoxia. Only a few of the mitochondria show matrical lucency and some swelling. The others are not markedly altered. (See also *Plate 56, Fig. 1*). ×23,000

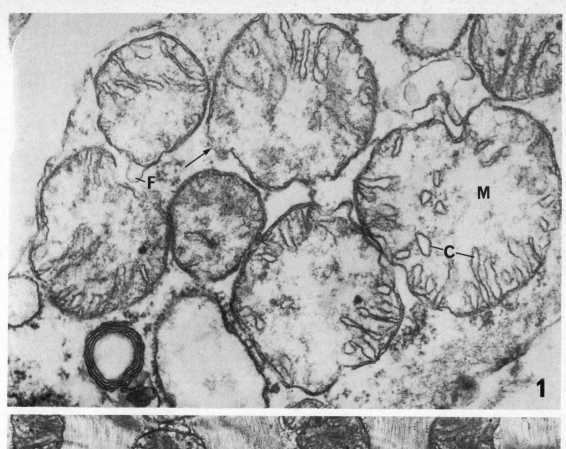

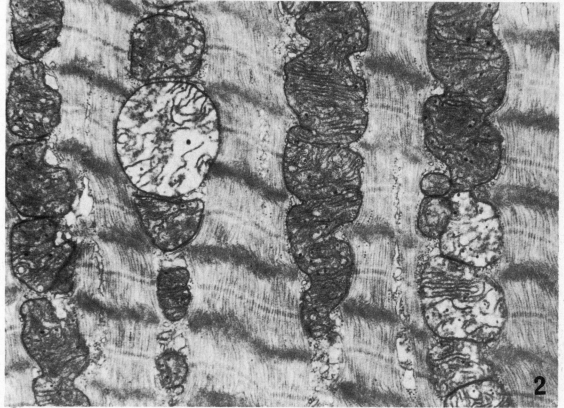

145

Mitochondrial enlargement due to hypertrophy is distinguishable from swelling or hydrops, because in the former there is no dilution of the matrix, and hence no reduction of matrix density. Also, in hypertrophied mitochondria the concentration of cristae is normal or increased, but in swollen mitochondria the cristae are lost or displaced to the periphery.

Examples of increase in the size (hypertrophy) and/or number (hyperplasia) of mitochondria have been observed in cardiac, uterine and skeletal muscle subject to various pathological and experimental states where an increased functional demand is made on the tissue. Thus the marked hypertrophy of the myometrium during pregnancy is matched not only by a great increase in the number and size of mitochondria but also by an increase in the number of cristae (Dessouky, 1968). Similar mitochondrial changes have also been observed in the myocardium after acute and exhaustive exercise (Laguens et al., 1966; Pelosi and Agliati, 1968) and in cardiac hypertrophy produced by natural disease or experimental situations (Meerson et al., 1964; McCallister and Brown, 1965; Bishop and Cole, 1969). Such studies show that mitochondrial hypertrophy commences during the early stages of cardiac hypertrophy, before the hypertrophy of myofibrils. During the final stage of exhaustion and cardiac failure there is a decrease in the mitochondrial mass, and also swelling of mitochondria.

A single non-lethal but toxic dose of digoxin has also been shown to produce a significant increase in the quantity of mitochondria and enhanced energy production by rat myocardial cells (Arcasoy and Smuckler, 1969). In the rat gastrocnemius muscle, Gustafsson et al. (1965) noted an increase in the size and number of mitochondria and an increase in the number and length of cristae after the administration of L-thyroxine under anabolic conditions. In these hypermetabolic rats, the enlargement of the mitochondrial apparatus amounted to an increase two and one-half times normal. No simple correlation, however, exists between the enhanced metabolic activity produced by thyroxine and mitochondrial hypertrophy and hyperplasia. Thyroidectomy also produces a smaller but definite enlargement of the mitochondrial apparatus, and even three weeks after cessation of thyroxine treatment, mitochondrial hypertrophy and hyperplasia persists although their elevated respiratory activity has returned to normal.

Perhaps the largest concentration of mitochondria known to occur is seen in cells called oncocytes. As is well known, these acidophilic cells with a markedly granular cytoplasm arise in tissues that have already attained histological maturity. For instance, in salivary glands, transition from normal epithelial cells to oncocytes is known to occur (Tandler, 1966). During such transformation a remarkable hyperplasia of mitochondria occurs. Oncocytes from various sites show certain common features, the most important being the abundance of mitochondria which invariably lack dense granules (*Plate 67*). Indeed, often the cytoplasm contains little besides mitochondria, but it is difficult to see what energy requirement so remarkable a collection of mitochondria is supposed to meet. A plausible explanation that has been offered is that these mitochondria are probably biochemically defective and that this is an example of compensatory hyperplasia occurring at the organelle level (Tandler and Shipkey, 1964; Tandler et al, 1970).

Plate 67

An oncocyte from a bronchial mucosal gland of man, showing cytoplasm packed with mitochondria. ×24,000

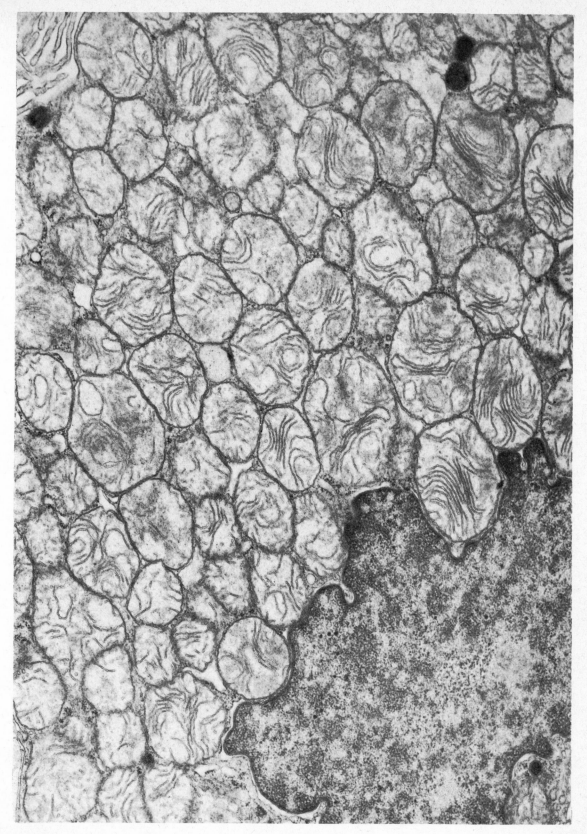

GIANT MITOCHONDRIA

Grossly enlarged mitochondria have been observed in a variety of tissues under diverse situations, and terms such as 'megamitochondria' and 'giant mitochondria' have been employed to describe them. Such organelles may evolve either by fusion of a number of mitochondria or by growth of a single mitochondrion, or both. Often such enlargement affects only one or two mitochondria in a cell, the size and number of the remainder being normal or even diminished. Giant mitochondria frequently show highly interesting alterations of internal structure (*Plates 68–72*), such as an increase in the number of cristae (often showing novel arrangements), myelin figures, prominent dense granules, and crystalline and lipidic inclusions. Some of these alterations, such as crystalline inclusions, are at times also seen in some of the remaining normal-sized mitochondria in the cell containing the giant forms. (See also page 170.)

A study of published electron micrographs and tissues containing giant mitochondria leads one to believe that in the evolution of these organelles there is a phase of enlargement followed by a phase of degeneration and disintegration of internal architecture. The former phase is characterized by an abundance of well preserved cristae, matrix and, at times, large, numerous matrical dense granules. The formation of myeline figures, granular amorphous debris and osmiophilic lipidic material may be regarded as regressive changes due to degeneration and disintegration within the enlarged organelle (*Plate 70*). Later, segmental or total dissolution of the inner mitochondrial membrane may occur, and a single-membrane-bound body containing membrane remnants and electron-dense material, morphologically acceptable as a cytolysosome, may develop (*Plate 70, Fig. 2*).

Plate 68

Fig. 1. A giant mitochondrion containing tubular cristae (C), crystalline inclusions (arrow) and large matrical dense granules (D) is seen in this liver cell. The remarkable increase in size of this organelle is well demonstrated by comparison with normal-sized mitochondria in the bottom right corner of the picture. From non-neoplastic human liver adjacent to a hepatoma. × 43,000 (*From Ghadially and Parry, 1966*)

Fig. 2. A small part of a golf-club-shaped giant mitochondrion is illustrated here. Numerous crystals, some cut longitudinally (L) and others transversely (T), can be seen in addition to transversely and obliquely cut cristae. From same specimen as *Fig. 1.* × 75,000 (*Ghadially and Parry, unpublished electron micrograph*)

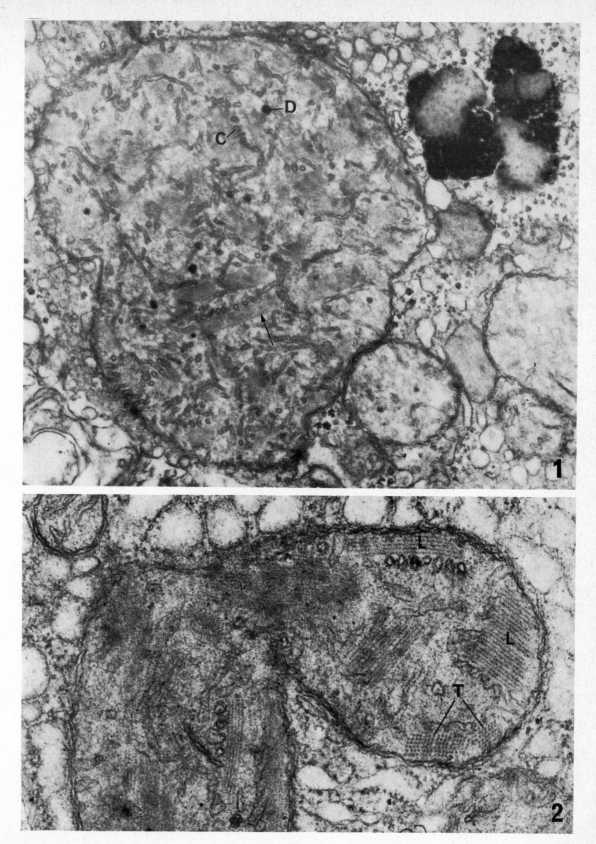

Mitochondrial abnormalities of the sort described above have been seen in various tissues under apparently unrelated conditions, and different theories regarding their genesis have been suggested.

Hormonal mechanisms have been held responsible for the giant mitochondria produced in some situations, as in : (1) rat adrenals (seen with greater frequency in female rats) after hypophysectomy (Sabatini et al., 1962; Volk and Scarpelli, 1966); (2) the foetal zone of the human adrenal cortex during the sixth and twelfth weeks of gestation (Luse, 1961; Ross, 1962); (3) rats given ACTH, and also in rats given aminoglutethimide which blocks steroid synthesis (Racela et al., 1969). However, other adrenal inhibitors such as dichlorodiphenyl-dichloroethane (DDD) and amphenone do not produce this effect (for references, see Racela et al., 1969). Hormonal stimuli may have also been responsible for the production of enlarged mitochondria found in the endometrium of mink during the phase of delayed implantation of early pregnancy (Enders et al., 1963).

Protein, vitamin and associated nutritional deficiencies seem to be responsible for another group of cases (seen mainly in the liver) where giant mitochondria and moderately enlarged mitochondria are found, although in some of these cases hormonal imbalance and toxic factors may also be involved. Thus, such mitochondria have been seen in : (1) the pancreas in kwashiorkor (Blackburn and Vinijchaikul, 1969); (2) the liver and adrenals of protein-deficient rats (Svoboda and Higginson, 1964; Svoboda et al., 1966); and (3) the liver of riboflavin-deficient mice (Tandler et al., 1968). Numerous giant mitochondria were found by us (Ghadially and Parry, 1966) in the liver tissue surrounding a large but well differentiated hepatoma which occurred in a woman (Plates 68–70). In this respect it is worth recalling that profound disturbances of protein metabolism also occur in the neoplastic state, and the cachexia and anaemia which occur in the tumour-bearing host are well recognized (Greenstein, 1954; Wiseman and Ghadially, 1958).

Plate 69

From non-neoplastic human liver adjacent to a hepatoma. A bipartite (fusion?) giant mitochondrion is seen in this hepatocyte. Abundant cristae and crystals are seen in the upper part of the organelle while the lower part is filled with granular matrix. × 50,000. (*Ghadially and Parry, unpublished electron micrograph*)

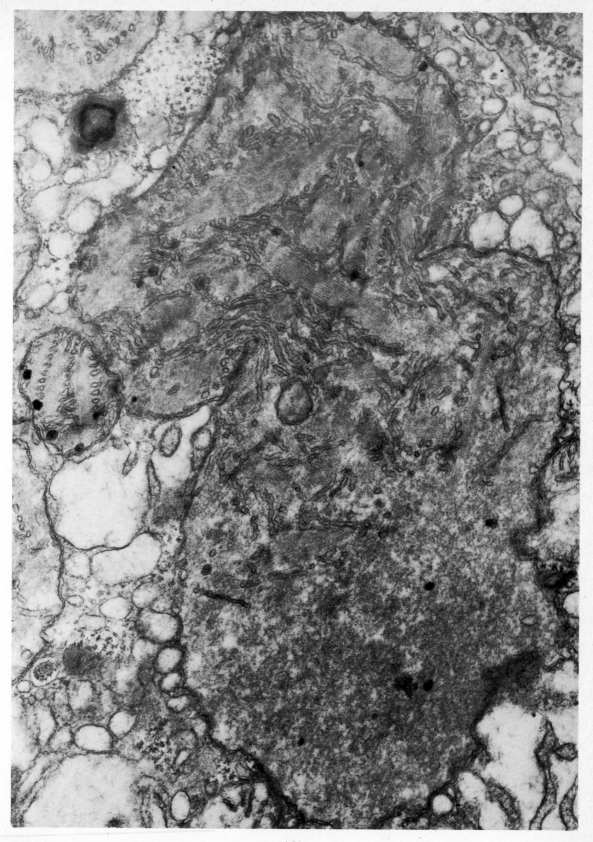

Chronic alcoholism, in which complex nutritional deficiencies may also be operative, provides another interesting example of megamitochondria. The Mallory bodies found in the liver of chronic alcoholics have long been the subject of much interest and discussion. One interpretation is that some or perhaps all of these eosinophilic hyaline bodies (Mallory bodies) are megamitochondria and their degenerate remains (Porta *et al.*, 1965). However, this view is not accepted by others, who regard Mallory bodies as areas of focal cytoplasmic degeneration involving other organelles besides mitochondria (Flax and Tisdale, 1964) or as compacted masses of non-membrane-bound fine filaments in the cytoplasm (Ma, 1972). Rats given special diets and alcohol also develop megamitochondria in their hepatocytes and it is claimed that these are homologous to the Mallory bodies seen in human liver (Porta *et al.*, 1969).

Giant mitochondria have also been observed in the liver of man in obstructive jaundice due to carcinoma of the bile duct, viral hepatitis (Jezequel, 1959) and amyloidosis (Thiery and Caroli, 1962). A moderate degree of mitochondrial enlargement with crystalline inclusions or normal-sized mitochondria with crystals have often been reported to occur in apparently normal human liver (Reppart *et al.*, 1963; Mugnaini, 1964; Svoboda and Manning, 1964; Wills, 1965; Lynn *et al.*, 1969), and regarding giant mitochondria in the liver, David (1964) states, 'We have been able to notice it in various non-characteristic diseases without any pathological–histological findings on the liver'. The view that mitochondria with crystalline inclusions can occur in normal human liver has been challenged recently by Bhagwat and his co-workers (Bhagwat and Ross, 1971; Bhagwat *et al.*, 1972), who point out that in such studies the normality of the livers can be seriously questioned and that, when stricter criteria are employed in selecting normal human liver, mitochondria with crystalline inclusions are not seen. (See also pages 170–172).

Plate 70

From non-neoplastic human liver adjacent to a hepatoma. (*Ghadially and Parry, unpublished electron micrographs*)

Fig. 1. The giant mitochondrion in the centre of this illustration shows early degenerative changes as evidenced by the presence of a lipid droplet (L) and disintegration of internal architecture. Compare with *Plates 68 and 69.* × 32,000

Fig. 2. A large, single-membrane-bound body, presumably derived from a giant mitochondrion, is seen in this electron micrograph. It contains amorphous granular material similar to that found in giant mitochondria, and paired membranous structures which could be derived from disintegrating cristae (arrows). A lipid droplet (L) is also present. × 40,000

152

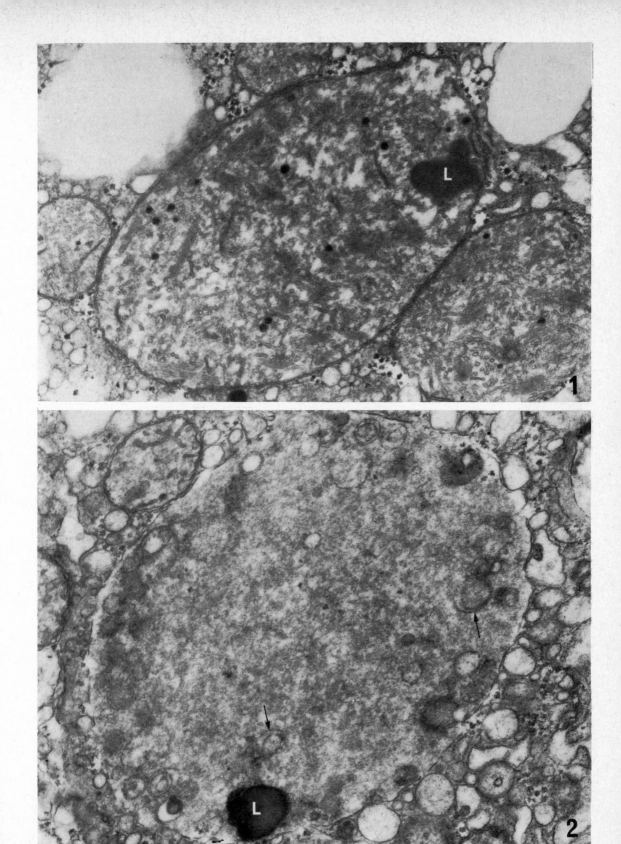

153

In *Plate 71* are illustrated two giant mitochondria found in the liver of an apparently normal dog; but, as can be seen, the internal architecture of these organelles is different from the giant mitochondria illustrated in the previous plates (*Plates 68 and 69*). Such mitochondria with an abundant matrix but sparse cristae are readily produced in the liver of mice fed cuprizone (Suzuki, 1969). Giant mitochondria with crystalline inclusions have been seen in dogs two and three-quarter hours after reversible hypovolaemic shock (Blair *et al.*, 1968), but these resembled more the giant mitochondria of human liver described earlier.

Giant mitochondria had not until recently been reported to occur in haemopoietic tissues but they have now been seen in: (1) bone marrow macrophages from a case of myeloid leukaemia (Bessis and Breton-Gorius, 1969); (2) bone marrow macrophages from a case of erythroleukaemia (Ghadially and Skinnider, 1974) (*Plate 72, Fig. 2*); and (3) plasma cells from a case of myeloma in which an acute leukaemia had developed (Skinnider and Ghadially, 1975).

The mitochondria of striated muscle appear to be singularly prone to fusion and formation of giant mitochondria. Even in apparently normal muscle, long mitochondria extending over several sarcomere lengths are encountered at times, and these are almost certainly due to end-to-end fusion of pre-existing mitochondria. This is in keeping with Fawcett's (1967) statement that 'the majority of mitochondria in muscle are 2 to 3 microns long but it is not uncommon to find a few 8 or even 10 microns in length'. Giant mitochondria, presumably produced by end-to-end fusion and also lateral fusion, can develop within a few minutes of myocardial hypoxia (*Plate 72*). Giant mitochondria in muscle tissue have been seen also in various pathological and experimental states, but in some instances they could equally well have been formed by the enlargement of solitary mitochondria.

Thus giant mitochondria (including long end-to-end fused mitochondria) have been seen in: (1) hypoxic myocardium of dogs (Lozada and Laguens, 1966) (*Plate 72, Fig. 1*); (2) myocardium of dogs with aortic stenosis (Wollenberger and Schulze, 1961); (3) hypoxic isolated perfused rat hearts (Sun *et al.*, 1969); (4) myocardium of rats maintained for long periods on small doses of thyroxine (Zaimis *et al.*, 1969); (5) myocardium of dogs treated with quinidine (Hiott and Howell, 1971); (6) myocardium of mouse, bat and dog after the administration of reserpine (Wilcken *et al.*, 1967; Sun *et al.*, 1968; Hagopian *et al.*, 1972); and (7) in various myopathies of man (Luft *et al.*, 1962; Gruner, 1963; Shy *et al.*, 1966; Shafiq *et al.*, 1967). Particularly interesting are the enlarged mitochondria found in some myopathies, for crystalline inclusions occur in the intracristal compartment and not as they usually do (e.g. liver) in the matrix compartment.

Plate 71

Figs. 1 and 2. Two giant mitochondria from the liver of an apparently normal dog. The remarkable increase in size is demonstrated by comparison with a normal-sized mitochondrion (M) in *Fig. 1*. These giant mitochondria show a paucity of cristae (arrow) but an abundance of granular matrix and intramatrical dense granules (G) of a similar size to that seen in the normal-sized mitochondrion. × 35.000; × 37.000

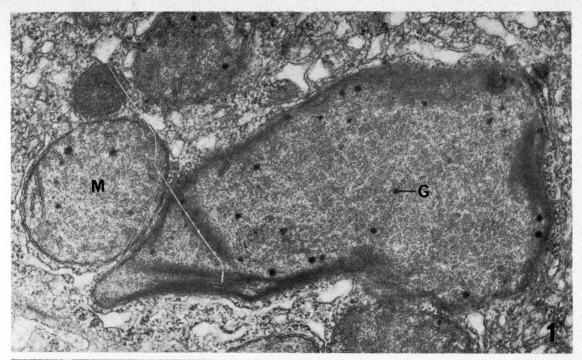

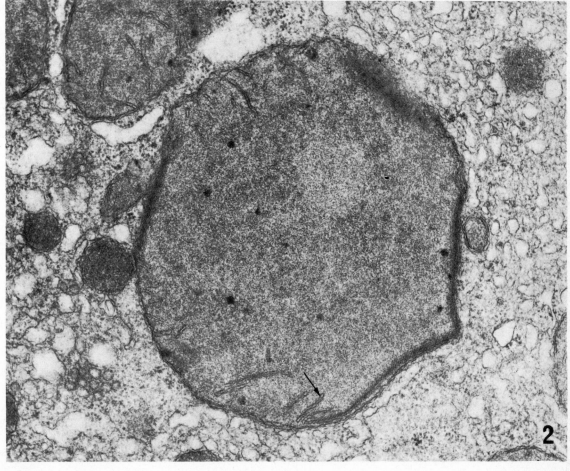

The occurrence of various mitochondrial abnormalities, particularly giant or enlarged mitochondria with or without crystalline and/or other inclusions, has led to the idea that such defects may be primarily responsible for the production of certain diseases of muscle in man. The idea of a mitochondrial disease was first put forward by Luft *et al.* (1962) and later developed by Gonatas and Shy (1966) and by Shy *et al.* (1966), who found mitochondrial abnormalities in two cases of slowly progressive muscular dystrophy. In one case there were enlarged and giant mitochondria; this condition they named 'megaconial myopathy'. In the other case the mitochondria were small but very numerous; this they described as 'pleoconial myopathy'. The term 'mitochondrial myopathy' has been employed by Spiro *et al.* (1970) and other workers to describe muscular disorders where abnormal mitochondria are found.

However, some 40 cases or more of a great variety of muscular disorders with mitochondrial alterations have now been described (for references, see Mair and Tomé, 1972) and it would appear that such changes are neither primary nor specific for a particular disease or group of diseases. The mitochondrial changes seen no doubt reflect deranged mitochondrial metabolism, but this is more likely to be a secondary change engendered by various disease processes and noxious influences. Thus, little aetiological significance can be attached to the finding of abnormal mitochondria in pathological muscle tissue of man (Peter *et al.*, 1970).

The precise manner in which giant mitochondria (in all sites) are born is debatable, but as suggested earlier this can be by enlargement of pre-existing mitochondria or by fusion of smaller organelles to form large ones. It is also conceivable that both these processes (which are not mutually exclusive) may be involved in any given instance.

Some giant mitochondria have a fairly regular margin and a round or ovoid shape. They also contain a fairly regular pattern of cristae within them and there is little need to postulate that anything more than an enlargement of a single organelle has occurred. More frequently, however, giant mitochondria have irregular contours, and show bipartite or lobular forms. This, taken in conjunction with the reduction in the number of mitochondria so often seen in their neighbourhood, suggests that a fusion process may also be involved. This seems clearly to be the case at least in some of the giant mitochondria found in muscular tissue, and is also probably the case in some of the enlarged mitochondria seen in hepatocytes (Ghadially and Parry, 1966). On the other hand in the case of erythroleukaemia studied by us (Ghadially and Skinnider, 1974), this morphological evidence suggested that giant mitochondria had been derived by enlargement rather than fusion of pre-existing mitochondria.

Crystalline inclusions are a common feature of giant mitochondria in various tissues, but particularly so in the liver. They are generally considered to be protein or lipoprotein in nature. Such crystals often bear a close relationship to the cristae and may at times appear to overlie them or even arise from them. Svoboda and Manning (1964) have interpreted this as a degenerative change in the cristae, leading to a release and subsequent crystallization of lipoproteins derived from the membranes of the cristae.

Plate 72

Fig. 1. Giant mitochondrion found in dog myocardium. Mitochondria from adjacent rows are seen in the process of fusing with the main mass forming the giant mitochondrion. × 20,000

Fig. 2. Giant mitochondrion found in a bone marrow macrophage from a case of erythroleukaemia. × 17,500 (*Ghadially and Skinnider, 1974*)

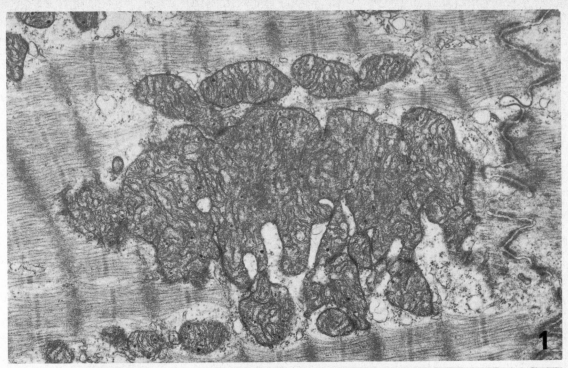

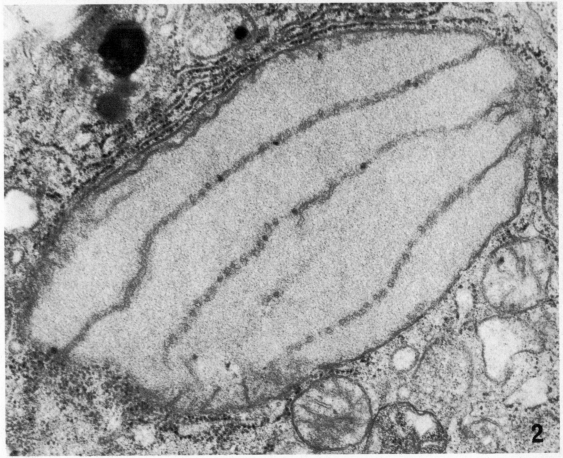

In ultrathin sections, mitochondria showing C-, U- and O-shaped configurations have at times been seen in normal and pathological tissues (*Plate 73*). It is now believed that in most instances such mitochondrial forms represent sections in various planes through cup-shaped organelles.

Mitochondria with the O-shaped configuration in section are often referred to as doughnut mitochondria or ring-shaped mitochondria. The 'hole' within such forms may be placed centrally or eccentrically, and usually contains cytoplasmic matrix and various structures such as ribosomes, rough endoplasmic reticulum or glycogen. The material, however, is clearly demarcated from the mitochondrion by the double membrane of the mitochondrial envelope and is akin in some ways to a pseudoinclusion. If, due to obliquity of sectioning, the membranes are not visualized, an erroneous impression of a mitochondrial inclusion could be created. Usually the 'hole' is quite small, but at times it can be quite large so that a long, slender, ring-shaped mitochondrion is seen surrounding a large volume of cytoplasm. At times two or more cup-shaped mitochondria may be stacked within one another so that in section they appear as concentric rings of mitochondria. Such an appearance is at times referred to as a chondrosphere.

It is conceivable that annular-shaped mitochondrial forms could represent a section through a genuine doughnut-shaped organelle produced perhaps by the fusion of the tips of a curved mitochondrion, and indeed such an interpretation has at times been favoured in the earlier literature. However, the chances of cutting a three-dimensionally doughnut-shaped structure so that it presents as a ring are small, and since such 'ring mitochondria' are almost invariably seen in company with C-shaped and U-shaped forms, it is now generally conceded that these forms (C, U and O) represent sections through mitochondria which, in fact, have a cup-shaped or dome-shaped configuration. It is also clear that at times the ring form represents sections through Y-shaped mitochondria and those with complex irregular forms such as that shown in *Plate 73, Fig. 2*. Yet another possibility is that a ring-shaped appearance may be created by a circularly arranged crista near the central part of the mitochondrion. We (Ghadially and Ailsby, unpublished observations) have seen this in an apparently normal cow adrenal (*Plate 74*) where such mitochondria were abundant but C- or U-shaped mitochondrial forms were absent. At times a single modified crista lined the central 'hole'; in other instances two or more cristae encircled this region. Also, at times mitochondria with two 'holes' were noted.

Ring-shaped mitochondria or mitochondria judged to be cup-shaped by the above-mentioned criteria have been seen in a variety of normal tissues, such as: (1) interstitial cells of rat testis; (2) opossum Leydig cells; (3) nurse cells of *Drosophila* testis; (4) grasshopper and scorpion testes

---

Plate 73

All illustrations except *Fig. 5* are from the livers of rats treated with carbon tetrachloride. *Fig. 5* was obtained from a normal dog liver.

Fig. 1. A U-shaped mitochondrion. × 37,000

Fig. 2. An irregular-shaped mitochondrion. One end of the mitochondrion is C-shaped, the other O-shaped. × 25,000

Fig. 3. A C-shaped mitochondrion. Note the narrow opening through which continuity of cytoplasmic structures is maintained × 29,000

Figs. 4 and 5. Ring forms with centrally placed 'holes'. × 34,000; × 48,000

Figs. 6 and 7. Ring forms with eccentrically placed 'holes'. × 29,000; × 40,000

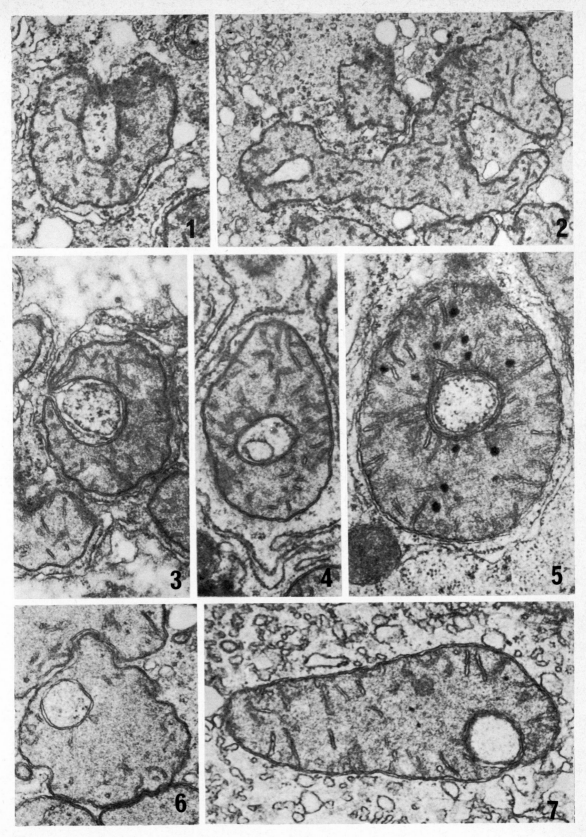

during spermatogenesis; (5) adrenal cortex of hamsters; (6) beta cells of the islets of embryonic mouse pancreas; (7) occasional hepatocytes in apparently normal rat liver (for references to the above-mentioned examples, see Stephens and Bils, 1965); (8) brown fat in rats (Suter, 1969); and (9) livers of four apparently normal dogs (*Plate 73, Fig. 5*).

The rat liver seems to be quite prone to the formation of such mitochondria, and this kind of mitochondrial transformation has been seen after the administration of various drugs, such as: (1) carbon tetrachloride (Reynolds, 1960) (*Plate 73, Figs. 1–4, 6 and 7*); (2) ammonium carbonate (David and Kettler, 1961); and (3) alcohol (Kiessling and Tobe, 1964; Porta *et al.*, 1965; Koch *et al.*, 1968). Such mitochondria have also been seen in the liver of foetal rats when the mothers received prednisolone during pregnancy (Hill and Blackburn, 1967).

Other situations in which these mitochondria have been seen include: (1) the great alveolar cells of oxygen-adapted rats exposed to 100 per cent oxygen (Rosenbaum *et al.*, 1969; Yamamoto *et al.*, 1970); (2) kidney of winter-starved frogs (Karnovsky, 1962, 1963); (3) rat brain tissue fixed by glutaraldehyde perfusion after a delay of 1 hour (Karlson and Schultz, 1966); (4) clear cell carcinoma of kidney (Seljelid and Ericsson, 1965); (5) oncocytoma (Askew *et al.*, 1971); (6) Fortner hamster melanoma (Wolff *et al.*, 1971); and (7) human leukaemia (Ghadially and Skinnider, unpublished observations; see page 116).

The significance of such transformation of mitochondrial morphology is obscure.

Since cup-shaped mitochondria have been seen in the liver after the administration of various toxic agents, and at times these organelles proceed to the formation of membranous whorls and myelin figures, one could argue that this is a degenerative phenomenon. On the other hand, such mitochondria were considered by Rosenbaum *et al.* (1969) to represent an adaptive change in the lungs of rats treated with various concentrations of oxygen, and evidence was presented that this change may be reversible. Others (Stephens and Bils, 1965) have seen an analogy between the cup-shaped mitochondrion and the mitochondria associated with lipid droplets. In the latter instance the mitochondrion spreads out over a lipid droplet and assumes a cup-shaped form, and this, as we have noted, seems to be a functionally meaningful relationship (see page 126). Hence, one can argue that, since in the cup-shaped mitochondrion there is an increase in the mitochondrial surface and a more extensive or close relationship between the mitochondrion and cytoplasmic structures, this may facilitate exchanges between the cytoplasm and the mitochondrion.

Plate 74

From the adrenal cortex of a normal cow. (*Ghadially and Ailsby, unpublished electron micrographs*)

Fig. 1. Numerous mitochondria with cresentic or concentric tubular cristae, demarcating a circular area of matrix, are evident. × 23,000

Fig. 2. Two 'doughnut' mitochondria (A and B) and a mitochondrion (C) with a cresentic crista are present. It is evident that in certain planes of sectioning C would present an image similar to that seen at A or B. × 35,000

Figs. 3 and 4. Another ring-shaped mitochondrion with a large central 'hole', and a mitochondrion with two 'holes'. × 53,000; × 46,000

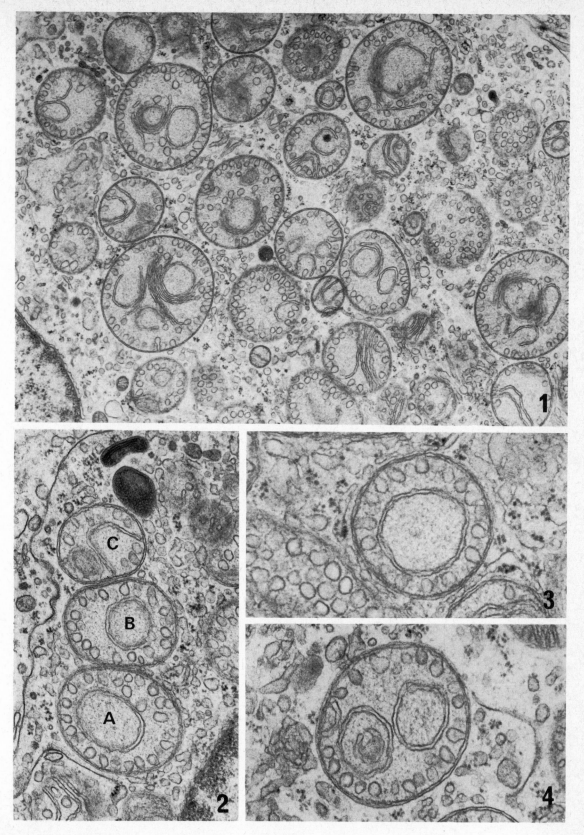

Glycogen inclusions in mitochondria appear morphologically similar to the common glycogen deposits that occur in the cytoplasm (see page 444). Usually such inclusions consist of mono-particulate glycogen (β-glycogen, 150–350 Å diameter), but in rare instances glycogen rosettes (α-glycogen, 600–900 Å diameter) are also seen. Both true and false inclusions occur. The latter are merely invaginations of the mitochondrial envelope, containing glycogen and other cyto-plasmic material, and they are distinguishable by the double membranes of the mitochondrial envelope demarcating them from the mitochondrial matrix.

True intramitochondrial glycogen inclusions present as: (1) small deposits of glycogen particles lying within expanded cristae or the intramembranous chamber; (2) larger deposits lying in a compartment enclosed by a single membrane; or (3) a collection of glycogen particles apparently lying in the matrix.

Numerous studies attest to the fact that glycogen is deposited in the intracristal space (*Plate 75*), and it seems that the single-membrane-limited type of deposit is a further stage of develop-ment of this process. It is tempting to speculate that deposits seen lying, or apparently lying, in the matrix are derived by dissolution or outward displacement of this limiting membrane till it is no longer identifiable. However, the possibility that true matrical deposits also some-times occur cannot be ruled out by such considerations.

Intramitochondrial glycogen has been seen in: (1) spermatozoa of pulmonates and sea-urchin (Personne and Andre, 1964; Andre, 1965; Anderson, 1968; Personne and Anderson, 1970); (2) prothoracic gland of silkworm (Beaulaton, 1964); (3) hypobranchial gland of molluscs (Fain-Manrel, 1966); (4) digestive cells of *Hydra* (Lentz, 1966); (5) Inter-renal (adrenocortical) cells of the spotted salamander (Picheral, 1968; Berchtold, 1969); (6) *Drosophila* heart (Burch *et al.*, 1970); (7) rat pinealocytes (Lin, 1965); (8) retinal receptor cells of rat (Ishikawa and Pei, 1965; Ishikawa and Yamada, 1969); (9) lumbar spinal ganglia of frog (Berthold, 1966); (10) axons in prelaminar optic nerve of normal monkeys, (Schutta *et al.*, 1970); (11) neurons of rats with bilirubin encephalopathy (Schutta *et al.*, 1970); (12) dystrophic axoplasm (Lampert, 1967); (13) mouse hepatocytes in riboflavin deficiency (Tandler *et al.*, 1968); (14) myopathy and cardio-myopathy in man (Hulsmann *et al.*, 1967; D'Agostino *et al.*, 1968; Hug and Schubert, 1970); and (15) human adenolymphoma, and oncocytoma (Tandler and Shipkey, 1964; Tandler, 1966; Hubner *et al.*, 1967; Tandler *et al.*, 1970).

Plate 75

Glycogen deposits in mitochondria from visual receptor cells of normal rat retina. Such deposits are not seen in new-born rats; they are first detectable at 3 months and are quite common in rats over 1 year old. (*From Ishikawa and Pei, 1965*)

Fig. 1. A mitochondrion in a synaptic spherule, showing a few glycogen particles lying in the intracristal space (arrow). × 41,000

Figs. 2 and 3. Intramitochondrial single-membrane-bound glycogen deposits are seen in these electron micrographs. × 41,000; × 41,000

Fig. 4. A large glycogen deposit is seen in a mitochondrion. The cristae are pushed to the periphery. × 38,000

Fig. 5. Mitochondrion from the inner segment of rat retina incubated with saliva. The clear area represents a zone from which glycogen was removed by this procedure. × 33,000

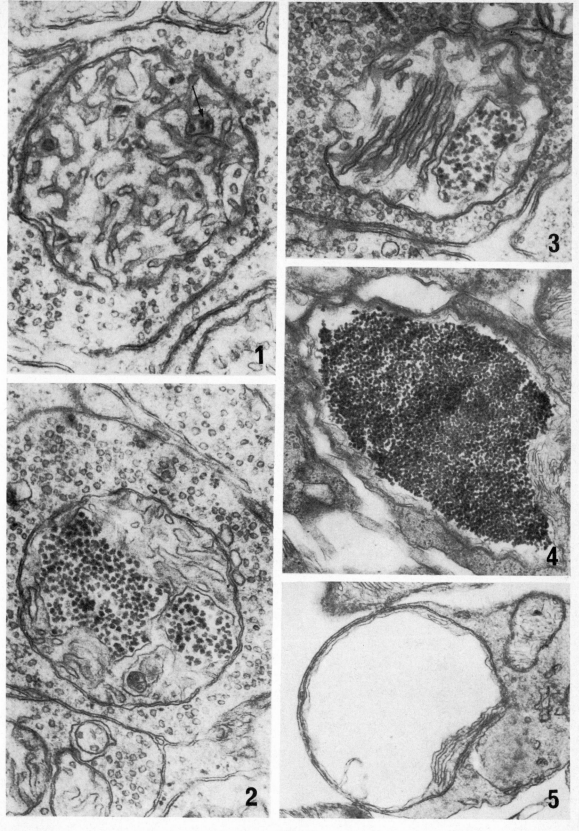

The manner in which glycogen appears in the mitochondrion and the significance of this phenomenon are difficult to evaluate. One may postulate that glycogen particles are taken in by some process akin to phagocytosis, or that glycogen is synthesized or at least polymerized from morphologically undetectable units (monomers or dimers) taken up via the mitochondrial membranes. For the former hypothesis (phagocytosis) there is no support, but for the latter some support may be found at least in the case of spermatocyte mitochondria of the type mentioned earlier. Here there is evidence (Anderson, 1968; Personne and Anderson, 1970) that enzymes for synthesis and degradation of glycogen exist in these organelles and that such deposits provide energy for metabolism and motility.

Such a situation, however, has not been demonstrated in mitochondria in other sites. Indeed, it is generally accepted, mainly on the basis of studies on isolated liver and muscle mitochondria, that the enzymes necessary for glycogenogenesis and glycogenolysis reside outside these organelles, and that any activity of this type seen in isolated mitochondrial fractions is due to contamination of the sample by enzymes derived from the cytoplasm or other cellular components.

Nevertheless, differences may exist between mitochondria in different sites, and there may also be differences engendered by altered physiological and pathological states. Certainly the notion that synthesis or at least polymerization of glycogen can occur in some mitochondria is compatible with morphological appearances. An observation made by Tandler et al. (1970) seems pertinent here. They found α-glycogen-containing mitochondria in oncocytes whose cytoplasm contained only β-glycogen, and they state, 'at a minimum oncocytoma mitochondria possess the enzymes necessary to convert β-glycogen to α-glycogen'.

Plate 76

Glycogen-containing mitochondria from an oncocytoma. (*From Tandler, Hutter and Erlandson, 1970*)
Fig. 1. Three glycogen-containing mitochondria. ×23,000
Fig. 2. A mitochondrion containing glycogen rosettes (α-glycogen). ×44,000
Fig. 3. A dividing mitochondrion (partition indicated by arrow). A single-membrane-bound glycogen deposit is present. ×52,000

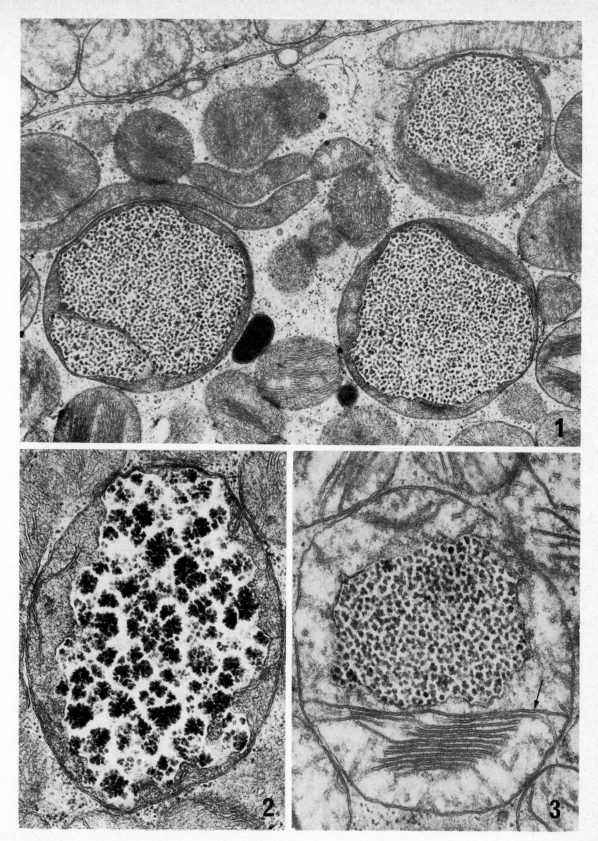

165

Intramitochondrial lipidic inclusions are characterized by the lack of a limiting membrane, an amorphous appearance, a medium to high electron density, and a rounded or irregular form. Either solitary or multiple inclusions can occur in a single mitochondrion. Morphologically, then, these inclusions are similar to the lipid inclusions found in the cytoplasm of various cells.

Nevertheless, confident diagnosis of lipid inclusions in mitochondria is beset by many difficulties. When a medium or high density inclusion, morphologically similar to a cytoplasmic lipid droplet, is sighted in a mitochondrion, it is difficult to rule out the possibility that it could be some entirely different material or that it may contain other constituents besides lipid. A small osmiophilic lipid droplet might be confused with a rather large matrical dense granule, and often the possibility that the inclusion comprises lipoprotein rather than lipid cannot be ruled out. Therefore in the electron microscopic literature, many examples of presumably lipidic inclusion have been referred to by the non-committal term 'dense inclusions'. Since such inclusions are smaller than mitochondria, histochemical analysis with the light microscope is hardly feasible, and unless numerous mitochondria in a sample of tissue contain such inclusions the effect of lipid solvents cannot be confidently assessed with the aid of the electron microscope.

Yet another source of difficulty stems from the close association which develops between mitochondria and cytoplasmic lipid droplets. It has already been noted (page 126) that in such an instance a lipid droplet may lie in a deep invagination of the mitochondrial envelope and that in certain planes of sectioning it may appear to lie within the mitochondrion. The situation here is analogous to pseudoinclusions of the nucleus, and one could contend that the lipid droplet is still in fact outside the mitochondrion. However, contact between the mitochondrion and lipid droplet is said at times to lead to the dissolution of the mitochondrial envelope, so one might also contend that a true intramitochondrial lipid inclusion could also be derived in this fashion.

Plate 77

Figs. 1 and 2. Mitochondria from the brown fat of a squirrel, showing lipid droplets (L) apparently lying in the mitochondrion. Many examples of close association of lipid and mitochondria were present in this tissue. This, combined with the fact that there is a dense halo around the droplets, suggests the presence of obliquely sectioned membranes in this region. It is therefore difficult to accept these as examples of true intramitochondrial lipid inclusions. ×39,000; ×26,000 (*Grodums, unpublished electron micrographs*)

Figs. 3 and 4. Mitochondria from the suprarenal cortex of a cow showing electron-dense lipid (L) inclusions. Small examples of these could be confused with enlarged matrical granules. ×39,000; ×41,000

Fig. 5. A swollen mitochondrion with sparse cristae containing a medium-density inclusion morphologically acceptable as lipid (L). From a human hepatoma. ×90,000 (*Ghadially and Parry, 1966*)

Fig. 6. A partitioned (dividing) mitochondrion from a rat liver in which an RD_3 sarcoma was transplanted. Note the lipidic inclusions (L) and virtual absence of cristae. ×32,000 (*Parry, unpublished electron micrograph*)

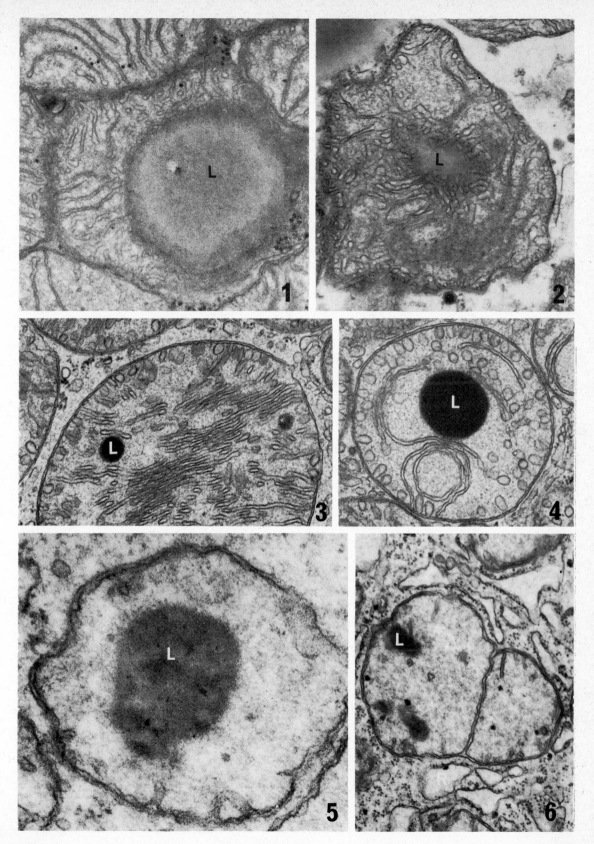

Besides the above-mentioned situation, intramitochondrial inclusions acceptable as lipidic in nature on morphological grounds have been seen in a variety of tissues. Occasional mitochondria of the suprarenal cortex of normal man and other animals contain one or two small osmiophilic lipidic droplets (*Plate 77*). Many mitochondria in the brown adipose tissue of neonatal rats also contain one or two electron-dense lipid droplets morphologically similar to those illustrated in the suprarenal cortex of the cow (*Plate 77, Figs. 3 and 4*), and Suter and Satbuli (1970) have shown that such inclusions are absent in isolated mitochondria treated with lipid solvents. Prolonged treatment with Pronase did not affect the inclusions, so they probably do not contain much protein. Since these intramitochondrial lipid inclusions disappear during early post-natal life, at a stage when the mitochondria in the brown fat enlarge in size, it has been suggested by these authors that the lipid is probably used for the synthesis of the lipoprotein membranes of the cristae.

In the above-mentioned examples, lipidic inclusions were noted in normal-looking mito-chondria with well formed cristae, where presumably the lipid has a physiological role. But there are other examples where lipidic inclusions have been seen in pathologically altered mito-chondria with sparse cristae, and it would appear that such lipid or lipoprotein inclusions are derived by breakdown or disintegration of the cristae (*Plate 77, Figs. 5 and 6; Plate 78*).

Such lipidic inclusions have often been noted in degenerating giant mitochondria (see *Plate 70*) and we (Ghadially and Parry, unpublished observations) have seen such intramitochondrial lipid or lipoprotein inclusions in the liver of rats bearing carcinogen-induced subcutaneous sarcomas, and also in a human hepatoma. Rat hepatocyte mitochondria with numerous irregular-shaped inclusions acceptable as lipid or lipoprotein were found by Parry (personal communica-tion), when an RD_3 sarcoma was transplanted into the livers of these animals (*Plate 78, Fig. 2*). Deposits of a similar morphology have also been noted in the mitochondria of stimulated rat adrenals (for references, see Giacomelli *et al.*, 1965) and other steroid-secreting cells in various experimental or pathological situations, and several workers have regarded them as intra-mitochondrial lipid accumulations (Lever, 1956; Gordon *et al.*, 1964).

Irregular-shaped electron-dense intramitochondrial inclusions were found in a great number of hepatocyte mitochondria of ethionine-fed rats by Minick *et al.* (1965), so they were able to trace the stages of development of these inclusions. Numerous mitochondria with centrally placed stacked cristae similar to those shown in *Plate 78, Fig. 1*, were seen, and they concluded that the inclusions were derived by breakdown of cristae of such altered mitochondria.

Plate 78

Fig. 1. Mitochondria from liver of a rat bearing a transplanted tumour in its flank. Note the centrally placed cristae (C) and irregular electron-dense deposit, presumably lipid or lipoprotein in nature (L). × 50,000

Fig. 2. A mitochondrion from a rat liver in which an RD_3 sarcoma was transplanted. Note the irregular masses of electron-dense material, presumed to be lipid or lipoprotein in nature (L). × 80,000 (*Parry, unpublished electron micrograph*)

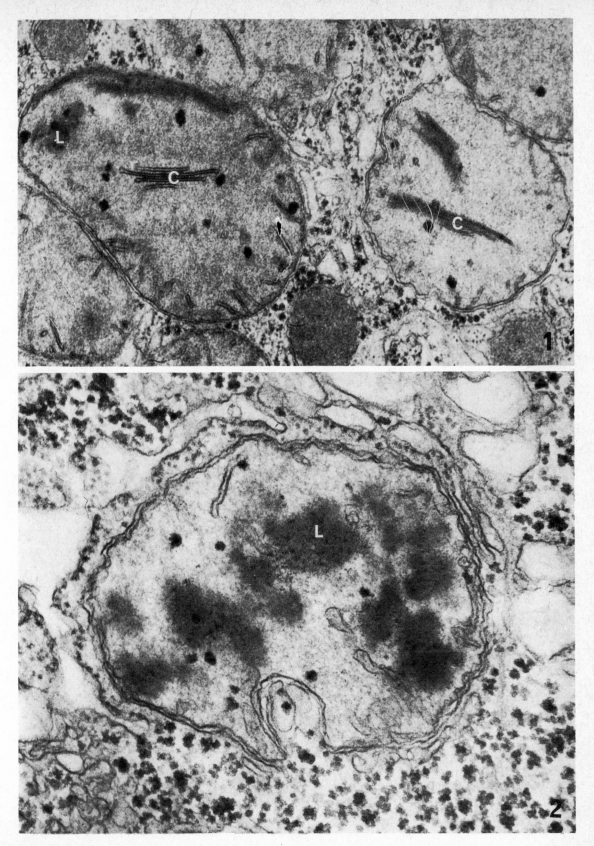

INTRAMITOCHONDRIAL CRYSTALLINE INCLUSIONS

Crystalline inclusions generally assumed to be protein have been noted in various cell compartments such as the nucleus (see page 62), cytoplasm (see page 452) and mitochondria. Details of structure vary, but the characteristic feature of crystals in all sites is that they have a highly ordered pattern of internal organization. Terms such as 'crystalloid' or 'paracrystalline' inclusions are employed when the ordered arrangement is less than the expected ideal. Obviously, many differences in fine structure exist between crystals found in various situations. However, certain general considerations about the appearance of crystals in electron micrographs are worth noting before dealing with intramitochondrial crystals.

The appearance of crystals in ultrathin sections depends, among other things, on the plane of sectioning with respect to the plane of the crystal lattice (*Plates 79 and 80*). Thus, in longitudinal sections a crystal may present as a system of closely spaced parallel 'lines', in transverse section as an ordered array of 'dots' and in oblique sections as a lattice (*Plate 31*) honeycomb pattern or reticular pattern (*Plate 79, Fig. 3*). The 'parallel line' pattern has been interpreted in some instances as representing longitudinal sections through filaments, rods, tubules or microtubules; in other instances it is quite clear that this 'parallel line' image is produced by an off-register superimposition of rows of spherical or short cylindrical units. Similarly the 'dot' pattern may be interpreted either as transverse sections through rods, filaments or tubules, or as representing macromolecular units of globular, granular or short cylindrical form. The lattice pattern could be produced by interlacing filaments, or again by off-register superimposed images of closely packed but highly ordered arrays of 'dots'. The true three-dimensional structure of most crystals still awaits clarification.

Intramitochondrial crystals or paracrystalline inclusions have been noted in various normal and pathological tissues, such as: (1) brown fat (Napolitano and Fawcett, 1958); (2) renal tubules of hibernating snakes (Kurosumi *et al.*, 1966); (3) renal tubules of frogs collected in the winter (*Plate 80, Fig. 3*); (4) renal tubules of rat (Osvaldo and Latta, 1966); (5) oöcytes of amphibians and certain cells in early embryogenesis (Ward, 1962; Karasaki, 1963); (6) epitheliomuscular cells of *Hydra* (Davis, 1967); (7) retinal rods of frog's eye (Yamada, 1959); (8) pinealocytes (Lin, 1965); (9) rat and domestic fowl adrenals fixed by glutaraldehyde perfusion (Kjaerheim, 1967); (10) chorioallantoric placenta of the rat (Ollerich, 1968); (11) thyroid follicular cells of rats treated with propylthiouracil and potassium iodide (Fujita and Machino, 1964); and (12) giant mitochondria in various tissues (see page 148).

In the liver of man, intramitochondrial crystals have been seen in giant mitochondria, and also at times in normal-sized mitochondria in various pathological states, such as carcinoma of the bile duct, obstructive jaundice, viral hepatitis, alcoholism, diabetes mellitus, Weil's disease,

---

Plate 79

Intramitochondrial crystals from the liver of a patient with hepatitis.
Fig. 1. Longitudinally sectioned crystal, presenting as a series of evenly spaced parallel lines. × 89,000
Fig. 2. Transversely sectioned crystal, showing discrete dot pattern. × 200,000
Fig. 3. Obliquely sectioned crystal, showing a reticular pattern. × 220,000

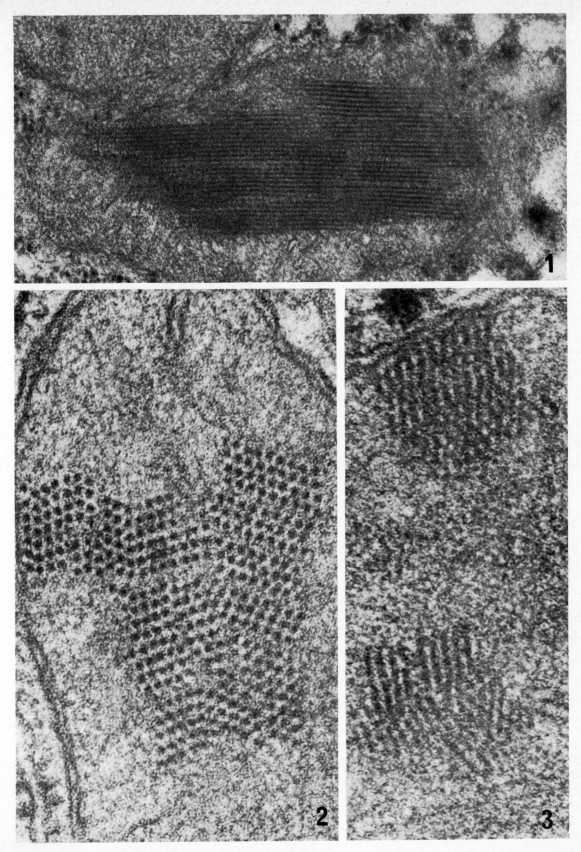

Waldenström's disease, bacterial infections, amyloidosis, congenital defects of bilirubin meta-bolism, hepatitis, mucopolysaccharidosis, type I hyperlipoproteinaemia, Wilson's disease, mushroom poisoning and after prolonged use of oral contraceptives. Such crystalline inclusions are also said to occur occasionally in the mitochondria of normal human liver, but this view has been challenged recently (for references, see David, 1964; Shiraki and Neustein, 1971; Bhagwat and Ross, 1971; Bhagwat *et al.*, 1972).

The mitochondria of human liver seem to be singularly prone to crystal formation. Reports dealing with such crystalloids in the liver of other animals are few except for the dog, where they have been reported to occur in: (1) protein deficiency (Ericsson *et al.*, 1966); (2) sulfame-thoxypyrazine administration (Stein *et al.*, 1966); (3) *in vivo* ischaemia (Swenson *et al.*, 1967); (4) hypovolaemic shock (Blair *et al.*, 1968); and (5) three apparently normal dogs (Shiraki and Neustein, 1971). Intramitochondrial crystalloids have also been noted in the liver of monkeys receiving alcohol (Voelz, 1968) and in the liver of pigs poisoned with lead (Watrach, 1964).

Rectangular intramitochondrial crystals have been observed in a variety of muscular diseases (for references, see Chou, 1969). These crystals seem to develop in the intracristal or intermem-branous compartment (*Plate 80, Fig. 1*), in contrast to the crystals in hepatocyte mitochondria mentioned above, which develop in the matrix compartment (*Plate 80, Figs. 2 and 3*). Some workers consider that the crystals are composed of spherical subunits 50–100 Å in diameter, but Chou (1969) considers that the subunits are filamentous structures arranged in a double helix.

Little is known about the chemistry or significance of intramitochondrial crystals. Such crystals in hibernating animals and oöcytes may well represent a form of protein storage, but those seen in human hepatocytes are generally regarded as a product of degenerative changes in the mitochondrion. Another possibility is that they might represent crystallized mitochondrial enzymic proteins. There is as yet little to support or refute such assumptions.

Plate 80

Fig. 1. A mitochondrion from an atrophic deltoid muscle showing rectangular paracrystalline inclusions lying in the intracristal space. Each crystal is surrounded by a membrane, derived from a crista. × 71,000 (*Ghadially and Ailsby, unpublished electron micrograph*)

Fig. 2. Most of the crystals in this hepatocyte mitochondrion from a case of hepatitis present as a highly ordered array of electron-dense dots. In one instance, however (arrow), the plane of sectioning is such that the dots are partially superimposed to form a pattern of dotted parallel lines. × 72,000

Fig. 3. A mitochondrion containing a crystalline inclusion, from a renal tubular cell of a winter-starved frog. × 107,000

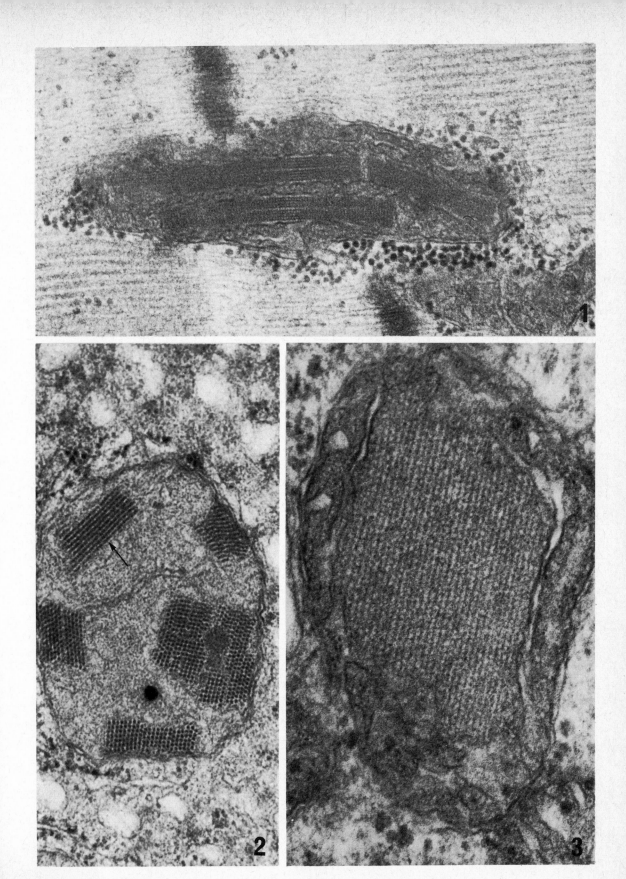

Small deposits of intracellular iron-containing electron-dense particles (ferritin and/or haemo-siderin) may normally be found in the reticuloendothelial system. Larger deposits occur locally in tissues after a haemorrhage (see page 320) or in the reticuloendothelial system, liver and other sites in conditions of iron overload produced by a variety of diseases and experimental pro-cedures. Such deposits take the form of fine electron-dense particles scattered diffusely in the cytoplasmic matrix and/or collection of particles in single-membrane-bound lysosomal bodies called siderosomes (Richter, 1957). In the early literature, before the lysosome concept had evolved, iron deposits were at times erroneously thought to be localized in mitochondria. How-ever, it is now clear that as a rule intramitochondrial iron deposits do not occur in such conditions (Kuff and Dalton, 1957; Bessis and Caroli, 1959).

Substantial deposits of intramitochondrial iron are, however, frequently observed in erythro-blasts and reticulocytes in sideroblastic anaemia (Bessis and Breton-Gorius, 1961; Sorenson, 1962; Heilmeyer *et al.*, 1962; Larizza and Orlandi, 1964; Tanaka, 1967), but even in this condition some iron is found in single-membrane-bound bodies acceptable as siderosomes.

Mollin and Hoffbrand (1968) define sideroblastic anaemia as 'a dyshaemopoietic anaemia in which there is defective synthesis of haemoglobin associated with an abnormal accumulation of ionizable iron granules in the erythroblasts, some of which show a ' "ring" or "collar" of iron granules around the nucleus'. Electron microscopy shows that the ring sideroblast owes its appearance to a perinuclear distribution of iron-containing mitochondria (*Plate 81, Fig. 1*). At higher magnifications it is abundantly clear that the iron deposits lie in the mitochondrial matrix between the cristae (*Plate 81, Fig. 2*; *Plate 82, Fig. 1*), and that the iron occurs in a much finer form than the occasional aggregates of ferritin found in the cytoplasm of these cells (*Plate 82, Fig. 2*).

Plate 81

From bone marrow of a case of sideroblastic anaemia secondary to Hodgkin's disease.
Fig. 1. Normoblast, showing perinuclear distribution of mitochondria containing iron deposits. × 19,000
Fig. 2. A group of iron-containing mitochondria found in the cytoplasm of a reticuloycte. × 78,000

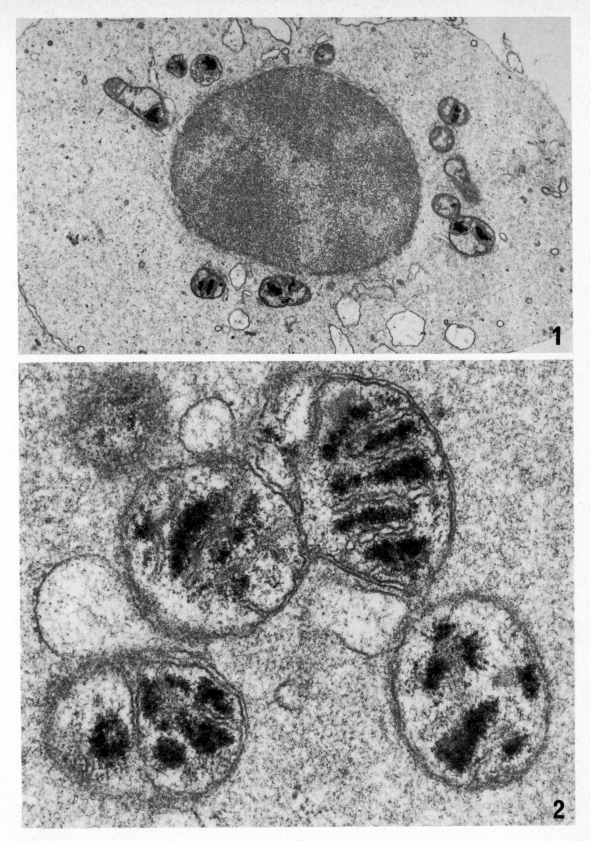

175

Tanaka (1967) has claimed that intramitochondrial iron is also seen in reticulum cells of the bone marrow in sideroblastic anaemia, but other workers (including ourselves—Ghadially and Skinnider) have not observed this in their material. Intramitochondrial iron has also been reported to occur in erythroid cells of apparently normal guinea-pigs and in thalassaemia (Bessis and Breton-Gorius, 1961), but this has not been reported by other workers. I can, however, confirm that the guinea-pig marrow does at times contain mitochondria with iron inclusions.

Sideroblastic anaemia is a chronic anaemia which is usually refractory to treatment and occurs despite the presence of adequate or large iron stores and high serum iron values. Two main varieties of this anaemia are known to occur. A primary or idiopathic variety which is sometimes hereditary, and a secondary variety associated with various disorders (for details, see Mollin and Hoffbrand, 1968) including malignancies such as Hodgkin's disease (*Plates 81 and 82*).

It would appear that the accumulation of iron in mitochondria is provoked by deficient porphyrin or haem synthesis. Mitochondria are known to be involved in the synthesis of porphyrin and the incorporation of iron into porphyrin to produce haem (Remington, 1957; Sano *et al.*, 1959). It is conceivable, therefore, that enzymatic defects in mitochondria may hinder such a synthesis and the iron destined for incorporation into haemoglobin would then accumulate in the mitochondrion.

Plate 82

From the same tissue as *Plate 81*.
Fig. 1. High power view of an iron-containing mitochondrion. The fine particulate nature of the deposit and the high electron density is clearly seen. The iron deposits lie in the matrix between the cristae. × 110,000
Fig. 2. The difference between the fine powdery intramitochondrial deposits of iron (A) and a ferritin deposit (B) in the cytoplasm is demonstrated in this electron micrograph. × 100,000

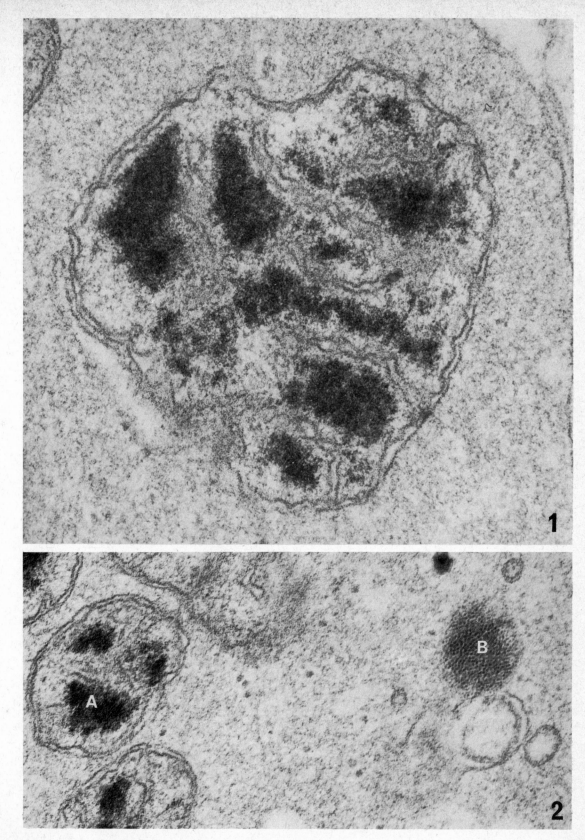

G

REFERENCES

Aho, A. J., Arstila, A. U., Ahonen, J. and Scheinin, T. M. (1970). 'The fine structural changes in intestinal epithelium cells in acute experimental mesenteric vascular occlusion.' *Scand. J. clin. Lab. Invest.* **25**, Suppl. 113, 58

Alpert, L., Pai, S. H., Zak, F. G. and Werthamer, S. (1972). 'Cardiomyopathy associated with a pheochromocytoma.' *Archs Path.* **93**, 544

Anderson, W. A. (1968). 'Cytochemistry of sea urchin gametes. I. Intramitochondrial localisation of glycogen, glucose-6-phosphatase, and adenosine triphosphatase activity in spermatozoa of *Paracentrotus lividus.*' *J. Ultrastruct. Res.* **24**, 398

—(1969). 'Nuclear and cytoplasmic DNA synthesis during early embryogenesis of *Paracentrotus lividus.*' *J. Ultrastruct. Res.* **26**, 95

André, J. (1962). 'Contribution à la connaissance du chondriome; étude de ses modifications ultrastructurales pendant la spermatogénèse.' *J. Ultrastruct. Res.* Suppl. 3

—(1965). 'Quelques données recentes sur la structure et la physiologie des mitochondries: glycogène, particules element-aires, acides nucleiques.' *Archs Biol., Liege,* **76**, 277

Arcasoy, M. M. and Smuckler, E. A. (1969). 'Acute effects of digoxin intoxication on rat hepatic and cardiac cells.' *Lab. Invest.* **20**, 190

Arhelger, R. B., Broom, J. S. and Boler, R. K. (1965). 'Ultrastructural hepatic alterations following tannic acid admini-stration to rabbits.' *Am. J. Path.* **46**, 409

Askew, J. B., Fechner, R. E., Bentinck, D. C. and Jenson, A. B. (1971). 'Epithelial and myoepithelial oncocytes. Ultra-structural study of a salivary gland oncocytoma.' *Archs Otolar.* **93**, 46

Barka, T., Scheuer, P. J., Schaffner, F. and Popper, H. (1964). 'Structural changes of liver cells in copper intoxication.' *Archs Path.* **78**, 331

Beams, H. W. and Tahmisian, T. N. (1954). 'Structure of the mitochondria in the male germ cells of Helix as revealed by the electron microscope.' *Expl Cell Res.* **6**, 87

Beaulaton, J. (1964) 'Sur l'accumulation intramitochondriale de glycogène dans la gland prothoracigne du ver à soie du chêne *Antheraea peruyi* (Guér) pendant les quatrième et cinquième stades larvaires.' *C.r. Acad. Sci. (D), Paris* **258**, 4139

Benda, C. (1902). 'Die mitochondria.' *Ergebn. Anat. Entw. Gesch.* **12**, 743

Berchtold, J. P. (1969). 'Contribution à l'étude ultrastructurale des cellules interrénales de *Salamandra salamandra L* (Amphibien urodèle). 1. Conditions normales.' *Z. Zellforsch. mikrosk. Anat.* **102**, 357

Berger, E. R. (1964). 'Mitochondria genesis in the retinal photoreceptor inner segment.' *J. Ultrastruct. Res.* **11**, 90

Bergeron, M. and Droz, B. (1969). 'Protein renewal in mitochondria as revealed by electron microscope radioauto-graphy'. *J. Ultrastruct. Res.* **26**, 17

Bernhard, W. and Rouiller, C. (1956). 'Close topographical relationship between mitochondria and ergastoplasm of liver cells in a definite phase of cellular activity.' *J. biophys. biochem. Cytol.* **2**, Suppl., 73

Berthold, C. H. (1966). 'Ultrastructural appearance of glycogen in the β-neurons of the lumbar spinal ganglia of the frog.' *J. Ultrastruct. Res.* **14**, 254

Bessis, M. and Breton-Gorius, J. (1961). 'Presence de fer dans les mitochondries des erythroblastes chez le cobaye normal.' *Nouv. Rev. franc. Hemat.* **1**, 356

— — (1969). 'Pathologie et asynchronisme de developpmente des organelles cellulaires au cours des leucemies aigues granulocytaires.' *Nouv. Rev. franc. Hemat.* **9**, 245

— and Caroli, J. (1959). 'A comparative study of hemachromatosis by electron microscopy.' *Gastroenterology* **37**, 538

Bhagwat, A. G. and Ross, R. C. (1971). 'Hepatic intramitochondrial crystalloids.' *Archs Path.* **91**, 70

— — and Currie, D. J. (1972). 'Ultrastructure of normal human liver.' *Archs Path.* **93**, 227

Bishop, S. P. and Cole, C. R. (1969). 'Ultrastructural changes in the canine myocardium with right ventricular hyper-trophy and congestive heart failure.' *Lab. Invest.* **20**, 219

Blackburn, W. R. and Vinijchaikul, K. (1969). 'The pancreas in kwashiorkor. An electron microscopic study.' *Lab. Invest.* **20**, 305

Blair, O. M., Stenger, R. J., Hopkins, R. W. and Simeone, F. A. (1968). 'Hepatocellular ultrastructure in dogs with hypovolemic shock.' *Lab. Invest.* **18**, 172

Boler, R. K. and Bibighaus, A. J. (1967). 'Ultrastructural alterations of dog livers during endotoxin shock.' *Lab. Invest.* **17**, 537

Bowman, R. W. (1967). 'Mitochondrial connections in canine Myocardium.' *Tex. Rep. Biol. Med.* **25**, 517

Brandt, P. W. and Pappas, G. D. (1959). 'The nuclear-mitochondrial relationship in *Pelomyxa carolinensis.*' *J. biophys. biochem. Cytol.* **6**, 91

Brown, R. A., Chiu, C., Scott, H. J. and Gurd, F. N. (1970). 'Ultrastructural changes in the canine ileal musosal cell after mesenteric arterial occlusion.' *Archs Surg., Chicago* **101**, 290

Burch, G. E., Sohal, R. and Fairbanks, L. D. (1970). 'Ultrastructural changes in Drosophila heart with age.' *Archs Path., Chicago* **89**, 128

Butler, W. H. and Judha, J. D. (1970). 'Ultrastructural studies on mitochondrial swelling.' *Biochem. J.* **118**, 883

Cameron, G. R. (1952). *Pathology of the Cell.* Edinburgh: Oliver and Boyd

Campiche, M. (1960). 'Les inclusions lamellaires des cellules alvéolaires dans le poumon du raton. Relations entre l'ultrastructure et la fixation.' *J. Ultrastruct. Res.* **3**, 302

Caulfield, J. B. and Schrag, P. E. (1964). 'Electron microscopic study of renal calcification.' *Am. J. Path.* **44**, 365

Chappell, J. B., Greville, G. D. and Bicknell, K. E. (1962). 'Stimulation of respiration of isolated mitochondria by manganese ions.' *Biochem. J.* **84**, 61p

178

Chou, S. M. (1969). '"Megaconial" mitochondria observed in a case of chronic polymyositis.' *Acta neuropath.* **12,** 68

Copeland, D. E. and Dalton, A. J. (1959). 'An association between mitochondria and the endoplasmic reticulum in cells of the pseudobranch gland of a Teleost.' *J. biophys. biochem. Cytol.* **5,** 393

Coupland, R. E. and MacDougall, J. D. B. (1968). 'The effect of hyperbaric oxygen on rat liver cells in organ culture: a light- and electron-microscope study.' *J. Path. Bact.* **96,** 149

D'Agostino, A. N. (1963). 'An electron microscopic study of skeletal and cardiac muscle of the rat poisoned by plasmocid.' *Lab. Invest.* **12,** 1060

— (1964). 'An electron microscopic study of cardiac necrosis produced by 9-α-fluorocortisol and sodium phosphate.' *Am. J. Path.* **45,** 633

— Ziter, F. A., Rallison, M. L. and Bray, P. F. (1968). 'Familial myopathy with abnormal muscle mitochondria.' *Archs Neurol., Chicago* **18,** 388

Dalton, A. J. and Felix, M. D. (1957). 'Electron microscopy of mitochondria and the golgi complex.' *Symp. Soc. exp. Biol.* **10,** 148

David, H. (1964). *Submicroscopic Ortho and Pathomorpology of the Liver.* Translated by H. G. Epstein. Berlin: Akademie-Verlag. (Oxford: Pergamon Press; New York: Macmillan)

— and Kettler, L. H. (1961). 'Degeneration von Lebermitochondrien nach ammonium-intoxikation.' *Z. Zellforsch. mikrosk. Anat.* **53,** 857

Davis, L. E. (1967). 'Intramitochondrial crystals in Hydra.' *J. Ultrastruct. Res.* **21,** 125

De Robertis, E. and Bleichmar, H. (1962). 'Mitochondriogenesis in nerve fibers of the infrared receptor membrane of pit vipers.' *Z. Zellforsch. mikrosk. Anat.* **57,** 572

— and Sabatini, D. (1958). 'Mitochondrial changes in the adrenocortex of normal hamsters.' *J. biophys. biochem. Cytol.* **4,** 667

Dessouky, D. A. (1968). 'Electron microscopic studies of the myometrium of the guinea pig.' *Am. J. Obstet. Gynec.* **100,** 30

Duffy, J. L., Suzuki, Y. and Churg, J. (1971). 'Acute calcium nephropathy. Early proximal tubular changes in the rat kidney.' *Archs Path.* **91,** 340

Enders, A. C., Enders, R. K. and Schlafke, S. (1963). 'An electron microscope study of the gland cells of the mink endometrium.' *J. Cell Biol.* **18,** 405

Engfeldt, B., Gardell, S., Hellstrom, J., Ivemark, B., Rhodin, J. and Strandh, J. (1958). 'Effect of experimentally induced hyperparathyroidism on renal function and structure.' *Acta endocr.* **29,** 15

Ephrussi, B. (1953). *Nucleocytoplasmic Relations in Microorganisms,* p. 124. London: Oxford University Press

Ericsson, J. L. E. and Biberfeld, P. (1967). 'Studies on aldehyde fixation. Fixation rates and their relation to fine structure and some histochemical reactions in liver.' *Lab. Invest.* **17,** 281

— Orrenius, S. and Holm, I. (1966). 'Alterations in canine liver cells induced by protein deficiency: ultrastructural and biochemical observations.' *Expl Molec. Path.* **5,** 329

Ernster, L. and Luft, R. (1963). 'Further studies on a population of human skeletal muscle mitochondria lacking respiratory control.' *Expl Cell Res.* **32,** 26

Fain-Manrel, M. A. (1966). 'Localisations intramitochondriale et intracisternale de glycogene monoparticulaire.' *C.r. Acad. Sci. (D), Paris* **263,** 1107

Fawcett, D. W. (1955). 'Observations on the cytology and electron microscopy of hepatic cells.' *J. natn. Cancer Inst.* **15,** (Suppl.), 1475

— (1959) In *Developmenta Cytology.* Chapter 8. Ed. by D. Rudnick. New York: Ronald Press

— (1967). *The Cell: Its Organelles and Inclusions.* Philadelphia and London: Saunders

— and McNutt, M. S. (1969). 'The ultrastructure of the cat myocardium. I. Ventricular papillary muscle.' *J. Cell Biol.* **42,** 1

Ferrans, V. J., Hibbs, R. G., Weily, H. S., Weilbaecher, D. G., Walsh, J. J. and Burch, G. E. (1970). 'A histochemical and electron microscopic study of epinephrine-induced myocardial necrosis.' *J. Molec. Cell. Cardiol.* **1,** 11

— Buja, L. M., Levitsky, S. and Roberts, W. C. (1971). 'Effects of hyperosmotic perfusate on ultrastructure and function of the isolated canine heart.' *Lab. Invest.* **24,** 265

Fisher, E. R. and Horvat, B. (1971). 'Experimental production of so-called spironolactone bodies.' *Archs Path.* **91,** 471

Fisher, E. R., Copeland, C. and Fisher, B. (1967). 'Correlation of ultrastructure and function following hypothermic preservation of canine kidneys.' *Lab. Invest.* **17,** 99

Flaks, B. (1968). 'Unusual aspects of ultrastructural differentiation in rat hepatoma cells.' *J. Cell Biol.* **38,** 230

Flax, M. H. and Tisdale, W. A. (1964). 'An electron microscopic study of alcoholic hyalin.' *Am. J. Path.* **44,** 441

Fujita, H. and Machino, M. (1964). 'Fine structure of intramitochondrial crystals in rat thyroid follicular cell.' *J. Cell Biol.* **23,** 383

Gansler, H. and Rouiller, C. (1956). 'Modifications physiologiques et pathologiques du chondriom. Étude au microscope électronique.' *Schweiz. Z. Path. Bact.* **19,** 217

Geren, B. B. and Schmitt, F. O. (1954). 'The structure of the Schwann cell and its relation to the axon in certain invertebrate nerve fibers.' *Nat. Acad. Sci. Proc.* **40,** 863

Gey, G. O. (1956). 'Some aspects of the constitution and behaviour of normal and malignant cells maintained in continuous culture.' *Harvey Lect.* **50,** 154

Ghadially, F. N. and Parry, E. W. (1965). 'Ultrastructure of the liver of the tumor-bearing host.' *Cancer* **18,** 485

— — (1966). 'Ultrastructure of a human hepatocellular carcinoma and surrounding non-neoplastic liver.' *Cancer* **19,** 1989

— and Skinnider, L. F. (1974). 'Giant mitochondria in erythroleukaemia. *J. Path.* **114,** 113

Ghidoni, J. J. and Thomas, H. (1969). 'Connection between a mitochondrion and endoplasmic reticulum in liver.' *Experientia* **25,** 632

Giacomelli, F., Wiener, J. and Spiro, D. (1965). 'Cytological alterations related to stimulation of the zona glomerulosa of the adrenal gland.' *J. Cell Biol.* **26,** 499

Glinsmann, W. H. and Ericsson, J. L. E. (1966). 'Observations on the subcellular organization of hepatic parenchymal cells. II. Evolution of reversible alterations induced by hypoxia.' *Lab. Invest.* **15**, 762

Gonatas, N. K. and Shy, G. M. (1966). 'Childhood myopathies with abnormal mitochondria.' *Proc. 5th Int. Congr. Neuropath.,* Zurich, 1965. Int. Congr. Ser. No. 100, p. 606. Amsterdam: Excerpta Medica

Gordon, E. E. and Bernstein, J. (1970). 'Effect of valinomycin on mitochondrial ultrastructure and function of intact Ehrlich ascites tumor cells.' *Biochim. biophys. Acta* **205**, 464

Gordon, G. B., Miller, L. R. and Bensch, K. G. (1964). 'Electron microscopic observations of the gonad in the testicular feminization syndrome.' *Lab. Invest.* **13**, 152

Grasse, P. P., Carasso, N. and Favard, P. (1956). 'Les ultrastructures cellulaires au cours de la spermiogenese de l'escargot (*Helix pomatia* L.).' *Annls sci. nat. Zool.* (*11*) **18**, 339

Greenawalt, J. W., Foster, G. V. and Lehninger, A. L. (1962). 'The observation of unusual membranous structures associated with liver mitochondria in thyrotoxic rats.' In *Electron Microscopy,* Vol. 2, p. 00–5. Ed. by S. S. Breese, Jr. New York: Academic Press

Greenstein, J. P. (1954). *Biochemistry of Cancer.* New York: Academic Press

Gruner, J. E. (1963). 'Sur quelques anomalies mitochondriales observées au cours affections musculaires variées.' *C.r. Soc. Biol., Strasbourg* 157, 181

Gustafsson, R., Tata, J. R., Lindberg, O. and Ernster, L. (1965). 'The relationship between the structure and activity of rat skeletal muscle mitochondria after thyroidectomy and thyroid hormone treatment.' *J. Cell Biol.* **26**, 555

Hackenbrock, C. R. (1968a). 'Ultrastructural bases for metabolically linked mechanical activity in mitochondria. II. Electron transport linked ultrastructural transformations in mitochondria.' *J. Cell. Biol.* **37**, 345

— (1968b). 'Chemical and physical fixation of isolated mitochondria in low-energy and high-energy states.' *Proc. natn. Acad. Sci., USA* **61**, 598

Hagopian, M., Gershon, M. D. and Nunez, E. A. (1972). 'An ultrastructural study of the effect of reserpine on ventricular cardiac muscle of active and hibernating bats *(Myotis lucifugus)*.' *Lab. Invest.* **27**, 99

Heggtveit, H. A., Herman, L. and Mishra, R. K. (1964). 'Cardiac necrosis and calcification in experimental magnesium deficiency.' *Am. J. Path.* **45**, 757

Heilmeyer, V. L., Merker, H., Molbert, E. and Neidhardt, M. (1962). 'Zur Mikromorphologie der hereditaren hypochromen sideroachrestischen Anamie.' *Acta Haemat.* 27, 78

Herdson, P. B., Sommers, H. M. and Jennings, R. B. (1965). 'A comparative study of the fine structure of normal and ischemic dog myocardium with special reference to early changes following temporary occlusion of a coronary artery.' *Am. J. Path.* **46**, 367

Hill, R. B. and Blackburn, W. R. (1967). 'Effect of prednisolone treatment of pregnant rats on fetal liver structure and metabolism.' *Lab. Invest.* **17**, 146

Himmelhoch, S. R. and Karnovsky, M. J. (1961). 'Oxidative and hydrolytic enzymes in the nephron of *Necturus maculosus.*' *J. biophys. biochem. Cytol.* **9**, 893

Hiott, D. W. and Howell, R. D. (1971). 'Acute electron microscopic changes in myocardial cells induced by high doses of quinidine.' *Toxic. appl. Pharmac.* **18**, 964

Hoffman, H. and Grigg, G. W. (1958). 'An electronmicroscopic study of mitochondria formation.' *Expl Cell Res.* **15**, 118

Horvath, E., Somogyi, A. and Kovacs, K. (1970). 'Histochemical study of the electrolyte-steroid-cardiopathy with necrosis (ESCN) in rats.' *Cardiovasc. Res.* **4**, 355

Howatson, A. F. and Ham, A. W. (1957). 'The fine structure of cells.' *Can. J. Biochem. Physiol.* **35**, 549

Hruban, Z., Swift, H. and Slesers, A. (1965). 'Effect of triparanol and diethanolamine on the fine structure of hepatocytes and pancreatic acinar cells.' *Lab. Invest.* **14**, 1652

Hübner, G. (1965). 'Elektronenmikroskopische Untersuchungen zur Allylalkoholvergiftung der Mäuseleber.' *Verh. deutsch. Ges. Path.* **49**, 256

— Paulussen, F. and Kleinsasser, O. (1967). 'Zur Feinstruktur und Genese der Onkocyten.' *Virchows Arch. path. Anat. Physiol.* **343**, 34

Hug, G. and Schubert, W. K. (1970). 'Idiopathic cardiomyopathy. Mitochondrial and cytoplasmic alterations in heart and liver.' *Lab. Invest.* **22**, 541

Hulsmann, W. C. (1962). 'Fatty acid synthesis in heart sarcosomes.' *Biochim. biophys. Acta* **58**, 417

— Bethlem, J., Meijer, A. E. F. H., Fleury, P. and Schellens, J. P. M. (1967). 'Myopathy with abnormal structure and function of muscle mitochondria.' *J. Neurol. Neurosurg. Psychiat.* **30**, 519

Ishikawa, T. and Pei, Y. F. (1965). 'Intramitochondrial glycogen particles in rat retinal receptor cells.' *J. Cell Biol.* **25**, 402

— and Yamada, E. (1969). 'Atypical mitochondria in the ellipsoid of the photoreceptor cells of vertebrate retinas.' *Invest. Ophthal.* **8**, 302

Jezequel, A. M. (1959). 'Dégénérescence myélinique des mitochondries de foie humain dans un épithélioma du cholédoque et un ictère viral.' *J. ultrastruct. Res.* 3, 210

Kagawa, Y., Racker, E. and Hauser, R. E. (1966). 'Partial resolution of the enzymes catalysing oxidative phosphorylation X: Correlation of morphology and function in submitochondrial particles.' *J. Biochem.* **241**, 2475

Karasaki, S. (1963). 'Studies on amphibian yolk. I. The ultrastructure of the yolk platelet.' *J. Cell Biol.* **18**, 135

Karlson, U. and Schultz, R. L. (1966). 'Fixation of the central nervous system for electron microscopy by aldehyde perfusion. III. Structural changes after exsanguination and delayed perfusion.' *J. Ultrastruct. Res.* **14**, 47

Karnovsky, M. J. (1962). 'Mitochondrial changes and cytochrome oxidase in the frog nephron.' In *Electron Microscopy,* Vol. 2, p. Q–9, Ed. by S. S. Breese, Jr. New York: Academic Press

— (1963). 'The fine structure of mitochondria in the frog nephron correlated with cytochrome oxidase activity.' *Expl Molec. Path.* **2**, 347

180

Kerr, J. F. R. (1969). 'An electron-microscope study of liver cell necrosis due to heliotrine.' *J. Path.* **97,** 557

Kiessling, K. H. and Tobe, U. (1964). 'Degeneration of liver mitochondria in rats after prolonged alcohol consumption.' *Expl Cell Res.* **33,** 350

Kjaerheim, A. (1967). 'Crystallized tubules in the mitochondrial matrix of adrenal cortical cells.' *Expl Cell Res.* **45,** 236

Koch, D. R., Porta, E. A. and Hartroft, W. S. (1968). 'A new experimental approach in the study of chronic alcoholism. III. Role of alcohol versus sucrose or fat-derived calories in hepatic damage.' *Lab. Invest.* **18,** 379

Kuff, E. L. and Dalton, A. J. (1957). 'Identification of molecular ferritin in homogenates and sections of rat liver.' *J. Ultrastruct. Res.* **1,** 62

Kurosumi, K., Matsuzawa, T. and Watari, N. (1966). 'Mitochondrial inclusions in the snake renal tubules.' *J. Ultrastruct. Res.* **16,** 269

Lafontaine, J. G. and Allard, C. (1964). 'A light and electron microscope study of the morphological changes induced in rat liver cells by the azo dye 2-ME-DAB.' *J. Cell. Biol.* **22,** 143

Laguens, R. P. and Bianchi, N. (1963). 'Fine structure of the liver in human idiopathic diabetes mellitus. 1. Parenchymal cell mitochondria'. *Expl Molec. Path.* **2,** 203

— Lozada, B. B., Gomez-Dumm, C. L. and Beramendi, A. R. (1966). 'Effect of acute and exhaustive exercise upon the fine structure of heart mitochondria.' *Experientia* **22,** 244

Laiho, K. U., Shelburne, J. D. and Trump, B. F. (1971). 'Obervations on cell volume, ultrastructure, mitochondrial conformation and vital dye uptake in Ehrlich ascites tumor cells: effects of inhibiting energy production and function of the plasma membrane.' *Am. J. Path.* **65,** 203

Lampert, P. W. (1967). 'A comparative electron microscopic study of reactive, degenerating, regenerating and dystrophic axons.' *J. Neuropath. Exp. Neurol.* **26,** 345

Larizza, P. and Orlandi, F. (1964). 'Electron microscopic observations on bone marrow and liver tissue in non-hereditary refractory sideroblastic anemia.' *Acta haemat.* **31** 9

Leduc, E. H., Bernhard, W. and Tournier, P. (1966). 'Cyclic appearance of atypical mitochondria containing DNA fibers in cultures of an adenovirus-12-induced hamster tumor.' *Expl Cell Res.* **42,** 597

Leeson, C. R. and Leeson, T. S. (1969). 'Mitochondrial organization in skeletal muscle of the rat soft palate.' *J. Anat.* **105,** 363

Lehninger, A. L. (1960). 'Energy transformation in the cell.' *Scientific American* Reprint No. 69

— (1961). 'How cells transform energy.' *Scientific American* Reprint No. 91

— (1962). 'Water uptake and extrusion by mitochondria in relation to oxidative phosphorylation.' *Physiol. Rev.* **42,** 467

— (1965). *The Mitochondrion. Molecular basis of structure and function.* New York and Amsterdam: W. A. Benjamin

— (1970). *Biochemistry. The molecular basis of cell structure and function.* New York: Worth

— Rossi, C. S. and Greenawalt, J. W. (1963). 'Respiration-dependent accumulation of inorganic phosphate and Ca^{++} by rat liver mitochondria.' *Biochem. Biophys. Res. Comm.* **10,** 444

Lentz, T. L. (1966). 'Intramitochondrial glycogen granules in digestive cells of hydra.' *J. Cell. Biol.* **29,** 162

— (1971). *Cell Fine Structure.* Philadelphia, London and Toronto: Saunders

Lever, J. D. (1956). 'Physiologically induced changes in adrenocortical mitochondria.' *J. biophys. biochem. Cytol.* **2,** Suppl 313

Lin, H. S. (1965). 'Microcylinders within mitochondrial cristae in the rat pinealocyte.' *J. Cell Biol.* **25,** 435

Linnane, A. W., Vitols, E. and Nowland, P. G. (1962). 'Studies on the origin of yeast mitochondria.' *J. Cell Biol.* **13,** 345

Lozada, B. B. and Laguens, R. P. (1966). 'Hypoxia and the heart ultrastructure with special reference to the protective action of the coronary drug Persantin.' *Cardiologia* **49,** Suppl., 1, 33

Luft, R., Ikkos, D., Palmieri, F. Ernster, L. and Afzelius, B. (1962). 'A case of severe hypermetabolism of non-thyroid origin with a defect in the maintenance of mitochondrial respiratory control: a correlated clinical, biochemical and morphological study.' *J. clin. Invest.* **41,** 1776

Luse, S. (1961). 'Electron microscopic observations on the adrenal gland.' In *The Adrenal Cortex,* Ed. by H. D. Moon, p. 46. New York: Hoeber

Lynn, J. A., Bailey, J. J., Willis, J. M. and Race, G. J. (1969). 'Hepatic ultrastructural variations in apparently "normal" humans.' *Lab. Invest.,* Abstr. **20,** 594

McCallister, B. D. and Brown, A. L. (1965). 'A quantitative study of myocardial mitochondria in experimental cardiac hypertrophy.' *Lab. Invest.* **14,** 692

MacKay, B., Moloney, P. J. and Rix, D. B. (1968). 'The use of electron microscopy in renal preservation and perfusion.' In *Organ Perfusion and Preservation,* p. 697. Ed. by J. C. Norman, J. Folkman, W. G. Hardison, L. E. Rudolf and F. J. Veith. New York: Appleton-Century-Crofts

McNutt, N. S. and Fawcett, D. W. (1969). 'The ultrastructure of the cat myocardium. II. Atrial muscle.' *J. Cell Biol.* **42,** 46

Ma, M. H. (1972). 'Ultrastructural pathologic findings of the human hepatocyte. 1. Alcoholic liver disease.' *Archs Path.* **94,** 554

Mair, W. G. P. and Tomé, F. M. S. (1972). *Atlas of the Ultrastructure of Diseased Human Muscle:* Edinburgh and London: Churchill Livingstone

Mannweiler, K. and Bernhard, W. (1957). 'Recherches ultrastructurales sur une tumeur rénale experimental du hamster.' *J. Ultrastruct. Res.* **1,** 158

Matthews, J. L., Martin, J. H., Arsenis, C., Eisenstein, R. and Kuettner, K. (1971). 'The role of mitochondria in intracellular calcium regulation.' In *Cellular Mechanisms for Calcium Transfer and Homeostasis,* p. 239. Ed. by G. Nichols and R. H. Wasserman. New York and London: Academic Press

Meerson, F. Z., Zaletayeva, T. A. Lagutchev, S. S. and Pshennikova, M. G. (1964). 'Structure and mass of mitochondria in the process of compensatory hyperfunction and hypertrophy of the heart.' *Expl Cell Res.* **36,** 568

181

Minick, O. T., Kent, G., Orfei, E. and Volini, F. I. (1965). 'Non-membrane enclosed intramitochondrial dense bodies.' *Expl Molec. Path.* **4**, 311

Mollin, D. L. and Hoffbrand, A. V. (1968). 'Sideroblastic anaemia.' In *Recent Advances in Clinical Pathology*, p. 273. Ed. by S. C. Dyke. Edinburgh and London: Churchill Livingstone

Moore, D. H. and Ruska, H. (1957). 'Electron microscope study of mammalian cardiac muscle cells.' *J. biophys. biochem. Cytol.* **3**, 261

Mugnaini, E. (1964). 'Filamentous inclusions in the matrix of mitochondria from human livers.' *J. Ultrastruct. Res.* **11**, 525

Napolitano, L. and Fawcett, D. (1958). 'The fine structure of brown adipose tissue in the newborn mouse and rat.' *J. biophys. biochem. Cytol.* **4**, 685

Nass, M. M. K. and Nass, S. (1963). 'Intramitochondrial fibers with DNA characteristics. I. Fixation and electron staining reactions. II. Enzymatic and other hydrolytic treatments.' *J. Cell Biol.* **19**, 593; 613

— — and Afzelius, B. A. (1965). 'The general occurrence of mitochondrial DNA.' *Expl Cell Res.* **37**, 516

Novikoff, A. B. (1961). 'Mitochondria (Chondriosomes).' In *The Cell*, Vol. 2, p. 299. Ed. by J. Brachet and A. E. Mirsky. New York and London: Academic Press

Ogura, M. and Furuta, Y. (1957). 'A study of fixation for electron microscopy (on the effect of osmotic pressure).' *Electron Microscopy* **5**, 15

Ollerich, D. A. (1968). 'An intramitochondrial crystalloid in element III of rat chorioallantoic placenta.' *J. Cell Biol.* **37**, 188

Osvaldo, L. and Latta, H. (1966). 'Interstitial cells of the renal medulla.' *J. Ultrastruct. Res.* **15**, 589

Palade, G. E. (1952). 'The fine structure of mitochondria.' *Anat. Rec.* **114**, 427

— (1953). 'An electron microscope study of the mitochondrial structure.' *J. Histochem. Cytochem.* **1**, 188

— (1959). In *Subcellular Particles*, p. 64. Ed. by T. Hagashi. New York: Roland Press

— and Schidlowsky, G. (1958). 'Functional association of mitochondria and lipid inclusions.' *Anat. Rec.* **130**, 352

Palay, S. L. (1956). 'Synapses in the central nervous system.' *J. biophys. biochem. Cytol.* **2**, Suppl., 193

Pappas, G. D. and Brandt, P. W. (1959). 'Mitochondria. I. Fine structure of the complex patterns in the mitochondria of *Pelomyxa carolinensis Wilson (Chaos chaos L.)*.' *J. biophys. biochem. Cytol.* **6**, 85

Parry, E. W. and Ghadially, F. N. (1966). 'Ultrastructural changes in the liver of tumour-bearing rats during the terminal stages of life.' *Cancer* **19**, 821

Pavel, I., Bonaparte, H. and Petrovici, A. (1971). 'Involution of liver mitochondria in viral hepatitis.' *Archs Path.* **91**, 294

Peachey, L. D. (1964). 'Electron microscopic observations on the accumulation of divalent cations in intramitochondrial granules.' *J. Cell Biol.* **20**, 95

Pelosi, G. and Agliati, G. (1968). 'The heart muscle in functional overload and hypoxia. A biochemical and ultrastructural study.' *Lab. Invest.* **18**, 86

Personne, P. and Anderson, W. (1970). 'Localization mitochondriale d'enzymes liées au metabolisme du glycogène dans le spermatozoid de l'escargot.' *J. Cell Biol.* **44**, 20

— and Andre, J. (1964). 'Existence de glycogene mitochondrial dans le spermatozoid de la testacelle.' *J. Microscopie* **3**, 643

Peter, J. B., Stempel, K. and Armstrong, J. (1970). 'Biochemistry and electron microscopy of mitochondria in muscular and neuromuscular diseases.' In *Proceedings of the International Congress on Muscle Diseases*. Int. Congr. Ser. No. 199, p. 228. Ed. by J. N. Walton, N. Canal and G. Scarlato. Amsterdam: Excerpta Medica

Picheral, B. (1968). 'Les tissues elaborateurs d'hormones steroides chez les amphibiens urodeles. II. Aspects ultra-structuraux de la glande interrenale— de *Salamandra salamandra* (L). Etude particulière du glycogène.' *J. Microscopie* **7**, 907

Polack, F. M., Kanai, A. and Hood, C. I. (1971). 'Light and electron microscopic studies of orbital rhabdomyosarcoma.' *Am. J. Ophthal.* **71**, 75

Porta, E. A., Hartroft, W. S. and de la Iglesia, F. A. (1965). 'Hepatic changes associated with chronic alcoholism in rats.' *Lab. Invest.* **14**, 1437

— Koch, O. R. and Hartroft, W. S. (1969). 'A new experimental approach in the study of chronic alcoholism. IV. Reproduction of alcoholic cirrhosis in rats and the role of lipotropes versus vitamins.' *Lab. Invest.* **20**, 562

Porter, K. R. and Hogeboom, G. (1964). Addendum to paper by Peachey, L. D. (1964): 'Electron microscopic observations on the accumulation of divalent cations in intramitochondrial granules.' *J. Cell Biol.* **20**, 109

Racela, A., Azarnoff, D. and Svoboda, D. (1969). 'Mitochondrial cavitation and hypertrophy in rat adrenal cortex due to aminoglutethimide.' *Lab. Invest.* **21**, 52

Racker, E. (1968). 'The membrane of the mitochondrion.' *Scientific American* **218**, 32 (Reprint 1101)

— (Ed.) (1969). *Structure and Function of Membranes of Mitochondria and Chloroplasts*. New York: Reinhold

Remington, C. (1957). 'Connaissances recentes sur la biosynthese des porphyrines et de l'heme.' *Revue Hémat.* **12**, 591

Reppart, J. T., Peters, R. L., Edmondson, H. A. and Baker, R. F. (1963). 'Electron and light microscopy of sclerosing hyaline necrosis of the liver.' *Lab. Invest.* **12**, 1138

Revel, J. P., Fawcett, D. W. and Philpott, C. W. (1963). 'Observations on mitochondrial structure. Angular configurations of the cristae.' *J. Cell Biol.* **16**, 187

Reynolds, E. S. (1960). 'Cellular localization of calcium deposition in liver of rat poisoned with carbon tetrachloride.' *J. Histochem. Cytochem.* **8**, 331

— (1963). 'The nature of calcium-associated electron-opaque masses in mitochondria of livers or carbon tetrachloride poisoned rats.' *J. Cell Biol.* **19**, 58A

Rhodin, J. A. G. (1963). *An Atlas of Ultrastructure*. Philadelphia and London: Saunders

Richter, G. W. (1957). 'A study of hemosiderosis with the aid of electron microscopy.' *J. Exp. Med.* **106**, 203

Rifkin, R. J. and Gahagan-Chase, P. A. (1970). 'Morphologic and biochemical effects of a chelating agent, α,α'-dipyridyl, on kidney and liver in rats.' *Lab. Invest.* **23**, 480

Rohr, H. P., Strebel, H., Henning, L. and Bianchi, L. (1970). 'Ultrastrukturell-morphometrische Untersuchungen, an der Rattenleberparenchymzelle in der Frühphase der Regeneration nach partieller Hepatektomie.' *Beitr. path. Anat.* **141,** 52

— Wirz, A., Henning, L. C., Riede, U. N. and Bianchi, L. (1971). 'Morphometric analysis of the rat liver cell in the perinatal period.' *Lab. Invest.* **24,** 128

Rosenbaum, R. M., Wittner, M. and Lenger, M. (1969). 'Mitochondrial and other ultrastructural changes in great alveolar cells of oxygen adapted and poisoned rats.' *Lab. Invest.* **20,** 516

Ross, M. H. (1962). 'Electron microscopy of the human foetal adrenal cortex.' In *The Human Adrenal Cortex,* p. 558. Ed. by A. R. Cumie. T. Symington and J. K. Grant. Edinburgh and London: Churchill Livingstone

Rouiller, C. (1957). 'Contribution de la microscopie électronique à l'étude du fore normal et pathologique.' *Annls Anat. path.* **2,** 548

— (1960). 'Physiological and pathological changes in mitochondrial morphology.' *Int. Rev. Cytol.* **9,** 227

— and Bernhard, W. (1956). 'Microbodies and the problem of mitochondrial regeneration in liver cells.' *J. biophys. biochem. Cytol.* **2,** Suppl., 355

— and Simon, G. (1962). 'Contribution de la microscopie electronique au progres de nos connaissances en cytologie et en histopathologie hepatique.' *Revue int. Hépat.* **12,** 167

Sabatini, D. D., DeRobertis, E. D. P. and Bleichmar, H. B. (1962). 'Submicroscopic study of the pituitary action on the adrenocortex of the rat.' *Endocrinology* **70,** 390

Sano, S., Inoue, S., Tanabe, Y., Sumiya, C. and Koike, S. (1959). 'Significance of mitochondria for porphyon and heme biosynthesis.' *Science* **129,** 275

Schaffner, F. and Felig, P. (1965). 'Changes in hepatic structure in rats produced by breathing pure oxygen.' *J. Cell Biol.* **27,** 505

Schutta, H. S., Johnson, L. and Neville, H. E. (1970). 'Mitochondrial abnormalities in bilirubin-encephalopathy.' *J. Neuropath. exp. Neurol.* **29,** 296

Seljelid, R. and Ericsson, J. L. E. (1965). 'An electronmicroscopic study of mitochondria in renal cell carcinoma.' *J. Microscopie* **4,** 759

Shafiq, S. A., Milhorat, A. T. and Gorycki, M. A. (1967). 'Giant mitochondria in human muscle with inclusions.' *Archs Neurol.* **17,** 666

Shiraki, K. and Neustein, H. B. (1971). 'Intramitochondrial crystalloids and amorphous granules. Occurrence in experimental hepatic ischemia in dogs.' *Archs Path.* **91,** 32

Shy, G. M., Gonatas, N. K. and Perez, M. (1966). 'Two childhood myopathies with abnormal mitochondria. I. Megaconial myopathy. II. Pleoconial myopathy.' *Brain* **89,** 133

Siekevitz, P. (1957). 'Powerhouse of the cell.' *Scientific American* Reprint No. 36

Sjostrand, F. S. (1956). 'The ultrastructure of cells as revealed by the electron microscope.' *Int. Rev. Cytol.* **5,** 455

Skinnider, L. E. and Ghadially, F. N. (1975). 'Ultrastructure of acute myeloid leukaemia arising in multiple myeoloma.' *Human Path.* In press

Slautterback, D. B. (1961). 'The fine structure of shrew *(Blarina)* cardiac muscle.' *Anat. Rec.* **139,** 274

— (1965). 'Mitochondria in cardiac muscle cells of the canary and some other birds.' *J. Cell Biol.* **24,** 1

Smith, D. S. (1961). 'The organization of the flight muscle in a dragonfly *Aeshna* Sp. *(Odonata).*' *J. biophys. biochem. Cytol.* **11,** 119

— (1963). 'The structure of flight muscle sarcosomes in the blowfly *Calliphora erythrocephala (Diptera).*' *J. Cell Biol.* **19,** 115

Sorenson, G. D. (1962). 'Electron microscopic observations of bone marrow from patients with sideroblastic anemia.' *Am. J. Path.* **40,** 297

Spiro, A. J., Prineas, J. W. and Moore, C. L. (1970). 'A new mitochondrial myopathy in a patient with salt craving.' *Archs Neurol., Chicago* **22,** 259

Stein, R. J., Richter, W. R. and Brynjolfsson, G. (1966). 'Ultrastructural pharmacopathology. I. Comparative morphology of the livers of the normal street dog and purebred beagle: a base-line study.' *Expl Molec. Path.* **5,** 195

Stenger, R. J. and Spiro, D. (1961). 'The ultrastructure of mammalian cardiac muscle.' *J. biophys. biochem. Cytol.* **9,** 325

Stephens, R. J. and Bils, R. F. (1965). 'An atypical mitochondrial form in normal rat liver.' *J. Cell Biol.* **24,** 500

Sulkin, N. M. and Sulkin, D. (1962). 'Mitochondrial alterations in liver cells following vitamin E deficiency.' In *Proceedings of the Fifth International Congress for Electron Microscopy,* Vol. 2, p. vv–8. Ed. by S. S. Breese. New York: Academic Press

Sulkin, D. F. and Sulkin, N. M. (1967). 'An electron microscopic study of autonomic ganglion cells of guinea pigs during ascorbic acid deficiency and partial inanition.' *Lab. Invest.* **16,** 142

Sun, S. C., Sohal, R. S., Colcolough, H. L. and Burch, G. E. (1968). 'Histochemical and electron microscopic studies of the effects of reserpine on the heart muscle of mice.' *J. Pharmac. exp. Ther.* **161,** 210

Sun, C. N., Dhalla, N. S. and Olson, R. E. (1969). 'Formation of gigantic mitochondria in hypoxic isolated perfused rat hearts.' *Experientia* **25,** 763

Suter, E. R. (1969). 'The fine structure of brown adipose tissue. III. The effect of cold exposure and its mediation in newborn rats.' *Lab. Invest.* **21,** 259

— and Staubli, W. (1970). 'An ultrastructural histochemical study of brown adipose tissue from neonatal rats.' *J. Histochem. Cytochem.* **18,** 100

Suzuki, K. (1969). 'Giant hepatic mitochondria: production in mice fed with cuprizone.' *Science* **163,** 81

Svoboda, D. J. and Higginson, J. (1963). 'Ultrastructural hepatic changes in rats on a necrogenic diet.' *Am. J. Path.* **43,** 477

— — (1964). 'Ultrastructural changes produced by protein and related deficiences in the rat liver.' *Am. J. Path.* **45,** 353

— and Manning, R. T. (1964). 'Chronic alcoholism with fatty metamorphosis of the liver—mitochondrial alterations in hepatic cells.' *Am. J. Path.* **44**, 645

— Grady, H. and Higginson, J. (1966). 'The effect of chronic protein deficiency in rats. II. Biochemical and ultrastructural changes.' *Lab. Invest.* **15**, 731

Swenson, O., Grana, L., Inouye, T. *et al.* (1967). 'Immediate and long-term effects of acute hepatic ischemia.' *Archs Surg., Chicago* **95**, 451

Tanaka, Y. (1967). 'Iron-laden mitochondria in reticulum cells of hypersiderotic human bone marrows.' *Blood* **29**, 747

Tandler, B. (1966). 'Warthin's tumor, electron microscopic studies.' *Archs Otolar.* **84**, 90

— and Shipkey, F. H. (1964). 'Ultrastructure of Warthin's Tumor. I. Mitochondria.' *J. Ultrastruct. Res.* **11**, 292

— Erlandson, R. A. and Wynder, E. L. (1968). 'Riboflavin and mouse hepatic cell structure and function. I. Ultrastructural alterations in simple deficiency.' *Am. J. Clin. Path.* **52**, 69

— — Smith, A. L. and Wynder, E. L. (1969). 'Riboflavin and mouse hepatic cell structure and function. II. Division of mitochondria during recovery from simple deficiency.' *J. Cell Biol.* **41**, 477

— Hutter, R. V. P. and Erlandson, R. A. (1970). 'Ultrastructure of oncocytoma of the parotid gland.' *Lab. Invest.* **23**, 567

Thiery, J. P. and Caroli, J. (1962). 'Etude comparative en microscopie electronique de l'amylose hepatique primaire humaine et de l'amylose experimentale de la souris.' *Revue int. Hépat.* **12**, 207

Threadgold, L. T. and Lasker, R. (1967). 'Mitochondrogenesis in integumentary cells of the larval sardine *(Sardinops caerulea)*.' *J. Ultrastruct. Res.* **19**, 238

Trump, B. F. and Bulger, R. E. (1967). 'Studies of cellular injury in isolated flounder tubules. I. Correlation between morphology and function of control tubules and observations of autophagocytosis and mechanical cell damage.' *Lab. Invest.* **16**, 453

— — (1968). 'Studies of cellular injury in isolated flounder tubules. III. Light microscopic and functional changes due to cyanide.' *Lab. Invest.* **18**, 721

— and Ginn, F. L. (1968). 'Studies of cellular injury in isolated flounder tubules. II. Cellular swelling in high potassium media.' *Lab. Invest.* **18**, 341

— Goldblatt, P. J. and Stowell, R. E. (1965a). 'Studies on necrosis of mouse liver *in vitro*: ultrastructural alterations in the mitochondria of hepatic parenchymal cells.' *Lab. Invest.* **14**, 343

— — — (1965b). 'Studies of necrosis *in vitro* of mouse hepatic parenchymal cells. Ultrastructural alterations in endoplasmic reticulum Golgi apparatus, plasma membrane and lipid droplets.' *Lab. Invest.* **14**, 2000

Voelz, H. (1968). 'Structural comparison between intramitochondrial and bacterial crystalloids.' *J. Ultrastruct. Res.* **25**, 29

Volk, T. L. and Scarpelli, D. G. (1966). 'Mitochondrial gigantism in the adrenal cortex following hypophysectomy.' *Lab. Invest.* **15**, 707

Wachstein, M. and Besen, M. (1964). 'Electron microscopy of renal coagulative necrosis due to *dl*-serine, with special reference to mitochondrial pyknosis.' *Am. J. Path.* **44**, 383

Walker, S. M. and Schrodt, G. R. (1966). 'Evidence for connections between mitochondria and the sarcoplasmic reticulum and evidence for glycogen granules within the sarcoplasmic reticulum.' *Am. J. Phys. Med.* **45**, 25

— — Truong, X. T. and Wall, E. J. (1965). 'Evidence for structural connections between mitochondria and intermediate elements of triads.' *Am. J. phys. Med.* **44**, 26

Warberg, O. (1956). 'The metabolism of tumors.' English translation, London, 1930.' *Science* **123**, 309

— (1962). 'Uber die fakultative anaerobiose der krebszellen und ihre amuendung auf die chemotherapie.' In *On Cancer and Hormones. Essays in Experimental Biology*, p. 29. Chicago: University of Chicago Press

Ward, R. T. (1962). 'The origin of protein and fatty yolk in *Rana pipiens*. II. Electron microscopical and cytochemical observations of young and mature oocytes.' *J. Cell Biol.* **14**, 309

Watrach, A. M. (1964). 'Degeneration of mitochondria in lead poisoning.' *J. Ultrastruct. Res.* **10**, 177

Watson, M. L. (1952). University of Rochester (New York) Atomic Energy Project, unclassified report. U.R. 185

Wilcken, D. E. L., Brender, D., Shorey, C. D. and MacDonald, G. J. (1967). 'Reserpine: effect on structure of heart muscle.' *Science* **157**, 1332

Wills, E. J. (1965). 'Crystalline structures in the mitochondria of normal human liver parenchymal cells.' *J. Cell Biol.* **24**, 511

Wiseman, G. and Ghadially, F. N. (1958). 'A biochemical concept of tumour growth infiltration and cachexia.' *Br. med. J.* **2**, 18

Wolff, H. H., Balda, B. R., Birkmayer, G. D. and Braun-Falco, O. (1971). 'Zur Ultrastruktur des Hamster-Melanoms A Mel 3 von Fortner.' *Arch. Derm. Forsch.* **240**, 192

Wollenberger, A. and Schulze, W. (1961). 'Mitochondrial alterations in the myocardium of dogs with aortic stenosis.' *J. biophys. biochem. Cytol.* **10**, 285

Wrigglesworth, J. M. and Packer, L. (1968). 'Optical rotary dispersion and circular dichroism studies on mitochondria: correlation of ultrastructure and metabolic state with molecular conformational changes.' *Archs Biochem. Biophys.* **128**, 790

Yamada, E. (1959). 'A crystalline body found in the rod inner segment of the frog's eye.' *J. biophys. biochem. Cytol.* **6**, 517

Yamamoto, E., Wittner, M. and Rosenbaum, R. M. (1970). 'Resistance and susceptibility to oxygen toxicity by cell types of the gas–blood barrier of the rat lung.' *Am. J. Path.* **59**, 409

Yotsuyanagi, Y. (1959). 'Etude au microscope electronique des coupes ultra-fines de la levure.' *Compt. Rend.* **248**, 274

Zacks, S. I. and Sheff, M. F. (1964). 'Studies on tetanus toxin. I. Formation of intramitochondrial dense granules in mice acutely poisoned with tetanus toxin,' *J. Neuropath. exp. Neurol.* **23**, 306

— Hall, J. A. S. and Sheff, M. F. (1966). 'Studies on tetanus. IV. Intramitochondrial dense granules in skeletal muscle from human cases of tetanus intoxication.' *Am. J. Path.* **48,** 811

Zaimis, E., Papadaki, I., Ash, A. S. F., Larbi, E., Kakari, S., Matthew, M. and Paradelis, A. (1969). 'Cardiovascular effects of thyroxine.' *Cardiovasc. Res.* **3,** 118

Zealander, T. (1959). 'Ultrastructure of the mouse adrenal cortex. An electron microscopical study in intact and hydro-cortisone-treated male adults.' *J. Ultrastruct. Res.* Suppl. **2,** 1

185

CHAPTER IV

Golgi Complex and Secretory Granules

INTRODUCTION

In 1898 Golgi reported the occurrence of a new organelle in nerve cells. He called it the 'internal reticular apparatus', but later workers dropped this appellation and adopted the term 'Golgi apparatus'. This term is also losing favour now; today the organelle is more frequently referred to as the 'Golgi complex'.

Heated controversy raged for many years regarding the significance and the very existence of this organelle in living cells, for the chief way in which it could be convincingly demonstrated was in tissues fixed for prolonged periods in solutions containing silver or osmium. It became clear that most cells contained an area of cytoplasm which could reduce silver and osmium salts, but whether this indicated the presence of a specific organelle in the living cell was doubted. With ordinary light microscopy it is, as a rule, not demonstrable in the living cell, nor can it be unequivocally demonstrated in routine histological preparations in most cell types. (For a critique on this old controversy, see Bensley, 1951, and Dalton, 1961.) However, it should be noted that in cells with a well developed Golgi complex a 'negative image' of the Golgi complex is discernible as a clear area in the juxtanuclear position. A well known example of this is the 'Hof', seen as a clear crescentic area adjacent to the nucleus of the plasma cell.

With the advent of phase-contrast microscopy, some of the doubts regarding the existence of this organelle in the living cell were removed, but the controversy was not truly settled until, with the electron microscope, Dalton and Felix (1954a, b) demonstrated that the silver or osmium deposits produced in the cell by the classical methods were associated with a membranous organelle of characteristic morphology.

The Golgi complex consists essentially of stacks of flattened sacs (it is not customary to refer to these as cisternae, which in fact they are) and also vacuoles and vesicles. Like the smooth endoplasmic reticulum, it is composed of smooth membrane, but as a rule it can be distinguished from the former because of the characteristic organization of its elements. Regions of specialization exist within this organelle, for with silver and osmium impregnation methods only the outer stacks (the forming face) show the characteristic 'staining'. It is said that no amount of prolonged fixation will stain all the elements of the Golgi complex (Fawcett, 1967).

Numerous studies have now shown that in many cells which produce a protein-rich secretion, the contents of the rough endoplasmic reticulum are transported to the Golgi where they are condensed, modified and packaged to form secretory granules. In cells that secrete glycoproteins or mucoproteins, much of the carbohydrate component is added to the protein (derived from the rough endoplasmic reticulum) in the Golgi complex. Sulphation of mucopolysaccharides also occurs in this organelle. Other roles of the Golgi include packaging of hydrolytic enzymes to form primary lysosomes and the repair and replenishment of the cell membrane and the glycoprotein coat of cells. The latter process is believed to be achieved by vacuoles arising from the Golgi which fuse with the cell membrane and discharge their contents on to the cell surface. The Golgi complex is also believed to be involved in the production of melanosomes (Chapter IX) and rod bodies (Chapter X). It is also involved in lipid and lipoprotein transport and secretion in certain cell types.

STRUCTURE AND FUNCTION

Although the Golgi complex is a pleomorphic organelle which shows some variations in morphology and distribution within various cell types, there is also a distinctiveness about its membranous formations which clearly allows its identification and establishes it as an organelle in its own right (*Plates 83–85*).

The Golgi complex is composed of three basic elements, the most characteristic part being a stack of flattened sacs the ends of which are often slightly dilated. The stack of sacs is occasionally straight but more often is slightly or markedly curved (*Plate 83*). On the convex or outer face of the stack (at times referred to also as the forming face or immature face) lie numerous vesicles. There is ample evidence now that these vesicles arise by a process of budding from the endoplasmic reticulum and bring with them not only products made in this organelle for processing and packaging in the Golgi complex but also add to the pool of Golgi complex membranes. On the inner or concave face (at times referred to as the mature or maturing face) of the stack are vacuoles of various dimensions containing secretory material which has been condensed and packaged and is leaving the Golgi complex.

The packaging of material into vacuoles involves the utilization of membranes from the Golgi stacks. This, however, is continually replenished by the membranes derived from the small vesicles (called 'intermediate vesicles') migrating from the endoplasmic reticulum to the Golgi complex. The alternate idea that the secretory products from the endoplasmic reticulum flow via 'permanent' connections between this organelle and the Golgi sacs is difficult to support on available evidence. Since ribosomes are essential for protein synthesis and the Golgi complex is composed only of smooth membranes, the most logical site for new lipoprotein membrane formation must be the rough endoplasmic reticulum, and one can therefore argue that the ultimate source of the Golgi membranes is also likely to be derived from this structure.

Plate 83

Mucus-secreting cell from human bronchial mucosa, showing a large Golgi complex comprising several stacks of flattened sacs (S) and numerous vacuoles and vesicles. Current concepts regarding the manner in which secretory granules containing mucin (a protein–polysaccharide which with water forms mucus) are made is illustrated with the aid of this electron micrograph. The protein part of the protein–polysaccharide complex is synthesized from the amino acids by the ribosomes of the rough endoplasmic reticulum, and travel along its cisternae (A). Some sugars may be added to the protein at this stage. Intermediate or transport vesicles containing the newly synthesized material bud off (B) from the margins of the cisternae and coalesce with the saccules of the Golgi complex. The completion of mucoprotein synthesis is achieved in the Golgi complex by the addition of other sugars and the fully formed mucoprotein then emerges as single-membrane-bound granules (at times called droplets) by a process of budding from the Golgi stacks (C). In merocrine glands the secretory granules (D) then travel to the apex of the cell where the membrane bounding the granule fuses with the cell membrane prior to discharge of its contents. Thus at no stage is the cell cytoplasm exposed to the exterior during merocrine secretion. × 23,000

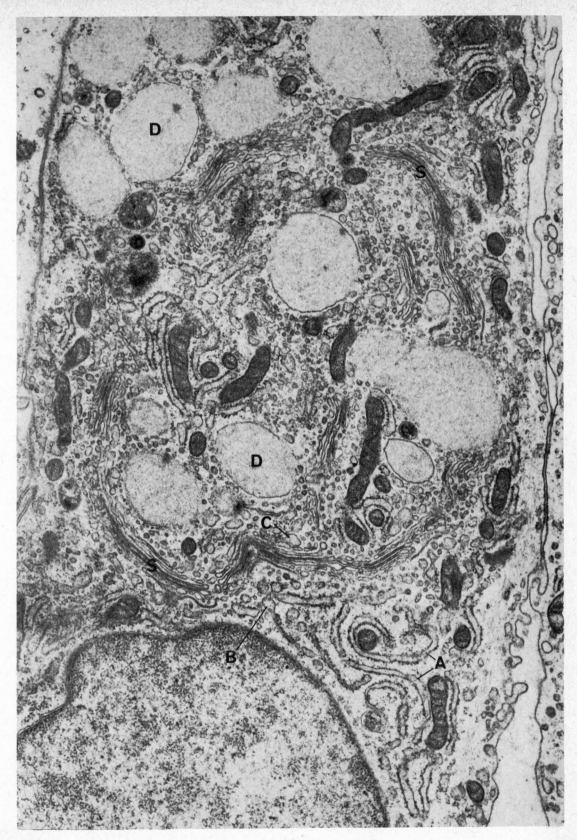

189

The above description depicts the basic unit of the Golgi complex and the probable mode of turn-over of its components. More often than not, several such Golgi units of curved packets of flattened sacs and associated vesicles and vacuoles are seen arranged in a circular, oval crescentic or cup-shaped configuration within the cytoplasm of a variety of cells (*Plates 83–85*). It would appear that the system of peripherally placed stacks is the equivalent of the 'dictyosome' of light microscopists, while the centrally placed vacuoles with the secretory contents correspond to the 'archoplasm'. In keeping with general practice, I have avoided using the perfectly appropriate term 'cisternae' for the flattened sacs of the Golgi complex. The reason for such reluctance generally is not clear but perhaps this attitude stems from a desire to avoid confusion with the cisternae of the rough endoplasmic reticulum.

The circular or oval configuration of the Golgi complex mentioned above is characteristic of many but not all cell types. In others the stacks appear somewhat randomly distributed, and at times groups of stacks with their associated vacuoles and vesicles placed quite far apart in the cytoplasm may be found in a cell. In such cases (particularly in pathological tissues) one is left wondering whether there are two or more Golgi complexes present or whether continuity between the two systems would be demonstrable by serial sectioning.

The Golgi complex generally occupies a juxtanuclear position. In secretory epithelia the position of the complex is in the juxtanuclear cytoplasm facing the apical portion of the cell. In hepatocytes the Golgi complex is usually represented by only a few rather slightly curved stacks adjacent to the cell membrane. Occasionally, however, it is seen extending from the nucleus to the cell membrane. In neurons the Golgi complex is quite diffuse and its components have a perinuclear distribution.

Although in most cells the Golgi complex is located in the apical portion of the cell, in the juxtanuclear zone there are instances in which this organelle occupies the basal part of the cell (see the review by Kirkman and Severinghaus, 1938), and examples have also been cited where the Golgi shifts from one pole of the cell to the other. Thus in ameloblasts the Golgi complex migrates from the apical to the basal pole prior to the production of the enamel matrix (Jasswoin, 1924; Beams and King, 1933). Two similar shifts in the position of the Golgi have also been noted to occur during the development of the chick corneal epithelium. The first is related to the formation of the primary corneal stroma and the second shift occurs when Bowman's membrane is forming beneath the epithelium (Trelstad, 1970).

The functions of the Golgi are many and varied. Its involvement in secretory processes had long been suspected by light microscopists, because of the prominence of this organelle in such cells and the presence of secretory droplets in the Golgi region. Thus, on the basis of such observation, in 1914 Cajal had already envisaged that in the goblet cells of intestinal epithelium mucus

---

Plate 84

A zone 3 chondrocyte from articular cartilage of a 9-month-old rabbit, showing characteristic glycogen deposits (G), intracytoplasmic filaments (F) and cell processes (P) extending into the matrix. The well developed Golgi complex shows many stacks and secretory vacuoles (V), the contents of which are remarkably similar in appearance to the cartilage matrix. × 31,000 (*From Ghadially and Roy, 1969*)

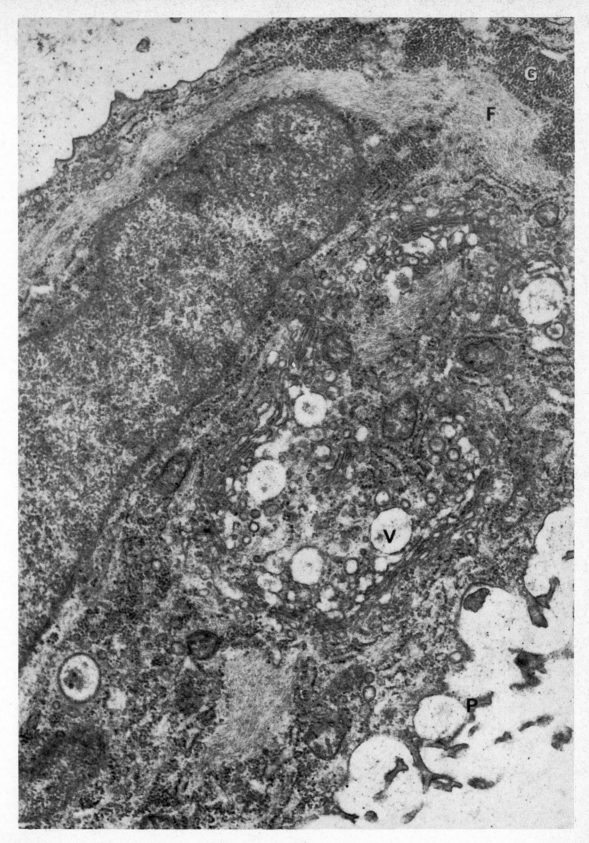

was synthesized within the Golgi complex. The remarkable clarity with which some light microscopists saw the involvement of the Golgi complex in secretory activity is demonstrated in a review by Bowen (1929) who wrote, 'Secretion is in essence a phenomenon of "granule" or droplet formation. Starting with a single such secretory droplet about to be expelled from the cell, we find it possible to trace its origin step by step to a minute vacuole, which has thus from the beginning served as a segregation center for a specific secretion material. The primordial vacuole is found to arise in that zone of the cell characterized by the presence of the Golgi apparatus, and the evidence indicates, if it does not demonstrate, that the primary vacuole arises through the activity of the Golgi substance and undergoes a part at least of its development in contact with, or embedded in, the Golgi apparatus.'

A series of studies employing electron microscopic, cytochemical and autoradiographic techniques have now established beyond doubt that the Golgi complex is involved in the production of virtually every exocrine and endocrine secretion. A few examples to illustrate this will now be considered, together with the techniques used in elucidating the function of the Golgi.

The first study of this kind was on the exocrine cells of the pancreas where, by using radioactive amino acids, it was shown that the newly formed labelled protein appears first in the rough endoplasmic reticulum and is then transported to the Golgi where it is packaged to form secretory granules. However, in most proteinaceous secretions the protein is combined with carbohydrate, to form protein polysaccharides designated as either mucoproteins or glycoproteins (the distinction between the two is somewhat tenuous and arbitrary; glycoproteins contain less than 4 per cent carbohydrate measured as hexosamine while mucoproteins contain more than this amount). The question then arose as to where the carbohydrate component was added to the protein. The presence of glycoprotein in the Golgi complex had long been demonstrated by histochemical methods, but it was the work of Leblond and his colleagues (Peterson and Leblond, 1964; Neutra and Leblond, 1966a, b) which convincingly demonstrated that it is the Golgi saccule where certain carbohydrates are added to the protein to form glycoprotein. These authors injected glucose-^{3}H into rats and found that the Golgi saccules of the goblet cells in the large intestine were labelled within 15 minutes. At 20 minutes the newly formed radioactive glycoprotein began to appear in the mucus droplets and by 40 minutes almost all the radioactive glycoprotein had migrated from the Golgi to the collection of mucus droplets in the goblet cells.

Plate 85

Fig. 1. Type A cell from human synovial membrane, showing Golgi stacks (G), vacuoles containing secretory material (V) and mitochondria (M). The scant rough endoplasmic reticulum and ribosomes lying free in the cytoplasm are barely discernible. × 25,000 (*From Ghadially and Roy, 1969*)

Fig. 2. Type A cell from rat synovial membrane, showing mitochondria (M) and sparse rough endoplasmic reticulum (R). A characteristic feature of the synovial cells of this species is the occurrence of numerous rather large secretory vacuoles which contain electron-lucent material surrounded by some medium-density material and a few electron-dense granules. A gradation in size of the vacuoles (A, B and C) is seen stemming from the Golgi region (G) to the cell surface which lay just beyond the top edge of the picture. × 26,000 (*From Roy and Ghadially, 1967a*)

192

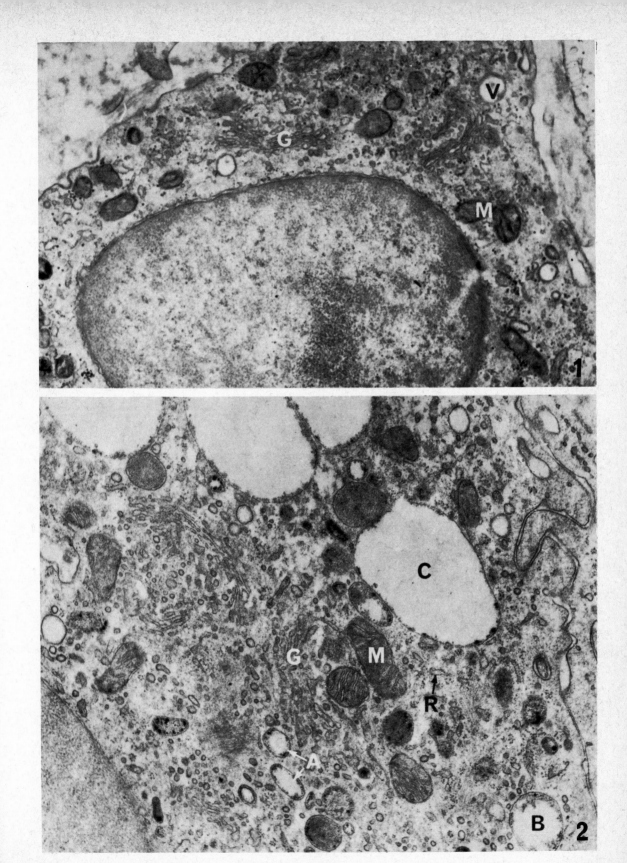

However, it is worth noting that the Golgi complex is not the sole site of uptake and coupling of sugars to protein (see review by Rambourg, 1971). For example, while tritiated mannose is taken up primarily by the Golgi complex of intestinal epithelial cells (Ito, 1969), in thyroid follicular cells its primary site of incorporation is the rough endoplasmic reticulum (Whur et al., 1969). Similarly, in plasma cells the autoradiographic reaction following the administration of tritiated glucosamine is first seen in the rough endoplasmic reticulum (Zagury et al., 1970).

Further interesting insights into the function of the Golgi complex spring from studies on cartilage and synovial membrane. The matrix of cartilage contains collagen fibres* and an interfibrillary matrix which, among other things, is rich in chondromucoproteins. Native chondromucoprotein is made up of chains of mucopolysaccharides (chondroitin sulphate and keratosulphate) combined with non-collagenous protein to form large complexes often referred to as protein–polysaccharide complexes (Barland et al., 1966). It would appear that the protein part of the complex is synthesized in the rough endoplasmic reticulum of the chondrocyte and that the synthesis of the carbohydrate (mucopolysaccharide) component and its combination with protein occur largely in the Golgi complex. Such protein polysaccharides at times present as characteristic angular granules in cartilage matrix and they can also at times be seen in the Golgi vacuoles (Plate 84).

The uptake of ^{35}S–sulphate into chondrocytes either in vivo or in vitro has been used as an indicator of the synthesis of sulphomucopolysaccharides (Dziewiatkowski, 1951; Bostrom and Aquist, 1952; Adams and Rienits, 1961). Electron microscopic observations on the autoradiographic localization of ^{35}S–sulphate in chondrocytes has shown (Fewer et al., 1964; Godman and Lane, 1964) that the radiosulphate is first localized in the Golgi complex. Later the radioactivity is seen over large Golgi-derived secretory vacuoles, which then seem to migrate to the surface and discharge their contents into the matrix (Plate 86). Such experiments indicate that sulphation of mucopolysaccharides also occur in the Golgi.

In the synovial membrane there is a somewhat different situation, for the mucopolysaccharide produced by the synovial intimal cells (hyaluronate or hyaluronic acid) and poured into the joint cavity as a part of the synovial fluid is not sulphated. Much of it occurs free (that is to say, not bound to protein), some in loose combination with plasma protein, and only a small amount is firmly bound to protein which is thought to be derived from synovial intimal cells.

* The manner in which tropocollagen is synthesized by the rough endoplasmic reticulum and released from the cell to form collagen fibres is discussed on page 214.

Plate 86

Fig. 1. Electron micrograph of an autoradiogram of a pair of chondrocytes 20 minutes after presentation of radiosulphate, illustrating the concentration of the grains over the vaculated Golgi regions. × 18,500 (From Godman and Lane, 1964)

Fig. 2. Electron micrograph of an autoradiogram of a chondrocyte 19 hours after presentation of radiosulphate. The grains now overlie the large smooth-walled vacuoles, some of which (arrows) seem to be in the process of discharging their contents into the matrix. Many other grains, presumably discharged at an earlier stage, are also seen in the matrix. × 21,000 (From Godman and Lane, 1964)

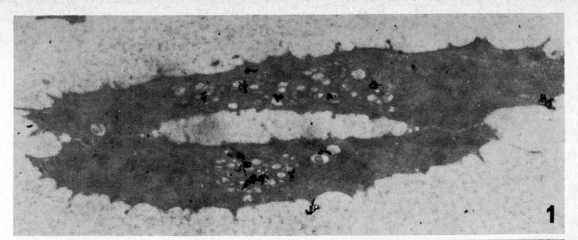

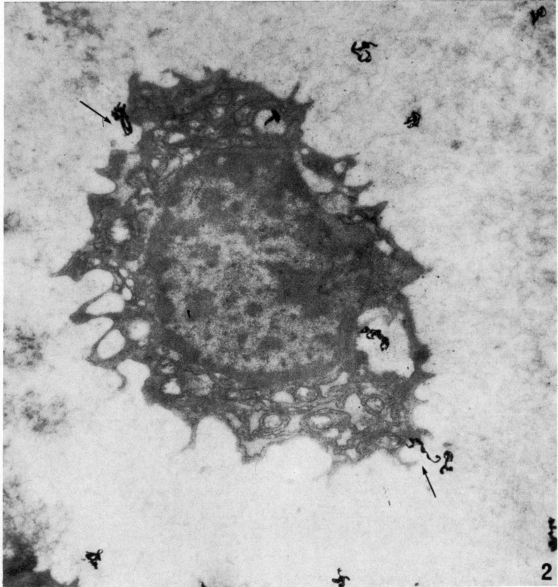

Almost all the protein in the synovial fluid is derived directly from the blood (plasma protein). Only about 2 per cent of the total protein of synovial fluid, which is distinct from plasma proteins, is firmly bound to hyaluronate, and there is evidence that this small amount of protein–polysaccharide complex is produced by the rough-endoplasmic-reticulum-rich type B synovial intimal cell (for references and more details, see Ghadially and Roy, 1969).

Thus here there is a tissue which produces much free mucopolysaccharide, and the morphology of the synovial intima seems to reflect how this is accomplished (*Plate 85*). In the synovial intima of all species studied to date two main cell types have been found: one called the type A cell, which contains abundant Golgi complexes and numerous vacuoles and vesicles but little or no rough endoplasmic reticulum, and another called the type B cell, which contains abundant rough endoplasmic reticulum but in which the Golgi complex by comparison is poorly represented, and vacuoles and vesicles are scanty. Intermediate forms also occur, clearly indicating that type A and B cells are not distinct cell lines but variants whose morphology reflects the kind of functional activity they are engaged in at a given moment. In normal synovial membrane many more type A cells are seen than type B cells.

In view of what is now known about the functions of the rough endoplasmic reticulum and Golgi complex, one may surmise that type A cells which have little or no rough endoplasmic reticulum for export protein synthesis but well developed Golgi complexes for polysaccharide synthesis, produce the hyaluronic acid of the synovial fluid; indeed this material has been demonstrated within the Golgi complex and secretory vacuoles by colloidal iron staining and enzyme digestion techniques (Roy and Ghadially, 1967b) (*Plate 87*). Similarly, one may argue that the source of the small amount of protein-bound hyaluronate lies in the small population of type B cells. Support for this view may also be found in the fact that in rheumatoid arthritis, where there is an increase in the hyaluronate-bound protein in the synovial fluid (Hamerman and Sandson, 1963), there is also a remarkable increase in the population of type B and intermediate type cells (Wyllie *et al.*, 1966; Ghadially and Roy, 1967). Much has been made of the role of type A cells in the removal of material from joints, while its role in the production of hyaluronic acid seems to have been largely overlooked; yet phagocytosed material may be found in both cell types and there is no reason to suppose that the major cell population of the synovial intima is devoted solely to scavenging activity.

Plate 87

The illustrations on this plate show the results obtained with the colloidal iron technique for localizing acid mucopoly-saccharides (hyaluronic acid) in synovial cells. Osmium-fixed tissue was treated with colloidal iron and embedded in araldite. Sections were not 'stained'. The black granular iron deposit is located at sites where acid mucopolysaccharide is present. In tissues pre-treated with hyaluronidase such deposits were not seen. (*From Roy and Ghadially. 1967b*)

Fig. 1. Normal rabbit synovial membrane, showing deposits of electron-dense iron particles on the surface of the synovial cell (S) facing the joint cavity (J). A large number of electron-dense particles can be seen localized in a large smooth-walled vacuole (V). A less intense but still fairly distinct localization of dense particles is seen in smaller vacuoles and vesicles (V). Dense particles can also be seen localized in the matrix (M) between the synovial cells. × 37,000

Fig. 2. Normal rabbit type A synovial cell, showing iron particles localized in Golgi vesicles (G) and a large smooth-walled vacuole (V). × 61,000

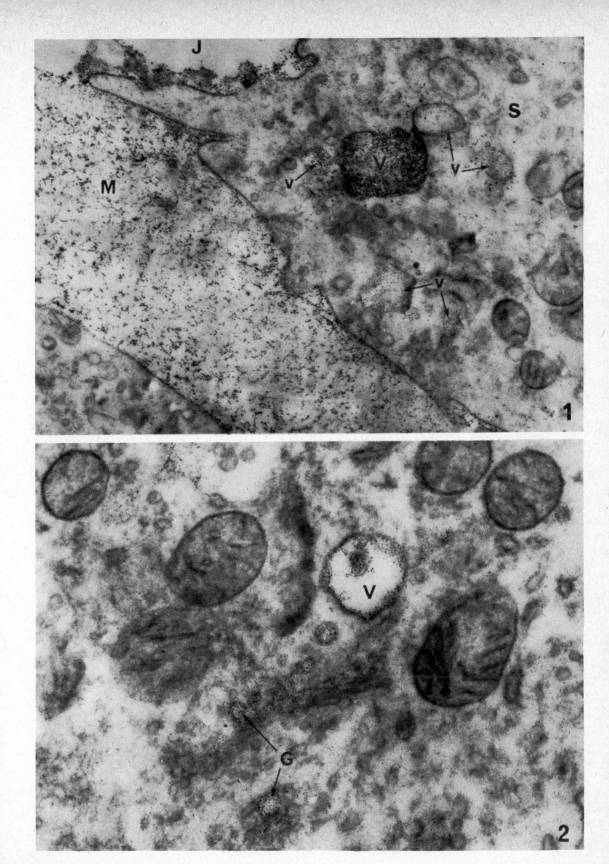

The Golgi complex is a specialized structure which performs many functions. Its activity may therefore be looked upon as an expression of cellular differentiation and functional maturity of the cell. In keeping with this is the oft-made observation that immature cells or undifferentiated cells (i.e. stem cells or blast cells) have a poorly developed Golgi complex as compared to their normal mature counterparts. Similarly, fast-growing cells such as cells in tissue culture and anaplastic tumour cells, where the accent is on growth and multiplication rather than on differentiation and function, also tend to have a poorly developed Golgi complex.

Exceptions or apparent exceptions to such generalizations are also easily found. Thus, in the erythroid series of cells, all organelles including the Golgi complex (which is not too prominent to begin with) are lost in the mature red blood cell. Similarly, in the mature granulocytes the Golgi complex is small or hard to find because once the various granules are formed, the Golgi complex disappears or becomes markedly atrophic.

Light microscopic studies on tumours (Ludford, 1929, 1952; Severinghaus, 1937; Dalton and Edwards, 1942; Bothe *et al.*, 1950) have shown many variations in size and distribution of the Golgi complex but none that can be considered specific for the neoplastic state. Electron microscopic studies have done little besides confirm and clarify these findings (Haguenau and Lacour, 1955; Haguenau and Bernhard, 1955; Howatson and Ham, 1955, 1957; Dalton and Felix, 1956; Selby *et al.*, 1956; Suzuki, 1957; Epstein, 1957a, b; Dalton, 1959, 1961; Oberling and Bernhard, 1961; Bernhard, 1969).

From a review of the literature and personal observations on tumours of man and experimental animals, the following tentative conclusions are drawn: (1) in fast-growing anaplastic tumours the Golgi complex is almost invariably poorly developed or difficult to identify; (2) there is a rough correlation between the degree of differentiation and the size of the Golgi complex in a given tumour type, the less differentiated tumours having poorer Golgi complexes; (3) relatively well differentiated malignant tumours and benign tumours usually have a well developed Golgi complex if the parent tissue of origin is also well endowed in this respect; and (4) marked hypertrophy, dilatation and distortion of the Golgi complex are, at times, found in some tumours.

We (Ghadially and Parry, 1966) have seen hypertrophy, dilatation and distortion of Golgi complexes in a human hepatoma (*Plate 88*) and such changes have also been reported by other workers in some examples of: (1) mouse and rat hepatomas (Dalton and Edwards, 1942; Bothe *et al.*, 1950; Dalton, 1961, 1964); (2) Rous sarcoma (Bernhard, 1969); and (3) experimentally produced pituitary adenomas (Severinghaus, 1937). It must, however, be stressed that as a general rule tumours are poorly endowed with Golgi complexes as compared to their cell of origin.

Most of the above-mentioned variations are easily reconciled with our concepts of cell differentiation and function on the one hand and the differentiation and loss or impairment of functional ability in the tumour cell on the other. The marked hypertrophy of Golgi complexes seen in some tumours is also not particularly surprising because excessive production of secretory materials is, at times, a feature of some tumours.

Plate 88

Figs. 1–3. Examples of hypertrophy, dilatation and distortion of Golgi complexes found in a singularly well differentiated human hepatoma. ×38,000; ×17,000; ×25,000 (*Figs. 1, from Ghadially and Parry, 1966; Figs. 2 and 3, Ghadially and Parry, unpublished electron micrographs*)

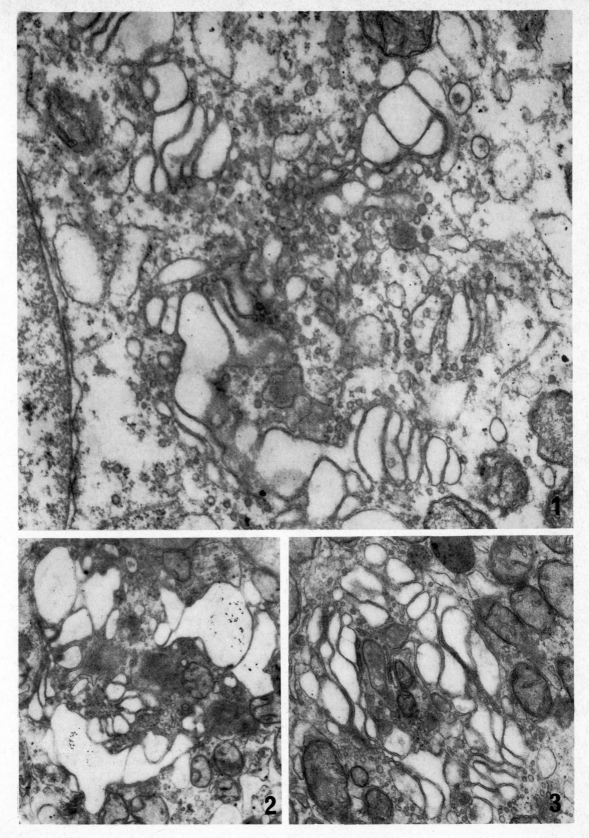

A variety of changes has been reported to occur in the Golgi complex in normal and pathological tissues. Such differences can be accounted for in terms of cell differentiation (already dealt with on page 198), physiological activity and pathological or toxic influences. The changes themselves comprise: (1) hypertrophy or atrophy of the Golgi complex; (2) dilatation or collapse of the Golgi elements; (3) changes in intracellular positions of the Golgi complex (page 190); and (4) quantitative and/or qualitative differences in the contents of the Golgi complex (page 202). So frequent are reports of slight alterations of Golgi complex morphology and contents that they cannot all be cited here; however, a few examples will be quoted which illustrate the significance of such changes.

Hypertrophy of the Golgi elements (i.e. stacks, vesicles and vacuoles), evidenced by an increase in the number of Golgi units (i.e. a set of stacks and associated vacuoles and vesicles) or by multiple Golgi complexes occupying larger areas of the cell cytoplasm, can usually be correlated with an increased secretory activity (i.e. work hypertrophy) or a compensatory hypertrophy (i.e. secondary to atrophy or malfunction in adjacent cells). Thus, during experimentally induced adrenal cortical regeneration in the rat there is a remarkable hypertrophy of the Golgi complexes in the ACTH-secreting cells of the adenohypophysis, presumably reflecting the increased synthesis of ACTH which ensues. When adrenal regeneration is nearing completion and the ACTH level falls, the Golgi complex is restored to normal size (Nakayama *et al.*, 1969). After the injection of papain there is a depletion of matrix from the rabbit ear cartilage and the ears become floppy. During the subsequent phase of restoration of the matrix and recovery of the ears to an erect position the actively synthesizing chondrocytes show a remarkable Golgi hypertrophy (Sheldon and Robinson, 1960; Sheldon and Kimball, 1962).

Marked atrophy or destruction and the disappearance of recognizable Golgi elements have been noted to occur in various situations; for example, in enucleate *Amoeba proteus* (Flickinger, 1970) where a suppression of lipoprotein synthesis necessary for the formation and maintenance of membranes may be responsible. In cases of osteoarthritis (Roy, 1967; Ghadially and Roy, 1969) marked atrophy of Golgi complexes is seen in many synovial intimal cells. This is evidenced by a smaller cell area being occupied by the organelle and by the small size and number of stacks and vesicles (*Plate 89*). In some neighbouring cells, however, there were a large number of Golgi units and a singularly large number of associated vesicles which occupied quite large areas of the cytoplasm. Nevertheless, in both instances, vacuoles containing secretory material were hard to find (*Plate 89*). Thus the appearance seen here suggests an attempt at compensatory hypertrophy in response to atrophy of this organelle in adjacent cells. Such changes are in keeping with the reduced amount of hyaluronic acid known to occur in the synovial fluid from osteoarthritic joints (Decker *et al.*, 1959; Castor *et al.*, 1966).

Atrophic changes and destruction and the disappearance of Golgi elements have also been noted in hepatocytes subject to a variety of toxic influences. In such instances the disturbance of lipoprotein synthesis and secretion which occurs is reflected also by alterations of the Golgi complex and endoplasmic reticulum contents (pages 202 and 248).

Plate 89

Synovial cells from an osteoarthritic human joint.
Fig. 1. A synovial cell showing a markedly atrophic Golgi complex. × 42,000 (*From Roy, 1967*)
Fig. 2. A synovial cell showing Golgi stacks and an unusually large number of associated vesicles. × 39,000 (*From Ghadially and Roy, 1969*)

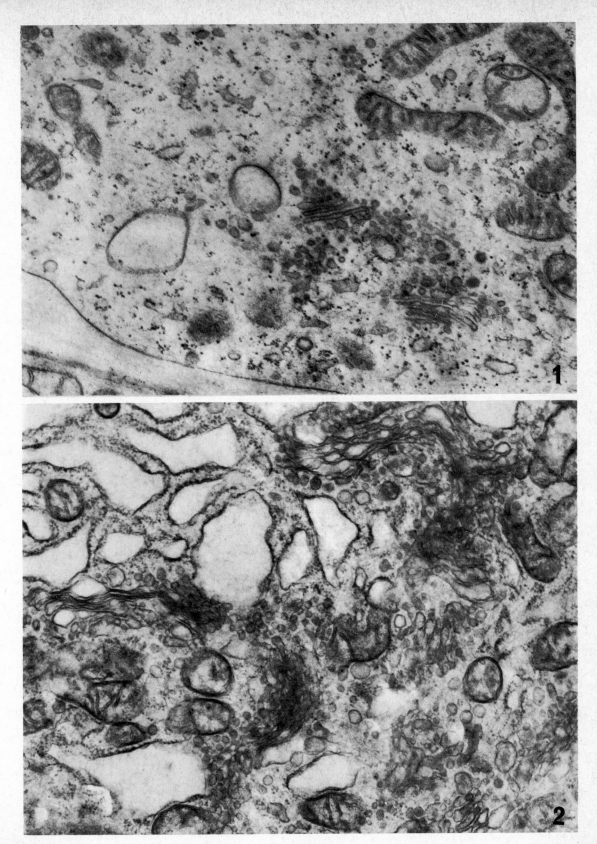

LIPID AND LIPOPROTEIN IN GOLGI COMPLEX

In certain cell types the Golgi complex has frequently been implicated in the transport and secretion of lipids and/or lipoproteins. The best-known example of this is the Golgi complex of rat hepatocytes where electron microcopists have long noted the occurrence of occasional electron-dense 'granules' (800–1,000 Å diameter) (*Plate 90, Fig. 1*). In animals such as the rabbit, where the lipid is saturated, electron-lucent 'granules' occur instead of electron-dense ones. It is now clear that such granules (both electron-lucent and electron-dense varieties) comprise very low-density lipoproteins. It would appear that such a difference in electron density between the very low-density lipoproteins reflects the saturated and unsaturated fatty acid content of the lipid in the diet and, hence, the lipoprotein.

Although the precise sites at which the steps in lipoprotein synthesis occur are debatable, the bulk of the evidence suggests that the synthesis occurs in the endoplasmic reticulum. The material is probably modified in the Golgi complex and then transported and secreted into the space of Disse and ultimately the blood stream.

A variety of hepatotoxic agents and experimental situations which ultimately produce a fatty liver also produce an increase in the size and number of lipid droplets in the endoplasmic reticulum. Such membrane-bound droplets are called liposomes, and the manner in which they are formed is dealt with later.* In such situations, however, alterations in the lipid or lipoprotein contents within the Golgi complex are also noted. For example, Reynolds (1963) has reported that 30 minutes after the administration of carbon tetrachloride to rats the Golgi complex is transformed into a cluster of dilated vacuoles devoid of coarse electron-dense particles. It is said that in rat livers perfused with free fatty acid for 90 minutes a few hepatocytes accumulate liposomes and that such cells appear to 'lack an organized system of membranes recognizable as the Golgi region' (Hamilton *et al.*, 1966, 1967). Similarly, in rat livers after administration of a choline-deficient diet (Amick and Stenger, 1964; Estes and Lombardi, 1969), puromycin (Jones *et al.*, 1967) and orotic acid (Jatlow *et al.*, 1965) disrupted or dilated particle-free Golgi complexes are found.

* The occurrence of lipid in endoplasmic reticulum is dealt with later (page 248). This topic is so closely linked with the subject dealt with here that it is recommended that both essays are read conjunctly.

Plate 90

Fig. 1. Numerous electron-dense granules, representing very low-density lipoproteins, are seen in Golgi vacuoles (arrows). From a normal suckling rat hepatocyte. × 29,000

Fig. 2. Numerous electron-lucent particles, representing very low-density lipoproteins, are seen in Golgi vacuoles (arrows). From a cortisone-treated rabbit hepatocyte. × 52,000 (*From Mahley, Gray, Hamilton and Lequire, 1968*)

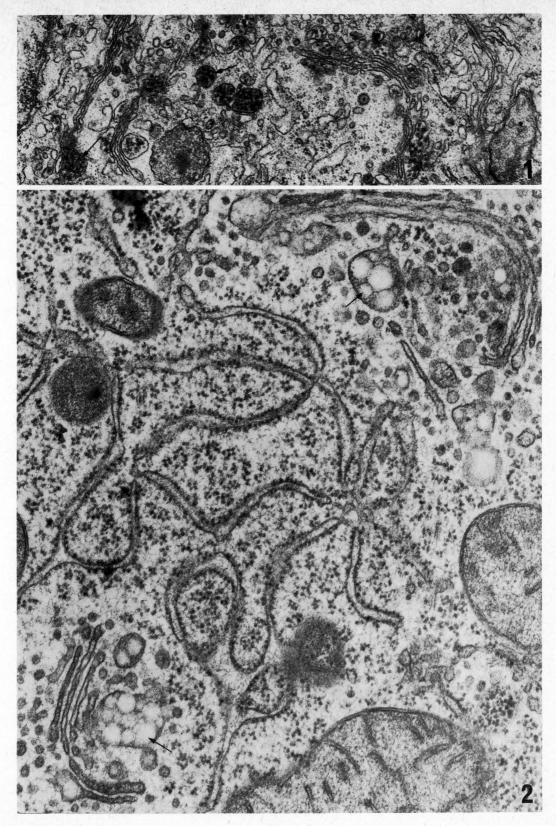

In the liver of cortisone-treated rabbits (*Plate 90, Fig. 2*), Mahley *et al.* (1968) found that by 2 days typical Golgi complexes were extremely rare or hard to find but by 4–6 days there was a dramatic increase in Golgi complexes containing electron-lucent particles. On the basis of their observation and a review of the literature they concluded that '(1) the appearance of liposomes in and near the hepatocyte Golgi apparatus is indicative of a degree of impaired very low density lipoprotein synthesis and/or secretion which, if not reversed, can lead to widespread accumulation of liposomes and development of fatty liver; and (2) that disappearance of typical Golgi apparatus, or Golgi apparatus devoid of any lipid particles, is indicative of a major or prolonged block in very low density lipoprotein synthesis and/or secretion.'

It is now well established that fatty acid esterification occurs in the endoplasmic reticulum of many cell types (Stein and Shapiro, 1959; Hultin, 1961; Tzur and Shapiro, 1964) and that during uptake of lipid, osmiophilic or non-osmiophilic lipid may be demonstrated in this system and also often in the Golgi complex. Perhaps the model studied most extensively here is the intestinal epithelial cell where, during lipid transport, lipid may be demonstrated both in the endoplasmic reticulum and in the Golgi complex (Palay and Karlin, 1959; Onoe and Ohno, 1963; Fawcett, 1967).* The concept that emerges from these studies and studies on lipid uptake by various other tissues such as adipose, mammary, hepatic, cartilage, cardiac and skeletal muscle (Stein and Stein, 1967a, b; Ghadially *et al.*, 1970; Scow, 1970; Mehta and Ghadially, 1973) is that, although some cells can pick up lipid droplets directly by a process of pinocytosis or micropinocytosis (e.g. Kupffer cells and polymorphonuclear neutrophils), generally and in the majority of instances the lipid is first hydrolysed and the component parts are picked up by the cell. The lipid is then resynthesized in the endoplasmic reticulum, and often at some stage of the process appears in the Golgi complex.

An example of this is seen in the chondrocytes of articular cartilage, where a few lipid droplets normally occur in the cytoplasm (Ghadially *et al.*, 1965, Collins *et al.*, 1965). In the rabbit, depot lipid is well saturated and hence usually presents in the chondrocytes and elsewhere as electron-lucent material. In this animal, if a lipid rich in unsaturated fatty acid (e.g. corn oil) is injected into the joint, electron-dense material (presumably lipidic in nature) soon appears in the Golgi complex and large osmiophilic lipid droplets accumulate in the cytoplasm (Mehta and Ghadially, 1973). On the other hand, if autologous fat (obtained from the omentum) rich in saturated fatty acids is injected into the joint, the Golgi complex becomes distended with lucent material and numerous electron-lucent lipid droplets are found in the cytoplasm (Ghadially *et al.*, 1970) (*Plate 91*). Besides the lipid in the Golgi complex, elongated electron-lucent areas were sometimes found in the cisternae of the rough endoplasmic reticulum, in the perinuclear cisternae and apparently lying free in the cytoplasm. It would therefore appear that resynthesis of the lipid was probably occurring within the endoplasmic reticulum.

---

* It is interesting to recall that a long while ago light microscopic studies had led Cramer and Ludford (1925) to conclude that the Golgi complex was in some way concerned with resynthesis of fat during intestinal lipid absorption.

Plate 91

Fig. 1. Chondrocyte from articular cartilage of a rabbit after the injection of corn oil into the joint. Electron-dense lipidic droplets are seen within Golgi vacuoles (arrow). Similar but larger electron-dense lipid droplets found in the cytoplasm are illustrated in *Plate 179.* ×22,000 (*From Mehta and Ghadially, 1973*)

Fig. 2. Chondrocyte from articular cartilage of a rabbit after the injection of autologous lipid into the joint, showing a large round electron-lucent lipid droplet (L). The contents of the dilated Golgi complex (G) are remarkably electron lucent and resemble the lipid droplet in the cytoplasm. ×31,000 (*From Ghadially, Mehta and Kirkaldy-Willis, 1970*)

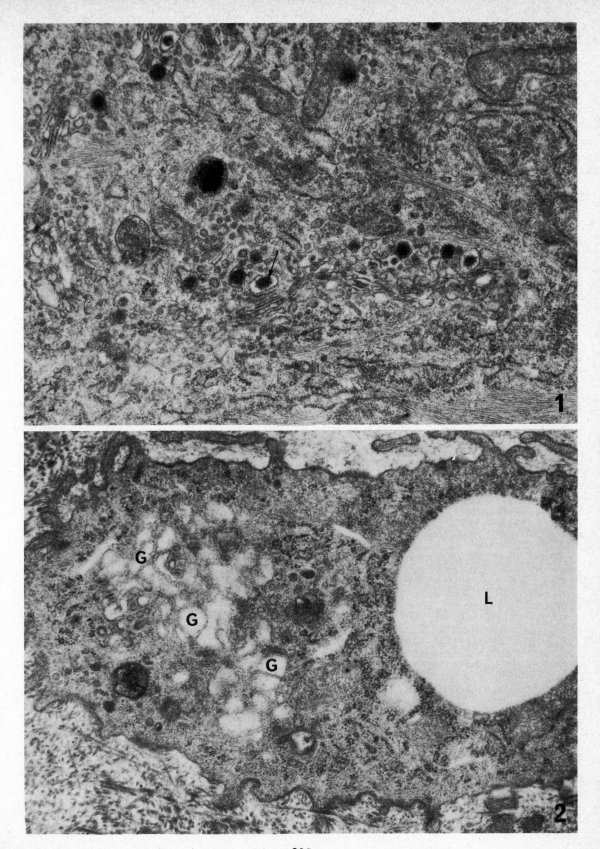

REFERENCES

Adams, J. B. and Rienits, K. G. (1961). 'The biosynthesis of chondroitin sulphates. Influence of nucleotides and hexosamines on sulphate incorporation.' *Biochem.. biophys. Acta* **51**, 567

Amick, C. J. and Stenger, R. (1964). 'Ultrastructural alterations in experimental acute hepatic fatty metamorphosis.' *Lab. Invest.* **13**, 128

Barland, P., Janis, R. and Sandson, J. (1966). 'Immunofluorescent studies of human articular cartilage.' *Ann. rheum. Dis.* **25**, 156

Beams, H. W. and King, R. L. (1933). 'The Golgi apparatus in the developing tooth, with special reference to polarity.' *Anat. Rec.* **57**, 29

Bensley, R. R. (1951). 'Facts versus artefacts in cytology: the golgi apparatus.' *Expl Cell Res.* **2**, 1

Bernhard, W. (1969). 'Ultrastructure of the cancer cell.' In *Handbook of Molecular Cytology*. Ed. by A. Lima-de-Faria. Amsterdam and London: North Holland Publ.

Bostrom, H. and Aquist, F. (1952). 'Utilization of S^{35}-labelled sodium sulphate in the synthesis of chondroitin sulphuric acid, taurine, methionine and cystine.' *Acta chem. Scand.* **6**, 1557

Bothe, A. E., Dalton, A. J., Hastings, W. S. and Zillessen, F. O. (1950). 'A study of Golgi material and mitochondria in malignant and benign prostatic tissue.' *J. natn. Cancer Inst.* **11**, 239

Bowen, R. H. (1929). 'The cytology of glandular secretion.' *Q. Rev. Biol.* **4**, 299

Cajal, R. Y. (1914). 'Algunas variaciones fisiologicas y pathologicas del aparato reticular de Golgi.' *Trab. Lab. Inv. Madrid* **12**, 127

Castor, C. W., Prince, R. K. and Hazelton, M. J. (1966). 'Hyaluronic acid in human synovial effusion.' *Arthritis Rheum.* **9**, 783

Collins, D. H., Ghadially, F. N. and Meachim, G. (1965). 'Intracellular lipids of cartilage.' *Ann. rheum. Dis.* **24**, 123

Cramer, W. and Ludford, R. J. (1925). 'On cellular changes in intestinal fat absorption.' *J. Physiol.* **60**, 342

Dalton, A. J. (1959). 'Organization in benign and malignant cells.' *Lab. Invest.* **8**, 510

— (1961). 'Golgi apparatus and secretion granules.' In *The Cell,* Vol. 2, p. 603. Ed. by J. Brachet and A. E. Mirsky. New York: Academic Press

— (1964). 'An electron microscopical study of a series of chemically induced hepatomas.' In *Cellular Control, Mechanisms and Cancer*, p. 211. Ed. by P. Emmelot and O. Muhlbock. New York: American Elsevier

— and Edwards, J. E. (1942). 'Mitochondria and Golgi apparatus of induced and spontaneous hepatomas in the mouse.' *J. Natn. Cancer Inst.* **2**, 565

— and Felix, M. D. (1954a). 'Cytologic and cytochemical characteristics of the Golgi substance of epithelial cells of the epididymis *in situ*, in homogenates and after isolation.' *Am. J. Anat.* **94**, 171

— — (1954b). In *The Fine Structure of Cells,* Proc. 8th Int. Congr. Cell Biol., Leiden, 1954, p. 274. New York: Interscience

— — (1956). 'A comparative study of the Golgi complex.' *J. biophys. biochem. Cytol.* **2**, 79

Decker, B., McGuckin, W. F., McKenzie, B. F. and Slocumb, C. H. (1959). 'Concentration of hyaluronic acid in synovial fluid.' *Clin. Chem.* **5**, 465

Dziewiatkowski, D. (1951). 'Isolation of chondroitin sulfate-S^{35} from articular cartilage of rats.' *J. biol. Chem.* **189**, 187

Epstein, M. A. (1957a). 'The fine structure of the cells in mouse sarcoma 37 ascitic fluids.' *J. biophys. biochem. Cytol.* **3**, 567

— (1957b). 'The fine structural organization of Rous tumor cells.' *J. biophys. biochem. Cytol.* **3**, 851

Estes, L. and Lombardi, B. (1969). 'Effect of choline deficiency on the Golgi apparatus of rat hepatocytes.' *Lab. Invest.* **21**, 374

Fawcett, D. W. (1967). *The Cell: Its Organelles ahd Inclusions*. Philadelphia and London: Saunders

Fewer, D., Threadgold, J. and Sheldon, H. (1964). 'Studies on cartilage. V. Electron microscopic observations on the autoradiographic localization of S^{35} in cells and matrix.' *J. Ultrastruct. Res.* **11**, 166

Flickinger, C. J. (1970). 'The fine structure of the nuclear envelope in amebae: alterations following nuclear transplantation.' *Expl Cell Res.* **60**, 225

Ghadially, F. N. and Parry, E. W. (1966). 'Ultrastructure of a human hepatocellular carcinoma and surrounding non-neoplastic liver.' *Cancer* **19**, 1989

— and Roy, S. (1967). 'Ultrastructure of synovial membrane in rheumatoid arthritis.' *Ann. rheum. Dis.* **26**, 426

— and Roy, S. (1969). *Ultrastructure of Synovial Joints in Health and Disease*. London: Butterworths

— Meachim, G. and Collins, D. H. (1965). 'Extracellular lipid in matrix of human articular cartilage.' *Ann. rheum. Dis.* **24**, 136

— Mehta, P. H. and Kirkaldy-Willis, W. H. (1970). 'Ultrastructure of articular cartilage in experimentally produced lipoarthrosis.' *J. Bone Jt Surg.* **52A**, 1147

Godman, G. C. and Lane, N. (1964). 'On the site of sulfation in the chondrocyte.' *J. Cell Biol.* **21**, 353

Golgi, C. (1898). 'Sur la structure des cellules nerveuses des ganglions spinaux.' *Archo ital. biol.* **30**, 278

Haguenau, F. and Bernhard, W. (1955). L'appareil de Golgi dans les cellules normales et cancereuses de vertèbres.' *Archs Anat. microsc. Morph. exp.* **44**, 27

— and Lacour, F. (1955). 'Cytologie electronique de tumeurs hypophysaires experimentals; leur appareil de Golgi.' In *The Fine Structure of Cells,* Proc. 8th Int. Congr. Cell Biol., Leiden, 1954, p. 361. New York: Interscience

Hamerman, D. and Sandson, J. (1963). 'Unusual properties of hyaluronate-protein isolated from pathological synovial fluids.' *J. clin. Invest.* **42**, 1882

Hamilton, R. L., Regen, D. M. and Lequire, V. S. (1966). 'Electron microscopic studies of lipoprotein transport in the perfused rat liver.' *Fedn Proc.* **25**, 361

206

— — Gray, M. E. and Lequire, V. S. (1967). 'Lipid transport in liver. I. Electron microscopic identification of very low density lipoproteins in perfused rat liver.' *Lab. Invest.* **16,** 305

Howatson, A. F. and Ham, A. W. (1955). 'Electron microscope study of sections of two rat liver tumors.' *Cancer Res.* **15,** 62

— — (1957). 'The fine structure of cells.' *Can. J. Biochem. Physiol.* **35,** 549

Hultin, T. (1961). 'On the functions of the endoplasmic reticulum.' *Biochem. Pharmac.* **5,** 359

Ito, S. (1969). 'Structure and function of the glycocalyx.' *Fedn. Proc.* **28,** 12

Jasswoin, G. (1924). 'On the structure and development of the enamel in mammals.' *Q. Jl microsc. Sci.* **69,** 97

Jatlow, P., Adams, W. R. and Handschumacher, R. E. (1965). 'Pathogenesis of orotic acid-induced fatty change in the rat liver. Light and electron microscopic studies.' *Am. J. Path.* **47,** 125

Jones, A. L., Rudermann, N. B. and Herrera, M. G. (1967). 'Electron microscopic and biochemical study of lipoprotein synthesis in the isolated perfused rat liver.' *J. Lipid. Res.* **8,** 429

Kirkman, H. and Severinghaus, A. E. (1938). 'A review of the Golgi apparatus.' *Anat. Rec.* **70,** 557

Ludford, R. J. (1929). 'Vital staining of normal and malignant cells; staining of malignant tumours with trypan blue.' *Proc. R. Soc., B* **104,** 493

— (1952). 'Pathological aspects of cytology.' In *Cytology and Cell Physiology,* 2nd ed., p. 373. Ed. by G. Bourne. London and New York: Oxford University Press

Mahley, R. W., Gray, M. E., Hamilton, R. L. and Lequire, V. S. (1968). 'Lipid transport in liver. II. Electron microscopic and biochemical studies of alterations in lipoprotein transport induced by cortisone in the rabbit.' *Lab. Invest.* **19,** 358

Mehta, P. N. and Ghadially, F. N. (1973). 'Articular cartilage in corn oil induced lipoarthrosis.' *Ann. rheum. Dis.* **32,** 75

Nakayama, I., Nickerson, P. A. and Skelton, F. R. (1969). 'An ultrastructural study of the adrenocorticotrophic hormone-secreting cell in the rat adenohypophysis during adrenal cortical regeneration.' *Lab. Invest.* **21,** 169

Neutra, M. and Leblond, C. P. (1966a). 'Synthesis of the carbohydrate of mucus in the Golgi complex as shown by electron microscope radioautography of goblet cells from rats injected with glucose-H³.' *J. Cell Biol.* **30,** 119

— — (1966b). 'Radioautographic comparison of the uptake of galactose-H³ and glucose-H³ in the Golgi region of various cells secreting glycoproteins or mucopolysaccharides.' *J. Cell Biol.* **30,** 137

Oberling, Ch. and Bernhard, W. (1961). 'The morphology of the cancer cells.' In *The Cell,* Vol. 5, p. 405. Ed. by J. Brachet and A. E. Mirsky. New York: Academic Press

Onoe, T. and Ohno, K. (1963). 'Role of endoplasmic reticulum in fat absorption.' In *Intracellular Membranous Structure,* Vol. 14. Ed. by S. Seno and E. V. Cowdry. Okayama: The Japan Society for Cell Biology

Palay, S. L. and Karlin, L. J. (1959). 'An electron microscopic study of the intestinal villus. II. The pathway of fat absorption.' *J. biophys. biochem. Cytol.* **5,** 373

Peterson, M. R. and Leblond, C. P. (1964). 'Uptake by the Golgi region of glucose labelled with tritium in the 1 or 6 position, as an indicator of synthesis of complex carbohydrates.' *Expl Cell Res.* **34,** 420

Rambourg, A. (1971). 'Morphological and histochemical aspects of glycoproteins at the surface of animal cells.' *Int. Rev. Cytol.* **31,** 57

Reynolds, E. S. (1963). 'Liver parenchymal cell injury. I. Initial alterations of the cell following poisoning with carbon tetrachloride.' *J. Cell Biol.* **19,** 139

Roy, S. (1967). 'Ultrastructure of synovial membrane in osteoarthritis.' *Ann. rheum. Dis.* **26,** 517

— and Ghadially, F. N. (1967a). 'Ultrastructure of normal rat synovial membrane.' *Ann. rheum. Dis.* **26,** 26

— — (1967b). 'Synthesis of hyaluronic acid by synovial cells.' *J. Path. Bact.* **93,** 555

Scow, R. O. (1970). 'Transport of triglyceride. Its removal from blood circulation and uptake by tissues.' In *Parenteral Nutrition,* p. 294. Ed. by H. C. Meng and D. L. Law. Springfield, Illinois: Charles C Thomas

Selby, C. C., Biesele, J. J. and Grey, C. E. (1956). 'Electron microscope studies of ascites tumor cells.' *Ann. N.Y. Acad. Sci.* **63,** 748

Severinghaus, A. E. (1937). 'Cellular changes in the anterior hypophysis with special reference to its secretory activities.' *Physiol. Rev.* **17,** 556

Sheldon, H. and Kimball, F. B. (1962). 'Studies on cartilage. III. The occurrence of collagen within vacuoles of the Golgi apparatus.' *J. Cell Biol.* **12,** 599

— and Robinson, R. A. (1960) 'Studies on cartilage. II. Electron microscope observations on rabbit ear cartilage following the administration of papain.' *J. Biophys. biochem. Cytol.* **8,** 151

Stein, O. and Shapiro, B. (1959). 'Assimilation and dissimilation of fatty acids by the rat liver.' *Am. J. Physiol.* **196,** 1238

— and Stein, Y. (1967a). 'Lipid synthesis, intracellular transport, storage and secretion. I. Electron microscopic radio-autographic study of the liver after injection of tritiated palmitate or glycerol in fasted and ethanol-treated rats.' *J. Cell Biol.* **33,** 319

— — (1967b). 'The role of the liver in the metabolism of chylomicrons, studied by electron microscopic autoradiography.' *Lab. Invest.* **17,** 436

Suzuki, T. (1957). 'Electron microscopic cytohistopathology. III. Electron microscopic studies on spontaneous mammary carcinoma of mice.' *Gann* **48,** 39

Trelstad, R. L. (1970). 'The Golgi apparatus in chick corneal epithelium: changes in intracellular position during development.' *J. Cell Biol.* **45,** 34

Tzur, R. and Shapiro, B. (1964). 'Dependence of microsomal lipid synthesis on added protein.' *J. Lipid Res.* **5,** 542

Whur, P., Herscovics, A. and Leblond, C. P. (1969). 'Radioautographic visualization of the incorporation of galactose 3H and mannose 3H by rat thyroids *in vitro* in relation to the stages of thyroglobulin synthesis.' *J. Cell Biol.* **43,** 289

Wyllie, J. C., Haust, M. D. and More, R. H. (1966). 'The fine structure of synovial lining cells in rheumatoid arthritis.' *Lab. Invest.* **15,** 519

Zagury, D. Uhr, J. W., Jamieson, J. D. and Palade, G. E. (1970). 'Immunoglobulin synthesis and secretion. II. Radio-autographic studies of sites of addition of carboydrate moieties and intracelluar transport.' *J. Cell Biol.* **46,** 52

CHAPTER V

Endoplasmic Reticulum

INTRODUCTION

The organelle now known as endoplasmic reticulum was first noted by Porter *et al.* (1945) in whole mounts of cultured cells examined with the electron microscope, where it presented as a network of tubular strands and vesicles of varying size and form. It was later named the endoplasmic reticulum (Porter and Thompson, 1948; Porter and Kallman, 1952) because it appeared confined to the main mass of the cell cytoplasm (endoplasm) and did not extend to the cell periphery (ectoplasm). However, such a distribution is not seen in sectioned material, nor is the reticular form easily appreciated. Nevertheless, it is now quite clear that the organelle does in fact often extend close to the cell membrane, and although one has at times to stretch the meaning of the word 'reticulum', this organelle, in its well developed form at least, consists of a system of inter-connected cavities and passages and not a series of isolated sacs or vesicles.

Numerous electron microscopic studies now attest to the fact that virtually all the cells of higher plants and vertebrates contain elements of the endoplasmic reticulum (see reviews by Palade, 1955, and Porter, 1961). In some cells the organelle is quite simple and is represented by a few vesicles, tubules or cisternae. In others it is quite large and complex and occupies a major volume of the cell cytoplasm.

Two main morphological types of endoplasmic reticulum are recognized: the granular or rough endoplasmic reticulum, and the agranular or smooth endoplasmic reticulum. The rough or granular endoplasmic reticulum is so named because its cytoplasmic surface is studded with loops, rows or spirals of ribosomes (called polyribosomes). The smooth endoplasmic reticulum or agranular endoplasmic reticulum, as its name implies, is not associated with ribosomes. This, however, is the main but not the only morphological difference because, while the rough endo-plasmic reticulum has a marked tendency to form lamellae and cisternae, the smooth endoplasmic reticulum tends to present as fine branching tubules and vesicles. Cell types which have abundant rough endoplasmic reticulum usually have little smooth endoplasmic reticulum and vice versa. An exception to this is the hepatocyte where both forms of endoplasmic reticulum are fairly well represented and continuities between the two can frequently be demonstrated.

It is generally accepted that the main function of the rough endoplasmic reticulum is the production of secretory or 'export' protein, and that the protein required for endogenous cellular needs is produced by polyribosomes lying free in the cytoplasm. No such common function can be ascribed to the smooth endoplasmic reticulum. It is believed to be involved in a variety of tasks such as: (1) the synthesis of steroid hormones in certain endocrine cells; (2) the detoxification of drugs and metabolism of cholesterol, lipoproteins and perhaps also glycogen in liver cells; (3) the release and recapture of calcium ions in muscle during contraction and relaxation; (4) the transport of ions in the chloride cells of fishes; (5) the secretion of chloride ions by oxyntic cells of the stomach; and (6) lipid transport in intestinal epithelium (Porter, 1961; Fawcett, 1967). It is worth noting, however, that some doubts exist regarding the nature of the smooth membrane systems seen in certain cells such as the chloride cells and intestinal epithelial cells, for it is thought that the tubules and vesicles seen here could be invaginations of the plasma membrane.

ROUGH ENDOPLASMIC RETICULUM

The term 'granular' or 'rough endoplasmic reticulum' is used to describe a system of ribosome-studded membranes found in the cytoplasm of many cells. The morphology of this organelle varies markedly in different cell types. In its well developed form, the rough endoplasmic reticulum may be looked upon as a system of vesicular and tubular elements which frequently expand to form flat saccular structures called 'cisternae'. Such cisternae may be solitary, occur in loosely arranged groups, as closely packed parallel stacks, or as gracefully curved or concentric arrays of evenly spaced lamellae. The rough endoplasmic reticulum creates a complex two-phase system in the cell separated by a membrane. Outside the system lies the cytoplasmic matrix, and within it the proteinaceous products elaborated by the ribosomes of the rough endoplasmic reticulum.

Since the membrane-bound passages of the rough endoplasmic reticulum have often been found to be continuous with the perinuclear cistern, and the outer membrane of the nuclear envelope (page 20) is frequently studded with some ribosomes, Porter (1961) has looked upon the nuclear envelope as a stable subdivision of the endoplasmic reticulum. He states, 'the nuclear envelope appears in section as a large lamellar or cisternal unit of the endoplasmic reticulum enclosing the nucleus'. Further support for such a concept comes from the observation that after mitosis the nuclear envelope seems to be re-formed from the endoplasmic reticulum. Annulate lamellae (page 283), which bear much resemblance to the nuclear envelope, have also been looked upon as a variety of endoplasmic reticulum.

The amount of rough endoplasmic reticulum and its morphology in various cell types are quite variable. The greatest development of this organelle is seen in cells which produce an abundant, protein-rich secretion. Some others contain a more modest amount of rough endoplasmic reticulum, while almost all cells contain at least a few elements of this organelle. In pancreatic acinar cells and plasma cells singularly well endowed with rough endoplasmic reticulum the cytoplasm is packed with arrays of closely stacked cisternae (*Plates 92 and 93*) but in synovial cells and chondrocytes (*Plate 94*) the not-so-abundant complement of rough endoplasmic reticulum is represented by a system of irregular sacs and vesicles.

Although the main functions of the rough endoplasmic reticulum is the production of secretory or export proteins, it also produces some which are used endogenously. Thus there is evidence that, when hypertrophy of the rough or smooth endoplasmic reticulum occurs, the lipoproteins

---

Plate 92

Fig. 1. Pancreatic acinar cells from a child with islet cell adenoma, showing the graceful arrays of rough endoplasmic reticulum (R) characteristic of this cell type. Note also the myelin figure (arrow). This is an artefact of glutaraldehyde fixation which has at times been mistaken for a pathological lesion. × 20,000

Fig. 2. A group of transversely cut cisternae (C) of the rough endoplasmic reticulum, showing ribosomes at irregular intervals along the cytoplasmic surface of the membranes. A group of polyribosomes (P) is seen in an area where the section has passed tangential to the membrane. From same case as *Fig. 1.* × 48,000

Fig. 3. Tangentially cut cisternae showing polyribosomes. From a plasma cell found in human bronchial mucosa. × 50,000

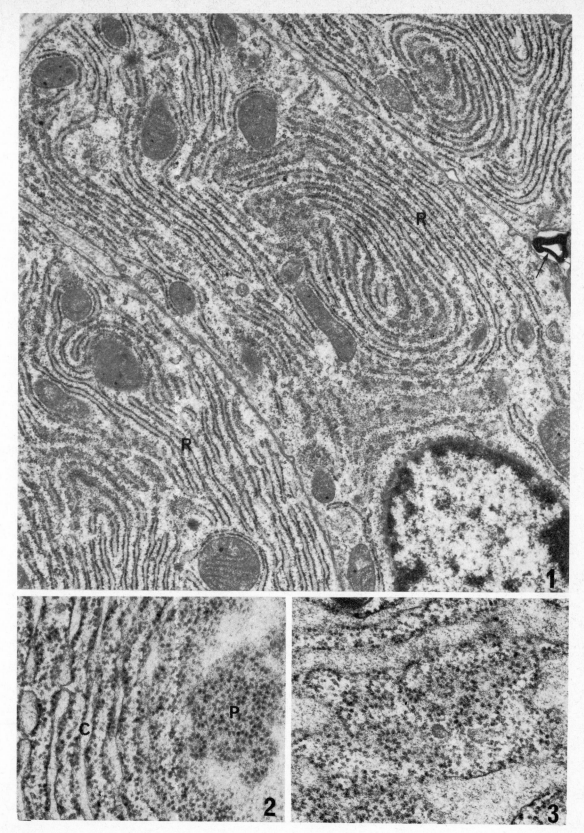

211

constituting the new membranes are produced by the rough endoplasmic reticulum. The hydrolytic enzymes of primary lysomes are also produced in the rough endoplasmic reticulum, as are the enzymes found in microbodies.

In transverse sections through the cisternae the ribosomes do not appear uniformly spaced along the membranes. The reason for this becomes apparent when tangential cuts revealing the surface of the cisternae are examined, for now most of the ribosomes are seen to occur in groups forming rosettes, linear arrays, loops or spirals (*Plate 92*). Such collections of ribosomes are spoken of as polysomes or polyribosomes. Ribosomes and polyribosomes occur not only on the membranes of the rough endoplasmic reticulum but also free in the cytoplasm. Polyribosomes consist of ribosomes (about 150 Å diameter) held together by a fine strand of messenger RNA (about 10–15 Å thick). (See page 230 for more details.)

It is now generally accepted that polyribosomes lying free in the cytoplasm are engaged in the synthesis of proteins for endogenous cellular needs, in contrast to those attached to the rough endoplasmic reticulum which, as can be seen, are concerned mainly with the production of export protein.

Cells which produce a protein-rich secretion (e.g. pancreatic cells and plasma cells) are well endowed with rough endoplasmic reticulum while fast-growing populations of cells, such as cells in culture, embryonic cells and tumour cells, are often characterized by numerous polyribosomes lying free in the cytoplasmic matrix. Similarly, in erythroblasts (normoblasts), where the haemoglobin produced is stored and not exported, numerous polyribosomes occur in the cytoplasm but rough endoplasmic reticulum is either absent or represented by an occasional small vesicle covered by sparse ribosomes.

Light microscopists have long known that the cytoplasm of all cells is not uniformly eosinophilic and that certain cell types contain basophilic material or discrete basophilic bodies in their cytoplasm. This has been referred to by various terms such as the 'chromidial substance', 'chromophilic substance' or 'ergastoplasm'. It is now clear that the electron microscopic equivalent of this is the rough endoplasmic reticulum and cytoplasmic ribosomes. Thus, the cytoplasmic basophilia and pyroninophilia of plasma cells reflect the abundant rough endoplasmic reticulum in these cells, while the Nissl bodies or Nissl substance of neurons, are revealed to be areas within the cytoplasm containing parallel arrays of rough endoplasmic reticulum and clusters of ribosomes in the intervening cytoplasmic matrix.

Plate 93

Plasma cells from the subsynovial tissue of a rheumatoid joint. (*From Ghadially and Roy, 1969*)

Fig. 1. Plasma cells showing abundant arrays of rough endoplasmic reticulum (R) which produces the cytoplasmic basophilia characteristic of this cell and a well developed juxtanuclear Golgi complex (G) which presents at light microscopy as a clear crescentic area called the 'Hof'. A lymphocyte (L) with scant cytoplasm and a small portion of a macrophage (M) containing lysosomes are also seen in this electron micrograph. × 11,000

Fig. 2. Plasma cell showing cisternae (C) of the rough endoplasmic reticulum which are moderately distended with proteinaceous secretory product. On the surface of the tangentially cut cisternae can be seen numerous polyribosomes (arrows). × 28,000

Fig. 3. A plasma cell showing vesiculation of the rough endoplasmic reticulum. Note that the vesicles (V) contain secretory product which is fairly electron dense. There is no evidence here that vesiculation has been produced by an ingress of water, for the contents appear neither diluted nor lucent. × 28,000

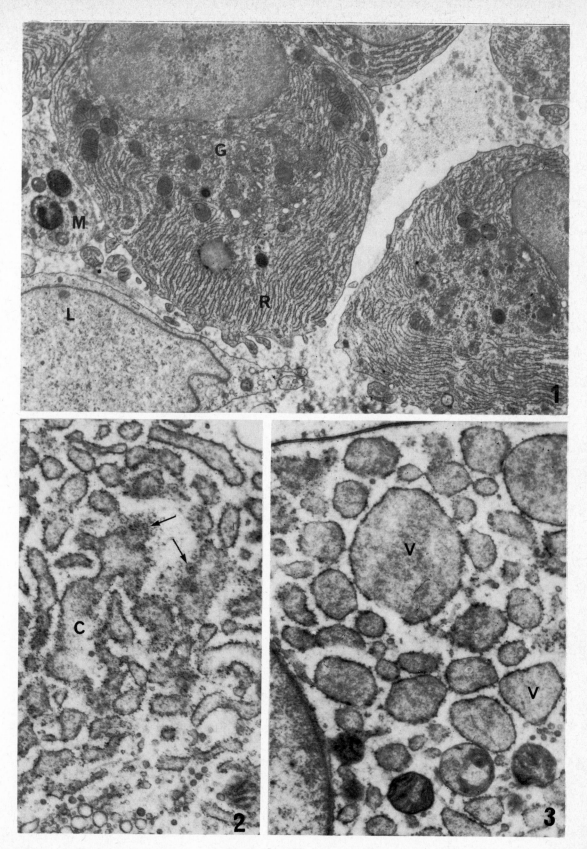

213

This basophilic reaction depends on the RNA in the ribosomes and is not related to the membranes themselves. Cells in which there is a paucity of rough endoplasmic reticulum and ribosomes show an eosinophilic cytoplasm at light microscopy. Since both the membranes of the smooth endoplasmic reticulum and the cytoplasm are eosinophilic the presence of modest amounts of smooth endoplasmic reticulum cannot be discerned by light microscopy. However, when the smooth membranes are abundant the cytoplasmic eosinophilia is quite intense. In instances where the smooth endoplasmic reticulum has a focal rather than a diffuse distribution within the cell, it may present as eosinophilic bodies in the cytoplasm.

In certain cells, such as hepatocytes and pancreatic acinar cells, the cisternae are quite narrow and often appear almost empty or contain but a sparse amount of medium-density material. In others, such as fibroblasts, chondrocytes and synovial cells, the sacs of the endoplasmic reticulum are invariably more distended. In plasma cells every conceivable variation may be found, but more often than not the cisternae are moderately distended. Occasionally, the rough endoplasmic reticulum in these cells is reduced to a collection of vesicles loaded with secretory products (*Plate 93*).

The manner in which secretory products leave the rough endoplasmic reticulum and the cell have been subject of much debate. The best-known and most widely held thesis is that material formed in the rough endoplasmic reticulum is transported to the Golgi complex where it is condensed and/or modified in various ways, and packaged into single-membrane-bound vacuoles which then travel to the cell membrane and the contents are discharged from the cell in a variety of ways.

At one time it was thought that connections existed between the rough endoplasmic reticulum and the cell membrane (Epstein, 1957a) and that secretory products were perhaps discharged via openings of the cisternae on the cell surface. This view has lost favour, for such openings are rarely if ever seen. However, line drawings of 'typical cells' showing such connections are commonly encountered in many elementary treatises on the cell.

Conflicting opinions have been expressed by workers who have studied the manner in which tropocollagen is secreted by fibroblasts and chondrocytes to form the matrical collagen fibres. The commonly held idea is that tropocollagen produced by the rough endoplasmic reticulum passes via the Golgi complex to the cell exterior as a merocrine secretion. However, Ross and Benditt (1965) have suggested that the rough endoplasmic reticulum approaches close to the cell membrane and discharges its contents into the matrix via vesicles budding from the cisternae. Other workers have proposed that a shedding of cell processes or segments of the cell containing rough endoplasmic reticulum and secretory material may occur to release tropocollagen into the matrix (Porter and Pappas, 1959; Godman and Porter, 1960; Chapman, 1962; Porter, 1964).

Plate 94

Fig. 1. Section through a human type B synovial cell, showing numerous profiles of rough endoplasmic reticulum, with moderately dilated cisternae (C) and a small Golgi complex (G). Although this cell is well endowed with rough endoplasmic reticulum as compared to the type A synovial cell (*Plate 85*) which contains only rare small vesicles studded with ribosomes, the endoplasmic reticulum here (type B cell) does not attain the level of development and organization found in plasma cells (*Plate 93*) or pancreatic acinar cells (*Plate 92*). × 30,000 (*From Ghadially and Roy, 1969*)

Fig. 2. A zone 2 chondrocyte from the articular cartilage of a rabbit. These cells are also fairly well endowed with rough endoplasmic reticulum. The cisternae (C) are moderately distended with medium-density material. × 37,000 (*From Ghadially and Roy, 1969*)

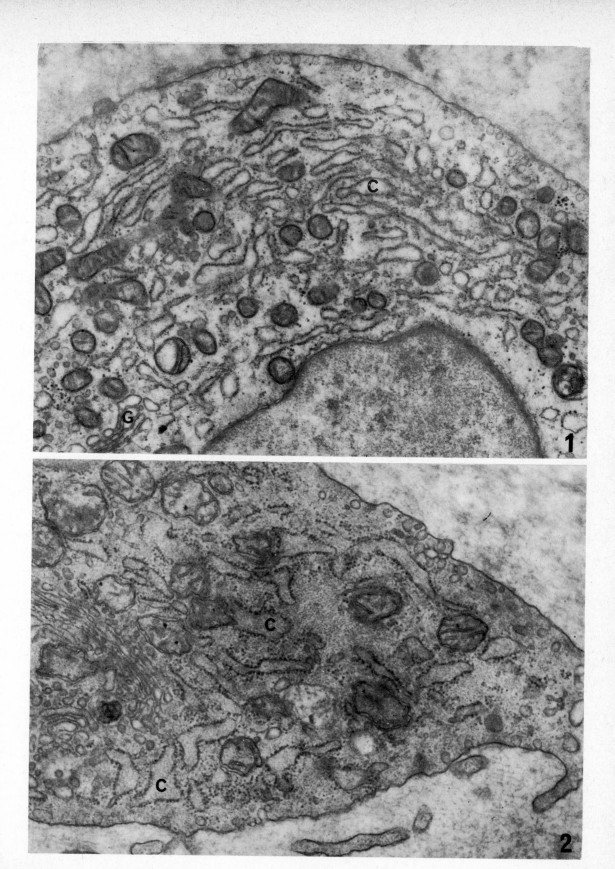

215

As its name implies, the agranular or smooth-surfaced endoplasmic reticulum is distinguished from the rough endoplasmic reticulum by the absence of attached ribosomes. Although continuities between the rough and smooth endoplasmic reticulum are frequently demonstrable in many cell types (*Plate 95, Fig. 1*; *Plate 124*), they are morphologically and functionally distinct (see reviews by Porter, 1961, and Fawcett, 1967). The smooth endoplasmic reticulum usually presents as a meshwork of branching tubules and/or vesicles. Relatively thick sections are needed to demonstrate the tubular pattern. Unlike the rough endoplasmic reticulum, the smooth endoplasmic reticulum rarely forms cisternae. It is worth noting that this is a delicate system which, at least in some cell types (e.g. steroid-producing cells), is easily affected by preparative procedures. Glutaraldehyde fixation is, as a rule, more likely to preserve the tubular formations while in osmium-fixed material the tubules tend to break up into vesicles. The smooth endoplasmic reticulum in hepatocytes, however, is not so sensitive to preparative procedures. In the tubular epithelial cells of rat kidney fixed by glutaraldehyde perfusion many focal aggregates of branching smooth-membrane-bound tubules are found (*Plate 95, Fig. 2*), but kidney tissue preserved by immersion in fixatives usually shows scant smooth endoplasmic reticulum (Newstead, personal communication).

Although the structure of the smooth endoplasmic reticulum is somewhat similar in most cell types, its enzyme content and functions differ. In the liver the smooth endoplasmic reticulum occupies focal areas of cytoplasm, usually in company with glycogen rosettes (*Plate 95, Fig. 1*). If the glycogen is abundant then the smooth endoplasmic reticulum is difficult to visualize. The smooth endoplasmic reticulum becomes somewhat more prominent and its association with glycogen more evident in animals fasted for a day or two. This close association of glycogen and smooth endoplasmic reticulum led Porter and Bruni (1959) and others to suggest that the smooth endoplasmic reticulum was perhaps involved in glycogenesis or glycogenolysis. Biochemical studies on isolated microsomal fraction have, however, failed to support this idea. It would appear that the main enzymes of glycogen metabolism lie in the cytoplasmic matrix or elsewhere, but not in the endoplasmic reticulum. (An exception to this is glucose-6-phosphatase, which is associated with the endoplasmic reticulum (Ernster *et al.*, 1962).) However, Rothschild (1963) has pointed out that enzymes may be detached from the endoplasmic reticulum and released into the 'soluble fraction' during isolation procedures. In any case, the significance of so distinct and constant an association between smooth endoplasmic reticulum and glycogen, which has been observed repeatedly in many species, still awaits clarification. That such an association is not a prerequisite of glycogen synthesis or breakdown is attested by the fact that in other situations such as brown adipose tissue and the glycogen body of birds (Revel *et al.*, 1960) the smooth endoplasmic reticulum is quite rudimentary. Simiarly, as noted elsewhere (pages 56 and 162), glycogen deposits are at times found in nuclei or mitochondria, and it has been suggested that glycogen may be synthesized in such sites without any obvious assistance from the smooth endoplasmic reticulum.

Plate 95

Fig. 1. Cow hepatocyte, showing cytoplasmic zones occupied by rough (R) and smooth (S) endoplasmic reticulum. Glycogen rosettes (G) occur almost exclusively in association with the smooth endoplasmic reticulum. Continuity between the rough and smooth endoplasmic reticulum can just be discerned at this low magnification (arrow). × 36,000

Fig. 2. Numerous smooth-membrane-bound ramifying tubules are seen in this tubular epithelial cell of a rat kidney perfused with glutaraldehyde. × 54,000 (*Newstead, unpublished electron micrograph*)

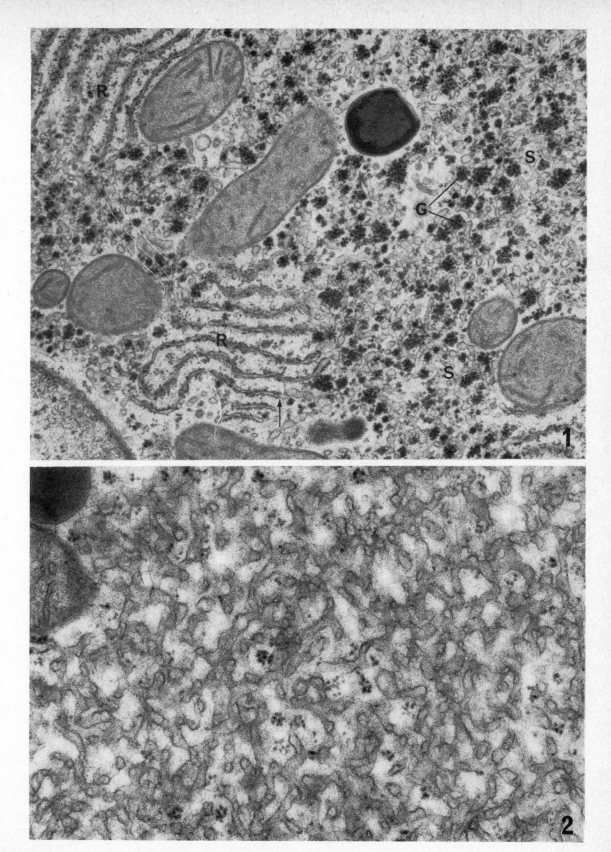

The smooth endoplasmic reticulum in the hepatocyte appears to be involved in cholesterol metabolism (Fawcett, 1964; Jones and Armstrong, 1965) and detoxification of drugs (page 272).

An extensively developed smooth endoplasmic reticulum occurs in cells engaged in the production and secretion of steroid hormones. Examples include: (1) the interstitial (Leydig) cells of the testis (Christensen and Fawcett, 1961; Christensen, 1965); (2) cells of the adrenal cortex (Brenner, 1966; Long and Jones, 1967a, b; McNutt and Jones, 1970); and (3) corpus luteum (Yamada and Ishikawa, 1960; Enders, 1962; Enders and Lyon, 1964). Biochemical studies have long indicated that cells of the above-mentioned organs synthesize steroid from acetate via chloesterol (Morris and Chaikoff, 1959; Werbin and Chaikoff, 1961; Armstrong *et al.*, 1964; Srere *et al.*, 1968). Christensen and Fawcett (1961) suggested that it was the smooth endoplasmic reticulum in such cells which was involved in the biosynthesis of cholesterol, and cell fractionation studies have since confirmed that the needed enzymes do reside in this organelle (Goldblatt, 1969).

Many interesting correlations exist between the amount of smooth endoplasmic reticulum and the biosynthesis of cholesterol by the adrenal cortex of different species. For example, the hamster adrenal cortex, which is poorly endowed with smooth endoplasmic reticulum, does not appear to use cholesterol as a precursor for steroid hormone production (Marks *et al.*, 1958; Schindler and Knigge, 1959). The guinea-pig adrenal cortex, which is richly endowed with smooth endoplasmic reticulum, is said to produce 40 per cent of the cholesterol used for steroid production but the rat adrenal cortex, with a relatively poorly developed smooth endoplasmic reticulum, depends almost entirely upon plasma cholesterol for steroid synthesis (Christensen, 1965; Jones and Fawcett, 1966).

In striated muscle the morphology and distribution of smooth endoplasmic reticulum (often called sarcoplasmic reticulum), shows many variations, depending upon species and type of muscle. Generally speaking, fast-acting muscle tends to have a well developed sarcoplasmic reticulum (*Plate 96*). Examples include: (1) the muscle of the swim bladder of the toad-fish (Fawcett and Revel, 1961; Fawcett, 1967); (2) the cricothyroid muscle of the bat (Revel, 1961); (3) the flight muscle of the dragon-fly (Smith, 1961); (4) the extrinsic eye muscle of *Fundulus heteroclitus* (Reger, 1961); and (5) the remotor muscle of the lobster (Rosenbluth, 1969).

In most skeletal muscles of mammals, the sarcoplasmic reticulum is not as abundant as in the examples stated above. Here it occurs as a sparse laciform network of fine tubules around each myofibril.* In the region of the A-bands the tubules of the system are longitudinally orientated (i.e. parallel to the myofibrils) but they are somewhat dilated and anastomose freely in the region of the H-bands (H-band sacs). At regular intervals along the myofibrils the longitudinally orientated tubules of the smooth endoplasmic reticulum join transversely orientated channels of the smooth endoplasmic reticulum called the terminal cisternae. In longitudinal sections of skeletal muscle fibres (*Plate 97*), three vesicular profiles (collectively referred to as a triad) are seen at regularly repeating intervals. The outer two represent sections through the transversely orientated cisternae of the smooth endoplasmic reticulum, while the inner, more slender, tubular or vesicular profile represents a section through a T-tubule.

* It is singularly difficult to explain the relationships of the sarcoplasmic reticulum without the aid of diagrams. Excellent drawings and a singularly lucid account of the subject may be found in Bloom and Fawcett, 1969

Plate 96

Flight muscle of dragon-fly, showing abundant smooth endoplasmic reticulum (S). (Compare with *Plate 97*.) Note also the close association of mitochondria with smooth endoplasmic reticulum and lipid droplets (L). × 20,000

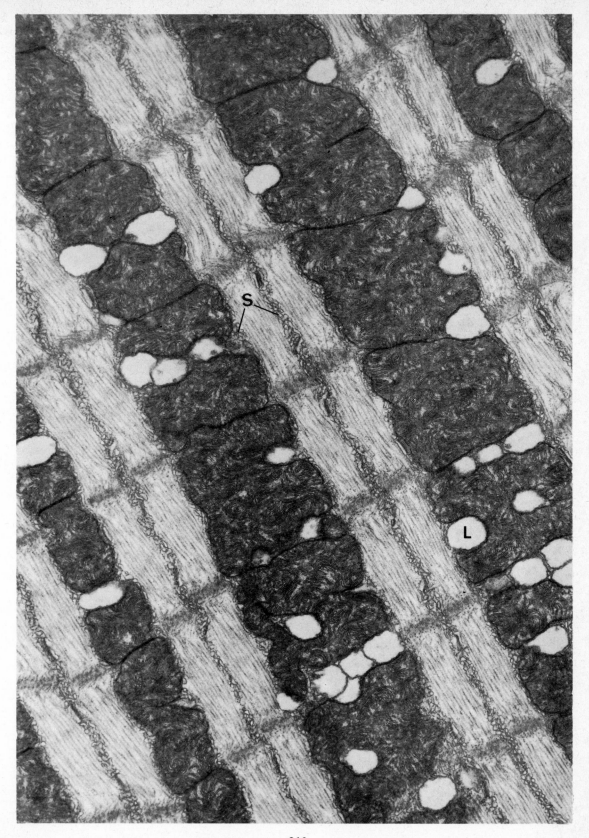

219

These T-tubules have now been demonstrated to be tubular invaginations of the plasma membrane into the muscle fibre of many species. The location of the triads with respect to the cross-banded pattern of the myofibrils varies from species to species. In mammals the triads occur at the junction of I- and A-bands. In the frog the triads are found at the Z-line.

Cardiac muscle is poorly endowed with smooth endoplasmic reticulum as compared to skeletal muscle (turtle heart is singularly deficient in this respect (Fawcett and Selby, 1958)), but the T-system tubules are much greater in diameter and run at the level of the Z-line. There are no terminal cisternae and hence no triads, but small expansions of the sarcoplasmic reticulum form a close association with the sarcolemma and T-tubules. The latter association presents as diads at the Z-line.

It is now clear that the coupling of excitation and contraction is mediated by the T-system tubules and the sarcoplasmic reticulum (Smith, 1966), but details of the sequence of events that occur during contraction and relaxation of muscle fibres has received various interpretations. It would appear that on arrival of an impulse a wave of depolarization is set up which spreads over the sarcolemma and into the T-system tubules. This explains why, on the arrival of an impulse, the myofibrils throughout the muscle fibre contract simultaneously. It is thought that in the resting state most of the calcium ions reside in the smooth endoplasmic reticulum, a point supported by the fact that electron-dense granular material is often seen there (*Plate 97*). When the depolarization wave reaches the triads, calcium ions diffuse out of the smooth endoplasmic reticulum and activate the dephosphorylation of ATP, with resultant muscle contraction (which is looked upon as a repetitive making and breaking of successive cross-links between myosin and actin).

In the apical cytoplasm of intestinal mucosa a fair amount of smooth endoplasmic reticulum is present. (There is argument as to whether the vesicles and tubules seen in this region truly represent smooth endoplasmic reticulum or whether they are pinocytotic vesicles and invaginations of the plasma membrane (Sjostrand, 1964).) During fat absorption, lipid droplets appear in this system of tubules and vesicles and are transported to the Golgi complex and thence to the lateral surface of the cell.

Teleosts living in the sea excrete via the gills large amounts of sodium chloride taken in with the sea-water. This is achieved by the activity of chloride cells which are well endowed with smooth endoplasmic reticulum. (Here also doubt exists as to whether these tubules and vesicles are derived from the plasma membrane.) The mechanisms involved are poorly understood, but both sodium (Mizuhira *et al.*, 1970) and chloride (Petrik, 1968) ions have been demonstrated in the smooth endoplasmic reticulum of the chloride cells of eel gills and it is thought that this organelle plays an important part in the transport of these ions.

Other cells in which a conspicuous amount of smooth endoplasmic reticulum is found include the retinal pigment cells (Porter and Yamada, 1960), gastric parietal cells (Ito, 1961) and cells of sebaceous glands (Palay, 1958).

Plate 97

Human skeletal muscle showing sparse, smooth endoplasmic reticulum (arrow). At the junction of the I- and A-bands lie the triads, consisting of a T-tubule (T) bounded on either side by the terminal cisternae or lateral sacs (S) of the smooth endoplasmic reticulum, containing moderately electron-dense material. × 65,000

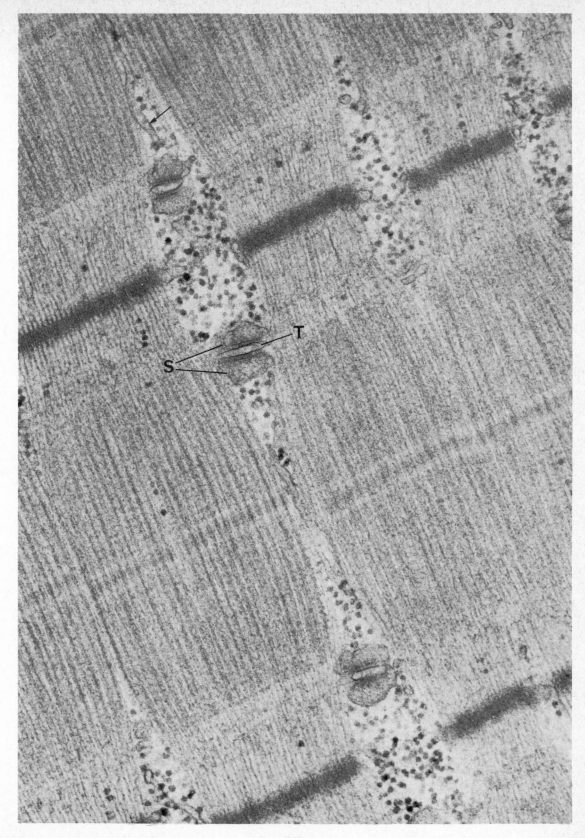

Ingress of water and solutes into the cell may lead to dilatation and vesiculation of various membrane-bound compartments, such as the rough and smooth endoplasmic reticulum, Golgi complex and mitochondria. It should be noted that when the rough endoplasmic reticulum suffers dilatation and vesiculation it tends to become degranulated and hence comes to resemble smooth endoplasmic reticulum; under similar circumstances the Golgi complex also loses its characteristic morphology and becomes indistinguishable from other membranous components.

Dilatation of the rough endoplasmic reticulum is often described as dilatation of the cisternae of the rough endoplasmic reticulum. Since not all the elements of the rough endoplasmic reticulum occur as cisternae, the shorter term 'dilatation of rough endoplasmic reticulum' seems more desirable. The term 'enlargement of the rough endoplasmic reticulum' is sometimes used (e.g. Pfeiffer *et al.*, 1971) but this seems undesirable as it might be confused with an increase in the amount of rough endoplasmic reticulum in the cell. Singularly confusing is the term 'cytoplasmic lakes' used by Ward *et al.* (1971) to describe dilated rough endoplasmic reticulum, for it could create the erroneous impression that cytoplasmic material is contained within dilated rough endoplasmic reticulum.

Dilatation of the rough endoplasmic reticulum may be quite modest in degree so that there is only a slight increase in width of the cisternae, or it may be quite marked so that the cell assumes a cribriform appearance (*Plate 98*). When the term 'dilated rough endoplasmic reticulum' is used, one assumes that the reticular nature of the organelle is not totally lost and that the enlarged cavities are still more or less continuous with each other. The term 'vesiculation' implies that the rough endoplasmic reticulum has broken up into numerous discrete vesicles (*Plate 99*) or somewhat larger vacuoles, pools or lakes. However, a clear distinction between dilatation and vesiculation is often not possible for, in another plane of sectioning, continuity might be demonstrable between such pools and lakes.

Dilatation and vesiculation of endoplasmic reticulum together with mitochondrial swelling are the main features of the change known to pathologists as cloudy swelling and hydropic degeneration. Since in this condition there is an ingress of water, the contents of endoplasmic reticulum are diluted and hence appear more electron lucent than normal. A similar situation can also result from improper handling and processing of tissue, such as the use of hypotonic fixatives.

On the other hand, it has already been noted that many cells, such as fibroblasts, chondrocytes, synovial cells and plasma cells, seem to have a tendency to store the secretory product awhile within the elements of the rough endoplasmic reticulum, so as a rule these tend to appear somewhat more dilated than, say, the rough endoplasmic reticulum of hepatocytes or pancreatic acinar cells. Cells with gross dilatation or vesiculation of rough endoplasmic reticulum but with normal-looking or not particularly diluted contents are also at times encountered (e.g. plasma cells, see *Plate 93, Fig. 3*). Here there is no reason to believe that an ingress of water and solutes has occurred, and one may postulate that some defect in the egress of secretory material might be responsible.

Plate 98

Human synovial intima two weeks after traumatic lipohaemarthrosis (fracture and separation of upper tibial epiphysis). This low power view shows an area of synovial membrane where there is marked dilatation (D) of the endoplasmic reticulum, which gives the cells a cribriform appearance. Joint space (J). × 12,000 (*From Ghadially and Roy, 1969*)

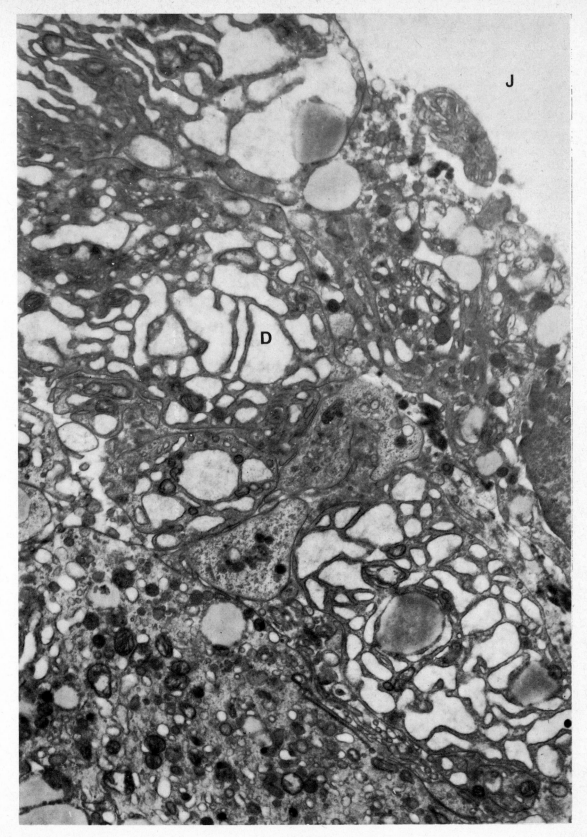

The tendency for secretions to tarry awhile in the rough endoplasmic reticulum may lead to a concentration of products within the cisternae, and the formation of proteinaceous bodies and crystals (page 242).

Consider now just dilatation and vesiculation of the endoplasmic reticulum due to ingress of water into the cell. As noted earlier, this is part and parcel of cloudy swelling, a ubiquitous change that occurs in cells subjected to various noxious influences. It therefore follows that dilatation of rough endoplasmic reticulum, like swollen mitochondria, will frequently be encountered. Vesiculation of rough endoplasmic reticulum which represents a more advanced lesion is encountered somewhat less frequently, but even so it is common enough. One of the finest examples of this lesion is seen in the liver, where the endoplasmic reticulum breaks up into numerous small vesicles (*Plate 99*).*

David (1964) lists various conditions where vesiculation of hepatocyte endoplasmic reticulum has been reported to occur. These include: starvation, kwashiorkor, choline deficiency, hormone administration, oxygen lack, scurvy, hepatitis, yellow fever, enteromelia, biliary obstruction, irradiation and administration of various drugs such as carbon tetrachloride, phosphorus, ethionine, dinitrophenol and dimethylnitrosamine.

Like mitochondrial swelling (page 140), dilatation of the rough endoplasmic reticulum can also be produced artefactually by poor techniques of tissue collection and processing, such as the use of hypotonic fixative solutions. Distinction between the two may at times be difficult or impossible. However, when cells showing dilated or vesiculated rough endoplasmic reticulum are found in company with others not so affected, one can be reasonably certain that it is not an artefact of tissue collection or preparation.

The vesicles produced by fragmentation of the rough endoplasmic reticulum in hepatocytes (*Plate 99*) are usually sparsely populated by ribosomes and vesicles without ribosomes are also seen. Such appearances are probably the result of degranulation of the rough endoplasmic reticulum (page 228) and also involvement of the smooth endoplasmic reticulum and Golgi complex in vesicle formation.

It has already been noted (page 216) that the smooth endoplasmic reticulum is a delicate structure easily affected by fixative procedures, and that in certain cells such as the steroid-secreting cells it usually presents as a collection of small smooth-walled vesicles rather than a system of ramifying tubules. Ingress of fluid in such cells results in the production of larger irregular-bordered vacuoles (*Plate 100*). Dilatation and vesiculation of the smooth endoplasmic reticulum has also been noted in a variety of pathologically altered muscle tissue (Mair and Tomé, 1972).

It was noted earlier that dilatation and vesiculation of the endoplasmic reticulum and mitocondrial swelling constitute the main change called cloudy swelling. This condition has been the subject of long-standing interest and controversy. Virchow (1858), in his classic studies on paren-chymatous inflammation, concluded that cells could absorb exudate from blood vessels and become swollen, cloudy and granular.

* It is interesting to note that the endoplasmic reticulum breaks up into small vesicles when cells are homogenized. The microsomal fraction prepared from normal hepatocytes contains ribosome-studded vesicles similar to those shown in *Plate 99*.

Plate 99

Marked mitochondrial swelling and vesiculation (V) of the rough endoplasmic reticulum is seen in one of the hepatocytes in this electron micrograph. An adjacent hepatocyte shows a more modest mitochondrial swelling and dilatation (D) of the rough endoplasmic reticulum. From the liver of a rat bearing a subcutaneous carcinogen-induced sarcoma. See also *Plate 53*. × 45,000 (*Ghadially and Parry, unpublished electron micrograph*)

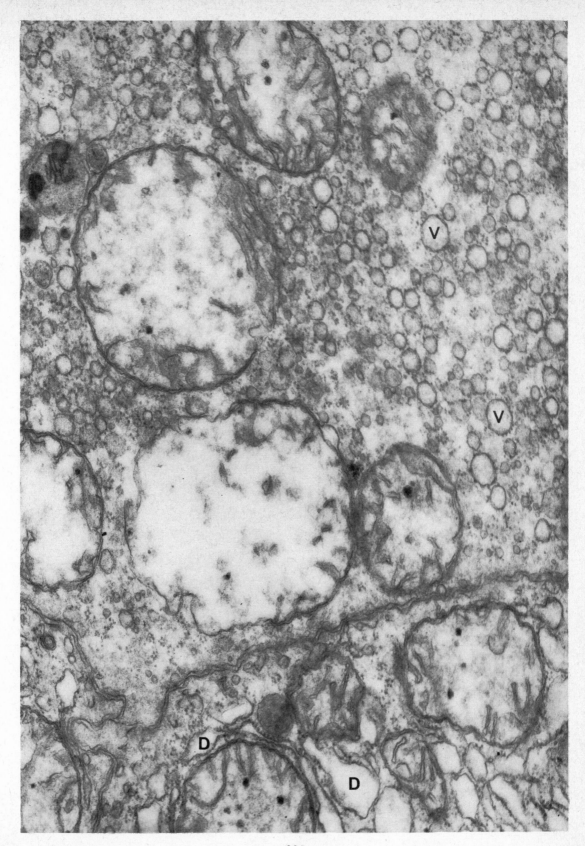

As early as 1914 at least three workers (Anitschkow, 1914; Ernst, 1914; Fahr, 1914) brought forward evidence in support of the idea that mitochondrial swelling was a factor responsible for the granularity of the cytoplasm, and this has since been reiterated by many light and electron microscopists. Remarkable were the careful observations of Anitschkow (1914) who noted that in cloudy swelling at first the mitochondria stained deeply with mitochondrial stain but, as swelling progressed, the mitochondria became sharp contoured spheres, where only the periphery appeared stained but the central portion took up no dye. The idea that other cytoplasmic constituents also participated in the formation of vesicles and granules was not denied; in fact, most workers subscribed to the idea that the granules were also derived from various other cytoplasmic structures, particularly the Golgi complex.

With the advent of the electron microscope and the discovery of the endoplasmic reticulum, it is now known that the 'other cytoplasmic structure' which gives rise to multiple vesicles is mainly the endoplasmic reticulum, but no doubt the Golgi complex also participates in this change. Indeed, one of the earliest studies on the endoplasmic reticulum (Fawcett and Ito, 1958) performed on spermatids *in vitro* showed that with the passage of time the lamellae of the endoplasmic reticulum break up into vesicles. This behaviour has since been observed in many cultured cells.

However, the time-hallowed controversies regarding the nature of the granules in cloudy swelling, and the mechanisms by which such changes are produced, have by no means ended. Some observers stress the importance of the mitochondria in the production of this phenomenon* while others consider dilatation and vesiculation of the endoplasmic reticulum more significant.

No simple generalization can be made, but certain points are worth considering. In hepatocytes vesiculation of the endoplasmic reticulum produces structures too small to be resolved by the light microscope. This probably contributes to the general cloudiness of the cytoplasm, but the marked granularity is probably due to the abundant swollen mitochondria. However, in cells not so richly endowed with mitochondria, and where the endoplasmic reticulum breaks up into quite sizable vacuoles (*Plate 100*), the swollen endoplasmic reticulum may well contribute to the granularity of the cytoplasm seen with the light microscope.

Regarding the sequence of events in cloudy swelling, it would perhaps be reasonable to generalize that in almost every example studied, some degree of dilatation of the endoplasmic reticulum precedes detectable mitochondrial swelling. Indeed, it is possible to have quite marked swelling of endoplasmic reticulum with mitochondria appearing almost normal in size or even pyknotic. However, the earliest change heralding cloudy swelling does seem to lie in the mitochondrion for there is a rapid loss of matrical dense granules (pages 138 and 140).

* Cloudy swelling is also discussed in the section on swollen mitochondria (pages 140–144)

Plate 100

Adrenal cortical cells from a case of Cushing's disease, showing many irregular-shaped vacuoles (V) derived from the smooth endoplasmic reticulum. Only occasional mitochondria (∗) show some swelling. The smooth-endoplasmic-reticulum-derived vacuoles are distinguished from lipid droplets (not present in this electron micrograph) which usually have a round smooth contour and electron-dense rims. ×9,000 (*Ghadially and Larsen, unpublished electron micrograph*)

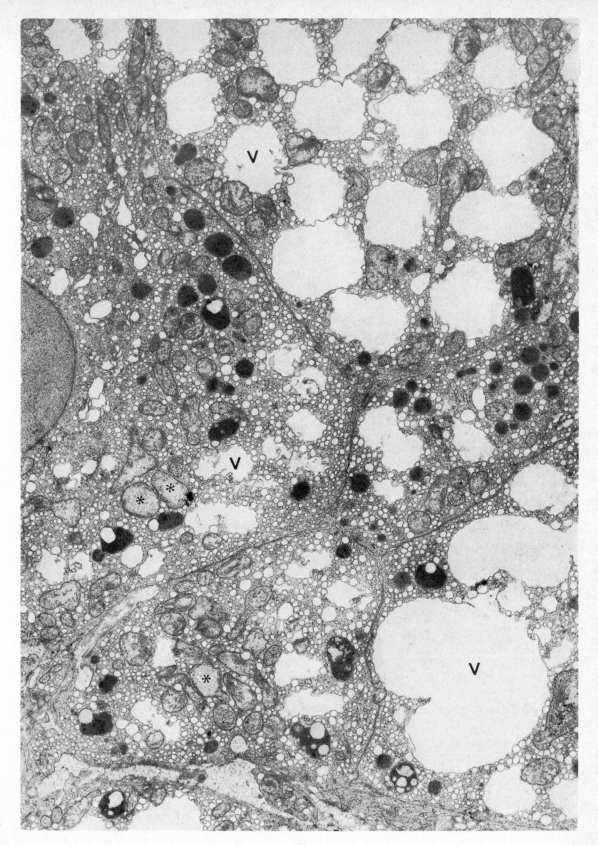

Degranulation of the rough endoplasmic reticulum is a distinct morphological change but it is usually accompanied by other morphological alterations, such as dilatation and vesiculation of the rough endoplasmic reticulum and disaggregation of polyribosomes (page 236). Collectively these changes are referred to as disorganization of rough endoplasmic reticulum. Such changes have been studied extensively in the hepatocytes of experimental animals subjected to various noxious influences.

In the phenomenon called 'degranulation of rough endoplasmic reticulum' the membranes of the rough endoplasmic reticulum appear sparsely populated by ribosomes. Since numerous ribosomes are often found lying free in the cytoplasm, it looks as though the ribosomes have dropped off the rough endoplasmic reticulum into the cytoplasmic matrix. Such an idea is supported by biochemical studies, for in the liver of carbon-tetrachloride-poisoned rats, where degranulation of rough endoplasmic reticulum is a prominent early change (*Plate 101*), there is a shift of RNA from the microsomal fraction (containing endoplasmic reticulum) into the supernatant fluid (containing cytoplasmic matrix) (Reynolds and Yee, 1967; Slater and Sawyer, 1969). Degranulation of the rough endoplasmic reticulum is associated with a loss of poly-ribosome configuration so that solitary ribosomes are seen in the cytoplasmic matrix (*Plate 101*).

Examples of degranulation of hepatocyte rough endoplasmic reticulum suggesting a dropping off of ribosomes are seen in rats after the administration of: (1) ethionine (Villa-Trevino *et al.*, 1964; Baglio and Farber, 1965a; Wood, 1965); (2) carbon tetrachloride (Smuckler *et al.*, 1962; Reynolds, 1963; Krishnan and Stenger, 1966); (3) α-naphthylisothiocyanate (Steiner and Baglio, 1963; puromycin and various other drugs (Reid *et al.*, 1970).

Degranulation of the type described above is an early, relatively mild lesion. The same noxious agent (e.g. carbon tetrachloride) can produce more drastic alterations of membrane structure such as vesiculation, fragmentation or dissolution of the membranes of the rough endoplasmic reticulum, accompanied by a general decrease in ribosomes, both attached to and lying free in the cytoplasm.

One would expect that changes of the type mentioned above would disturb protein synthesis, and there is ample biochemical evidence that protein synthesis is in fact impaired by drugs which produce this change. For example, it has now been shown that after carbon tetrachloride poison-ing the synthesis of several export proteins is depressed (Smuckler *et al.*, 1962), and cell frac-tionation studies show that the defect is related to polyribosome disaggregation and a decreased capacity to incorporate amino acids (Smuckler and Benditt, 1963).

Plate 101

Fig. 1. Rat hepatocyte 1 hour after the administration of carbon tetrachloride, showing vesiculation (V) of rough endo-plasmic reticulum and numerous solitary ribosomes, no doubt derived from disaggregated polyribosomes. Most of these ribosomes can be interpreted as lying free in the cytoplasm but some, seen on a dense background, could still be attached to tangentially cut membranes. × 34.000

Fig. 2. Normal rat hepatocyte, showing numerous polyribosomes (arrows) on tangentially cut cisternae of the rough endoplasmic reticulum. Note the paucity of free ribosomes in the cytoplasmic matrix as compared to *Fig. 1.* × 29,000

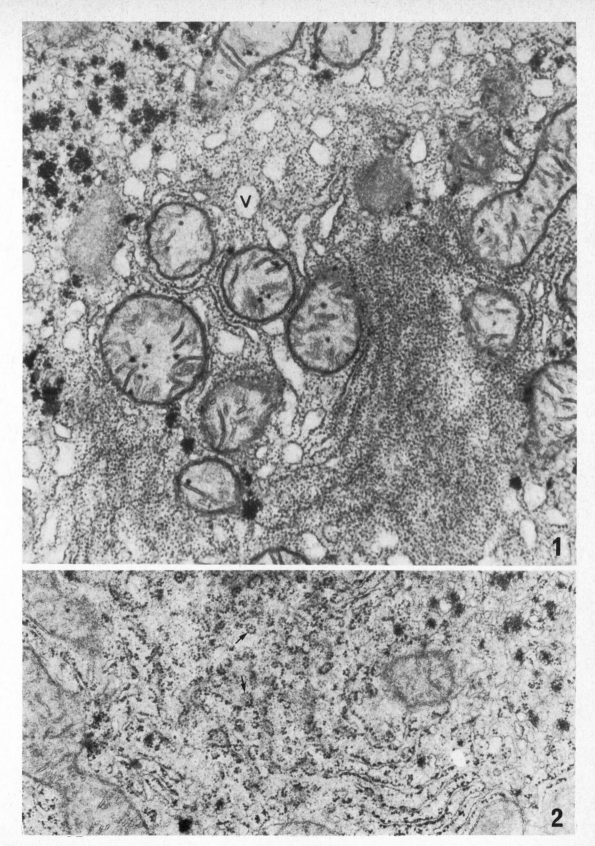

DISAGGREGATION OF POLYRIBOSOMES

As already noted (page 212), ribosomes lying free in the cytoplasm or attached to the membrane of the rough endoplasmic reticulum may occur either as solitary particles or in groups showing various configurations. Such aggregates of ribosomes, which usually present as rosettes, loops or spirals, are referred to as polyribosomes. It is now well established that such polyribosomes comprise ribosomes attached to a fine strand (single molecule) of messenger RNA. The number of ribosomes in a polyribosome is approximately proportional to the number of amino acid residues in the polypeptide chain that is to be synthesized. Thus the peptide chains of haemoglobin which contain only about 150 amino acid residues are synthesized by polyribosomes possessing 5 or 6 ribosomes; but much larger polyribosomes composed of 60–100 ribosomes synthesize the major chains of myosin which contain about 1,800 amino acid residues.

Current concepts envisage that protein synthesis is accomplished by polyribosomes. The ribosomes are believed to be attached to specific sites on a strand of messenger RNA that has the encoded information which determines the amino acid sequence for the specific protein being synthesized. The ribosomes are thought to move along the length of the messenger RNA and to be released when the specific polypeptide chain has been completed. Many studies on various mammalian and other cells now support the concepts stated above (Jacob and Monod, 1961; Goodman and Rich, 1963; Hardesty et al., 1963; Marks et al., 1963; Rich et al., 1963; Staehelin and Noll, 1963; Warner et al., 1963).

In the phenomenon variously referred to as loss of 'polyribosomal configuration', 'disaggregation of polyribosomes' and 'disaggregation of ribosomes', it is believed that polyribosomes break up and/or are not re-formed, so that one finds many solitary ribosomes in the cell but few or no characteristic polyribosomal forms. Two well known models where disaggregation of polyribosomes bound to the rough endoplasmic reticulum occur are the carbon-tetrachloride-poisoned rat hepatocyte and the fibroblast of vitamin-C-deficient guinea-pigs. In both instances there is a disaggregation of membrane-bound polyribosomes, but while in the former instance the ribosomes drop off the membranes (degranulation) in the latter instance they do not.

It will be recalled (page 228) that a prominent, widespread, early alteration of hepatocyte morphology after carbon tetrachloride administration is a degranulation of rough endoplasmic reticulum and a disaggregation of polyribosomes (*Plate 101*). It has now been shown that after carbon tetrachloride poisoning the synthesis of several 'export' proteins is depressed (Smuckler et al., 1962) and this is believed to be related to the disaggregation of hepatocellular polyribosomes (Smuckler and Benditt, 1963).

Plate 102

Disaggregation of polyribosomes produced in synovial cells by immobilizing a rabbit knee joint is illustrated here. *Fig. 1* is from the control joint, and *Fig. 2* from the contralateral immobilized (in a plaster cast) joint of the same animal

Fig. 1. Numerous polyribosomes (P) showing various configurations are seen on the surface of tangentially cut membranes of the rough endoplasmic reticulum. × 70,000

Fig. 2. The polyribosomes have disaggregated (as evidenced by the lack of characteristic configurations as seen in *Fig. 1*) to form solitary ribosomes (R), but they are still attached to the vesiculated (V) rough endoplasmic reticulum. × 65,000

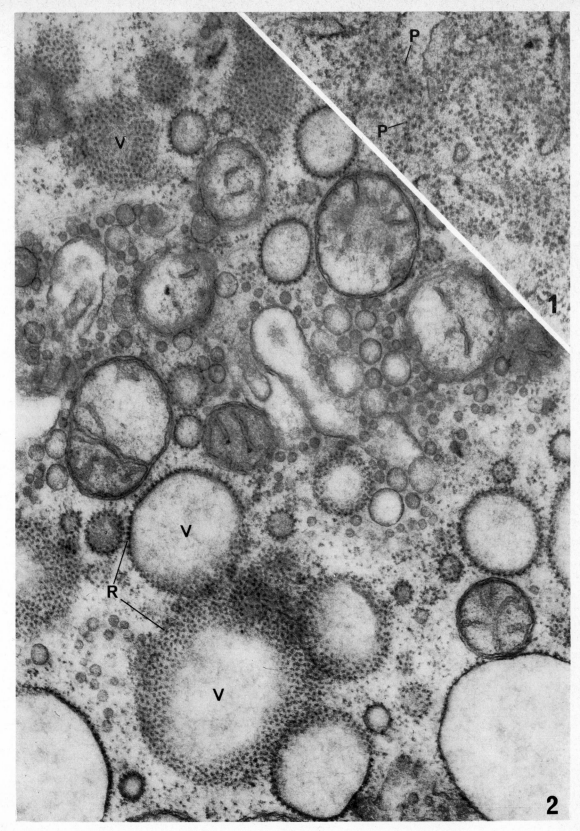

Singularly interesting also is the situation seen in the scorbutic guinea-pig where there is a pathological alteration of connective tissue associated with an impaired tropocollagen synthesis in fibroblasts and a paucity of collagen fibres in the matrix. (Details of biochemical changes that occur in the scorbutic fibroblast are beyond the scope of this text; the reader should refer to Schubert and Hamerman, 1968.) Ultrastructural studies on the fibroblasts from the healing wounds of such animals have shown that the characteristic lesion seen is a disaggregation of polyribosomes (Ross and Benditt, 1964). In healthy guinea-pigs numerous polyribosomes showing spiral and parallel linear configurations abound on the surface of the rough endoplasmic reticulum, but in the scorbutic animal this characteristic configuration is lost and numerous solitary ribosomes, still attached to the membranes, are seen. Vesiculation of the rough endoplasmic reticulum also occurs, but such vesicles are well populated by solitary ribosomes. Thus in the scorbutic fibroblast, disaggregation of polyribosomes is not accompanied by degranulation of the rough endoplasmic reticulum, as is the case in the carbon-tetrachloride-injured hepatocyte.

A similar disaggregation of poyribosomes without degranulation of the vesiculated rough endoplasmic reticulum is found (*Plate 102*) in the synovial membrane of the immobilized rabbit knee joint (Ghadially, unpublished). This correlates well with the marked synovial atrophy and regressive changes that occur in the immobilized joint.

It can be shown that, just as disaggregation of polyribosomes attached to the rough endoplasmic reticulum indicates an impaired 'export' protein production, disaggregation of polyribosomes lying free in the cytoplasm is associated with depressed endogenous protein production.

For example, in normoblasts and young reticulocytes where active haemoglobin synthesis is in progress, numerous polyribosomes occur in the cytoplasm, but as the cell matures such ribosomal clusters are replaced by solitary ribosomes (*Plate 103, Figs. 1 and 2*), and by the time the mature, well haemoglobinized erythrocyte has evolved even these disappear from the cytoplasm (Hardesty *et al.*, 1963; Marks *et al.*, 1963; Warner *et al.*, 1963). Similarly, cells in culture show numerous polyribosomes in their cytoplasm which presumably produce cytoplasmic proteins to keep pace with cell division. In virus-infected cells where cell division is halted a disaggregation of polyribosomes occurs and the cytoplasm is at times filled with innumerable solitary ribosomes (Rich *et al.*, 1963).

Numerous studies, including autoradiographic ones on cultured cells, have shown that there is a marked depression of protein synthesis during mitosis, and under such circumstances there is also a disaggregation of polyribosomes (Scharff and Robbins, 1966) (*Plate 103, Fig. 3*). These authors have also noted a disaggregation of polyribosomes in cells arrested in metaphase by colchicine.

Thus it is now well established that disaggregation of polyribosomes is a useful morphological indicator of depressed or arrested protein synthesis.

Plate 103

Fig. 1. A late normoblast from human bone marrow, showing numerous polyribosomes (arrow) in its cytoplasm. × 50,000

Fig. 2. Cytoplasm of a late reticulocyte from peripheral blood, showing numerous solitary ribosomes (arrow). × 50,000

Fig. 3. Ehrlich ascites tumour cell in mitosis, showing chromosomes (C) and numerous solitary ribosomes (arrow) in the cytoplasm. Compare with *Plate 106*, which shows an Ehrlich ascites tumour cell with abundant polyribosomes in the cytoplasm. × 50,000

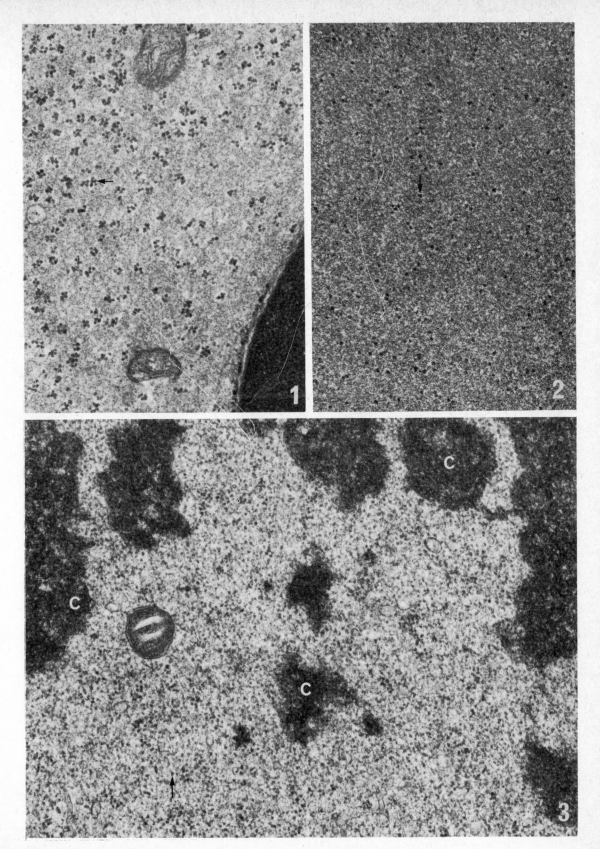

As pointed out earlier (pages 212 and 230), polyribosomes usually present as linear, spiral, or rosette-like formations. In some instances, however, polyribosomes showing a helical configuration have been found, and in rarer instances ribosomes arranged in crystalline arrays have also been noted. Ribosome crystals have at times been seen in company with helical polyribosomes, so it is convenient to consider these together.

Helical polyribosomes have been seen in: (1) developing mother pollen cells of *Ipomoea purpurea* (L) Roth (Echlin, 1965); (2) cotton embryo (Jensen, 1968); (3) *Entamoeba invadens* (Siddiqui and Rudzinska, 1963, 1965); (4) *E. histolytica* (Rosenbaum and Wittner, 1970); (5) intestinal cells of rat foetus (Behnke, 1963); (6) muscle cells of *Rana pipiens* embryo (Waddington and Perry, 1963); (7) follicular cells and oöcytes of rat ovary (Ghiara and Taddei, 1966); (8) chick embryo cells subjected to hypothermia (Byers, 1967; Maraldi and Barbieri, 1969); (9) cultures of chick embryo liver cells treated with vinblastine and subjected to hypothermia (Maraldi *et al.*, 1970); (10) HeLa cells in culture (Scharff and Robbins, 1966); (11) green monkey kidney cells in culture infected with herpesvirus (*Plate 104*); (12) fibroblast cultures treated with vincristine (Krishan and Hsu, 1969); (13) a mutant of *Escherichia coli* treated with vinblastine (Kingsbury and Voelz, 1969); (14) *in vitro* single beating rat myocardial cells (Cedergren and Harary, 1964); (15) ribosome pellets isolated from normal rat liver (Benedetti *et al.*, 1966); and (16) intact or regenerating rat liver after administration of lasiocarpine or aflatoxin (Monneron, 1969).

In intact rat liver helical polyribosomes have not been seen, and in ribosomal pellets obtained after fractionation only an occasional example of such polyribosomes has been recorded. Therefore it is particularly interesting to note the observation made by Monneron (1969) that within 10 minutes after administration of lasiocarpine or aflatoxin numerous helical polyribosomes develop and that they disappear within a few hours. Since the time required by the normal liver to make a ribosome is much longer than 10 minutes and since administration of actinomycin D at a dose level sufficient to block synthesis of 45 S RNA does not prevent the formation of helical polyribosomes by lasiocarpine, it would appear that a change in the nature of messenger RNA linking the ribosomes together is probably responsible for the helical form of the polyribosome rather than an alteration in the ribosomes. Monneron therefore suggests that under these experimental conditions a transient (perhaps abnormal) messenger RNA is produced. Similarly, Jensen (1968) also suggests that helical polyribosomes produced during cotton embryogenesis are related to the production of a special transient messenger RNA (informosome).

Plate 104

Green monkey kidney cells in culture, infected with herpesvirus (V) showing helical polyribosomes (arrows). × 67,000

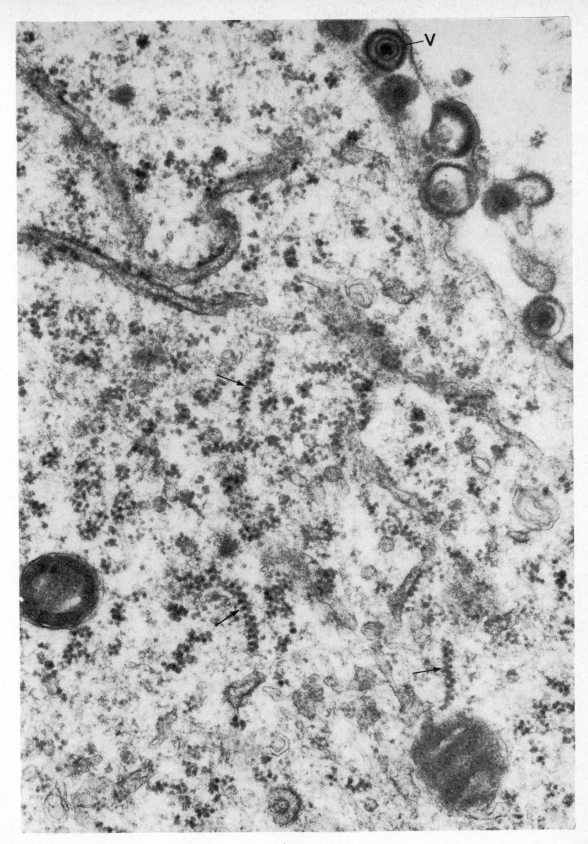

In various species of *Entamoeba* studied so far, classically formed mitochondria, Golgi complex and rough endoplasmic reticulum have not been found but helical polyribosomes and crystalline arrays of helical polyribosomes occur (these large ribonucleoprotein-containing bodies are the equivalent of the chromatid bodies seen in *Entamoeba* with the light microscope). Regarding this situation, Rosenbaum and Wittner (1970) state that 'the absence in *E. histolytica* of most of the usual cytoplasmic organelles and the presence of highly organized and apparently dynamic RNP material in helical form suggests the possibility that these structures may have a multifaceted and extremely labile role in the economy of amoeba'. Furthermore, since many helical poly-ribosomes were seen in close association with autophagic and phagocytic vacuoles which demonstrated acid phosphatase activity, they suggest that 'enzymic protein synthesis may be occurring in association with the larger bodies themselves and that the newly synthesized protein may be carried via the short helices to digestive vacuoles'. Thus, the helical polyribosome of *E. histolytica* becomes analogous to a primary lysosome of man and other animals, which transports hydrolytic enzymes made in the rough endoplasmic reticulum to the autophagic vacuole.

In *Entamoeba*, ribosomal crystals appear to be derived by parallel alignment of helical poly-ribosomes but other forms of ribosomal crystals not derived in this manner also seem to occur. Thus in chick embryos subjected to hypothermia (Byers, 1967; Maraldi and Barbieri, 1969) and in cultures of embryonic chick hepatocytes subjected to hypothermia (Barbieri *et al.*, 1970), square tetramer ribosome crystals are readily produced but helical polyribosomes rarely occur (*Plate 105*). However, in chick hepatocyte cultures treated with vinblastine and then subjected to hypothermia, numerous helical polyribosomes and square tetramer crystals were found, although it was noted that while the number of helical polyribosomes increased with increasing doses of vincristine the population of ribosome crystals remained constant. Maraldi *et al.* (1970) therefore concluded that 'these data which demonstrate a different ribosome behaviour owing to the same treatments (neoformation of polyribosome helices and ribosome crystallization) may suggest the existence at least of two distinct ribosome classes, the one functionally active in protein synthesis, the other inactive'.

Recently, Byers (1971) has isolated intracellular ribosome crystals from hypothermic chick embryos and also succeeded in producing such crystals and tetramers of ribosomes from solitary ribosomes *in vitro*. He states that 'the polypeptide synthesizing activity of these ribosomes was found to be unimpaired by their constraint in the tetrameric configuration'.

Plate 105

From the liver of a 9-day-old chick embryo subjected to 12 hours of hypothermia.

Figl 1. Hepatocyte showing a short helical polyribosome (H) and ribosome crystals (C). The square tetramer arrangement of ribosomes can just be discerned. × 58,000

Fig. 2. Ribosomes showing square tetramer arrangement. × 84,000

Fig. 3. The square tetramer configuration of ribosomes (arrow) in the crystal is evident only in a certain plane of sectioning. × 84,000

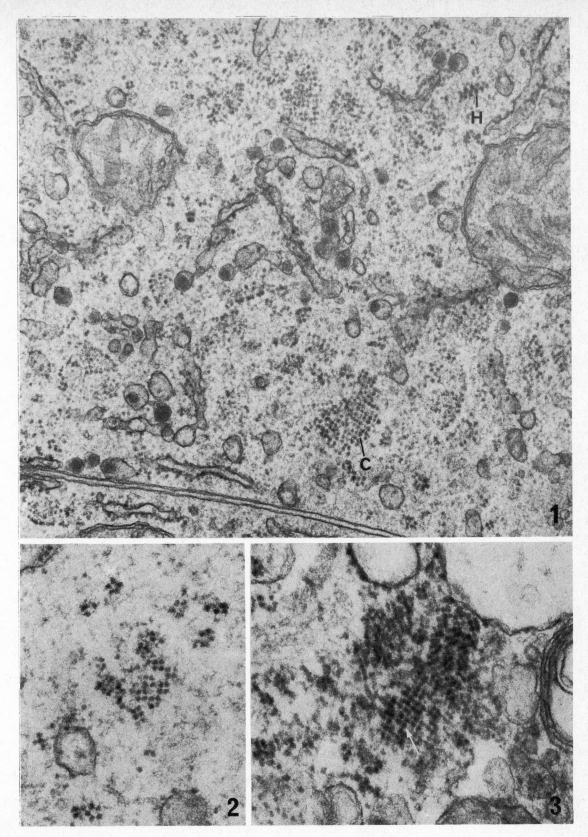

ENDOPLASMIC RETICULUM AND RIBOSOMES IN CELL DIFFERENTIATION AND NEOPLASIA

The endoplasmic reticulum is a highly specialized structure which performs many distinct functions. Hence a well developed endoplasmic reticulum may be looked upon as an expression of cell differentiation and functional activity. Innumerable examples support this concept (see review by Porter, 1961). It is also now abundantly clear that immature or undifferentiated cells such as stem cells, blast cells, embryonic cells, and cells in culture have, as a rule, a poor complement of endoplasmic reticulum as compared to their normal, mature· functioning counterparts. Such immature cells, particularly fast-growing populations of cells, generally also have an abundance of free polyribosomes in the cytoplasm. This presumably reflects the active synthesis of endogenous proteins needed for cell growth and division. The above-mentioned concepts also apply to tumours (*Plates 106 and 107*), where an inverse relationship has often been noted between the amount of rough endoplasmic reticulum present and the growth rate and malignancy of the tumour (Oberling and Bernhard, 1961; Bernhard, 1969).

One of the fastest-growing transplantable tumours is the Ehrlich ascites carcinoma. This highly anaplastic tumour derived from a mouse breast carcinoma is now grown as a free cell suspension in the peritoneal cavity of mice. The cells of this tumour contain scant rough endoplasmic reticulum but abundant polyribosomes in the cytoplasm (*Plate 106*).

Perhaps the most frequently studied model illustrating the above-mentioned concept is the rat hepatoma (Dalton, 1964; Hruban *et al.*, 1965a; Ma and Webber, 1966; Flaks, 1968). Here, the cells of very well differentiated slow-growing examples of this tumour have been found to contain a well developed rough endoplasmic reticulum resembling that found in normal hepatocytes, but in highly anaplastic fast-growing variants only an occasional vesicle of rough endoplasmic reticulum is seen and the cytoplasm contains little besides some mitochondria and innumerable polyribosomes. In extreme examples of this kind there is little difficulty in drawing meaningful positive correlations between signs of ultrastructural dedifferentiation and growth rate or malignancy, but when intermediate examples of tumours with moderate degrees of dedifferentiation and differences in growth rates are compared exceptions or apparent exceptions to our concepts are soon found. Such differences may be real or may be due to the small sample examined with the electron microscope not being truly representative of the whole tumour mass.

Plate 106

Ehrlich ascites tumour cell, showing scant lamellae of rough endoplasmic reticulum and numerous polyribosomes in the cytoplasm. × 32,000

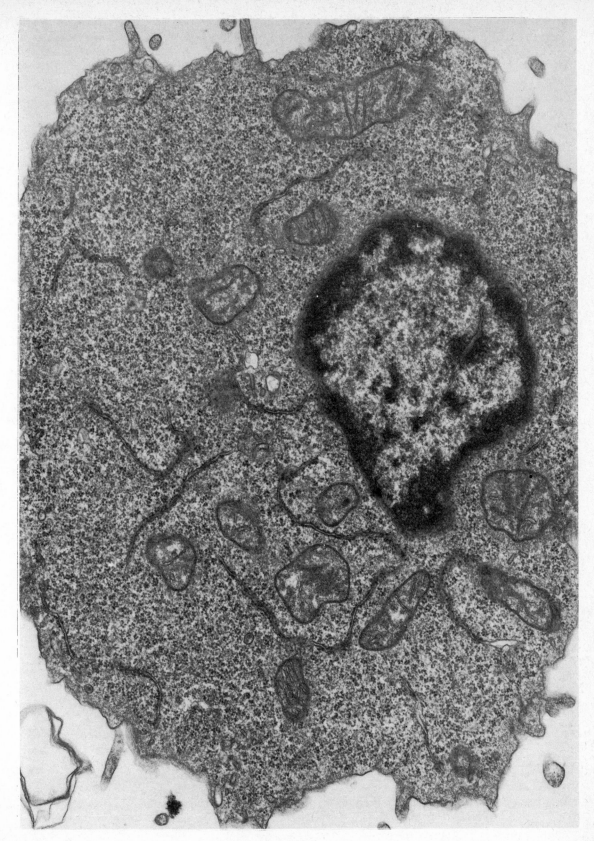

It is said that the rough endoplasmic reticulum is developed to a greater degree in the keratino-cytes of the keratoacanthoma as compared to the cells of the normal hair follicle from which such tumours arise (Prutkin, 1967). Similarly, Lipetz (1970) reports that 'crown gall cells of several plant species contain considerably more endoplasmic reticulum than their normal or hyper-plastic counterparts' and that 'this characteristic appears to be stable even in crown gall tissues grown *in vitro* for many years'. The significance of this situation in tumour tissue of plants is not clear but some crown gall cells, such as those of *Parthenocissus tricuspidata*, produce impressive amounts of peroxidase, presumably from the rough endoplasmic reticulum of the tumour cells (Lipetz and Galston, 1959).

The rough endoplasmic reticulum in animal tumours (particularly adenomas and well dif-ferentiated examples of malignant tumours) can also be functionally active and form products characteristic of the cell of origin. There are numerous examples of this ; for instance, the milk-producing mouse mammary tumours and thyroid tumours which contain abundant rough endoplasmic reticulum and actively produce secretory proteins (for references, see Bernhard, 1969). One of the best-known examples of this in man is the multiple myeloma (Skinnider and Ghadially, 1975) where the neoplastic cells (*Plate 107*) are usually well endowed with rough endo-plasmic reticulum and produce immunoglobulins or fragments thereof (e.g. Bence-Jones protein) in abundance. However, here also there is much variation in the morphology and amount of rough endoplasmic reticulum present, and one cannot correlate this too closely with the type or amount of immunoglubulin produced. (For discussion and references, see Zucker-Franklin. 1964.) Yet this may again reflect no more than the inescapable limitation imposed by the small samples that can be examined with the electron microscope.

In concluding, it is worth pointing out that, despite some claims to the contrary, none of the alterations seen in the endoplasmic reticulum of neoplastic cells can be regarded as characteristic of the neoplastic state. As a rule, such changes are similar to those found in embryonic tissues and reflect merely the well known increased growth rate, and poor functional capacity of tumour cells as a class.

Plate 107

Plasma cells from a case of multiple myeloma. These neoplastic cells are well endowed with rough endoplasmic reticulum. × 20,000 (*Ghadially and Skinnider, unpublished electron micrograph*)

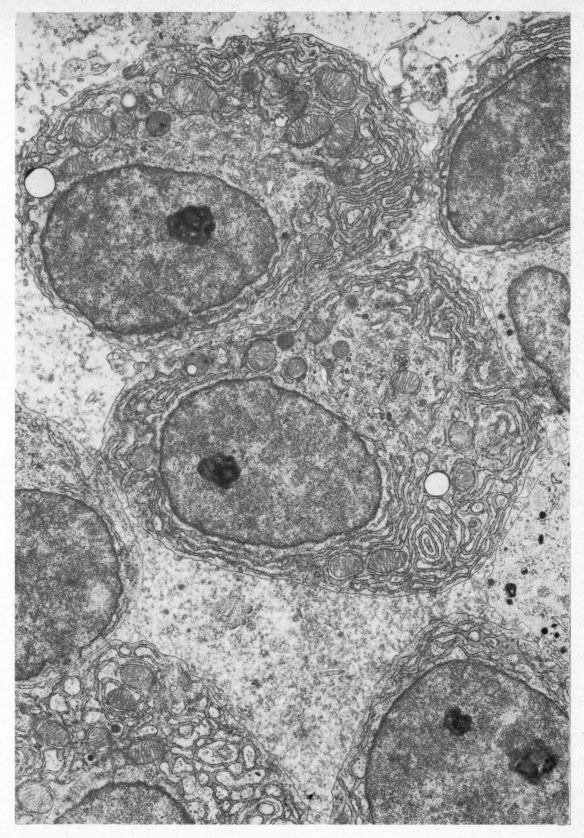

241

PROTEINACEOUS GRANULES AND CRYSTALLINE INCLUSIONS IN ROUGH ENDOPLASMIC RETICULUM

As a rule, the contents of the rough endoplasmic reticulum are fairly homogeneous and usually of medium to low electron density. One therefore gets the impression that the proteinaceous section in the rough endoplasmic reticulum exists in a fairly dilute state. The power to concentrate this material into the more electron-dense secretory granules is thought to lie in the Golgi complex and not in the rough endoplasmic reticulum itself.

However, exceptions to these generalizations exist and it is clear that in some circumstances the secretory products can become concentrated in the rough endoplasmic reticulum and the proteinaceous material then presents as medium- or high-density granules or bodies within the dilated cisternae (*Plates 108, 109 and 110, Fig. 1*). In some instances the proteinaceous material separates out not as amorphous granules but as crystals (*Plate 110, Fig. 2*). In most instances the composition of these granules is a matter of conjecture. Since they occur in the rough endoplasmic reticulum there is strong presumptive evidence that they contain protein. In some situations, however, they could represent glycoprotein or mucoprotein (e.g. Russell bodies in plasma cells, see below). Hence the term 'proteinaceous granules' is used here.

An interesting example of this phenomenon is seen in the pancreatic acinar cells. Here, normally, the protein-rich secretion produced in the rough endoplasmic reticulum is transported to the Golgi and condensed to form zymogen granules. However, in some animals, such as the guinea-pig, dog and cat, small electron-dense granules resembling zymogen granules are also found in occasional dilated cisternae of the rough endoplasmic reticulum (Palade, 1956; Ichikawa, 1965; Fawcett, 1967; Brown and Still, 1970). Intracisternal dense granules have also been noted in the pancreas of rats kept on a protein-free diet or following the administration of ethionine (Herman *et al.*, 1964). The situation in normal human pancreas is not known but intracisternal granules have been seen in a human pancreas in the Zollinger–Ellison syndrome (Brown and Schatzki, 1971) and in the neoplastic cells of a giant cell tumour of the pancreas (Rosai, 1968). The proteinaceous nature of the granules in the pancreatic tumour was confirmed by their sensitivity to pepsin.

The true significance of these pancreatic intracisternal granules is not clear. At one time it was thought (Siekevitz and Palade, 1958) that this might be an intermediate step in zymogen granule formation in some species where a condensation of proteinaceous material occurred not only in the Golgi but also in the rough endoplasmic reticulum. However, autoradiographic studies have

---

Plate 108

Figs. 1 and 2. Tumour cells from a well differentiated osteogenic sarcoma of man, showing dilated and vesiculated rough endoplasmic reticulum containing numerous electron-dense granules (G) thought to be proteinaceous in nature. ×32,000; ×27,000 (*Fig. 1, Ghadially and Mehta, unpublished electron micrograph; Fig. 2, from Ghadially and Mehta, 1970*)

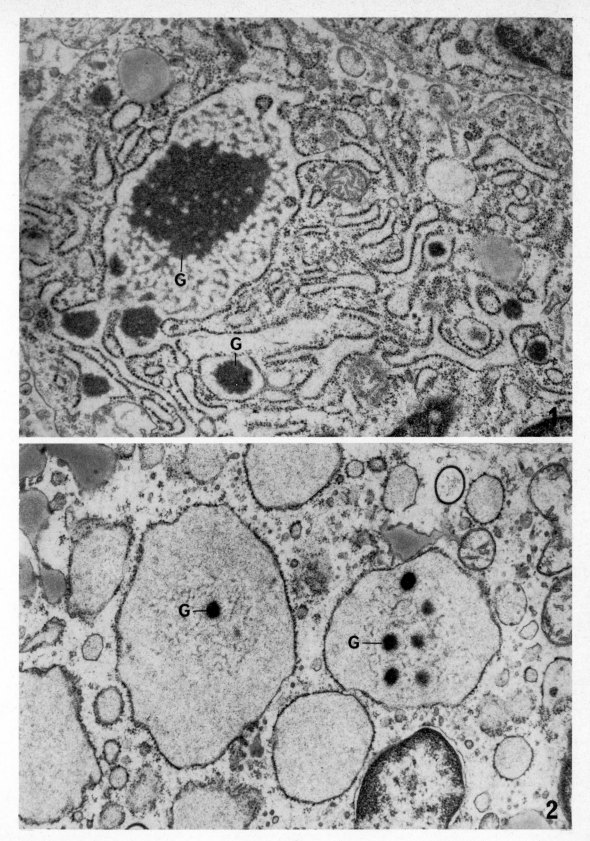

cast doubt on this thesis because no significant labelling of these intracisternal granules was found during zymogen granule production (Caro and Palade, 1964). This, taken in conjunction with the fact that intracisternal granules are seen in ethionine-treated but not normal rats, has led to the idea that they could be the result of blockage of transport within the rough endoplasmic reticulum and subsequent concentration of products therein.

Such a concept is also supported by the fact that intracisternal dense granules have been seen in pathological tissues, particularly tumours, where one can with some justification also speculate that the rough endoplasmic reticulum may be malformed and the passage of substances impeded.

As already noted, intracisternal dense granules have been seen in a giant cell tumour of the pancreas. Somewhat larger medium-density granules were also seen in the stromal cells of this tumour (Rosai, 1968). Dense granules morphologically similar to those in the pancreatic tumour cells have been seen by Hollman (1959) in a case of breast carcinoma and by Ghadially and Mehta (1970) in well differentiated osteogenic sarcoma of man (*Plate 108*), but they are not known to occur in normal mammary tissue or osteocytes. Dense granules have also been seen in glomerular endothelial cells in a boy with hereditary renal disease but not in normal glomeruli (Sengel and Stoebner, 1971). Larger but not so dense granules have been seen in the type B cells of rheumatoid synovial membrane (Ghadially and Roy, 1969) (*Plate 110, Fig. 1*). Other examples of intracisternal granules include those found in: (1) Paneth cells of the rat (Behnke and Moe, 1964); (2) crayfish oöcytes (Beams and Kessel, 1962, 1963); (3) endosperm of barley grain (Buttrose *et al.*, 1960); and (4) secretory cells of the venom gland of the South American rattlesnake (Warshawsky *et al.*, 1973). Autoradiographic studies on venom production have led Warshawsky *et al.* (1973) to conclude that 'the interstitial granules are not a part of the main sequence in the secretion of venom protein' and that 'they may represent a storage form of immature protein which condenses out of the otherwise flocculent content of the distended rough endoplasmic reticulum cisternae'.

However, the best-known intracisternal dense granule is the one that occurs in plasma cells (*Plate 109*) and has long been known to light microscopists as the Russell body (Russell, 1890; Stich *et al.*, 1955; Welsh, 1960; Sorenson, 1964; Zucker-Franklin, 1964). Although Russell thought that this body was a fungus and an aetiological agent of cancer, it is now well known that this glycoprotein-rich body may be found in both reactive and neoplastic plasma cells and that its formation can be induced by immunization (White, 1954; Ortega and Mellors, 1957). Here, too, the idea that excessive production of secretory material and/or a disordered secretory mechanism is responsible appears tenable.

Plate 109

Figs. 1 and 2. Plasma cells showing dilated and vesiculated rough endoplasmic reticulum, containing numerous Russell-type bodies (R). The bodies shown here are somewhat small and would be difficult to discern with the light microscope, but larger bodies of the type shown would present as classical Russell bodies. From bronchial mucosa adjacent to a bronchial carcinoma. × 18,000; × 45,000

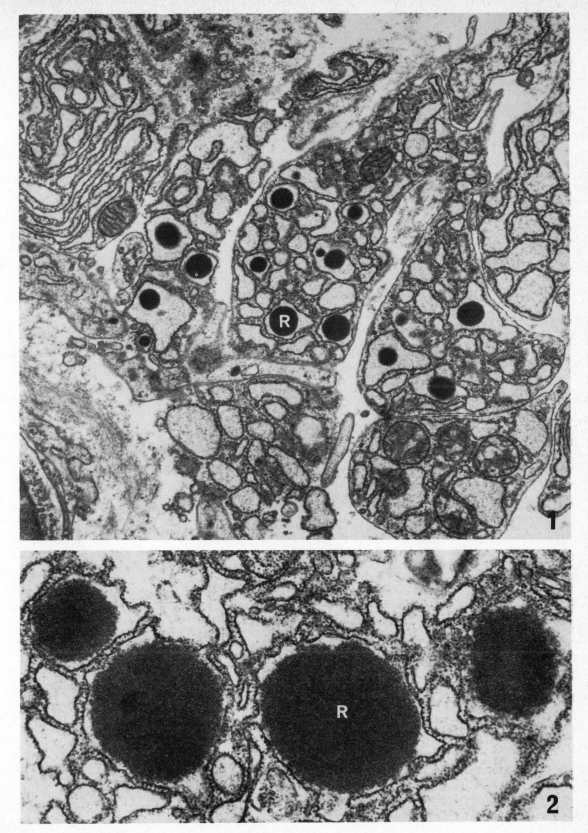

Much confusion exists in the literature regarding the ultrastructural equivalents of the many morphological (light microscopic) variations of the plasma cells, variously referred to as thesaurocytes, flame cells, Mott cells, morula cells and grape cells. An extended discussion on this point and the ultrastructural differences between these varieties of plasma cells is beyond the scope of this text (see instead Thiery, 1960). It would appear, however, that the above-mentioned variants reflect no more than the highly pleomorphic character of the rough endoplasmic reticulum and its contents in plasma cells. Illustrations in this chapter (*Plates 93, 109 and 110, Fig. 2*) demonstrate this point; the cisternae can be collapsed, dilated or vesiculated and their contents can vary from electron-lucent to quite dense. At the end of this scale is the compact, rounded, electron-dense Russell body. In rare instances the proteins separate out to form crystals (*Plate 110, Fig. 2*) which are detectable by the light microscope and are clearly seen by electron microscopy to lie within the rough endoplasmic reticulum (for references, see Sanel and Lepore, 1968). According to Sanel and Lepore (1968) such crystals in plasma cells 'have been invariably associated with dysproteinemia (i.e. cryoglobulinemia, macroglubulinemia of Waldenstrom's disease, or the hyperglobulinemia of multiple myeloma plasmacytoma or hyperimmune states)'.

Besides the example mentioned above, crystalline inclusions in the endoplasmic reticulum have been seen in: (1) Paneth cells of the rat (Behnke and Moe, 1964); (2) dog hepatocytes (Gueft and Kikkawa, 1962); (3) liver of slender salamander (Hamilton *et al.*, 1966); (4) submucosal gland cells of the fowl proventriculus (Toner, 1963); (5) root cells of radish (Bonnett and Newcomb, 1965); (6) spinal cord of lung-fish (*Polypterus enlicheri*) and the aquarium guppy (*Poecila reticulata*) (Marquet and Sobel, 1969). In the last example it was noted that the frequency of crystalline inclusions was greater in lordotic than normal guppies, and it was postulated that 'the volume of protein produced exceeds the volume which the Golgi apparatus can package and which the cell can utilize, and that subsequent accumulation and crystallization of this material occur in the nuclear envelope and dilated sacs of endoplasmic reticulum'. In some instances, however, intracisternal crystals may have a physiological role in the economy of the organism. Such a view is expressed by Fawcett (1967) regarding the protein crystals in the liver of the slender salamander; he states that 'they are presumed to be the storage form of a protein synthesized by the cell'.

Plate 110

Fig. 1. A type B synovial cell from a case of rheumatoid arthritis, showing medium-density proteinaceous granules (G) in dilated rough endoplasmic reticulum. × 50,000 (*Ghadially and Roy, unpublished electron micrograph*)

Fig. 2. Part of the cytoplasm of a plasmacytoid cell from a case of Hodgkin's disease, showing crystalline inclusions (C) lying within the cisternae (between arrows) of the rough endoplasmic reticulum. × 110,000 (*From Sanel and Lepore, 1968*)

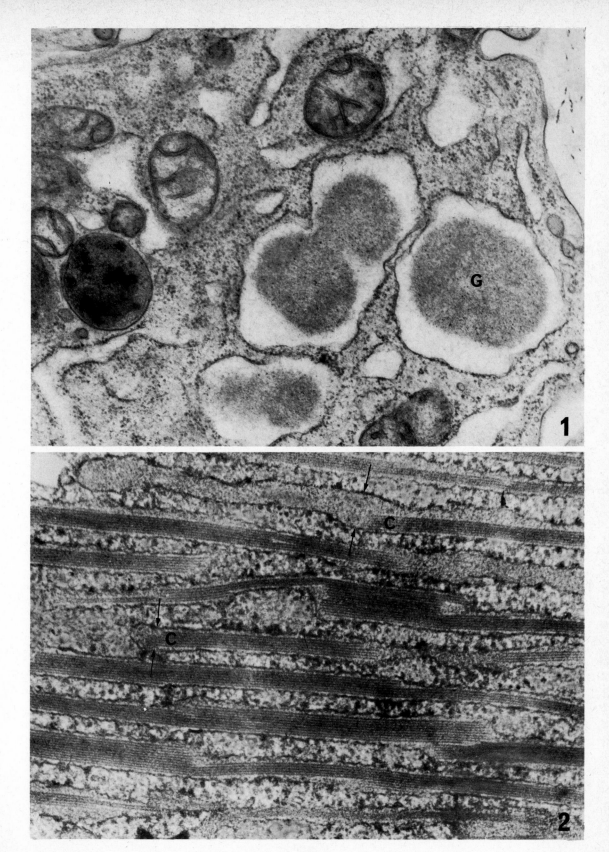

Lipids (triglycerides) generally occur as non-membrane-bound droplets lying free within the cytoplasm of various cell types. Occasionally, however, lipid droplets may be found in the endoplasmic reticulum (*Plates 111 and 112*), and also in the Golgi complex.* Such deposits may present in various ways, such as lipid droplets lying within: (1) dilated cisternae of the rough endoplasmic reticulum (*Plate 112*), (2) ribosome-studded vesicles clearly derived from the rough endoplasmic reticulum; or (3) smooth membrane-bound vesicles and tubules representing or derived from the Golgi complex, smooth endoplasmic reticulum or degranulated rough endoplasmic reticulum (*Plate 111*).

Such membrane-bound lipidic bodies, particularly those encountered in the liver, are often called liposomes—a term first introduced by Baglio and Farber (1965b) to describe these bodies in rat hepatocytes.

A few liposomes may be found in the livers of fasted but otherwise normal rats (Baglio and Farber, 1965b; Stein and Stein, 1965). Liposomes in great number, however, are characteristic of fatty livers where an abnormal accumulation of triglycerides is occurring. Since a large number of drugs, dietary regimens and experimental procedures can produce fatty livers, liposomes have frequently been observed and studied (for details and references, see Schlunk and Lombardi, 1967; Stenger, 1970).

Thus, shortly after the administration of agents such as carbon tetrachloride, ethionine, orotic acid or yellow phosphorus, membrane-bound lipidic material collects in the hepatocytes (*Plate 111*). Later much larger non-membrane-bound lipidic droplets appear in the cytoplasm of the hepatocyte but it is not clear how these evolve from the membrane-bound liposomes. One can only speculate that a dissolution of membranes and fusion of smaller droplets to form larger ones probably occurs.

The lipidic nature of liposomes was indicated by the histochemical studies of Novikoff *et al.* (1964), and this has now been amply confirmed by isolation and chemical characterization studies such as those of Schlunk and Lombardi (1967), which show that isolated liposomes contain mainly neutral fat.

Many theories have been advanced to explain the occurrence of liposomes and fatty livers, and it is clear that not all drugs produce this change in precisely the same fashion. However, one

---

* The occurrence of lipid and lipoprotein in the Golgi complex has already been discussed on page 202. This topic is so closely linked with the subject dealt with in this section that it is recommended that both sections are read conjunctly.

Plate 111

Liver of a rat given yellow phosphorus, showing numerous liposomes (L) which have collected mainly near the vascular pole of the hepatocytes. There was a marked hypertrophy of the smooth endoplasmic reticulum in this liver. This, combined with the fact that the liposomes are covered with a smooth membrane, and many show a tubular profile, suggests that the lipid accumulated in the smooth endoplasmic reticulum. In hepatocytes the Golgi complex is often located adjacent to the cell membrane in the same position as some of the liposomes. Hence one may speculate that some of the liposomes could also have been derived from the Golgi complex. Some of the liposomes (arrows) appear to have lost lipid during processing. This permits a good demonstration of the membrane covering liposomes. × 27,000

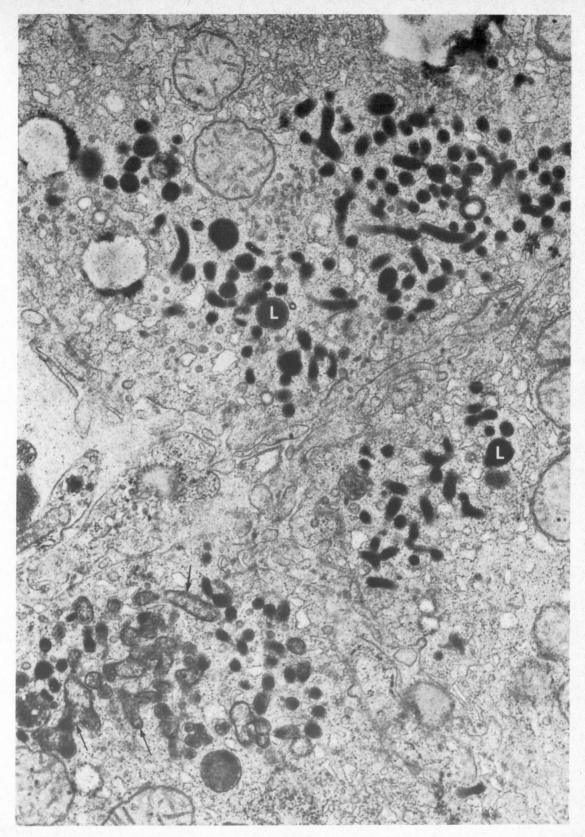

concept that seems applicable in many instances and has gained wide acceptance is that lipid accumulation is secondary to depressed protein synthesis, a point supported by the disorganization of rough endoplasmic reticulum which is so commonly seen in such livers (page 228). It is believed that in the normal situation a lipid acceptor protein is produced by the rough endoplasmic reticulum and this combines with triglycerides to form very low-density lipoproteins which are then released in the blood. It has hence been argued by many workers that any toxic agent which damages the rough endoplasmic reticulum and depresses the synthesis of this protein but not the synthesis of triglyceride will lead to a pathological accumulation of fat in the liver (for references, see Stenger, 1970). Other mechanisms that have been evoked to explain fat accumulation in the liver include: (1) ineffective coupling of lipid and acceptor protein; (2) impaired release of lipoproteins from liver to blood; (3) hypermobilization of free fatty acids from fat stores; and (4) enhanced lipogenesis.

However, as already indicated, liposome formation is not necessarily a pathological phenomenon. It may be no more than a morphological expression of fatty acid esterification in the endoplasmic reticulum. Membrane-enclosed lipids acceptable as liposomes have been described and isolated by Sheldon (1964) and by Angel and Sheldon (1965) from adipose tissue cells engaged in active triglyceride synthesis, and it is now well known that the endoplasmic reticulum of intestinal epithelial cells comes to contain lipid droplets during fat absorption (Palay and Karlin, 1959; Onoe and Ohno, 1963; Fawcett, 1967).

Since, in the latter example, lipid can be demonstrated in pinocytotic vesicles, argument has raged as to whether this is how the bulk of the lipid is picked up and the endoplasmic reticulum merely transports the lipid or whether most of the lipid is first hydrolysed and the component parts are picked up and resynthesized into triglycerides within the endoplasmic reticulum. There is now much evidence to support the latter concept.

The role of the microsomal fraction (derived from endoplasmic reticulum) in fatty acid esterification is now well established (Stein and Shapiro, 1959; Hultin, 1961; Tzur and Shapiro, 1964) and considerable evidence has also accumulated which shows that, although some cells (e.g. neutrophils and Kupffer cells) can pick up lipid by a process of pinocytosis or phagocytosis generally in the majority of instances, the lipid is first hydrolysed and the component parts are picked up and the lipid is resynthesized in the endoplasmic reticulum. Such a concept has been evoked to explain lipid uptake in many tissues, such as adipose, mammary, hepatic, cartilage, cardiac and skeletal muscle (Stein and Stein, 1967; Scow, 1970; Ghadially et al., 1970; Mehta and Ghadially, 1973).

Plate 112

Figs. 1 and 2. These electron micrographs show lipid droplets (L) found in the dilated endoplasmic reticulum of the hepatocyte of a rat bearing a carcinogen-induced tumour in its flank. This is not a feature of the condition; in fact this phenomenon was seen in the liver of only one animal. × 11,000; × 50,000 (*Ghadially and Parry, unpublished electron micrographs*)

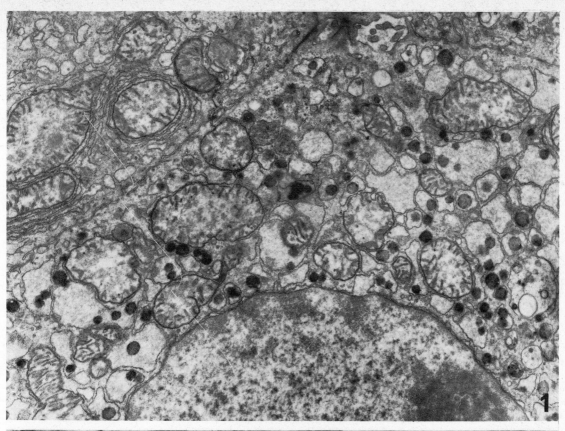

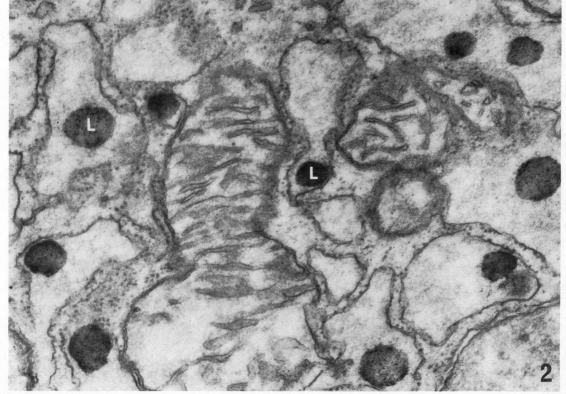

Several types of viruses have been observed lying in or budding from walls of cytoplasmic vacuoles. Such vacuoles may represent section through invaginations of the cell membrane (plasma membrane), or they could be derived from the endoplasmic reticulum or Golgi complex (intracytoplasmic membranes). Both phenomena are known to occur, and in some instances the virus particles have also been clearly demonstrated to lie in relatively unaltered cisternae of the rough endoplasmic reticulum or elements of the Golgi complex. Only a brief review of some of the instances where virus particles have been seen in such circumstances can be dealt with in the space available.

It has already been noted (page 24) that herpesvirus nucleocapsids assembled in the nucleus acquire one or two membranous coats from the nuclear envelope. In their subsequent passage through the cell they may acquire another coat by budding into vacuoles probably derived from intracytoplasmic membranes. The same phenomenon may also occur at the cell membrane as the virus leaves the cell.

Several RNA viruses have been found in the endoplasmic reticulum and Golgi complex, or in vacuoles derived from them. For example, the cores of rubella virus and some arboviruses assembled in the cytoplasm or close to intracytoplasmic membranes acquire their membranous coat by budding into these structures (Murphy *et al.*, 1968, 1970; Holmes *et al.*, 1969; Grimley and Friedman, 1970; Zlotnik and Harris, 1970; Boulton and Webb, 1971; Whitfield *et al.*, 1971).

Murine leukaemia viruses and avian tumour viruses are usually formed at the plasma membrane of the tumour cells by a process of budding; however, in some instances, they have been seen within vacuoles derived from intracytoplasmic membranes. A different situation, however, prevails in the megakaryocytes of such leukaemic mice. These cells do not become neoplastic but harbour many virus particles. Here the virus particles do not form and bud from the plasma membrane but into the endoplasmic reticulum, Golgi complex and numerous interconnecting channels and vacuoles clearly derived from these structures.

Viruses are now known to be associated with many transplantable mouse carcinomas and sarcomas. A well known example of this is the Ehrlich ascites carcinoma, which shows many virus particles within smooth-membraned tubules and vesicles derived from the rough endoplasmic reticulum and at times also in the region of the Golgi complex (*Plate 113*). This virus, however, is not the causative agent of this particular tumour, for cell-free extracts of this tumour injected into newborn mice produce a high incidence of leukaemias but not Ehrlich ascites carcinoma. It is therefore thought that this and other transplantable mouse tumours harbour a latent leukaemogenic virus. (The extensive literature on oncogenic viruses cannot be adequately quoted here. For references supporting the statements made, the reader is referred to Dalton and Haguenau, 1962, and Gross, 1970.)

Plate 113

Ehrlich ascites tumour cells showing many virus particles budding into the endoplasmic reticulum and vesicles derived therefrom. The probable sequence of events is indicated by letters A to D. ×92,000

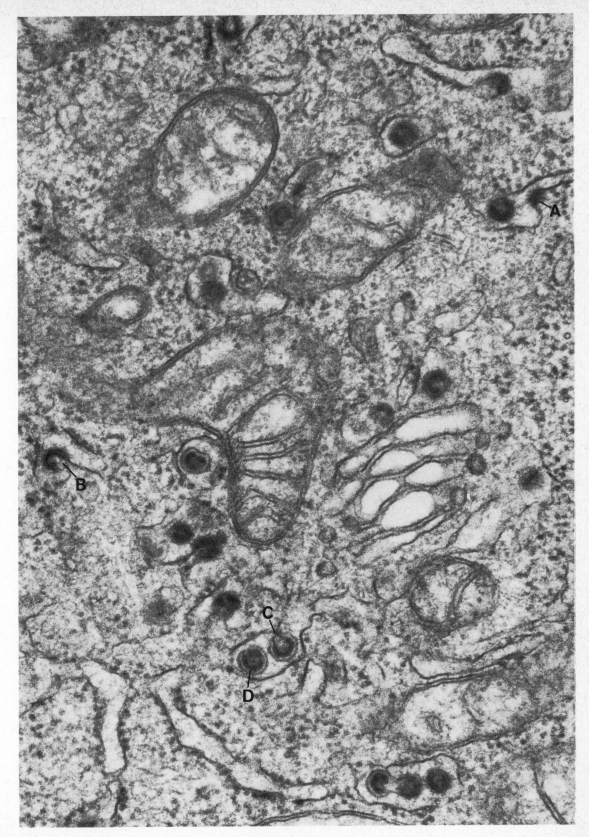

253

Many studies indicate that the endoplasmic reticulum is a dynamic labile organelle which can readily undergo hypertrophy or atrophy, and this usually reflects a state of altered functional activity. Atrophy or involution of the rough endoplasmic reticulum and hypertrophy of smooth endoplasmic reticulum are dealt with later (pages 256 and 272). Here are examined only a few of the many instances where an increase in the amount of rough endoplasmic reticulum has been noted to occur. Such an increase always raises the question as to whether the increased rough endoplasmic reticulum is produced in existing cells or whether the existing cells are replaced by a new population of rough-endoplasmic-reticulum-rich cells. Of course, each example has to be evaluated on its own merits, but at times the speed at which the change occurs and the absence of signs of any undue cellular proliferative activity leads one to conclude that the former mechanism may be operative.

Ultrastructural morphometric studies on the pregnant rat liver (Hope, 1970) have shown that an increase in the volume proportion of rough endoplasmic reticulum occurs in hepatocytes, and this is also evident as an increase in RNA biochemically and as an increase in basophilia histologically. An important function of the rough endoplasmic reticulum in the liver is the synthesis of plasma proteins. Therefore, it would appear that the increased rough endoplasmic reticulum reflects the increased demand for plasma proteins known to occur during pregnancy as a result of the increased blood volume (hydraemia of pregnancy).

Atrophy of the rough endoplasmic reticulum occurs in the submaxillary gland of the rat when the duct is ligated. Removal of the ligatures and resumption of secretory activity is accompanied by a reappearance of the rough endoplasmic reticulum. It has been noted (Tamarin, 1971a, b) that there is no evidence of overt cell proliferation and that the rough endoplasmic reticulum undergoes these changes within the existing population of cells.

Phagocytic cells such as macrophages are generally poorly endowed with rough endoplasmic reticulum, but when these cells become actively phagocytic they are said to develop much rough endoplasmic reticulum and hence come to resemble fibroblasts. Such an increase in rough endoplasmic reticulum probably reflects the increased production of acid hydrolases to form primary lysosomes (see page 354).

As noted earlier (pages 194–196), two main types of synovial cells have been found in the synovial membrane of all species studied to date: a type A cell where the rough endoplasmic reticulum is scanty or virtually absent, and a type B cell which is well endowed with rough endoplasmic reticulum. In normal synovial membrane there is a marked preponderance of type A cells, but in various pathological states such as traumatic arthritis, haemarthrosis and rheumatoid arthritis this situation is reversed; that is to say, there is a predominance of type B and intermediate cells well endowed with rough endoplasmic reticulum. In such situations there is usually an increased volume of synovial fluid, rich in certain protein. So here also one may correlate the relative and absolute increase of protein in the fluid with the rough endoplasmic reticulum hypertrophy seen in the synovial intimal cells (Ghadially and Roy, 1969).

Plate 114

Synovial cells showing marked hypertrophy of the rough endoplasmic reticulum. Long parallel arrays of cisternae (C) are seen. Such an arrangement is rarely, if ever, found in normal synovial intimal cells (compare with *Plates 85 and 94*). × 8,500 (*From Ghadially and Roy, 1969*)

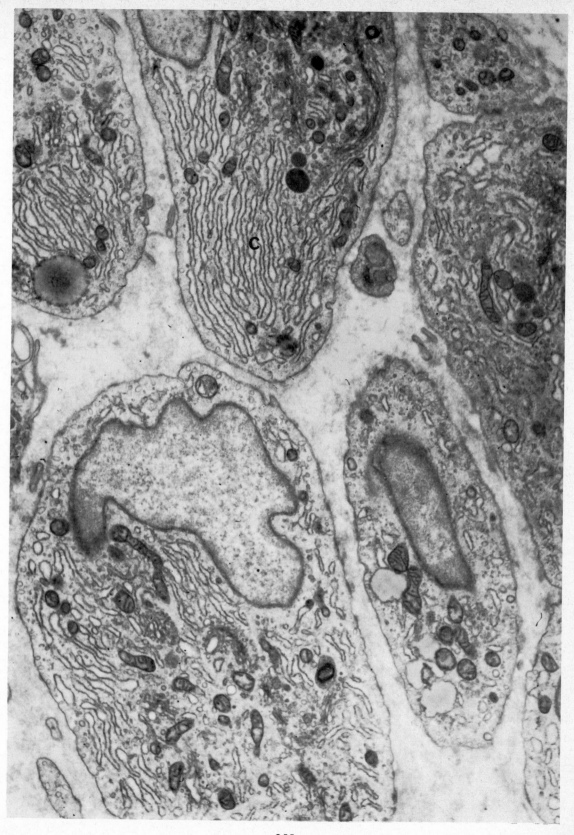

'Intracisternal sequestration' or 'microsequestration' are terms used to describe a pattern of organization of the rough endoplasmic reticulum where vesicular profiles of rough endoplasmic reticulum are seen lying within dilated cisternae. It is thought that the primary stage of this process is the formation of papillary processes from the wall of a dilated cistern. Later such processes may be pinched off to form vesicular structures which come to lie free within the cisternae (*Plate 115*). When such a change is extensive, so that numerous vesicular profiles of rough endoplasmic reticulum are seen lying in a few grossly dilated but perhaps not too well visualized cisternae, one may at a casual glance confuse this change with vesiculation of the rough endoplasmic reticulum— quite a different phenomenon, which has already been described (page 222). This point is well illustrated and discussed by Blackburn and Vinijchaikul (1969), who point out that in vesiculation of the rough endoplasmic reticulum the ribosomes line the outside of the vesicles, but, since intracisternal sequestration represents an invagination of the rough endoplasmic reticulum into the cistern, the ribosomes line the inner surface of the vesicles in this condition. Such vesicles may contain only the cytoplasmic matrix, but at times they also contain other structures such as lipid droplets, mitochondria and microbodies (*Plate 115*).

The vesicular profiles seen within the dilated cisternae may in some instances represent transverse sections through papillary processes, but there is often quite a preponderance of vesicular profiles over papillary forms, suggesting that these are portions of the invaginated rough endoplasmic reticulum which have indeed become detached from the wall of the cistern and are now lying free within it. Such a concept is further supported by evidence of regressive or degenerative changes in the sequestrated material.

The formation of papillary projections from ductal and surface epithelia has long been linked in the minds of histiopathologists with proliferative processes, and it could be argued that here, also, one is witnessing a similar process and that intracisternal sequestration could be a type of hypertrophy of the rough endoplasmic reticulum. However, the situations in which this phenomenon occurs militate against this view. Thus one of the most marked examples of intracisternal sequestration has been noted in the pancreatic acinar cells in kwashiorkor (Blackburn and Vinijchaikul, 1969) where there is a marked diminution in the quantity of rough endoplasmic

---

Plate 115

Fig. 1. Papilliferous (P) and vesicular (V) profiles of rough endoplasmic reticulum containing cytoplasmic matrix are seen within the dilated cisternae (arrow) of a human hepatocyte. From non-neoplastic liver adjacent to a hepatoma. ×51,000 (*From Ghadially and Parry, 1966*)

Fig. 2. Within the dilated cisternae of the rough endoplasmic reticulum of a hepatocyte are seen papillary (P) and vesicular structures (arrows) containing cytoplasmic matrix and microbodies (M). Note that the ribosomes line the inner surface of these vesicules. From an ill canary which had refused food for many days. ×28,000

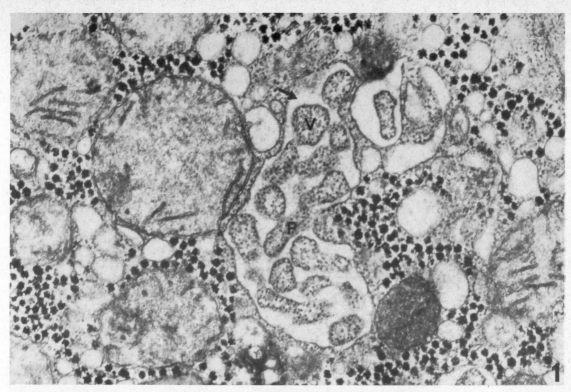

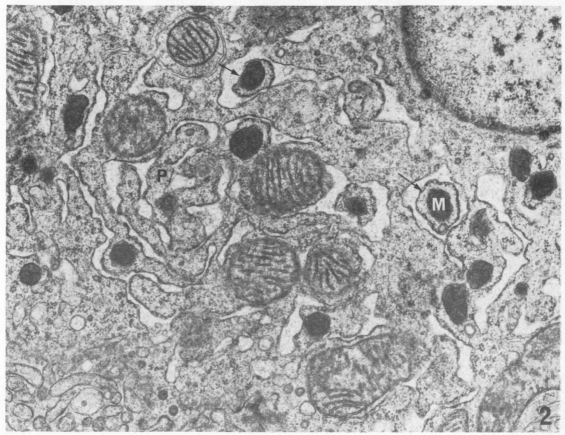

257

reticulum and much of what remains shows intracisternal sequestration. These authors have therefore suggested that intracisternal sequestration is a mechanism by which cytoplasmic atrophy may occur in cells with abundant rough endoplasmic reticulum. In other words, this is a process by which 'excess' rough endoplasmic reticulum is disposed of by the cell. It is postulated that such disposal may be achieved by degradation of the sequestrated rough endoplasmic reticulum and transport of this material to the Golgi and then into lysosomes. Svoboda and Higginson (1964) noted intracisternal sequestration (which they called microsequestration) in protein-deficient rats and considered this arrangement of the rough endoplasmic reticulum as a non-specific reaction of the cell to injury, leading to the formation of cytolysosomes.

We (Ghadially and Parry, unpublished observations) have observed occasional cells showing intracisternal sequestration in a wide variety of situations and, since such cells have shown other regressive changes also, we are inclined to agree with these hypotheses. For example, we have found cells showing intracisternal sequestration in the atrophic liver of starving canary and from the liver tissue surrounding a hepatoma (*Plate 115*). It is our experience that senescent cells in culture and regressing or dying tumour cells adjacent to an area of necrosis also show this change.

Recently, we (Ghadially and Larsen, unpublished observations) have observed a somewhat different pattern of intracisternal sequestration in the pancreas of a child who had an islet cell adenoma. Here occasional pancreatic acinar cells showed quite sizeable masses of rough endoplasmic reticulum and mitochondria sequestrated within focal vacuolar dilatations of rough endoplasmic reticulum. Support for the idea that such sequestrated material suffers disintegration was also seen (*Plate 116*).

The manner in which cytolysosomes (also called autophagic vacuoles, or autolysosomes) form and how the acid hydrolases arrive in these structures is not too clearly established, but various ideas have been put forward (see discussion on pages 298–300). Intracisternal sequestration is thought to be one of the ways in which a cytolysosome forms, the necessary enzymes being synthesized by the ensheathing rough endoplasmic reticulum.

Plate 116

From a case of islet cell adenoma of the pancreas. (*Ghadially and Larsen, unpublished electron micrographs*)

Fig. 1. Pancreatic acinar cell showing a rounded mass of rough endoplasmic reticulum (R) and a mitochondrion (M) lying within a vacuole clearly lined by ribosome-studded rough endoplasmic reticulum (arrow). × 25,000

Fig. 2. Appearances seen in this illustration are thought to represent a further stage of evolution of the type of lesion shown in *Fig. 1*. Here the sequestrated material (presumably rough endoplasmic reticulum) appears disorganized, clumped and electron dense. × 37.500

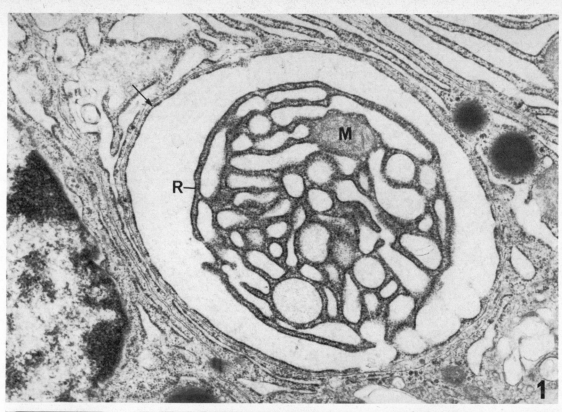

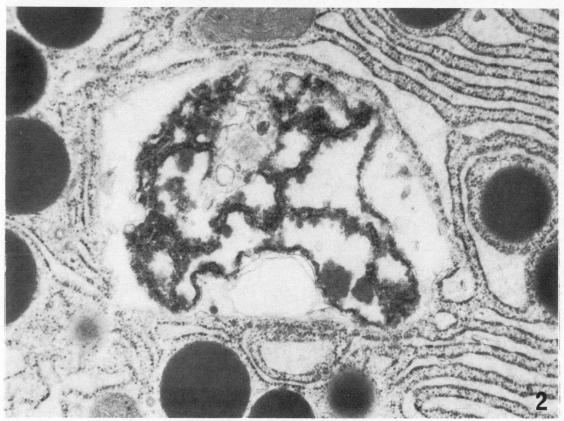

UNDULATING TUBULES

A system of tubular structures referred to as undulating tubules, tubular arrays or tubular aggregates have been seen in or associated with the endoplasmic reticulum in a large number and variety of pathological tissues and also at times in some normal or apparently normal cells. There is much controversy regarding the nature and significance of such formations, a most important point being whether at least in some instances such tubular arrays are viral in nature. In most studies such tubules have been reported to be between 200 and 300 Å in diameter, and it is with arrays of tubules of such dimensions that we are concerned here.

It is easy to appreciate that in sectioned material a system of undulating tubules will present a bewildering variety of appearances. The sectioning geometry of such formations was first dealt with by Bassot (1966), who studied the luminous cells of the polynoid worm elytra in which the photogenic grains are composed of well ordered undulating tubules. Connections with the endoplasmic reticulum were demonstrated and this structure was considered to be a specialized form of endoplasmic reticulum.

Chandra (1968) studied undulating tubules in cultured cell lines derived from normal and pathological tissues (*Plate 117*) and gave a convincing explanation of how the various appearances seen in sectioned material could be correlated with different planes of sectioning through systems of undulating tubules oriented in various ways. Since such structures occurred in cells irrespective of the presence or absence of virus, Chandra concluded that such endoplasmic-reticulum-associated tubules were not viral in nature.

Undulating tubules present in thin sections in various ways (*Plates 117–119*). In some examples the tubules are loosely arranged and their undulating form is easily recognized. When the tubules are obliquely cut and densely packed they tend to present as aggregates of small dense

---

Plate 117

Fig. 1. Undulating tubules found in the cytoplasm of a cell from a human embryonic kidney culture infected with HRV. The undulating nature of the tubules is well illustrated in one part of this tubular aggregate (T), while in another part images resembling virus particles are formed by these tubules (arrows). × 110,000. (*Chandra, unpublished electron micrograph*)

Fig. 2. The undulating tubules seen in this illustration present as thick-walled circular profiles about 240 Å in diameter. They are surrounded by a membrane which appears continuous (arrows marked X) with the endoplasmic reticulum (ER). × 110,000 (*From Chandra, 1968*)

Fig. 3. An area in the cytoplasm of a cell from Burkitt lymphoma culture, showing undulating tubules continuous with closely packed lamellae (L) of rough endoplasmic reticulum.* × 21,000. (*Chandra, unpublished electron micrograph*)

* Similar closely packed cisternae of the endoplasmic reticulum have at times been seen in fast-growing populations of cells such as tumour cells, embryonal cells, and cells in culture. They are referred to as 'intracytoplasmic confronting cisterna'. (For references, see Kelley, 1971.)

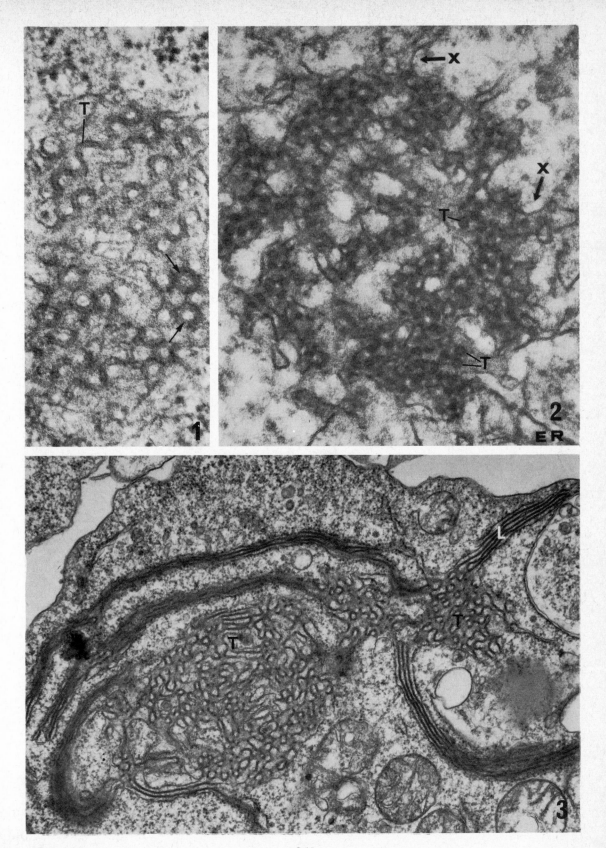

granules, or thick-walled tubules. Undulating tubules may also present as an interwoven mesh-work of strands or appear as double-membrane-bound bodies resembling virus particles. Crystalline arrays may also be formed, and at times the resemblance to viral crystals can be quite striking. Yet such appearances (double-membrane-bound bodies) can be produced by a superimposition of images of two parallel, overlying, undulating tubules where the crest of one lies opposite the trough of another (Chandra, 1968). At times undulating tubules are seen to lie within the endoplasmic reticulum; in other instances they appear to lie in the cytoplasm, often connected to or continuous with the endoplasmic reticulum system.

So many papers have now been published illustrating formations acceptable as undulating tubules that it would be impossible to list them here. Fortunately, the subject has been well reviewed recently by Uzman *et al.* (1971), who list the many situations where such formations have been sighted and they give ample references to the literature. I shall therefore give only a brief summary of the situations in which these structures have been found and comment on some points of interest. A full list of references is not presented.

Although such formations have occasionally been reported in normal or apparently normal mammalian cells, most examples come from tissues of diseased individuals, particularly from cases of viral infections, leukaemias and lymphomas, and autoimmune diseases.

These structures have been found in tissues of man, monkey, pig, dog, horse, rabbit, squirrel and mink (*Plate 118, Fig. 1*) but they seem to be of infrequent occurrence in tissues of common laboratory rodents. We (Ghadially and Bhatnagar, unpublished observations) have seen a rather unusual example of undulating tubules or lamellae in a hamster treated with pheno-barbitone (*Plate 118, Fig. 2*).

A singularly large number of reports have dealt with the occurrence of undulating tubules in cultured cells, particularly tumour cells, cells from the spleen and thymus, and white blood cells obtained from patients with a variety of disorders, including tumours such as melanoma, carcinoma of the pancreas, carcinoma of the colon and multiple myeloma.

Plate 118

Fig. 1. A macrophage showing dense tubular aggregates in the endoplasmic reticulum. From the olfactory bulb of a squirrel (*Citellus lateralis*) 7 days after a subcutaneous injection of Coxsackie virus. × 90,000 (*Grodums, unpublished electron micrograph*)

Fig. 2. Undulating tubules or lamellae set in an area of smooth endoplasmic reticulum hypertrophy found in the hepato-cyte of a phenobarbitone-treated hamster. Confident interpretation of this unusual formation, of which only one example was found, is difficult. It is not clear whether the material apparently lying within these narrow channels (arrows) represents smooth endoplasmic reticulum contents or cytoplasmic matrix. In the former instance this formation would be regarded as a tubular or lamellar extension of the smooth endoplasmic reticulum, while in the latter instance one would have to postulate that the narrow channels are formed by closely apposed walls of tightly packed smooth endoplasmic reticulum distended by electron-lucent material (L). × 70,000 (*Ghadially and Bhatnagar, unpublished electron micrograph*)

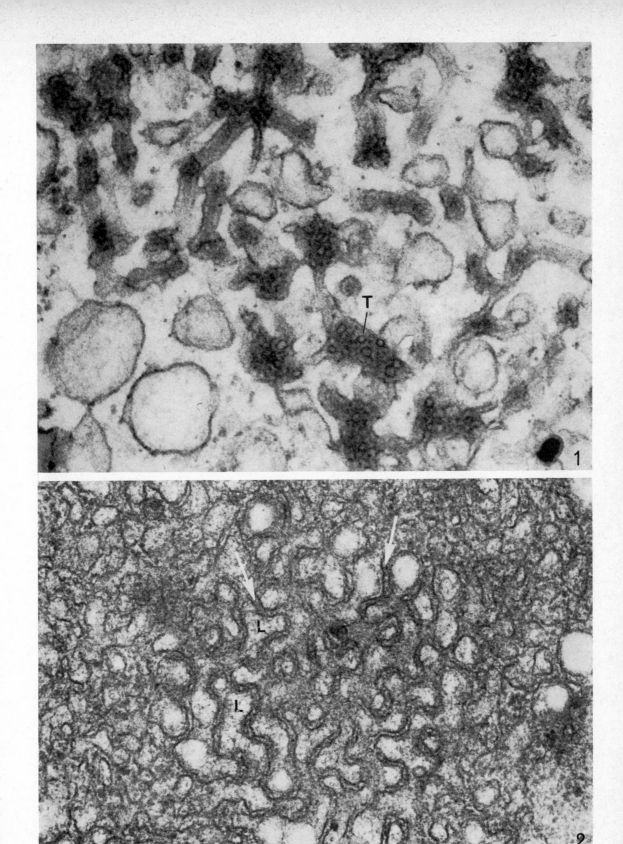

Such tubular formations have been seen in various tissues and organs such as kidney, skin, muscle, myocardium, synovium, brain, lymph node, liver, jejunum and blood. The cells (in tissues or in culture) in which they have been seen include endothelium, fibroblasts, glial cells, lymphoid cells, mononuclear cells, macrophages and tumour cells.

Perhaps the most intriguing and controversial group of undulating tubules are those which have now been frequently reported to occur in the vascular endothelium of kidneys from cases of systemic lupus erythematosus (for references, see Bloodworth and Shelp, 1970; Uzman *et al.*, 1971; Gyorkey *et al.*, 1972). Here some workers have pointed out that the morphology is comparable to crystalline arrays of virus particles, or the nucleoprotein strands of paramyxoviruses. Against the viral hypothesis is the failure to isolate a virus from inclusion-bearing tissue (Norton, 1969; Feorino *et al.*, 1970) and the immunofluorescence and tissue culture studies by Pincus *et al.* (1970) who point out that the strands of paramyxoviruses are smaller in size and occur in the cytoplasm and not in the endoplasmic reticulum.

To this one may add that such bodies have been seen in kidney biopsies from various other diseases and also apparently from normal kidney. Nevertheless, these bodies or inclusions do seem to occur much more frequently in lupus nephritis. Thus Norton (1969) found that such inclusions were 'present in 100% of active lesions of SLE', while an incidence of '62% was noted in lupus biopsies as opposed to 2·4% of non-lupus biopsies' by Bloodworth and Shelp (1970).

The viral nature of tubular arrays remains not proven even in the case of systemic lupus erythematosus and the alternative explanation offered for undulating tubules seen in most situations is that this is a response of the endoplasmic reticulum to a variety of pathological situations, including viral diseases, and neoplastic states. The true significance of this change remains obscure.

Plate 119

Undulating tubules or tubular aggregates found in vascular endothelial cells (glomerular capillaries) from the kidney of a case of systemic lupus erythematosus. (*Ghadially and Larsen, unpublished electron micrographs*)

Fig. 1. Glomerular capillary showing tubular aggregates (T). × 25,000

Figs. 2–6. At higher magnifications these structures show various forms, such as a collection of loosely arranged tubules (*Fig. 2*), thick-walled tubules (*Fig. 3*) or a collection of rounded electron-dense granules (*Fig. 6*). Sometimes they appear to be within dilatations of the endoplasmic reticulum (*Figs. 3, 5 and 6*) and in other instances, where the surrounding membrane is absent or not clearly visualized, they appear to lie in the cytoplasmic matrix (*Fig. 4*). × 54,000; × 115,000; × 62,000; × 62,000; × 62,000

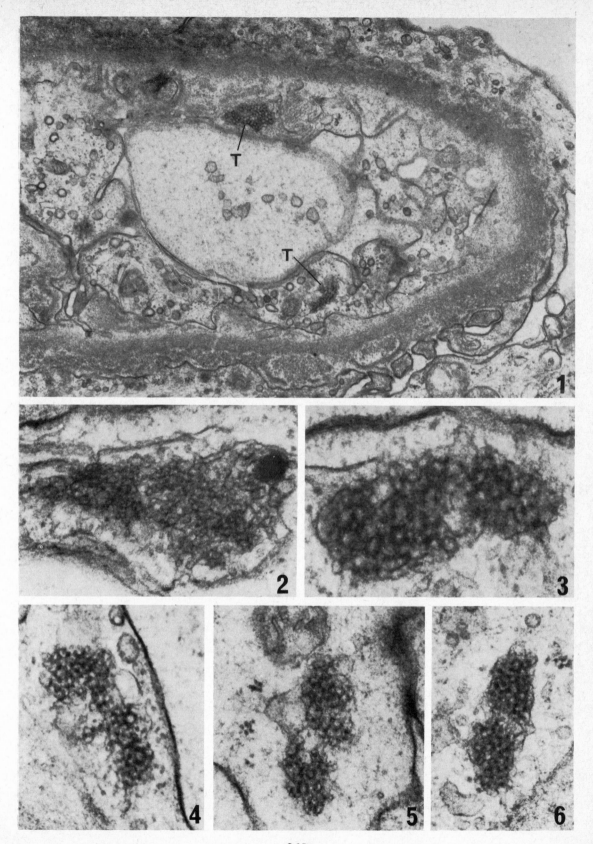

CONCENTRIC LAMELLAR BODIES

Concentric lamellar bodies derived from the endoplasmic reticulum and usually composed of paired membrane arrays have been observed in some normal cells and in a variety of pathologically altered cells. Sequestered at the centre of such bodies there often lies a portion of cytoplasm containing some organelles and inclusions, particularly common being lipid droplets and mitochondria (*Plates 120–122*).

On a morphological basis, one might divide these concentric lamellar bodies into three varieties: (1) those composed of rough endoplasmic reticulum; (2) those composed of smooth membranes; and (3) those composed of membranes in association with glycogen. However, intermediate forms occur which are difficult to classify in this fashion.

Terms such as 'ergastoplasmic Nebenkern' (Haguenau, 1958) or 'Nebenkern' may aptly be applied to those concentric lamellar bodies composed of ribosome-studded membranes, for they are likely to present as juxtanuclear basophilic bodies at light microscopy. Terms such as 'myelin figures', 'myelinoid figures', and 'finger-prints' have been used to describe concentric lamellar structures devoid of particles (i.e. ribosomes or glycogen). These are likely to present as eosinophilic bodies at light microscopy. The term 'glycogen body' was coined by Steiner *et al.* (1964) to describe the lamellar bodies which contain both membrane and glycogen.

Most of the above-mentioned terms are acceptable, but terms such as 'myelin figures' and 'myelinoid figures' or 'bodies' should be avoided, for they relate to highly electron-dense membranous whorls found in certain lysosomes (see pages 310–314). However, the situation is complicated somewhat by the fact that the lamellar bodies may suffer degenerative changes and be converted into cytolysosomes (autolysosomes) and myelinoid bodies (i.e. lysosomes containing myelin figures, see page 310).

It is said that concentric lamellar bodies do not occur in normal liver (Steiner *et al.*, 1964) but they have often been observed in hepatocytes altered by disease or experimental procedure. Thus they have been seen in: (1) viral infections and viral hepatitis of man and mouse (Albot and Jezequel, 1962; Leduc and Bernhard, 1962; Miyai *et al.*, 1963; McGavran and Easterday, 1963); (2) guinea-pig hepatocytes after the administration of diphtheria toxin (Caesar and Rapaport, 1963); (3) hepatomas of man, rat and mouse (Fawcett and Wilson, 1955; Rouiller, 1957; Driessens *et al.*, 1959; Ghadially and Parry, 1966; Flaks, 1968; and Moyer *et al.*, 1970) (*Plate 122*). Such bodies have also been seen in rat hepatocytes after the administration of: (4) DL-ethionine (Herman *et al.*, 1962; Steiner *et al.*, 1964; Shinozuka *et al.*, 1970; (5) thiocetamide (Salomon, 1962a, b; Rouiller and Simon, 1962; Thoenes, 1962; Thoenes and Bannasch, 1962); (6) α-naphthylisothiocyanate (Steiner and Baglio, 1963); (7) dimethylnitrosoamine (Benedetti and Emmelot,

---

Plate 120

From a hepatocyte of a rat treated with yellow phosphorus. The membranes of the rough endoplasmic reticulum have formed a whorl in the cytoplasm enclosing mitochondria and lipid droplets. ×21,000 (*Ganote and Otis, unpublished electron micrograph*)

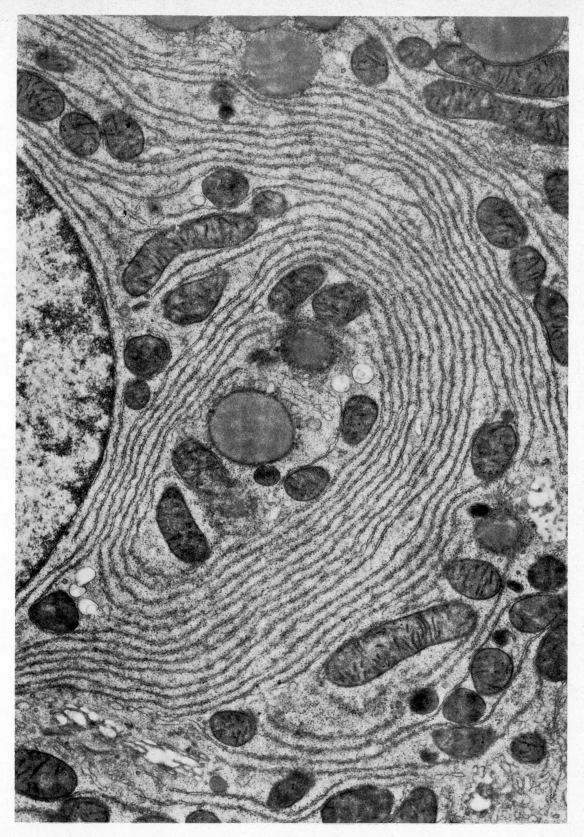

1960; Emmelot and Benedetti, 1960, 1961); (8) thiohydantoin compound (Bax 4222) (Herdson *et al.*, 1964a; Herdson and Kaltenbach, 1965); (9) N-2-fluorenyldiacetamide (Mikata and Luse, 1964); (10) aflatoxin B_1 (Svoboda *et al.*, 1966); (11) carbon tetrachloride (Stenger, 1964, 1966); (12) yellow phosphorous (Ganote and Otis, 1969) (*Plate 120*); (13) dichlorodiphenyltrichloroethane (DDT) (Ortega *et al.*, 1956); (14) phenobarbitone (Herdson *et al.*, 1964b; Burger and Herdson, 1966) (*Plate 121, Fig. 1*); (15) toxic fat (Norback and Allen, 1969); and (16) fructose (Phillips *et al.*, 1970).

Besides altered hepatocytes, a variety of other normal and pathologically altered cells have shown concentric lamellar bodies in their cytoplasm. These include: (1) germinal epithelial cells of the testes of guinea-pigs (Fawcett and Ito, 1958); (2) testicular interstitial cells of 28-day-old mice (Ichihara, 1970); (3) spermatocytes of *Ascaris megalocephala* (Favard, 1958); (4) oöcyte of *Spicula solidissima* (Rebhun, 1961); (5) parietal endoderm cells of guinea-pig yolk sac (King, 1971); (6) acinar cells of salivary gland in *Chironomus* larvae (Haguenau, 1958); (7) transitional epithelium of urinary bladder of mouse (Walker, 1960); (8) sympathetic ganglion cells of the rat (Palay and Palade, 1955); (9) sensory nerve fibres of cat muscle spindles (Corvaja *et al.*, 1971); (10) ciliated epithelium of rabbit fallopian tube (Le Beux, 1969); (11) adrenal cortical cells of cat, guinea-pig and hamster (Cotte, 1959); (12) oxyphil cells of parathyroid in monkey (Trier, 1958); (13) pancreatic acinar cells of the rat after DL-ethionine (Herman and Fitzgerald, 1962; Herman *et al.*, 1962), and of the mouse after fasting and re-feeding (Weiss, 1953); (14) argyrophil cells of gastric mucosa of mouse after fasting and water deprivation (Helander, 1961); (15) Rous sarcoma cells (Epstein, 1957b); (16) oestrogen-induced pituitary adenoma (Haguenau, 1958); (17) Ehrlich ascites tumour cells infected with Newcastle virus (Adams and Prince, 1959); and (18) 9:10-dimethyl-1:2-benzanthracene-induced subcutaneous sarcoma of rat (*Plate 121, Fig. 2*).

A study of the literature shows that the most common type of lamellar body is that composed of smooth membranes only. The glycogen body, although rare by comparison, has attracted much attention and its morphology and distribution in various situations have been reviewed in recent publications (Le Beux, 1969; Corvaja *et al.*, 1971). It is also evident that all three types of bodies can at times be seen in a single disease state or be produced by a single agent. A variety of structures such as lipid droplets, mitochondria, and microbodies appear at the centre of these

Plate 121

Fig. 1. From a hepatocyte of a hamster treated with phenobarbitone. A smooth-membraned lamellar body is seen enclosing a portion of cytoplasm containing numerous mitochondria and two microbodies, one of which contains glycogen. The significance of this unusual finding (glycogen in a microbody) is obscure. (See page 376 for further details.) × 18,000 (*Bhatnagar and Ghadially, unpublished electron micrograph*)

Fig. 2. A membranous body found in a tumour cell. From a fibrosarcoma produced in the flank of a rat by injection of 9:10-dimethyl-1:2-benzanthracene × 12,000 (*Ghadially and Parry, unpublished electron micrograph*)

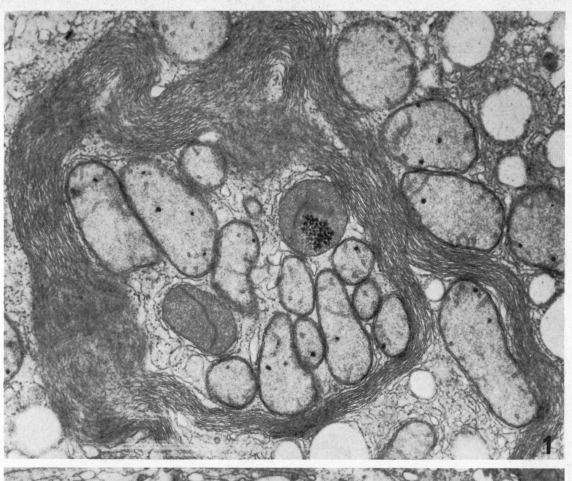

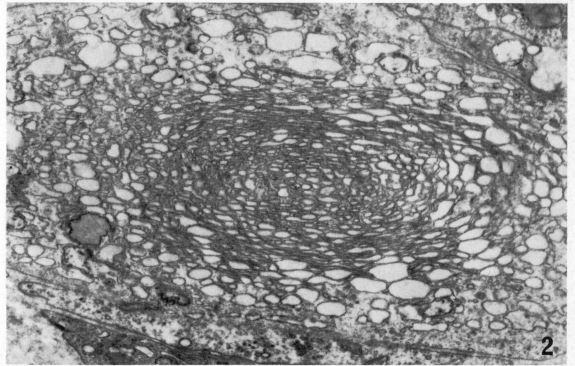

lamellar bodies. A reasonable assumption would be that this is fortuitous and not meaningful. However, Stenger (1964) has speculated that the membranes may be derived from the centrally placed lipid.

Since continuities between the peripheral membranes of smooth-membraned lamellar bodies and adjacent endoplasmic reticulum in the cell have been observed, it has been proposed that these lamellar bodies represent either (1) a new formation of smooth endoplasmic reticulum, or that (2) they are produced by a degranulation of pre-existing rough endoplasmic reticulum. Both mechanisms are probably operative but often the amount of membranous material is so abundant that it is difficult to reconcile this as being derived solely by degranulation of pre-existing rough endoplasmic reticulum. There is now much evidence indicating that the biogenesis of the membranes of the smooth endoplasmic reticulum occurs in the rough endoplasmic reticulum where the necessary protein synthesis and the incorporation of lipid involved is achieved (Dallner et al., 1966; Jones and Fawcett, 1966). Thus, the concentric membranes of the lamellar body could be regarded as modified smooth endoplasmic reticulum arising from the rough endoplasmic reticulum, as does the normal smooth endoplasmic reticulum in the hepatocyte.

Broadly speaking, two views have been expressed regarding the nature of concentric lamellar bodies: (1) that they represent a degenerative change or an elaborate autophagic vacuole; and (2) that this is a regenerative change leading to a specialized type of hypertrophy of the endoplasmic reticulum which may have a functional significance. Since cytomembranes clearly in excess of normal occur at least in the larger concentric membranous bodies, and since no limiting membrane is apparent, the second hypothesis seems more attractive.

The concentric smooth membrane arrays produced as a result of drugs may then be looked upon as a specialized type of smooth endoplasmic reticulum hypertrophy and one may speculate that this probably helps in the detoxication of drugs, as does the smooth endoplasmic reticulum in the hepatocyte. The association of glycogen with some of these membrane systems is reminiscent of its close association with the smooth endoplasmic reticulum in the hepatocyte.

Since the rough endoplasmic reticulum is involved in the production of secretory proteins, one may speculate that the ribosome-studded lamellar bodies may indicate enhanced protein secretory activity. This seems to be so at least in the spermatocytes of *Ascaris megalocephala* (Favard 1958).

The significance of the occurrence of lamellar bodies in hepatomas and other neoplasms is obscure, but one may speculate that it represents yet another example of atypical or exaggerated growth associated with the neoplastic state.

Plate 122

A glycogen body found in a human hepatoma. × 23,000 (*Ghadially and Parry, unpublished electron micrograph*)

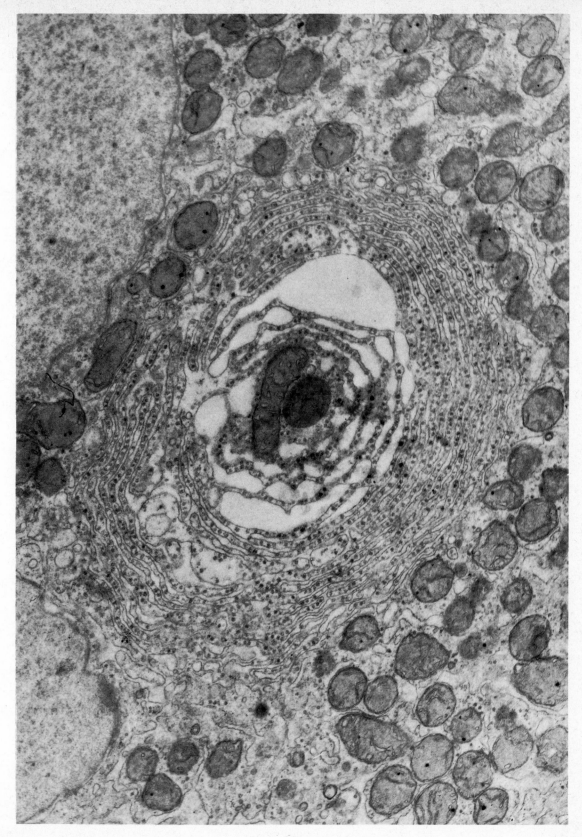

271

HYPERTROPHY OF SMOOTH ENDOPLASMIC RETICULUM IN HEPATOCYTES

Perhaps the most extensively studied example of smooth endoplasmic reticulum hypertrophy is that seen in the hepatocytes of phenobarbitone-treated rats and hamsters, where after a few doses of the drug almost every nook and cranny of the cell may be filled with a ramifying network of smooth-membraned branching tubules and vesicles. This change is associated with an increase in liver weight, an increase in the size of the microsomal fraction (in this case composed mainly of smooth endoplasmic reticulum membranes) and a concomitant rise in drug-metabolizing enzymes. Smooth endoplasmic reticulum hypertrophy (*Plates 123 and 124*) has now come to be regarded as an adaptive response (drug tolerance) by which an animal develops an enhanced ability to handle doses of drugs which would be fatal to normal animals.

Smooth endoplasmic reticulum hypertrophy shows many interesting morphological variations, dependent on the drug used and the amount, frequency and duration of its administration. It may also at times be related to the species, age and sex of the animal. One can find a spectrum of changes varying from obvious degranulation of rough endoplasmic reticulum followed by a barely discernible or modest new smooth endoplasmic reticular formation (e.g. after administration of some hepatocarcinogens) to overt hypertrophy of smooth endoplasmic reticulum without a marked reduction in the amount of rough endoplasmic reticulum (e.g. after administration of phenobarbitone; *Plate 124*). Phosphorus poisoning provides a further interesting variation, for here marked hypertrophy of the rough endoplasmic reticulum with concentric ribosome-studded membrane formations is seen prior to smooth endoplasmic reticulum hypertrophy (*Plates 120 and 123*). Furthermore, one may observe that smooth endoplasmic reticulum hypertrophy may be diffuse and occur as large areas of branching tubules almost filling the cytoplasm (*Plate 123*), or it can be focal and present as small rounded aggregates of vesicular smooth endoplasmic reticulum in the cell.

With light microscopy focal zones of smooth endoplasmic reticulum hypertrophy may present as hyaline eosinophilic inclusions in the cytoplasm. Many of the drugs that produce this change also yield concentric membranous whorls of smooth membranes in the cytoplasm (*Plate 121, Fig. 1*). Smooth endoplasmic reticulum hypertrophy has occasionally been noted in a few pathological states such as viral hepatitis (Schaffner, 1966) and extrahepatic cholestasis (Steiner *et al.*, 1962), but it has mainly been observed after the administration of a large variety of drugs, including many hepatocarcinogens. There is ample evidence that such changes occur not only in a variety of laboratory animals but also in man.

Drugs which have produced smooth endoplasmic reticulum hypertrophy in the liver include: (1) aflatoxin (Svoboda *et al.*, 1966); (2) allylisopropylacetamide (Posalaki and Barka, 1968; Moses *et al.*, 1970; Biempica *et al.*, 1971); (3) β-3-furylalanine (Hruban *et al.*, 1965b); (4) β-3-thienylalanine (Hruban *et al.*, 1963); (5) butylated hydroxytoluene (Lane and Lieber, 1967); (6) carbon tetrachloride (Bassi, 1960; Ganote and Otis, 1969); (7) dicholorodiphenyltrichloroethane (DDT) (Ortega, 1966); (8) dieldrin (Hutterer *et al.*, 1968); (9) dimethylnitrosamine (Emmelot and Benedetti, 1960, 1961; Svoboda and Higginson, 1963, 1966); (10) ethanol (Rubin *et al.*, 1968); (11) ethionine (Wood, 1964, 1965; Meldolesi *et al.*, 1967) (12) N-2-fluorenyldiacetamide (Mikata and

---

Plate 123

Two hepatocytes are seen in this electron micrograph. The cytoplasm of one of these (A) is packed with smooth endoplasmic reticulum, but the other (B) is not so affected. From the liver of a rat given yellow phosphorus. × 20,000 (*Ghadially and Bhatnagar, unpublished electron micrograph*)

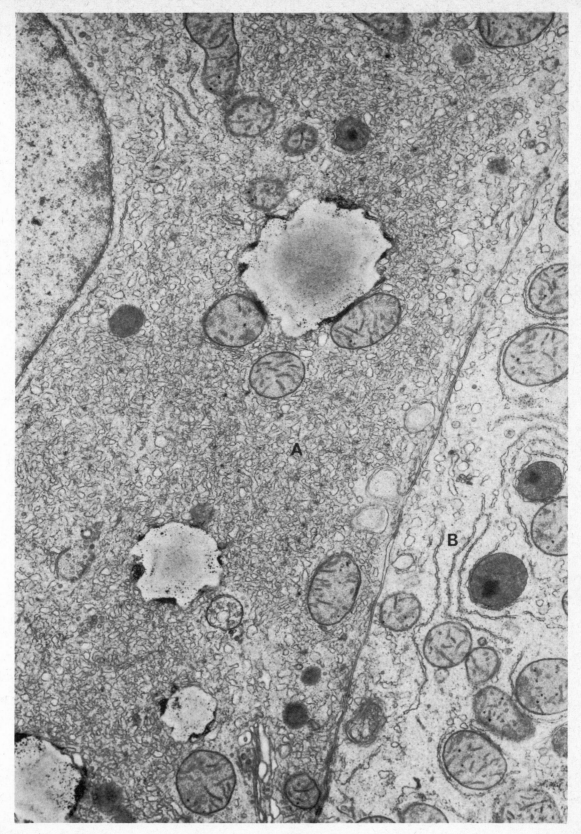

Luse, 1964); (13) 2-methyl-4-dimethylaminoazobenzene (Lafontaine and Allard, 1964); (14) 3-methyl-4-dimethylaminoazobenzene (butter yellow) (Porter and Bruni, 1959; Arcasoy et al., 1968; Hutterer et al., 1969); (15) naphthylisothiocyanate (Steiner and Baglio, 1963); (16) phenobarbitone (Remmer and Merker, 1963; Orrenius et al., 1965; Orrenius and Ericsson, 1966a, b; Burger and Herdson, 1966; Jones and Fawcett, 1966; Chiesara et al., 1967); (17) lasiocarpine (Svoboda and Higginson, 1963); (18) reserpine (Winborn and Seelig, 1970); (19) tannic acid (Arhelger et al., 1965); (20) thioacetamide (Ashworth et al., 1965; Kendrey, 1968); and (21) yellow phosphorus (Ganote and Otis, 1969).

An examination of the above-mentioned list of compounds shows that drugs with diverse pharmacological properties and chemical structure can produce smooth endoplasmic reticulum hypertrophy. However, most of these compounds are lipid soluble and since large doses of progesterone can also produce this change it has been suggested (Jones and Fawcett, 1966) that enzymes of the smooth endoplasmic reticulum are responsible for the degradation of both endogenous and exogenous lipid-soluble compounds. Such a concept is further supported (see review by Conney, 1965) by the observation that the liver of phenobarbitone-treated rats have a several-fold increased ability to hydroxylate testosterone, androsterone, oestradiol, progesterone and cortisone and that the hydroxylases involved are located in the microsomal fraction (Kuntzman and Jacobson, 1965; Orrenius et al., 1965). Smooth endoplasmic reticulum hypertrophy has been noted in viral hepatitis (Schaffner, 1966) and in extrahepatic cholestasis (Steiner et al. 1962). This may indicate an adaptive response to deal with endogenously produced toxic material (Barka and Popper, 1967).

Proliferation of smooth endoplasmic reticulum is now regarded as the morphological expression of drug-induced enzyme production in the liver. The newly formed smooth endoplasmic reticulum has frequently been seen to arise from the rough endoplasmic reticulum (*Plate 124*). This is in keeping with the idea that the lipoproteins needed for new membrane synthesis are produced by the rough endoplasmic reticulum, as are the associated drug-metabolizing enzymes. The expanded smooth endoplasmic reticulum may then be looked upon as providing the surface for interaction of drugs and enzymes.

Recent studies (Barka and Popper, 1967; Arcasoy et al., 1968; Hutterer et al., 1969) show that three stages may be identified in the response of the liver to drugs which produce smooth endoplasmic reticulum hypertrophy. The first stage (induction) is associated with liver enlargement, smooth endoplasmic reticulum hypertrophy, increase in microsomal protein fraction and formation of drug-handling enzymes. This is followed by a steady state of increased drug tolerance, the length of which may be fairly long as in the case of phenobarbitone and dieldrin, or quite short as in the case of 3-methyl-4-dimethylaminoazobenzene. Finally, a third stage (decompensation) may be reached where the activity of the drug-handling enzymes diminishes and the smooth endoplasmic reticulum is seen as focal clusters of tightly packed vesicles in the cell cytoplasm.

Plate 124

An area of smooth endoplasmic reticulum hypertrophy from the liver of a hamster that had received phenobarbitone. Note the continuity between the rough and the smooth endoplasmic reticulum (arrows). ×48,000 (*Ghadially and Bhatnagar, unpublished electron micrograph*)

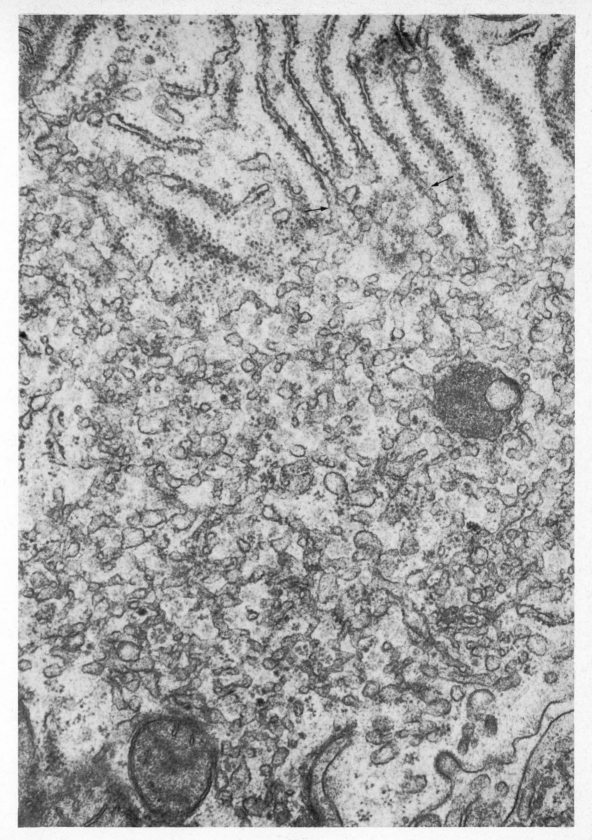

REFERENCES

Adams, W. R. and Prince, A. M. (1959). 'Cellular changes associated with infection of the Ehrlich ascites tumor with Newcastle disease virus.' *Ann. N. Y. Acad. Sci.* **81**, 89

Albot, P. M. G. and Jezequel, A. M. (1962). 'Ultrastructure du foie et pathogenie de l'ictere au cours des hepatites virales.' *Archs. Mal. Appar. dig.* **51**. 38

Angel, A. and Sheldon, H. (1965) 'Adipose cell organelles: isolation, morphology and possible relation to intracellular lipid transport.' *Ann. N.Y. Acad. Sci.* **131**, 157

Anitschkow, N. (1914). 'Zur Frage der tropfigen Entmischung.' *Verh. deutsch. Ges. Path.* **17**, 103

Arcasoy, M., Smuckler, E. A. and Benditt, E. P. (1968). 'Acute effects of 3-methyl-4-dimethyl aminoazobenzene intoxication on rat livers. Structural and functional changes in the endoplasmic reticulum and NADPH-related electron transport.' *Am. J. Path.* **62**, 841

Arhelger, R. B., Broom, S. and Boler, R. K. (1965). 'Ultrastructural hepatic alterations following tannic acid administration to rabbits.' *Am. J. Path.* **46**, 409

Armstrong, D. T., O'Brien, J. and Greep, R. O. (1964). 'Effects of luteinizing hormone on progestin biosynthesis in the luteinized rat ovary.' *Endocrinology* **75**, 488

Ashworth, C. T., Werner, D. J., Glass, M. D. and Arnold, N. J. (1965). 'Spectrum of fine structural changes in hepato-cellular injury due to thioacetamide.' *Am. J. Path.* **47**, 917

Baglio, C. M. and Farber, E. (1965a). 'Correspondence between ribosome aggregation patterns in rat liver homogenates and in electron micrographs following administration of ethionine.' *J. molec. Biol.* **12**, 466

—— (1965b). 'Reversal by adenine of the ethionine-induced lipid accumulation in the endoplasmic reticulum of the rat liver.' *J. Cell. Biol.* **27**, 591

Barbieri, M., Simonelli, L., Simoni, P. and Maraldi, N. M. (1970). 'Ribosome crystallization. II. Ultrastructural study on nuclear and cytoplasmic ribosome crystallization in hypothermic cell cultures.' *J. Submicr. Cytol.* **2**, 33

Barka, T. and Popper, H. (1967). 'Liver enlargement and drug toxicity.' *Medicine, Baltimore* **46**, 103

Bassi, M. (1960). 'Electron microscopy of rat liver after carbon tetrachloride poisoning.' *Expl Cell. Res.* **20**, 313

Bassot, J. M. (1966). 'Une forme microtubulaire et paracristalline de reticulum endoplasmique dans les photocytes des annelides polynoinae.' *J. Cell. Biol.* **31**, 135

Beams, H. W. and Kessel, R. (1962). 'Intracisternal granules of the endoplasmic reticulum in the crayfish oocyte.' *J. Cell. Biol.* **13**, 158

—— (1963). 'Electron microscope studies on developing crayfish with special reference to the origin of yolk.' *J. Cell Biol.* **18**, 621

Behnke, O. (1963). 'Helical arrangement of ribosomes in the cytoplasm of differentiating cells of the small intestine of rat foetuses.' *Expl Cell Res.* **30**, 597

— and Moe, H. (1964). 'An electron microscope study of mature and differentiating Paneth cells in the rat, especially of their endoplasmic reticulum and lysosomes.' *J. Cell Biol.* **22**, 633

Benedetti, E. L. and Emmelot, P. (1960). 'Changes in the fine structure of rat liver cells brought about by dimethyl-nitrosamine.' In *Proceedings of the European Regional Conference on Electron Microscopy, Delft,* Vol. 2, p. 875. Ed. by A. L. Henwick and B. J. Spit. Uppsala: Almqvist and Wiksell

— Bont, W. S. and Bloemendal, H. (1966). 'Electron microscopic observation on polyribosomes and endoplasmic reticulum fragments isolated from rat liver.' *Lab. Invest.* **15**, 196

Bernhard, W. (1969). 'Ultrastructure of the cancer cell.' In *Handbook of Molecular Cytology.* Ed. by A. Lima-De-Faria. Amsterdam and London: North Holland Publ.

Biempica, L., Kosower, N. S. and Roheim, P. S. (1971). 'Cytochemical and ultrastructural changes in rat liver in experimental porphyria. II. Effects of repeated injections of allylisopropylacetamide.' *Lab. Invest.* **24**, 110

Blackburn, W. R. and Vinijchaikul, K. (1969). 'The pancreas in kwashiorkor. An electron microscopic study.' *Lab. Invest.* **20**, 305

Bloodworth, J. M. B. and Shelp, W. D. (1970). 'Endothelial cytoplasmic inclusions.' *Archs Path.* **90**, 252

Bonnett, H. T. and Newcomb, E. H. (1965). 'Polyribosomes and cisternal accumulations in root cells of radish.' *J. Cell Biol.* **27**, 423

Boulton, P. S. and Webb, H. E. (1971). 'An electron microscopic study of Langat virus encephalitis in mice.' *Brain* **94**, 411

Brenner, R. M. (1966). 'Fine structure of adrenocortical cells in adult male rhesus monkeys.' *Am. J. Anat.* **119**, 429

Brown, R. E. and Schatzki, P. F. (1971). 'Intracisternal granules in the human pancreas.' *Archs Path.* **91**, 351

— and Still, W. J. S. (1970). 'Acinar-islet cells in the exocrine pancreas of the adult cat.' *Am. J. dig. Dis.* **15**, 327

Burger, P. C. and Herdson, P. B. (1966). 'Phenobarbital-induced fine structural changes in rat liver.' *Am. J. Path.* **48**, 793

Buttrose, M. S., Frey-Wyssling, A. and Muhlethaler, K. (1960). 'Intracisternal granules in the endosperm cell of the barley grain.' *J. Ultrastruct. Res.* **4**, 258

Byers, B. (1967). 'Structure and formation of ribosome crystals in hypothermic chick embryo cells.' *J. molec. Biol.* **26**, 155

— (1971). 'Chick embryo ribosome crystals: analysis of bonding and functional activity *in vitro*.' *Proc. natn Acad. Sci., U.S.A.* **68**, 440

Caesar, R. and Rapaport, M. (1963). 'Elektronenmikroskopische Untersuchung des Leberzellschadens bei der Diphtherietoxinvergiftung.' *Frankfurt. Ztschr. Path.* **72**, 517

Caro, L. G. and Palade, G. E. (1964). 'Protein synthesis, storage, and discharge in the pancreatic exocrine cell—an autoradiographic study.' *J. Cell. Biol.* **20**, 473

Cedergren, B. and Harary, I. (1964). '*In vitro* studies on single beating rat heart cells. VI. Electron microscopic studies of single cells.' *J. Ultrastruct. Res.* **11**, 428

Chandra, S. (1968). 'Undulating tubules associated with endoplasmic reticulum in pathologic tissues.' *Lab. Invest.* **18**, 422

Chapman, J. A. (1962). 'Fibroblasts and collagen.' *Br. med. Bull.* **18**, 233

Chiesara, E., Clementi, F., Conti, F. and Meldolesi, J. (1967). 'The induction of drug-metabolizing enzymes in rat liver during growth and regeneration.' *Lab. Invest.* **16**, 254

Christensen, A. K. (1965). 'The fine structure of testicular interstitial cells in guinea pigs.' *J. Cell Biol.* **26**, 911

— and Fawcett, D. W. (1961). 'The normal fine structure of opossum testicular interstitial cells.' *J. biophys. biochem. Cytol* **9**, 653

Conney, A. H. (1965). 'Enzyme induction and drug toxicity. In *Proceedings of the Second International Pharmacological Meeting*, Vol. 4, *Drugs and Enzymes*, p. 277. Ed. by B. B. Brodie. Oxford: Pergamon Press

Corvaja, N., Magherini, P. C. and Pompeiano, O. (1971). 'Ultrastructure of glycogen-membrane complexes in sensory nerve fibres of cat muscle spindles.' *Z. Zellforsch. mikrosk. Anat.* **121**, 199

Cotte, G. (1959). 'Quelques problèmes posés par l'ultrastructure des lipides de la cortico-surrenale.' *J. Ultrastruct. Res.* **3**, 186

Dallner, G., Siekevitz, P. and Palade, G. E. (1966). 'Biogenesis of endoplasmic reticulum membranes. I. Structural and chemical differentiation in developing rat hepatocyte.' *J. Cell Biol.* **30**, 73

Dalton, J. A. (1964). 'An electron microscopical study of a series of chemically induced hepatomas.' In *Cellular Control, Mechanisms and Cancer*, p. 211. Ed. by P. Emmelot and O. Muhlbock. New York: American Elsevier

— and Haguenau, F. (1962). *Tumors Induced by Viruses: Ultrastructural Studies*. New York and London: Academic Press

David, H. (1964). *Submicroscopic Ortho- and Pathomorphology of the Liver*. Oxford: Pergamon Press

Driessens, J., Dupont, A. and Demaille, A. (1959). 'L'hepatome experimental azoique du rat examine au microscope electronique.' *C.r. Soc. Biol.* **153**, 788

Echlin, P. (1965). 'An apparent helical arrangement of ribosomes in developing pollen mother cells of *Ipomoea purpurea* (*L.*) Roth.' *J. Cell Biol.* **24**, 150

Emmelot, P. and Benedetti, E. L. (1960). 'Changes in the fine structure of rat liver cells brought about by dimethylnitrosamine.' *J. biophys. biochem. Cytol.* **7**, 393

— — (1961). 'Some observations on the effect of liver carcinogens on the fine structure and function of the endoplasmic reticulum of rat liver cells.' In *Protein Biosynthesis*, p. 99. Ed. by R. J. C. Harris. London and New York: Academic Press

Enders, A. C. (1962). 'Observations on the fine structures of lutein cells.' *J. Cell Biol.* **12**, 101

— and Lyon, W. R. (1964). 'Observations on the fine structure of lutein cells. II. The effects of hypophysectomy and mammotrophic hormones in the rat.' *J. Cell Biol.* **22**, 127

Epstein, M. A. (1957a). 'The fine structure of the cells in mouse sarcoma 37 ascitic fluids.' *J. biophys. biochem. Cytol.* **3**, 567

— (1957b). 'The fine structural organization of Rous tumor cells.' *J. biophys. biochem. Cytol.* **3**, 851

Ernst, P. (1914). *Verh. deutsch. Ges. Path.* **17**, 43. (Quoted by Cameron, G. R. (1952).) *Pathology of the Cell.* Edinburgh: Oliver and Boyd

Ernster, L., Siekevitz, P. and Palade, G. E. (1962). 'Enzyme-structure relationships in the endoplasmic reticulum of rat liver. A morphological and biochemical study'. *J. Cell Biol.* **15**, 541

Fahr, R. (1914). 'Zur Frade der sogenannten hyalintropfigen Zelldegeneration'. *Verh. deutsch. Ges. Path.* **17**, 119

Favard, P. (1958). 'L'origine ergastoplasmique des granules proteiques dans les spermatocytes d'Ascaris.' *C. r. Acad. Sci.* **247**, 531

Fawcett, D. W. (1964). 'Morphological considerations of lipid transport in the liver.' In *Proceedings of the International Symposium on Lipid Transport*, p. 1. Springfield, Illinois: Charles C Thomas

— (1967). *The Cell. An Atlas of Fine Structure*. Philadelphia and London: W. B. Saunders

— and Ito, S. (1958). 'Observations on the cytoplasmic membranes of testicular cells examined by phase contrast and electron microscopy.' *J. biophys. biochem. Cytol.* **4**, 135

— and Revel, J. P. (1961). 'The sarcoplasmic reticulum of a fast-acting fish muscle.' *J. biophys. biochem. Cytol.* **10**, Suppl., 89

— and Selby, C. C. (1958). 'Observations on the fine structure of the turtle atrium.' *J. biophys. biochem. Cytol.* **4**, 63

— and Wilson, J. W. (1955). 'A note on the occurrence of virus-like particles in the spontaneous hepatomas of C3H mice.' *J. natn. Cancer Inst.* **15**, 1505

Feorino, P. M., Hierholzer, J. C. and Norton, W. L. (1970). 'Viral isolation studies of inclusion positive biopsy from human connective tissue diseases.' *Arthritis Rheum.* **13**, 378

Flaks, B. (1968). 'Formation of membrane-glycogen arrays in rat hepatoma cells.' *J. Cell Biol.* **36**, 410

Ganote, C. E. and Otis, J. B. (1969) 'Characteristic lesions of yellow phosphorus-induced liver damage.' *Lab. Invest.* **21**, 207

Ghadially, F. N. and Mehta, P. N. (1970). 'Ultrastructure of osteogenic sarcoma.' *Cancer* **25**, 1457

— and Parry, E. W. (1966). 'Ultrastructure of a human hepatocellular carcinoma and surrounding non-neoplastic liver.' *Cancer* **19**, 1989

— and Roy, S. (1969). '*Ultrastructure of Synovial Joints in Health and Disease*. London: Butterworths

— Mehta, P. N. and Kirkaldy-Willis, W. H. (1970). 'Ultrastructure of articular cartilage in experimentally produced lipoarthrosis.' *J. Bone Jt Surg.* **52A**, 1147

Ghiara, G. and Taddei, C. (1966). 'Dati citologici e ultrastrutturali su di un particolare tipo di constituenti basofili del citoplasma di cellule follicolari e di ovociti ovarisi di rettili.' *Boll. Soc. ital. Biol. sper.* **42**, 784

Godman, G. and Porter, K. R. (1960). 'Chondrogenesis, studied with the electron microscope.' *J. biophys. biochem. Cytol.* **8**, 719

Goldblatt, P. J. (1969). 'The endoplasmic reticulum'. In *Handbook of Molecular Cytology*, p. 1101. Ed. by A. Lima-de-Faria. Amsterdam and London: North Holland Publ.

Goodman, H. M. and Rich, A. (1963). 'Mechanism of polyribosome action during protein synthesis.' *Nature, Lond.* **199**, 318

277

Grimley, P. M. and Friedman, R. M. (1970). 'Development of Semliki Forest virus in mouse brain: an electron microscopic study.' *Expl Molec. Path.* **12**, 1

Gross, L. (1970). *Oncogenic Viruses,* 2nd ed. Oxford: Pergamon Press

Gueft, B. and Kikkawa, Y. (1962). 'The periodic structure of nuclear and cytoplasmic crystals of dog liver cells.' In *Electron Microscopy,* Fifth International Congress on Electron Microscopy, Vol. 2, p. T-5. Ed. by S. Breese, Jr. New York: Academic Press

Gyorkey, F., Sinkovics, J. G., Min, K. W. and Gyorkey, P. (1972). 'A morphologic study on the occurrence and distribution of structures resembling viral nucleocapsids in collagen diseases.' *Am. J. Med.* **53**, 148

Haguenau, F. (1958). 'The ergastoplasm. Its history, ultrastructure and biochemistry.' *Int. Rev. Cytol.* **7**, 425

Hamilton, D. W., Fawcett, D. W. and Christensen, A. K. (1966). 'The liver of the slender salamander *Batrachoseps attenuatus*. I. The structure of its crystalline inclusions.' *Z. Zellforsch. mikrosk. Anat.* **70**, 347

Hardesty, B., Miller, R. and Schweet, R. (1963). 'Polyribosome breakdown and hemoglobin synthesis.' *Proc. natn. Acad. Sci.* **50**, 924

Helander, H. F. (1961). 'A preliminary note on the ultrastructure of the argyrophile cells of the mouse gastric mucosa.' *J. Ultrastruct. Res.* **5**, 257

Herdson, P. B. and Kaltenbach, J. P. (1965). 'Electron microscope studies on enzyme activity and the isolation of thiohydantoin induced myelin figures in rat liver.' *J. Cell Biol.* **25**, 485

— Garvin, P. J. and Jennings, R. B. (1964a). 'Reversible biological and fine structural changes produced in rat liver by a thiohydantoin compound.' *Lab. Invest.* **13**, 1014

— — — (1964b). 'Fine structural changes in rat liver induced by phenobarbital.' *Lab. Invest.* **13**, 1032

Herman, L. and Fitzgerald, P. J. (1962) 'Restitution of pancreatic acinar cells following ethionine.' *J. Cell Biol.* **12**, 297

— Eber, L. and Fitzgerald, P. J. (1962). 'Liver cell degeneration with ethionine administration.' In *Proceedings of the Fifth International Congress for Electron Microscopy,* Vol. 2, p. vv-6. Ed. by S. S. Breese, Jr. New York: Academic Press.

— Sato, T. and Fitzgerald, P. J. (1964). 'The pancreas.' In *Electron Microscopic Anatomy,* p. 72. Ed. by S. M. Kurtz. New York: Academic Press

Hollmann, K. H. (1959). L'ultrastructure de la glande mammaire normale de la souris en lactation—étude au microscope electronique., *J. Ultrastruct. Res.* **2**, 423

Holmes, I. H., Wark, M. C. and Warburton, M. F. (1969). 'Is rubella an arbovirus? II. Ultrastructural morphology and development.' *Virology* **37**, 15

Hope, J. (1970). 'Stereological analysis of the ultrastructure of liver parenchymal cells during pregnancy and lactation.' *J. Ultrastruct. Res.* **33**, 292

Hruban, Z., Swift, H. and Wissler, R. W. (1963). 'Alterations in the fine structure of hepatocytes produced by β-3-thienylalanine.' *J. Ultrastruct. Res.* **8**, 236

— — and Rechcigl, M. Jr. (1965a). 'Fine structure of transplantable hepatomas of the rat'. *J. natn. Cancer Inst.* **35**, 459

— — Dunn, F. W. and Lewis, D. E. (1965b). 'Effects of β-3-furylalanine on the ultrastructure of the hepatocytes and pancreatic acinar cells.' *Lab. Invest.* **14**, 70

Hultin, T. (1961). 'On the functions of the endoplasmic reticulum.' *Biochem. Pharmac.* **5**, 359

Hutterer, F., Schaffner, F., Klion, F. M. and Popper, H. (1968). 'Hypertrophic hypoactive smooth endoplasmic reticulum: a sensitive indicator of hepatotoxicity exemplified by dieldrin.' *Science* **161**, 1017

— Klion, F., Wengraf, A., Schaffner, F. and Popper, H. (1969). 'Hepatocellular adaptation and injury—structural and biochemical changes following dieldrin and methyl butter yellow.' *Lab. Invest.* **20**, 455

Ichihara, I. (1970). 'The fine structure of testicular interstitial cells in mice during postnatal development.' *Z. Zellforsch. mikrosk. Anat.* **108**, 475

Ichikawa, A. (1965). 'Fine structural changes in response to hormonal stimulation of the perfused canine pancreas.' *J. Cell Biol.* **24**, 369

Ito, S. (1961). 'The endoplasmic reticulum of gastric parietal cells.' *J. biophys. biochem. Cytol.* **11**, 333

Jacob, F and Monod, J. (1961). 'Genetic regulatory mechanisms in the synthesis of proteins.' *J. molec. Biol.* **3**, 318

Jensen, W. A. (1968). 'Cotton embryogenesis.' *J. Cell Biol.* **36**, 403

Jones, A. L. and Armstrong, D. T. (1965). 'Increased cholesterol biosynthesis following phenobarbital induced hypertrophy of agranular endoplasmic reticulum in liver.' *Proc. Soc. exp. Biol. Med.* **119**, 1136

— and Fawcett, D. W. (1966). 'Hypertrophy of the agranular endoplasmic reticulum in hamster liver induced by phenobarbital (with a review of the functions of this organelle in the liver).' *J. Histochem. Cytochem.* **14**, 215

Kelley, R. O. (1971). 'Ultrastructural comparisons of paired cisternae in leukemic and mesenchymal cells during mitosis.' *Anat. Rec.* **171**, 559

Kendrey, G. (1968). 'Fine structural changes in rat liver cells in response to prolonged thioacetamide.' *Path. europ.* **3**, 96

King, B. F. (1971). 'Differentiation of parietal endoderm cells of the guinea pig yolk sac with particular reference to the development of endoplasmic reticulum.' *Devl. Biol.* **26**, 547

Kingsbury, E. W. and Voelz, H. (1969). 'Induction of helical arrays of ribosomes by vinblastine sulfate in *Escherichia coli.*' *Science* **166**, 768

Krishan, A. and Hsu, D. (1969). 'Observations on the association of helical polyribosomes and filaments with vincristine-induced crystals in Earle's L-cell fibroblasts.' *J. Cell Biol.* **43**, 553

— and Stenger, R. J. (1966). 'Effects of starvation on the hepatotoxicity of carbon tetrachloride. A light and electron microscopic study.' *Am. J. Path.* **49**, 239

Kuntzman, R. and Jacobson, M. (1965). 'Effect of drugs on the metabolism of progesterone by liver microsomal enzymes from various animal species.' *Fedn Proc.* **24**, 152

Lafontaine, J. G. and Allard, C. (1964). 'A light and electron microscope study of the morphological changes induced in rat liver cells by the azo dye 2-Me-DAB.' *J. Cell Biol.* **22**, 143

278

Lane, B. P. and Lieber, C. S. (1967). 'Effects of butylated hydroxytoluene on the ultrastructure of rat hepatocytes.' *Lab. Invest.* **16**, 342

Le Beux, Y. J. (1969). 'An unusual ultrastructural association of smooth membranes and glycogen particles: the glycogen body.' *Z. Zellforsch mikrosk. Anat.* **101**, 433

Leduc, E. H. and Bernhard, W. (1962). 'Electron microscope study of mouse liver infected by ectromelia virus.' *J. Ultrastruct. Res.* **6**, 466

Lipetz, J. (1970). 'The fine structure of plant tumours. I. Comparison of crown gall and hyperplastic cells.' *Protoplasma* **70**, 207

— and Galston, A. W. (1959). 'Indole acetic acid oxidase and peroxidase activities in normal and crown gall tissues of *Parthenocissus tricuspidata*.' *Am. J. Bot.* **46**, 193

Long, J. A. and Jones, A. L. (1967a). 'Observations on the fine structure of the adrenal cortex of man.' *Lab. Invest.* **17**, 355

——(1967b). 'The fine structure of the zona glomerulosa and the zona fasciculata of the adrenal cortex of the opossum.' *Am. J. Anat.* **120**, 463

McGavran, M. H. and Easterday, B. C. (1963). 'Rift valley fever virus hepatitis. Light and electron microscopic studies in the mouse.' *Am. J. Path.* **42**, 587

McNutt, N. S. and Jones, A. L. (1970). 'Observations on the ultrastructure of cytodifferentiation in the human fetal adrenal cortex.' *Lab. Invest.* **22**, 513

Ma, M. H. and Webber, A. J. (1966). 'Fine structure of liver tumours induced in the rat by 3'-methyl-4-dimethylaminoazobenzene.' *Cancer Res.* **26**, 935

Mair, W. G. P. and Tomé, F. M. S. (1972). *Atlas of the Ultrastructure of Diseased Human Muscle*. Edinburgh and London: Churchill Livingstone

Maraldi, N. M. and Barbieri, M. (1969). 'Ribosome crystallization. I. Study on electron microscope of ribosome crystallization during chick embryo development.' *J. Submicr. Cytol* **1**, 159

— Simonelli, L., Pettazzoni, P. and Barbieri, M. (1970). 'Ribosome crystallization. III. Ribosome and protein crystallization in hypothermic cell cultures treated with vinblastine sulfate.' *J. Submicr. Cytol.* **2**, 51

Marks, B. H., Alpert, M. and Kruger, F. A. (1958). 'Effect of amphenone upon steroidogenesis in adrenal cortex of the golden hamster.' *Endocrinology* **63**, 75

Marks, P. A. Rifkind, R. A. and Danon, D. (1963). 'Polyribosomes and protein synthesis during reticulocyte maturation in vitro.' *Proc. natn. Acad. Sci.* **50**, 336

Marquet, E. and Sobel, H. J. (1969). 'Crystalline inclusions in the nuclear envelope and granular endoplasmic reticulum of the fish spinal cord.' *J. Cell Biol.* **41**, 774

Mehta, P. N. and Ghadially, F. N. (1973). 'Articular cartilage in corn oil induced lipoarthrosis.' *Ann. Rheum. Dis.* **32**, 75

Meldolesi, J., Clementi, F., Chiesara, E., Conti, F. and Fanti, A. (1967). 'Cytoplasmic changes in rat liver after prolonged treatment with low doses of ethionine and adenine. An ultrastructural and biochemical study.' *Lab. Invest.* **17**, 265

Mikata, A. and Luse, S. A. (1964). 'Ultrastructural changes in the rat liver produced by N-2-fluorenyldiacetamide.' *Am. J. Path.* **44**, 455

Miyai, K., Slusser, R. J. and Ruebner, B. H. (1963). 'Viral hepatitis in mice: electron microscopic study.' *Expl Molec. Path.* **2**, 464

Mizuhira, V., Amakawa, T., Yamashina, S., Shirai, N. and Utida, S. (1970). 'Electron microscopic studies on the localization of sodium ions and sodium-potassium activated adenosinetriphosphatase in chloride cells of eel gills.' *Expl Cell Res.* **59**, 346

Monneron, A. (1969). 'Experimental induction of helical polysomes in adult rat liver.' *Lab. Invest.* **20**, 178

Morris, M. D. and Chaikoff, I. L. (1959). 'The origin of cholesterol in liver, small intestine, adrenal gland, and testis of the rat: dietary versus endogenous contributions.' *J. Biochem.* **234**, 1095

Moses, H. L., Stein, J. A. and Tschudy, D. P. (1970). 'Hepatocellular changes associated with allylisopropylacetamide-induced hepatic porphyria in rats.' *Lab. Invest.* **22**, 432

Moyer, G. H. Murray, R. K., Khairallah, L. H., Suss, R. and Pitot, H. C. (1970). 'Ultrastructural and biochemical characteristics of endoplasmic reticulum fractions of the Morris 7800 and Reuber H-35 hepatomas.' *Lab. Invest.* **23**, 108

Murphy, F. A. Halonen, P. E. and Harrison, A. K. (1968). 'Electron microscopy of the development of rubella virus in BHK-21 cells.' *J. Virol.* **2**, 1223

— Harrison, A. K., and Collin, W. K. (1970). 'The role of extraneural arbovirus infection in the pathogenesis of encephalitis.' *Lab. Invest.* **22**, 318

Norback, D. H. and Allen, J. R. (1969). 'Morphogenesis of toxic fat-induced concentric membrane arrays in rat hepatocytes.' *Lab. Invest.* **20**, 338

Norton, W. L. (1969). 'Endothelial inclusions in active lesions of systemic lupus erythematosus.' *J. lab. clin. Med.* **74**, 369

Novikoff, A. B., Roheim, P. S. and Quintana, N. (1964). 'Lipid in the liver cells of rats fed orotic acid and adenine.' *Fedn Proc.* **23**, 126

Oberling, Ch. and Bernhard, W. (1961) 'The morphology of the cancer cells'. In *The Cell*, Vol. 5, p. 405. Ed. by J. Brachet and A. E. Mirsky. New York and London: Academic Press

Onoe, T. and Ohno, K. (1963). 'Role of endoplasmic reticulum in fat absorption.' In *Intracellular Membranous Structure*, Vol. 14. Ed. by S. Seno and E. V. Cowdry. Okayama, Japan: Japan Society for Cell Biology

Orrenius, S. and Ericsson, J. L. E. (1966a). 'Enzyme–membrane relationship in phenobarbital induction of synthesis of drug-metabolizing enzyme system and proliferation of endoplasmic membranes.' *J. Cell Biol.* **28**, 181

——(1966b). 'On the relationship of liver glucose-6-phosphatase to the proliferation of endoplasmic reticulum in phenobarbital induction.' *J. Cell Biol.* **31**, 243

—— and Ernster, L. (1965). 'Phenobarbital induced synthesis of microsomal drug-metabolizing enzyme system and its relationship to the proliferation of endoplasmic membranes. A morphological and biochemical study.' *J. Cell Biol.* **25**, 627

Ortega, P. (1966). 'Light and electron microscopy of dichlorodiphenyltrichloroethane (DDT) poisoning in the rat liver.' *Lab. Invest.* **15**, 657

Ortega, L. G. and Mellors, R. C. (1957). 'Cellular sites of formation of gamma globulin.' *J. exp. Med.* **106**, 627

Ortega, P., Hayes, W. J. Jr., Durham, W. F. and Mattson, A. (1956). *DDT in the Diet of the Rat; its effect on DDT storage, liver function and cell morphology.* Public Health Monograph, No. 43. Washington DC: US Government Printing Office

Palade, G. E. (1955). 'Studies on the endoplasmic reticulum. II. Simple dispositions in cells *in situ.*' *J. biophys. biochem. Cytol.* **1**, 567

— (1956). 'Intracisternal granules in the exocrine cells of the pancreas.' *J. biophys. biochem. Cytol.* **2**, 417

Palay, S. (1958). 'The morphology of secretion.' In *Frontiers of Cytology,* p. 305. New Haven, Conn: Yale University Press

— and Karlin, L. J. (1959). 'An electron microscopic study of the intestinal villus. II. The pathway of fat absorption.' *J. biophys. biochem. Cytol.* **5**, 373

— and Palade, G. E. (1955). 'The fine structure of neurons.' *J. biophys. biochem. Cytol.* **1**, 69

Petrik, P. (1968). 'The demonstration of chloride ions in the "chloride cells" of the gills of eels (*Anguilla anguilla L.*) adapted to sea water.' *Z. Zellforsch. mikrosk. Anat.* **92**, 422

Pfeiffer, C. J., Weibel, J., Bair, J. W., Jr. and Roth, J. L. A. (1971). 'Aspirin-induced damage to the gastric mucosa.' *29th Ann. Proc. Electron Microscopy Soc. Amer.,* Boston, Mass. Ed. by C. J. Arceneaux

Phillips, M. J., Hetenyi, G. and Adachi, F. (1970). 'Ultrastructural hepatocellular alterations induced by *in vivo* fructose infusion.' *Lab. Invest.* **22**, 370

Pincus, T., Blacklow, N. R., Grimley, P. M. and Bellanti, J. A. (1970). 'Glomerular microtubules of systemic lupus erythematosus.' *Lancet* **2**, 1058

Porter, K. R. (1961). 'The ground substance; observations from electron microscopy.' In *The Cell,* Vol. 2, p. 621. Ed. by J. Brachet and A. E. Mirsky. New York and London: Academic Press

— (1964). 'Cell fine structure and biosynthesis of intercellular macromolecules.' In *Connective Tissue: Intercellular Macromolecules,* New York Heart Ass. Symp., p. 167. Edinburgh and London: Churchill Livingstone

— and Bruni, C. (1959). 'An electron microscope study of the early effects of 3'-Me-DAB on rat liver cells.' *Cancer Res.* **19**, 997

— and Kallman, F. L. (1952). 'Significance of cell particulates as seen by electron microscopy.' *Ann. N. Y. Acad. Sci.* **54**, 882

— and Pappas, G. D. (1959). 'Collagen formation by fibroblasts of the chick embryo dermis.' *J. biophys. biochem. Cytol.* **5**, 153

— and Thompson, H. P. (1948). 'A particulate body associated with epithelial cells cultured from mammary carcinomas of mice of a milk-factor strain.' *J. exp. Med.* **88**, 15

— and Yamada, E. (1960). 'Studies on the endoplasmic reticulum. V. Its form and differentiation in pigment epithelium cells of the frog retina.' *J. biophys. biochem. Cytol.* **8**, 181

— Claude, A. and Fullam, E. F. (1945). 'A study of tissue culture cells by electron microscopy. Methods and preliminary observations.' *J. exp. Med.* **81**, 233

Posalaki, Z. and Barka, T. (1968). 'Alterations of hepatic endoplasmic reticulum in porphyric rats.' *J. Histochem. Cytochem.* **16**, 337

Prutkin, L. (1967). 'An ultrastructure study of the experimental keratoacanthoma.' *J. Invest. Derm.* **48**, 326

— and Bogart, B. (1970) 'The uptake of labelled vitamin A acid in keratoacanthoma'. *J. Invest. Derm.* **55**, 249

Rebhun, L. I. (1961). 'Some electron microscope observations on membranous basophilic elements of invertebrate eggs.' *J. Ultrastruct. Res.* **5**, 208

Reger, J. F. (1961). 'The fine structure of neuromuscular junctions and the sarcoplasmic reticulum of extrinsic eye muscles of *Fundulus heteroclitus.*' *J. biophys. biochem. Cytol.* **10**, No. 4 Suppl., 111

Reid, I. M., Shinozuka, H. and Sidransky, H. (1970). 'Polyribosomal disaggregation induced by puromycin and its reversal with time. An ultrastructural study of mouse liver.' *Lab. Invest.* **23**, 119

Remmer, H. and Merker, H. J. (1963). 'Enzyminduktion und Vermehrung von endoplasmatischem Reticulum in der Leberzelle wahrend der Behandlung mit phenobarbital (Luminal).' *Klin. Wschr.* **41**, 276

Revel, J. P. (1961). 'Electron microscopic study of the bat cricothyroid muscle.' *Anat. Rec.* **139**, 267 (abstract)

— Napolitano, L. and Fawcett, D. W. (1960). 'Identification of glycogen in electron micrographs of thin tissue sections'. *J. biophys. biochem. Cytol.* **8**, 575

Reynolds, E. S. (1963). 'Liver parenchymal cell injury. I. Initial alterations of the cell following poisoning with carbon tetrachloride.' *J. Cell Biol.* **19**, 139

— and Yee, A. G. (1967). 'Liver parenchymal cell injury. V. Relationships between patterns of chloromethane-C incorporation into constituents of liver *in vivo* and cellular injury.' *Lab. Invest.* **16**, 591

Rich, A. Penman, S., Becker, Y., Darnell, J. and Hall, C. (1963). 'Polyribosomes: size in normal and polio-infected HeLa cells.' *Science* **142**, 1658

Rosai, J. (1968). 'Carcinoma of pancreas simulating giant cell tumor of bone. Electron-microscopic evidence of its acinar cell origin.' *Cancer* **22**, 333

Rosenbaum, R. M. and Wittner, M. (1970). 'Ultrastructure of bacterized and axenic trophozoites of *Entamoeba histolytica* with particular reference to helical bodies.' *J. Cell Biol.* **45**, 367

Rosenbluth, J. (1969). 'Sarcoplasmic reticulum of an unusual fast-acting crustacean muscle.' *J. Cell Biol.* **42**, 534

Ross, R. and Benditt, E. P. (1964). 'Wound healing and collagen formation. IV. Distortion of ribosomal patterns of fibroblasts in scurvy.' *J. Cell Biol.* **22**, 365

— — (1965). 'Wound healing and collagen formation. V. Quantitative electron microscope radioautographic observations of proline H^3 utilisation by fibroblasts.' *J. Cell Biol.* **27**, 83

Rothschild, J. (1963). 'The isolation of microsomal membranes.' *Biochem. Soc. Symp.* **22**, 4

Rouiller, Ch. (1957). 'Contribution de la microscopie electronique a l'etude du foie normal et pathologique.' *Annls Anat. path.* **2**, 548

— and Simon, G. (1962). 'Contribution de la microscopie electronique au progres de nos connaissances en cytologie et en histo-pathologie hepatique.' *Revue int. Hépat.* **12**, 167

Rubin, E., Hutterer, F. and Lieber, C. S. (1968). 'Ethanol increases hepatic smooth endoplasmic reticulum and drug metabolizing enzymes.' *Science* **159**, 1469

Russell, W. (1890). 'An address on a characteristic organism of cancer.' *Br. med. J.* **2**, 1356

Ruthmann, A. (1958), 'Basophilic lamellar systems in the crayfish spermatocyte.' *J. biophys. biochem. Cytol.* **4**, 267

Salomon, J. C. (1962a). 'Modifications ultrastructurales des hepatocytes au cours de l'intoxication chronique par la thioacetamide.' In *Electron Microscopy*, Vol. 7. Fifth Int. Congress for Electron Microscopy. Ed. by S. S. Breese, Jr. New York: Academic Press

— (1962b). 'Modifications des cellules du parenchyme hepatique du rat sous l'effet de la thioacetamide. Etude au microscope électronique des lesions observées a la phase tardive d'une intoxication chronique.' *J. Ultrastruct. Res.* **7**, 293

Sanel, F. T. and Lepore, M. J. (1968). 'Granular and crystalline deposits in perinuclear and ergastoplasmic cisternae of human lamina propria cells'. *Expl Molec. Path.* **9**, 110

Schaffner, F. (1966). 'Intralobular changes in hepatocytes and the electron microscopic mesenchymal response in acute viral hepatitis. *Medicine, Baltimore* **45**, 547

Scharff, M. D. and Robbins, E. (1966). 'Polyribosome disaggregation during metaphase.' *Science* **151**, 992

Schindler, W. J. and Knigge, K. M. (1959). 'Adrenal cortical secretion by the golden hamster.' *Endocrinology* **65**, 739

Schlunk, F. F. and Lombardi, B. (1967). 'Liver liposomes. 1. Isolation and chemical characterization.' *Lab. Invest.* **17**, 30

Schubert, M. and Hamerman, D. (1968). *A Primer on Connective Tissue Biochemistry*. Philadelphia, Pa: Lea & Febiger

Scow, R. O. (1970). 'Transport of trygliceride. Its removal from blood circulation and uptake by tissues.' In *Parenteral Nutrition*, p. 294. Ed. by H. C. Meng and D. H. Law. Springfield, Illinois: Charles C. Thomas

Sengel, A. and Stoebner, P. (1971). 'Intracisternal granules in endothelial cells of human pathologic glomeruli.' *Virchows Arch. Abt. B. Zellpath.* **7**, 157

Sheldon, H. (1964). 'The fine structure of the fat cell.' In *Fat as a Tissue*, p. 41. Ed. by K. Rodahl and B. Issekutz. New York: McGraw-Hill

Shinozuka, H., Reid, I. M., Shull, K. H., Liang, H. and Farber, E. (1970). 'Dynamics of liver cell injury and repair. 1. Spontaneous reformation of the nucleolus and polyribosomes in the presence of extensive cytoplasmic damage induced by ethionine.' *Lab. Invest.* **23**, 253

Siddiqui, W. A. and Rudzinska, M. A. (1963). 'A helical structure in ribonucleoprotein bodies of *Entamoeba invadens*.' *Nature, Lond.* **200**, 74

— — (1965). 'The fine structure of axenically-grown trophozoites of *Entamoeba invadens* with special reference to the nucleus and helical ribonucleoprotein bodies.' *J. Protozool.* **12**, 448

Siekevitz, P. and Palade, G. E. (1958). 'A cytochemical study on the pancreas of the guinea pig. II. Functional variations in the enzymatic activity of microsomes.' *J. biophys. biochem. Cytol.* **4**, 309

Sjostrand, F. S. (1964). 'The endoplasmic reticulum.' In *Cytology and Cell Physiology*, 3rd edn., p. 311. Ed. by G. H. Bourne. New York: Academic Press

Skinnider, L. F. and Ghadially, F. N. (1975). 'Ultrastructure of acute myeloid leukemia arising in multiple myeloma.' *Human Path.* **6**, 379

Slater, T. F. and Sawyer, B. C. (1969). 'The effects of carbon tetrachloride on rat liver microsomes during the first hour of poisoning *in vivo*, and the modifying actions of promethazine.' *Biochem. J.* **111**, 317

Smith, D. S. (1961). 'The organization of the flight muscle in a dragonfly, *Aeshna sp.* (*Odonata*).' *J. biophys. biochem. Cytol.* **11**, 119

— (1966). 'The organization and function of the sarcoplasmic reticulum and T-system of muscle cells.' *Prog. Biophys. mol. Biol.* **16**, 109

Smuckler, E. A. and Benditt, E. P. (1963). 'Carbon tetrachloride poisoning in rats: alteration in ribosomes of the liver.' *Science* **140**, 308

— Iseri, O. A. and Benditt, E. P. (1962). 'An intracellular defect in protein synthesis induced by carbon tetrachloride.' *J. exp. Med.* **116**, 55

Sorenson, G. D. (1964). 'Electron microscopic observations of bone marrow from patients with multiple myeloma.' *Lab. Invest.* **13**, 196

Srere, P. A., Chaikoff, I. L. and Dauben, W. B. (1968). 'The *in vitro* synthesis of cholesterol from acetate by surviving adrenal cortical tissue.' *J. biol. Chem.* **176**, 829

Staehelin, W. and Noll, H. (1963). 'Breakdown of rat-liver ergosomes *in vivo* after actinomycin inhibition of messenger RNA synthesis.' *Science* **140**, 180

Stein, O. and Shapiro, B. (1959). 'Assimilation and dissimilation of fatty acids by the rat liver.' *Am. J. Physiol.* **196**, 1238

— and Stein, Y. (1965). 'Fine structure of ethanol induced fatty liver in the rat.' *Israel J. Med. Sci.* **1**, 378

— — (1967). 'The role of the liver in the metabolism of chylomicrons, studied by electron microscopic autoradiography.' *Lab. Invest.* **17**, 436

Steiner, J. W. and Baglio, C. M. (1963). 'Electronmicroscopy of the cytoplasm of parenchymal liver cells in α-napthyl-iosthiocyanate-induced chirrosis'. *Lab. Invest.* **12**, 765

— Carruthers, J. S. and Kalifat, R. S. (1962). 'Observations on the fine structure of rat liver cells in extrahepatic cholestasis.' *Z. Zellforsch. mikrosk. Anat.* **58**, 141

— Miyai, K. and Phillips, M. J. (1964). 'Electron microscopy of membrane-particle arrays in liver cells of ethionine-intoxicated rats.' *Am. J. Path.* **44**, 169

Stenger, R. J. (1964). 'Regenerative nodules in carbon tetrachloride induced cirrhosis. A light and electron microscopic study of lamellar structures encountered therein.' *Am. J. Path.* **44**, 31A

— (1966). 'Concentric lamellar formations in hepatic parenchymal cells of carbon tetrachloride-treated rats.' *J. Ultrastruct. Res.* **14**, 240

— (1970). 'Progress in gastroenterology. Organelle pathology of the liver. The endoplasmic reticulum.' *Gastroenterology* **58**, 554

Stich, M. H., Swiller, A. I. and Morrison, M. (1955). 'The grape cell of multiple myeloma.' *Am. J. clin. Path.* **25**, 601

— and Higginson, J. (1963). 'Ultrastructural changes in liver cells during carcinogenesis.' *Am. J. Path.* **4**, 70

— — (1964). 'Ultrastructural changes produced by protein and related deficiencies in rat liver.' *Am. J. Path.* **45**, 353

— Grady, H. J. and Higginson, J. (1966). 'Aflatoxin B_1 injury in rat and monkey liver.' *Am. J. Path.* **49**, 1023

Tamarin, A. (1971a). 'Submaxillary gland recovery from obstruction. I. Overall changes and electron microscopic alterations of granular duct cells.' *J. Ultrastruct. Res.* **34**, 276

— (1971b). 'Submaxillary gland recovery from obstruction. II. Electron microscopic alterations of acinar cells.' *J. Ultrastruct. Res.* **34**, 288

Thiery, J. P. (1960). 'Microcinematographic contributions to the study of plasma cells.' In *Cellular Aspects of Immunity*, p. 59. Ed. by G. E. W. Wolstenholme and M. O'Connor. Ciba Foundation Symposium. Boston, Mass: Little, Brown

Thoenes, W. (1962). 'Zur kenntnis des glatten endoplasmatischen retikulums der leberzelle.' *Verhand. deutsch. Ges. Path.* **46**, 202

— and Bannasch, P. (1962). 'Elektronen- und lichtmikroskopische untersuchungen am cytoplasma der Leberzellen nach akuter und chronischer thioacetamid-vergiftung.' *Virchows Arch. path. Anat. Physiol.* **335**, 556

Toner, P. G. (1963). 'The fine structure of resting and active cells in the submucosal glands of the fowl proventriculus.' *J. Anat.* **97**, 575

Trier, J. S. (1958). 'The fine structure of the parathyroid gland.' *J. biophys. biochem. Cytol.* **4**, 13

Tzur, R. and Shapiro, B. (1964). 'Dependence of microsomal lipid synthesis on added protein.' *J. Lipid Res.* **5**, 542

Uzman, B. G., Saito, H. and Kasac, M. (1971). 'Tubular arrays in the endoplasmic reticulum in human tumor cells.' *Lab. Invest.* **24**, 492

Villa-Trevino, S., Farber, R., Staehelin, T., Wettstein, F. O. and Noll, H. (1964). 'Breakdown and reassembly of rat liver ergosomes after administration of ethionine or puromycin.' *J. biol. Chem.* **239**, 3826

Virchow, R. (1858). *Die Cellularpathologie.* Berlin

Waddington, C. H. and Perry, M. M. (1963). 'Helical arrangement of ribosomes in differentiating muscle cells.' *Expl Cell Res.* **30**, 599

Walker, B. E. (1960). 'Electron microscopic observations on transitional epithelium of the mouse urinary bladder.' *J. Ultrastruct. Res.* **3**, 345

Ward, A. M., Shortland, J. R. and Darke, C. S. (1971). 'Lymphosarcoma of the lung with monoclonal (IgM) gammopathy.' *Cancer* **27**, 1009

Warner, J. R., Knof, P. M. and Rich, A. (1963). 'A multiple ribosomal structure in protein synthesis.' *Proc. natn. Acad. Sci., U.S.A.* **49**, 122

Warshawsky, H., Haddad, A., Goncalves, R. P., Valeri, V. and de Lucca, F. L. (1973). 'Fine structure of venom gland epithelium of the South American rattlesnake and radioautographic studies of protein formation by the secretory cells.' *Am. J. Anat.* **138**, 79

Weiss, J. M. (1953). 'The ergastoplasm. Its fine structure and relation to protein synthesis as studied with the electron microscope in the pancreas of the Swiss albino mouse.' *J. exp. Med.* **98**, 607

Welsh, R. A. (1960). 'Electron microscopic localization of Russel bodies in the human plasma cell.' *Blood* **16**, 1307

Werbin, H. and Chaikoff, I. L. (1961). 'Utilization of adrenal gland cholesterol for synthesis of cortisol by the intact normal and ACTH-treated guinea pig.' *Archs Biochem.* **93**, 476

White, R. G. (1954). 'Observations on the formation and nature of Russel bodies.' *Br. J. exp. Path.* **35**, 365

Whitfield, S. G., Murphy, F. A. and Sudia, W. D. (1971). 'Eastern equine encephalomyelitis virus: an electron microscopic study of *Aedes triseriatus* (*Say*) salivary gland infection.' *Virology* **43**, 110

Winborn, W. B. and Seelig, L. L. (1970). 'Cytologic effects of reserpine on hepatocytes. An ultrastructural study of drug toxicity.' *Lab. Invest.* **23**, 216

Wood, R. L. (1964). 'Morphological changes in hepatic cells during recovery from ethionine poisoning.' *Anat. Rec.* **148**, 352

— (1965). 'The fine structure of hepatic cells in chronic ethionine poisoning and during recovery'. *Am. J. Path.* **46**, 307

Yamada, E. and Ishikawa, T. M. (1960). 'The fine structure of the corpus luteum in the mouse ovary as revealed by electron microscopy.' *Kyushu J. med. Sci.* **11**, 235

Zlotnik, I. and Harris, W. J. (1970). 'The changes in cell organelles of neurons in the brains of adult mice and hamsters during Semliki forest virus and Louping ill encephalitis.' *Br. J. exp. Path.* **51**, 37

Zucker-Franklin, D. (1964). 'Structural features of cells associated with the paraproteinemias.' *Semin. Hemat.* **1**, 165

CHAPTER VI

Annulate Lamellae

INTRODUCTION

The term 'annulate lamellae' is used to describe an intracytoplasmic membrane system composed of parallel arrays of cisternae bearing at regular intervals small annuli or fenestrae. On rare occasions annulate lamellae have also been found in the nucleus. Other names that have been used to describe this organelle include 'pitted membranes', 'fenestrated lamellae' and 'periodic lamellae'.

Probably the first observations on annulate lamellae were made by McCulloch (1952) and Lansing *et al.* (1952) in oöcytes of marine animals. Palade (1955) described this organelle as fenestrated cisternae in the rat spermatocyte and considered it to be a local differentiation of the endoplasmic reticulum. The term 'annulate lamellae' was coined by Swift (1956) to describe this organelle in the pancreatic acinar cells of the larval salamander, oöcytes of snail and clam, and rat spermatids.

The occurrence of this organelle in vertebrate and invertebrate germ cells, embryonic cells and some tumour cells has frequently been documented. More recent work shows that this organelle may also be found occasionally in some adult somatic cells. The structure and distribution of this organelle in various cell types is dealt with in great detail in an excellent review by Kessel (1968). The functional significance of this organelle is still unknown but, since it is better developed and found more frequently in embryonic and tumour cells than in adult somatic cells, it is speculated that it has a role in cell growth and differentiation.

This membrane system, which is now regarded as an organelle in its own right is usually found in the cytoplasm but it is sometimes also seen in the nucleus (*Plates 125 and 126*).

Cytoplasmic annulate lamellae (*Plates 125 and 126, Figs. 1 and 2*) usually present as stacks of cisternae, the edges of which tend to be slightly or markedly dilated. In some cases the cisternae of the annulate lamellae have been reported to be continuous with the cisternae of the rough endoplasmic reticulum. Regular periodic fusion of the paired membranes of the cisternae produces structures reminiscent of nuclear pores.

Indeed, annulate lamellae bear a close resemblance to the structure of the nuclear envelope. The appearance created is that of segments of nuclear envelope stacked in parallel arrays in the cytoplasm. Such stacks may be scattered in the cytoplasm or lie in the juxtanuclear position. In the latter instance such stacks are usually orientated parallel to the nuclear envelope, but examples of annulate lamellae lying at right angles to the nuclear envelope are also known to occur (*Plate 125, Fig. 2*). The number of stacks and the number of lamellae per stack seen in various cells studied to date are also very variable. Kessel (1968) has stated that 'In general, cytoplasmic annulate lamellae in somatic cells are much less extensively developed than in germ cells, especially oöcytes'.

Intranuclear annulate lamellae (*Plate 126, Fig. 3*) have not as yet been observed to occur in stacked parallel arrays. They usually present as solitary lamellae showing straight, branched, curved or circular profiles.

Annulate lamellae have been observed in a variety of cells, including the following: (1) oöcytes of echinoderms (Afzelius, 1955; Gross *et al.*, 1960; Kane, 1960; Kessel, 1964a), snail and clam (Rebhun, 1956, 1961; Swift, 1956), sand dollar (Merriam, 1959), tunicates (Hsu, 1963; Kessel, 1964b, 1965) (*Plate 126, Figs. 2 and 3*), necturus (Kessel, 1963a, b), Drosophila (Okada and Waddington, 1959), teleosts (Yamamoto and Onozato, 1965; Kessel, 1968), amphibia (Wischnitzer, 1960; Balinsky and Devis, 1963) and man (Wartenberg and Stegner, 1960; Hertig and Adams, 1967); (2) spermatocytes or spermatids of crayfish (Ruthmann, 1958; Kaye *et al.*, 1961), locust (Barer *et al.*, 1960) and rat (Swift, 1956); (3) salivary gland cells (Gay, 1955), and blastoderm of Drosophila (Mahowald, 1962, 1963); (4) pancreatic acinar cells of ambystoma larva (Swift, 1956); (5) adrenal cortical cells of embryo rat (Ross, 1962), alligator and sea-gull (Harrison, 1966); (6) myocardial cells of chick embryo incubated at abnormal temperatures (Merkow and

---

Plate 125

The annulate lamellae shown in these electron micrographs were found in ciliated columnar cells of bronchial mucosa of patients with pulmonary tuberculosis or bronchial carcinoma. However, the specimens were collected some distance from the lesions in the lung where the mucosa appeared normal. (*From Frasca, Auerbach, Parks and Stockenius, 1967*)

Fig. 1. A large stack of annulate lamellae (arrow) is seen in the cytoplasm of a ciliated columnar cell. × 7,000

Fig. 2. Orientated perpendicular to the nuclear envelope lie some 50 cisternae of annulate lamellae. Many of the 'pores' in the stack are in register and an ill-defined, probably fibillar, material is seen extending through them. × 26,000

Fig. 3. Apparent continuity of the cisternae of rough endoplasmic reticulum and annulate lamellae is seen here. Note also the fibrillar substance extending across the 'pores' in the cisternae and nuclear pore (between arrows). × 52,000

Fig. 4. The cisternae of the rough endoplasmic reticulum are well aligned with the cisternae of the annulate lamellae. The images seen here indicate a continuity between the two cisternal systems. × 72,000

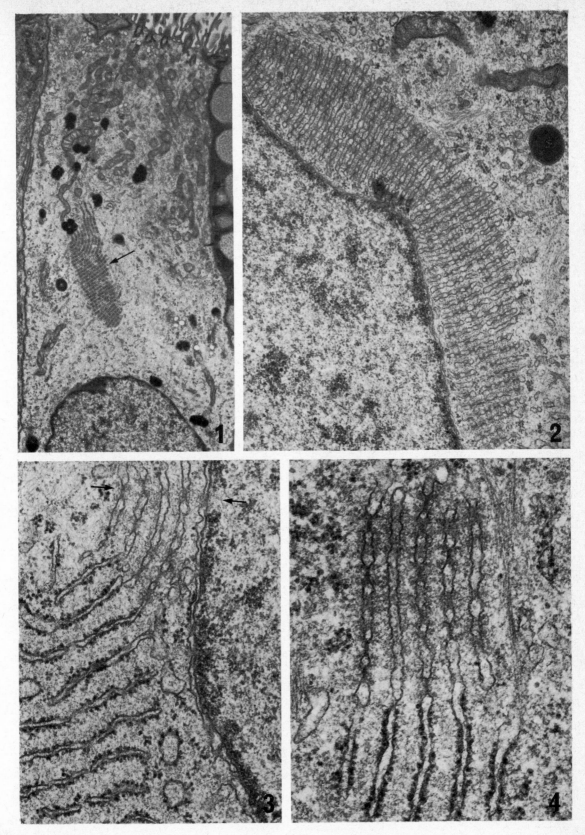

285

Leighton, 1966); (7) intestinal epithelial cells of a rat bearing a subcutaneous sarcoma (Ghadially and Parry, unpublished) (*Plate 126, Fig. 1*); (8) hepatocytes of a rat injured by azaserine, or 2-fluorenylacetamide or β-3-furylalanine (Hruban *et al.*, 1965a, b, and Merkow *et al.*, 1967); (9) Sertoli cells of human testis (Bawa, 1963); (10) ciliated columnar cells of human bronchial mucosa (Frasca *et al.*, 1967) *Plate 125*); (11) axillary apocrine gland cells of man (Gross, 1966); (12) neoplastic cells of apocrine adenoma (Gross, 1965), adenolymphoma (Tandler, 1966) and parathyroid adenomas of man (Elliott and Arhelger, 1966); and (13) cells of a variety of malignant tumours (Wessel and Bernhard, 1957; Epstein, 1957, 1961; Binggeli, 1959; Hoshino, 1963; Chambers and Weiser, 1964; Svoboda, 1964; Ma and Webber, 1966; Locker *et al.*, 1969; Ghadially and Parry, 1974).

The morphological similarity between annulate lamellae and the nuclear envelope has led most workers to conclude that this organelle is in some way derived from the nuclear envelope. It has been suggested that annulate lamellae may be formed: (1) from fragments of nuclear envelope left behind after mitosis; (2) by delamination from nuclear envelope with the nuclear envelope serving as a mould or template; or (3) from a large evagination of the outer membrane of the nuclear envelope which later becomes infolded to form the cisternae of the annulate lamellae.

Kessel (1968), however, has found that in tunicate oöcytes annulate lamellae are derived from the nuclear envelope by a process of blebbing. He presents convincing morphological evidence that the vesicles derived by this process subsequently fuse and flatten out to form the cisternae of the annulate lamellae. At each 'point' of fusion between two vesicles a 'pore' develops. Cytoplasmic annulate lamellae are thought to develop by blebbing of the outer membranes of the nuclear envelope, while the intranuclear ones are thought to be derived in a similar fashion from the inner membrane of the nuclear envelope. Harrison (1966) found a similar mechanism operating in alligator adrenal cortical tissue, but in the sea-gull annulate lamellae appeared to originate as sheets delaminated from the nuclear membranes, as suggested by Swift (1956).

However, the idea that the nuclear membrane serves as a template for the production of annulate lamellae is not too attractive, for recent studies on the newt oöcyte show that, although there are remarkable morphological similarities between the pores on both these structures, there are about twice as many pores on the annulate lamellae as on the corresponding nuclear envelope (Scheer and Franke, 1969).

Despite numerous studies the significance and function of annulate lamellae is unknown. Some of the speculations about their function are that they: (1) carry 'information' or 'genetic substance' from the nucleus to the cytoplasm; (2) provide a framework for the collection and assembly of specific substances required during certain stages of development; and (3) provide membrane material for subsequent morphogenetic activities.

Plate 126

Fig. 1 Annulate lamellae found in the small intestinal epithelial cell of a rat bearing a carcinogen-induced (9:10-dimethyl-1:2-benzanthracene) subcutaneous sarcoma in its flank. × 32,000

Fig. 2. Tangential section through the annulate lamellae of a tunicate oöcyte, showing numerous annulae with a dense central granule. × 25,000

Fig. 3. Both stacked cytoplasmic annulate lamellae (C) and solitary intranuclear annulate lamellae (N) are seen in this electron micrograph from a tunicate oöcyte. × 17,000

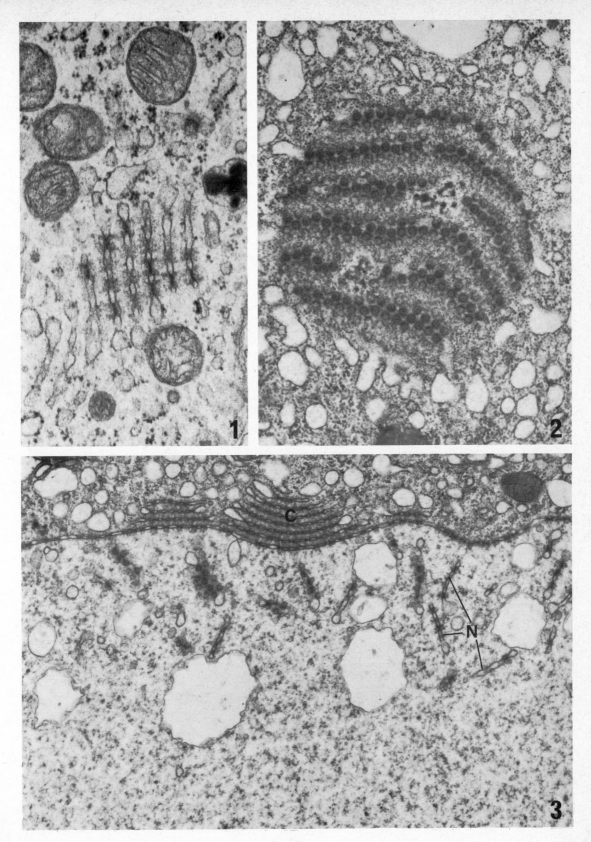

REFERENCES

Afzelius, B. A. (1955). 'The ultrastructure of the nuclear membrane of the sea urchin oocyte as studied with the electron microscope.' *Expl Cell Res.* **8**, 147

Balinsky, B. I. and Devis, R. J. (1963). 'Origin and differentiation of cytoplasmic structures in the oocytes of *Xenopus laevis.*' *Acta embryol. morphol. Exp. Palermo* **6**, 55

Barer, R., Joseph, S. and Meek, G. A. (1960). 'The origin and fate of the nuclear membrane in meiosis.' *Proc. R. Soc. B.* **152**, 353

Bawa, S. R. (1963). 'Fine structure of the Sertoli cell of the human testis.' *J. Ultrastruct. Res.* **9**, 459

Binggeli, M. F. (1959). 'Abnormal intranuclear and cytoplasmic formations associated with a chemically induced transplantable chicken sarcoma.' *J. biophys. biochem. Cytol.* **5**, 143

Chambers, V. C. and Weiser, R. S. (1964). 'Annulate lamellae in sarcoma I cells.' *J. Cell Biol.* **21**, 133

Elliott, R. L. and Arhelger, R. B. (1966). 'Fine structure of parathyroid adenomas with special reference to annulate lamellae and septate desmosomes.' *Archs Path.* **81**, 200

Epstein, M. A. (1957). 'The fine structure of the cells in mouse sarcoma 37 ascitic fluids.' *J. biophys. biochem. Cytol.* **3**, 567

— (1961). 'Some unusual features of fine structure observed in HeLa cells.' *J. biophys. biochem. Cytol.* **10**, 153

Frasca, J. M., Auerbach, O., Parks, V. R. and Stoeckenius, W. (1967). 'Electron microscopic observations of bronchial epithelium. I. Annulate lamellae.' *Expl Molec. Path.* **6**, 261

Gay, H. (1955). 'Nucleo-cytoplasmic relations in salivary-gland cells of Drosophila.' *Proc. natn. Acad. Sci., U.S.A.* **41**, 370

Ghadially, F. N. and Parry, E. W. (1974). 'Intranuclear annulate lamellae in Ehrlich ascites tumour cells.' *Virchows Archs.* **15**, 131

Gross, B. G. (1965). 'The apocrine hidrocystoma. An electron microscope study.' *Fedn Proc.* **24**, 432

— (1966). 'Annulate lamellae in the axillary apocrine glands of adult man.' *J. Ultrastruct. Res.* **14**, 64

Gross, P. R., Philpott, D. E. and Nass, S. (1960). 'Electron microscopy of the centrifuged sea urchin egg, with a note on the structure of the ground cytoplasm.' *J. biophys. biochem. Cytol.* **7**, 135

Harrison, G. A. (1966). 'Some observations on the presence of annulate lamellae in alligator and sea gull adrenal cortical cells.' *J. Ultrastruct. Res.* **14**, 158

Hertig, A. T. and Adams, E. C. (1967). 'Studies on the human oocyte and its follicle. I. Ultrastructural and histochemical observations on the primordial follicle stage.' *J. Cell Biol.* **34**, 647

Hoshino, M. (1963). 'Submicroscopic characteristics of four strains of Yoshida ascites hepatoma of rats: a comparative study.' *Cancer Res.* **23**, 209

Hruban, Z., Swift, H. and Slesers, A. (1965a). 'Effect of azaserine on the fine structure of the liver and pancreatic acinar cells.' *Cancer Res.* **25**, 708

— — Dunn, F. W. and Lewis, D. E. (1965b). 'Effects of β-3-furylalanine on the ultrastructure of the hepatocytes and pancreatic acinar cells.' *Lab. Invest.* **14**, 70

Hsu, W. S. (1963). 'The nuclear envelope in the developing oocytes of the tunicate *Boltenia villosa.*' *Z. Zellforsch. mikrosk. Anat.* **58**, 660

Kane, R. E. (1960). 'The effect of partial protein extraction on the structure of the eggs of the sea urchin, *Arbacia punctulata.*' *J. biophys. biochem. Cytol.* **7**, 21

Kaye, G. I., Pappas, G. D., Yasuzumi, G. and Yamamoto, H. (1961). 'The distribution of the endoplasmic reticulum during spermatogenesis in the crayfish *Cambaroides japonicus.*' *Z. Zellforsch. mikrosk. Anat.* **53**, 159

Kessel, R. G. (1963a). 'The formation and subsequent differentiation of cytoplasmic vesicles in oocytes of Necturus.' *Anat. Res.* **145**, 363

— (1963b). 'Electron microscope studies on the origin of annulate lamellae in oocytes of Necturus.' *J. Cell Biol.* **19**, 391

— (1964a). 'Electron microscopic studies on oocytes of an echinoderm, *Thyone briareus,* with special reference to the origin and structure of the annulate lamellae.' *J. Ultrastruct. Res.* **10**, 498

— (1964b). 'Intranuclear annulate lamellae in oocytes of the tunicate, *Styela partita.*' *Z. Zellforsch. mikrosk. Anat.* **63**, 37

— (1965). 'Intranuclear and cytoplasmic annulate lamellae in tunicate oocytes.' *J. Cell Biol.* **24**, 471

— (1968). 'Annulate lamellae.' *J. Ultrastruct Res.* Supp. 10.

Lansing, A. I., Hillier, J. and Rosenthal, T. B. (1952). 'Electron microscopy of some marine egg inclusions.' *Biol. Bull.* **103**, 294 (Abstract)

Locker, J., Goldblatt, P. J. and Leighton, J. (1969). 'Hematogenous metastasis of Yoshida ascites hepatoma in the chick embryo liver: ultrastructural changes in tumor cells.' *Cancer Res.* **29**, 1244

McCulloch, D. (1952). 'Fibrous structures in the ground cytoplasm of the Arbacia egg.' *J. expl Zool.* **119**, 47

Ma, M. H. and Webber, A. J. (1966). 'Fine structure of liver tumors induced in the rat by 3'-methyl-4-dimethylamino-azobenzene.' *Cancer Res.* **26**, 935

Mahowald, A. P. (1962). 'Fine structure of pole cells and polar granules in *Drosophila melanogaster.*' *J. exp. Zool.* **151**, 201

— (1963). 'Ultrastructural differentiations during formation of the blastoderm in the *Drosophila melanogaster* embryo.' *Devl Biol.* **8**, 186

Merkow, L. and Leighton, J. (1966). 'Increased numbers of annulate lamellae in myocardium of chick embryos incubated at abnormal temperatures.' *J. Cell Biol.* **28**, 127

— Epstein, S. M., Caito, B. J. and Bartus, B. (1967). 'The cellular analysis of liver carcinogenesis: ultrastructural alterations within hyperplastic liver nodules induced by 2-fluorenylacetamide.' *Cancer Res.* **27**, 1712

Merriam, R. W. (1959). 'The origin and fate of annulate lamellae in maturing sand dollar eggs.' *J. biophys. biochem. Cytol.* **5**, 117

Okada, E. and Waddington, C. H. (1959). 'The submicroscopic structure of the Drosophila egg.' *J. embryol. expl Morphol.* **7**, 583

Palade, G. E. (1955). 'Studies on the endoplasmic reticulum. II. Simple dispositions in cells *in situ*.' *J. biophys. biochem. Cytol.* **1**, 567

Rebhun, L. I. (1956). 'Electron microscopy of basophilic structures of some invertebrate oocytes. I. Periodic lamellae and the nuclear envelope.' *J. biophys. biochem. Cytol.* **2**, 93

— (1961). 'Some electron microscope observations on membranous basophilic elements of invertebrate eggs.' *J. Ultrastruct. Res.* **5**, 208

Ross, M. H. (1962). 'Annulate lamellae in the adrenal cortex of the fetal rat.' *J. Ultrastruct. Res.* **7**, 373

Ruthmann, A. (1958). 'Basophilic lamellar systems in the crayfish spermatocyte.' *J. biophys. biochem. Cytol.* **4**, 267

Scheer, U. and Franke, W. W. (1969). 'Negative staining and adenosine triphosphatase activity of annulate lamellae of newt oocytes.' *J. Cell Biol.* **42**, 519

Svoboda, D. J. (1964). 'Fine structure of hematomas induced in rats with p-Dimethylaminoazobenzene.' *J. natn Cancer Inst.* **33**, 315

Swift, H. (1956). 'The fine structure of annulate lamellae.' *J. biophys. biochem. Cytol.* **2**, 415

Tandler, B. (1966). 'Warthin's tumor, electron microscopic studies.' *Archs Otolar.* **84**, 68

Wartenberg, H. and Stegner, H. E. (1960). 'Uber die Electronenmikroskopische Feinstruktur des Menschlichen ovarialeies.' *Z. Zellforsch. mikrosk. Anat.* **52**, 450

Wessel, W. and Bernhard, W. (1957). 'Vergleichende elektronenmikroskopische Untersuchung von Ehrlichund Yoshida-Ascitestumorzellen.' *J. Krebsforsch.* **62**, 140

Wischnitzer, S. J. (1960). 'Observations on the annulate lamellae of immature amphibian oocytes.' *J. biophys. biochem. Cytol.* **8**, 558

Yamamoto, K. and Onozato, H. (1965). 'Electron microscope study on the growing oocyte of the goldfish during the first growth phase.' *Mem. Fac. Fisheries, Hokkaido Univ.* **13**, 69. (Quoted by Kessel, R. G. (1968). *J. Ultrastruct. Res.* Supp. 10)

CHAPTER VII

Lysosomes

INTRODUCTION (HISTORY, CLASSIFICATION AND NOMENCLATURE)

The term 'lysosome' is used to describe a group of membrane-bound particles which contain acid hydrolases. These organelles are now considered to be the main part of an intracellular digestive system (sometimes referred to as the vacuome or vacuolar apparatus) capable of digesting or degrading a variety of endogenous and exogenous substances (de Duve and Wattiaux, 1966). The other parts of the system include structures such as pinocytotic and micropinocytotic vesicles and phagocytic vacuoles which transport exogenous substances into the cell.

The classical cell organelles were discovered by morphologists long before they could be isolated and studied by biochemists; but the existence of lysosomes was predicted from biochemical studies on isolated cell fractions (rat liver) before they were identified with the electron microscope (for a historical review, see de Duve, 1969). This simple historical fact is of more than academic interest, for while most organelles are characterized by their morphological features, the identification of a structure as a lysosome rests on the demonstration of acid hydrolases within it. It thus becomes necessary to review briefly the historical aspects of this subject.

The lysosome concept began with the work of Christian de Duve and his colleagues in Louvain. During the course of certain unrelated experiments they observed that the acid phosphatase activity of rat liver homogenates and certain fractions thereof (particularly the mitochondrial fraction) was about seven to nine times lower in freshly prepared fractions than in those stored for a few days in the refrigerator.

This led to the suspicion that in freshly prepared fractions the enzyme might be located in a membrane-bound structure and was hence not available for reaction with the substrate (structure-linked latency), but, on storage, rupture of the membrane occurred, releasing the enzyme into the medium. Further fractionation of the 'mitochondrial fraction' into light and heavy components showed that most of the acid phosphatase activity resided in the light fraction, while the cytochrome oxidase activity occurred predominantly in the heavy fraction. Thus it became evident that the enzyme (acid phosphatase) did not reside in mitochondria but in a hitherto unidentified membrane-bound structure or organelle smaller than the mitochondrion.

Biochemical studies next revealed that at least four other acid hydrolases showed the same kind of structure-linked latency and sedimented out in company with the particles believed to contain acid phosphatase. Thus the idea of a membrane-bound organelle containing a battery of acid hydrolases was born and the term 'lysosome' (meaning 'lytic body') was coined by de Duve *et al.* (1955) to describe it.

The morphological identification of these particles was accomplished by Novikoff who examined with the electron microscope the lysosome-rich fraction from rat liver prepared by de Duve and his co-workers (Novikoff *et al.*, 1956). From this it became apparent that lysosomes of rat liver were single-membrane-bound particles with electron-dense contents morphologically identical to the peribiliary dense bodies described earlier by Rouiller (1954) (*Plate 127*).

The development and application of cytochemical methods for the *in situ* demonstration of acid phosphatase activity in ultrathin sections of tissues (for references, see the review by Novikoff, 1961) not only confirmed the presence of acid phosphatase in the peribiliary dense bodies but also led to the discovery of lysosomes in a variety of cells. Despite criticisms from de Duve, who considered that a battery of acid hydrolases should be demonstrated before a structure was labelled a lysosome, acid phosphatase came to be accepted as a marker for identifying lysosomes (*Plate 128*). It also soon became evident that these versatile organelles were involved in a variety of cellular functions.

Acid phosphatase activity has now been demonstrated in a variety of diverse structures long known to morphologists. Besides the peribiliary dense bodies, these include various others such as some of the granules in neutrophil leucocytes, the granules in eosinophil leucocytes, hyaline droplets in kidney tubules, haemosiderin granules in macrophages and other cells, and lipofuscin granules in heart, brain and various other tissues. Indeed, lysosomes have been found in virtually all animal cells examined to date, including even mature erythrocytes (page 326). They are also known to occur in many plant cells. Lysosomes are frequently encountered in pathological tissues, at times in greatly increased numbers as in the case of the lupus kidney illustrated in *Plate 127, Fig. 1* and in other situations described later in this chapter.

The enzyme content of lysosomes has been the subject of numerous investigations. Variations in enzyme content have been noted between lysosomes obtained from different tissues, but all contain a battery of hydrolases. About 40 enzymes capable of acting on almost every type of chemical bond have now been described (de Duve, 1970). Tappel (1969) gives a detailed list of enzymes discovered in lysosomes. He states that 'data on the enzyme content of lysosomes and other information support the present concept that the following polymeric or complex compounds are hydrolyzed in the lysosome; proteins and peptides, DNA, RNA, polysaccharides, the oligosaccharide portion of glycoproteins and glycolipids, lipids and phosphates.' However, many workers have pointed out (Wattiaux, 1969; see also page 308 for further discussion on this point) that lysosomes as a class are somewhat deficient in lipases, and this is one of the reasons why they turn into residual bodies containing lipofuscin.

Many functional and morphological forms of lysosomes have been identified and named (de Duve 1963; de Duve and Wattiaux, 1966). One such is the primary lysosome (also called 'virgin', 'true', 'pure' or 'original lysosome' and 'protolysosome') which is, in essence, a vesicle containing a battery of acid hydrolases. Here, the contents are usually of a medium or low electron density so that it cannot be unequivocally distinguished by morphological features alone from other vesicular structures in the cell and cytochemical methods have to be employed for its identification. However, certain primary lysosomes such as some of the granules in the neutrophil leucocyte (which are in fact storage granules containing acid hydrolases) are recognizable by their morphological features. Primary lysosomes are thought to be produced in a manner akin to zymogen granules and other secretory granules. The hydrolytic enzymes, being proteins or glycoproteins, are believed to be elaborated by the ribosomes on the rough endoplasmic

---

Plate 127

Fig. 1. Normal rat hepatocytes, showing a bile canaliculus (B), some microbodies (M) and peribiliary dense bodies now known to be lysosomes (L). ×21,000

Fig. 2. Disorganized tubular epithelial cells from the kidney of a patient with systemic lupus erythematosus, showing a markedly increased number of lysosomes (L). Similar but far fewer lysosomes are also found in the normal kidney. ×8,000

292

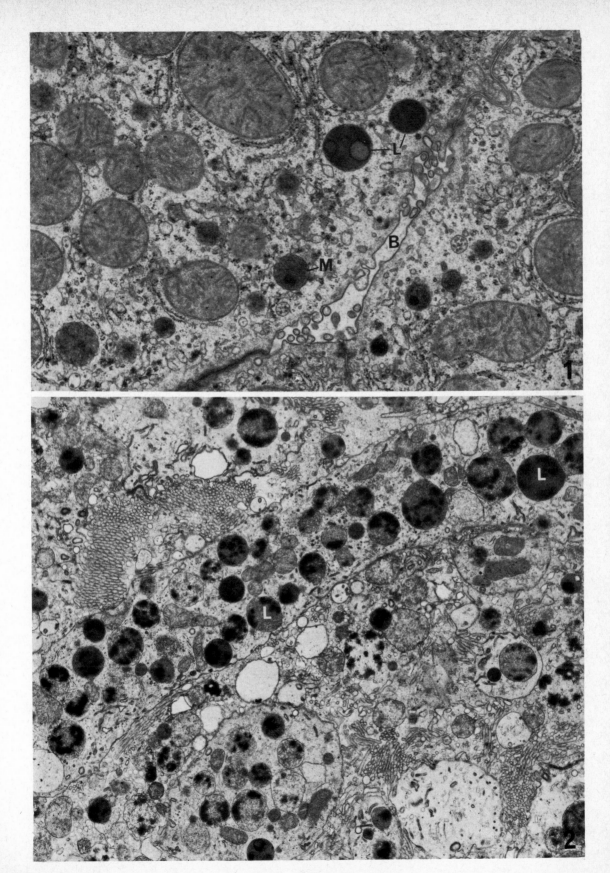

293

reticulum. Subsequent stages of primary lysosome formation are, however, debatable. In some sites the classical route from rough endoplasmic reticulum to Golgi complex is probably taken, followed by packaging into smooth membrane-lined vesicles. In others, it is suggested that the primary lysosomes are formed by a pinching-off process directly from the rough endoplasmic reticulum or that the hydrolases are first transported to the smooth endoplasmic reticulum and the primary lysosomes originate from this structure. The role of the endoplasmic reticulum and Golgi-associated vesicles in the formation of primary lysosomes is stressed in the GERL (Golgi, endoplasmic reticulum, lysosomes) concept of Novikoff *et al.* (1964).

The primary lysosomes, however derived, contain hydrolytic enzymes but no substrate to act upon. Structures in which the enzymes confront substrates and digestion ensues are called secondary lysosomes. Since the substrate may be derived exogenously or endogenously, two main types of secondary lysosomes are possible, namely phagolysosomes (heterolysosomes) and cytolysosomes (autolysosomes, autophagic vacuoles, cytosegrosomes, sites of focal cytoplasmic degeneration or degradation). (Phagolysosomes and cytolysosomes are discussed in greater detail on page 296.) At times exogenous and endogenous material may occur in the same secondary lysosome, when the term 'ambilysosome' may be employed.

The term 'residual body' (telolysosome) is employed to describe late forms of secondary lysosomes, however derived, where digestion is nearing completion or is completed and enzymic activity is scant or absent. Such bodies are loaded with undigested electron-dense residues of various kinds. Lipofuscin granules and haemosiderin granules (siderosomes) of light microscopy are now regarded as examples of residual bodies.

Certain enzyme-less members of the vacuolar system are called prelysosomes. These contain sequestrated material destined for lysosomal digestion. The only clear-cut example of this is the phagosome renamed by de Duve and Wattiaux (1966) as a heterophagosome. This is a single-membrane-bound structure containing material taken up by a process of pinocytosis, micropinocytosis or phagocytosis. Digestion ensues when fusion with a primary lysosome converts a heterophagosome into a heterolysosome. To allow for the possible existence of prelysosomes of the autophagic line the term 'autophagosome' has been coined, and to allow for the possible existence of prelysosomes containing exogenous and endogenous material the term 'ambiphagosome' has been suggested.

In concluding, it is worth noting that the lysosome concept has played an important role in our understanding of many physiological and pathological processes. An understanding of lysosome function and dysfunction is now essential to the understanding of various topics of interest to pathologists, as will become evident on perusal of this chapter.

Plate 128

The manner in which acid phosphatase activity is demonstrated in lysosomes is illustrated here with the aid of material from rheumatoid joints. See also *Plates 153 and 154*, which show the marked increase in lysosomes that occurs in this condition.

For the demonstration of acid phosphatase activity, thin slices of tissue or cells are incubated with Gomori medium which contains sodium-β-glycerophosphate and lead nitrate. At sites of acid phosphatase activity the glycerophosphate is hydrolysed and the phosphate combines with the lead ions, to produce a precipitate of electron-opaque lead phosphate (arrows). Thus the coarse black granular deposits seen in these electron micrographs represent sites of acid phosphatase activity.

Fig. 1. Type A synovial cell from a case of rheumatoid arthritis, showing acid phosphatase activity localized in organelles interpreted as lysosomes. × 21,000 (*From Barland, Novikoff and Hamerman, 1964*)

Figs. 2–5. Synovial fluid neutrophils from patients with rheumatoid arthritis, showing acid phosphatase activity in a variety of lysosomal bodies. × 52,000; × 41,000; × 32,000; × 34,000 (*From Coimbra and Lopes-Vaz, 1967*)

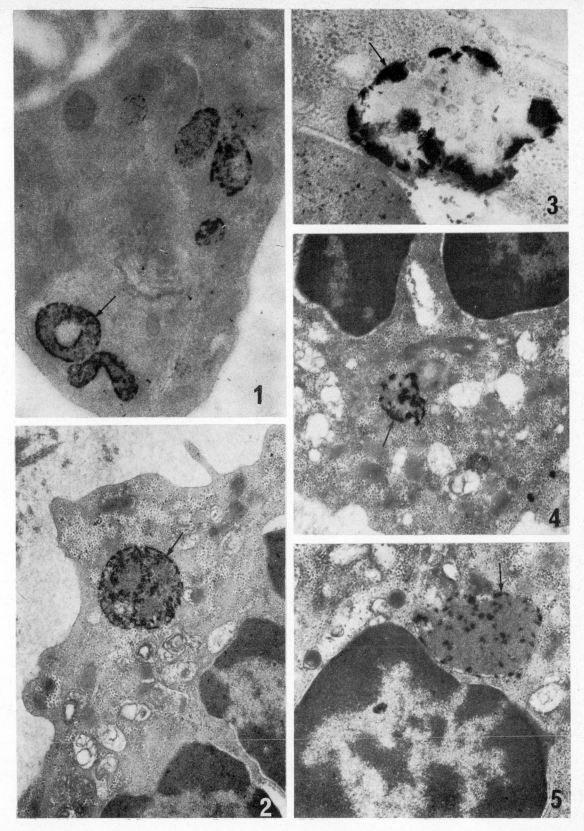

PHAGOLYSOSOMES (HETEROLYSOSOMES) AND CYTOLYSOSOMES (AUTOLYSOSOMES)

One of the important features of the masterly classification of lysosomes by de Duve and Wattiaux (1966) is that it clearly divides secondary lysosomes into two main classes: (1) heterolysosomes where exogenous material is digested; and (2) autolysosomes where endogenous material suffers digestion. Although the concept is admired and accepted, most authors still continue to use older terms such as 'phagolysosome' instead of heterolysosome, 'cytolysosome' or 'autophagic vacuole' instead of autolysosome and 'residual body' instead of telolysosome.

The reason for this is not evident, but one has to agree that there is no overwhelming need for an entire set of new names. In practice it is difficult to classify all secondary lysosomes as heterolysosomes or autolysosomes. For example, the multivesicular body (page 302), which is a special type of secondary lysosome of characteristic morphology, can be involved in the digestion of either exogenous or endogenous material. To divide these into two varieties, to call them heterolysosomes and autolysosomes and to group them with the others mentioned above seems hardly feasible or desirable.

In practice the distinction between phagolysosomes (*Plate 129*) and cytolysosomes (*Plates 130 and 131*) may be simple, difficult or impossible. The cytolysosome is characterized chiefly by sequestrated cell organelles and cytomembranes within its substance, yet such membranes may at times be exogenously derived by phagocytosis of a fragment of another cell. Further partial breakdown of ingested mitochondria or other membranous organelles may render their identification within the lysosome difficult. Despite such problems, in most instances there is little difficulty in distinguishing between these two varieties of secondary lysosomes. More details on this point and on the genesis and evolution of phagolysosomes and cytolysosomes form the subject of this section.

Phagolysosome formation has been studied in a variety of cell types. It is now clear that as a result of phagocytosis, pinocytosis or micropinocytosis (collectively referred to as cytosis or endocytosis), ingested material comes to lie within a single-membrane-bound structure called a phagosome. In each instance, the limiting membrane of this phagosome is derived from the cell membrane. Fusion of primary lysosomes (containing hydrolytic enzymes) with a phagosome leads to the formation of a phagolysosome where enzyme meets substrate and digestion of the ingested material ensures in most instances.*

A clear demonstration of this phenomenon was provided by the studies of Straus (1958, 1964) on kidney and liver tissue. He showed that ingested, cytochemically detectable foreign protein (horseradish peroxidase) first accumulates in cytoplasmic vacuoles (phagosomes) which stain negatively for acid phosphatase but positively for peroxidase. Later these phagosomes fuse with acid phosphatase containing primary lysosomes to form phagolysosomes which stain positively for both acid phosphatase and peroxidase.

* Enzymic digestion may be impeded for a variety of reasons, including a relative or absolute deficiency of enzymes, and ingestion of indigestible material or of a substance that inactivates lysosomal enzymes.

Plate 129

Neutrophil leucocytes containing phagocytosed bacteria (probably *E. coli*) found in the ascitic fluid of a patient with a perforation of the large bowel.

Fig. 1. Many phagolysosomes containing bacteria (∗) are seen in this neutrophil. One of these contains recognizable neutrophil granules (G); others contain granule-derived material in a dispersed form at times aligned against (arrow) the limiting membrane of the phagolysosome. × 27,000

Fig. 2. The bacteria in the neutrophil shown in *Fig. 1* do not appear markedly altered but the one (∗) seen in the phagolysosome of this neutrophil seems to be breaking down. × 30,000

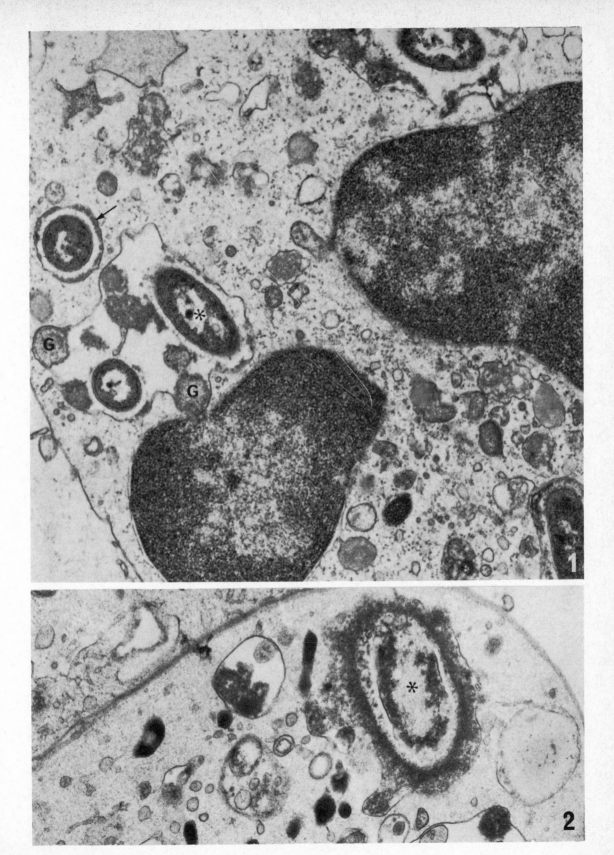

297

Later studies have shown that when various other substances such as inert colloids, enzymes, haemoglobin and ferritin are taken up by kidney tubule cells, a similar mechanism of phagosome and phagolysosome formation operates. The same mechanism operates when neutrophils ingest bacteria (*Plate 129*), and macrophages and cells of the reticuloendothelial system ingest red blood cells (page 316). Synovial intimal cells have a remarkable capacity for endocytosis. They can take up small particulate substances such as ferritin, gold, Thorotrast, iron dextran and carbon, or larger particulate matter such as entire erythrocytes, cell fragments and masses of fibrin and joint detritus (for references, see Ghadially and Roy, 1967b). Here, also, phagosome and phagolysosome formation is evident. Protozoa rely on the same method for dealing with ingested material in their food vacuoles (for more references to the above-mentioned studies, see de Duve and Wattiaux, 1966; Cohn and Fedorko, 1969; Daems *et al.*, 1969).

Cytolysosomes usually present as single-membrane-bound bodies containing a portion of cytoplasm bearing organelles such as mitochondria and endoplasmic reticulum and also inclusions such as glycogen and lipid (*Plate 130, Figs. 1 and 2*). The sequestrated material may be well preserved and easily identifiable or in various states of breakdown and degradation, until a point is reached when one cannot confidently assert whether a given lysosome started out as a cytolysosome or phagolysosome. Finally, a residual body containing undigested electron-dense lipidic residues (lipofuscin) is produced (*Plate 130, Figs. 3 and 4*).

Although cytolysosomes are usually bound by a single membrane, at times a double-membrane-bound cytolysosome or a structure mimicking a cytolysosome may be encountered. Thus, a double-membrane-bound structure may result from a sequestrated membranous structure (e.g. endoplasmic reticulum) lining up against the wall of the cytolysosome. Another possibility is that one may be witnessing an early stage in the formation of a cytolysosome where a lamellar extension of the endoplasmic reticulum or a double-membraned cup-shaped structure derived from the endoplasmic reticulum or Golgi complex may wrap around organelles to form cytolysosomes (see below for more details, and *Plate 131*). At least two further possibilities must be considered when such double-membrane-bound structures are sighted: (1) that this is a phagocytosed cell fragment; or (2) that it is a transverse section of a finger-like projection of one cell into another. Obviously, in such instances one would expect the structure to be lined by two membranes, one derived from the cell in which the structure lies and the other from the phago-cytosed fragment or the invaginating cell process.

A problem that has vexed many workers regarding the genesis of cytolysosomes is how sequestration occurs and how the acid hydrolases gain access into cytolysosomes. In the case of phagosomes, fusion with primary lysosomes has frequently been observed but this is not evident in many cases of cytolysosome formation where the enzymes seem to be present from the very

---

Plate 130

From a subcutaneous sarcoma of the rat produced by injection of 9:10-dimethyl-1:2-benzanthracene.

Fig. 1. Cytolysosomes with included mitochondria found in a tumour cell. ×36,000 (*Parry and Ghadially, unpublished electron micrograph*)

Fig. 2. This tumour cell contains numerous bodies interpreted as cytolysomes. In one of these (A) the cytomembranes are easily discerned, but in others where lysosomal digestion is more advanced cytomembrane remnants are barely discernible. ×32,000 (*From Parry and Ghadially, 1965*)

Figs. 3 and 4. Lipofuscin-containing residual bodies thought to be produced from cytolysosomes of the type shown in *Figs. 1 and 2*. Note the basic similarity between these lipofuscin granules and those illustrated in *Plates 134 and 135*. ×45,000; ×93,000 (*Fig. 3 from Parry and Ghadially, 1965*; *Fig. 4 Parry and Ghadially, unpublished electron micrograph*)

298

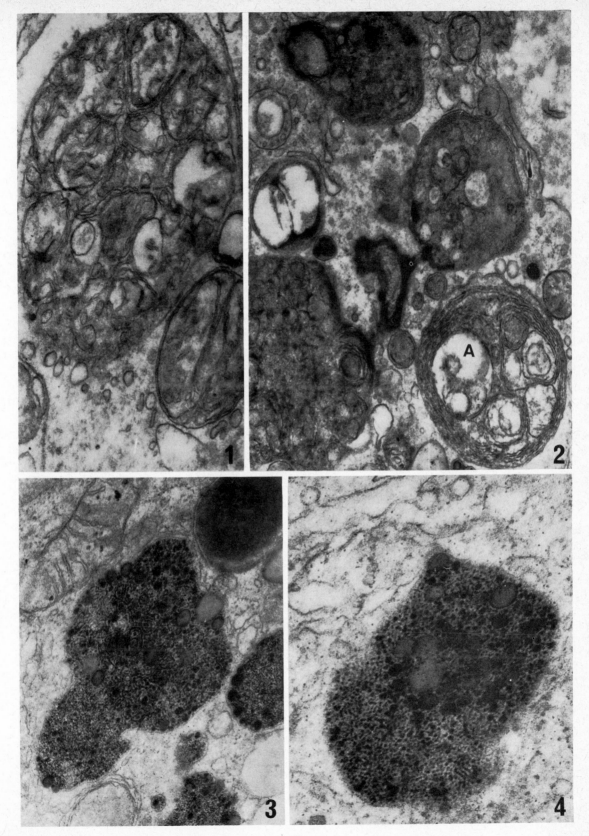

299

beginning of cytolysosome formation. In such cases a clear-cut stage which could be called an autophagosome (i.e. a vacuole containing sequestrated cellular material but no acid hydrolases) is either lacking or difficult to demonstrate.

Of the many possibilities, the one that is most acceptable is that a lamellar cup-shaped structure derived from the endoplasmic reticulum or Golgi region wraps around the organelle to be sequestrated (Moe *et al.*, 1965). It is likely that the hydrolytic enzymes would already be present in such a structure and either dissolution of the inner membrane or fusion of membranes would release the hydrolytic enzymes to form the cytolysosome. Certainly images which could be interpreted in this fashion (see Ericsson, 1969, for more details and references) have been seen in situations where cytolysosome formation is in progress (*Plate 131*). Only slightly different from this is the concept of intracisternal sequestraton where organelles 'drop in' dilated cisternae of the rough endoplasmic reticulum. Such a process could be looked upon as one of the ways in which a cytolysosome might be formed (*Plates 115 and 116*), the required enzymes being produced by the ribosomes lining the ensheathing membrane.

However, the possibility that structures containing sequestrated cell organelles may obtain the necessary hydrolytic enzymes by fusion with primary or secondary lysosomes in the cell can by no means be ruled out. For example, it has been reported (for references, see Ericsson, 1969) that in Thorotrast- or iron-treated rats the peribiliary-dense bodies become loaded with these electron-dense markers. If now cytolysosome formation is induced by partial hepatectomy or glucagon administration, then lysosomal bodies containing both mitochondria and the electron-dense marker are produced, and images are seen which suggest that structures containing sequestrated organelles are fusing with pre-existing secondary lysosomes containing the electron-dense marker.

Occasional cytolysosomes may be found in a variety of normal tissues; they are now regarded as a normal mechanism by which old and effete organelles are disposed of by the cell. An increased number of cytolysosomes generally indicates a sublethal intracellular focal injury caused by some noxious agent. A very large number of agents can induce cytolysosome formation in various tissues. These include mechanical trauma, x-rays, ultraviolet radiation, innumerable chemical agents including carcinogens and various antimetabolites, hypoxia, endotoxin shock and virus infections. (For further examples and references, see Ericsson, 1969; de Duve and Wattiaux, 1966.)

The lysosome content of tumours, particularly malignant tumours, is very variable. We have seen a human hepatoma where not a single structure morphologically acceptable as a lysosome was found (Ghadially and Parry, 1966a); on the other hand, a singularly large number of cytolysosomes were seen by us in rat sarcomas (Parry and Ghadially, 1965).

Plate 131

Fig. 1. A probable mode of cytolysosome formation is depicted here. Cup-shaped bodies (A) are seen lying free in the cytoplasm or wrapping around mitochondria (B) and other structures (C). Various images suggesting the breakdown of enclosed mitochondria and ultimate formation of single-membrane-bound dense bodies (D) are seen. From the megakaryocyte of a 6-month-old infant. (Same case as-*Plate 149.*) ×72,000 (*Ghadially and Skinnider, unpublished electron micrograph*)

Fig. 2. A double-membrane-bound body (arrow) which may be interpreted as (1) an early cytolysosome, (2) a phagocytosed cell fragment or (3) a finger-like evagination from an adjacent cell. From a case of malenosis coli (page 340). ×29,000 (*Ghadially and Parry, unpublished electron micrograph*)

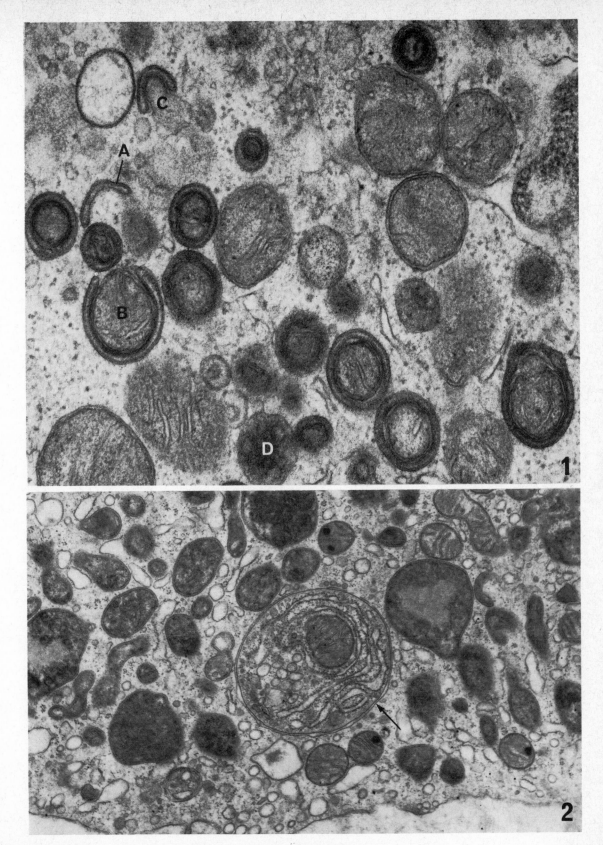

301

The term 'multivesicular body' is employed to describe a vacuole containing vesicles set in a lucent or dense matrix (*Plates 132 and 133*). Depending upon the density of the matrix, the body is referred to as either a light or a dark multivesicular body. Since acid phosphatase has been demonstrated in multivesicular bodies from various sites they are considered to be a variety of lysosome.

These bodies have been studied in: (1) oöcytes (Rebhun, 1960); (2) duodenal epithelium of foetal rats (Moe *et al.*, 1965); (3) HeLa cells (Robbins *et al.*, 1964); (4) neurons (Rosenbluth and Wissig, 1964); (5) adrenal medulla of rats (Holtzman and Dominitz, 1968); (6) anterior pituitary of rat (Smith and Farquhar, 1966); (7) fibroblasts in culture (Gordon *et al.*, 1965); (8) glomerular epithelial cells (Farquhar and Palade, 1962); (9) *Leishmania donovani* (Djaczenko *et al.*, 1969); (10) various tissues of an insect during moult–intermoult cycle (Locke and Collins, 1967); (11) epithelium of vas deferens and epididymis of rat (Friend and Murray, 1965; Sedar, 1966; Friend and Farquhar, 1967; Friend, 1969); (12) choroid plexus of chicken embryo (Meller and Breiphol, 1971); (13) proximal convoluted tubules of rat kidney (Spors, 1971); (14) human monocytic cells (*Plate 132, Figs. 1 and 2*); and (15) vascular endothelial cells (*Plate 170*).

Somewhat larger than usual multivesicular bodies were found by Fedorko (1968) in rat myelocytes incubated with chloroquine, while we (Ghadially and Parry, 1966b) have seen quite large and numerous multivesicular bodies in the colonic mucosa of a patient with melanosis coli (*Plate 132, Fig. 3*). Very large multivesicular bodies have also been noted in reticulosarcoma cells (Vasquez *et al.*, 1963) and myeloma (Sorensen, 1961).

Some of the above-mentioned studies have demonstrated that exogenous substances commonly employed as tracers, such as horseradish peroxidase and ferritin, are picked up in coated vesicles and are transported to multivesicular bodies, which then evolve into dense structures acceptable as lysosomes and residual bodies. In such instances the multivesicular body may be regarded as a variety of heterolysosome. In other instances, however, multivesicular bodies have been found to behave as autophagic vacuoles or autolysosomes and digest endogenous material such as secretory granules and thus regulate secretory processes within certain cells.

Several investigators believe that the vesicles within multivesicular bodies are primary lysosomes derived from the Golgi region (e.g. Novikoff *et al.*, 1964). In the rat epididymis, however, Friend (1969) has reported that acid phosphatase activity is seen in the matrix of the multivesicular body but not in the vesicles. According to him, the vesicles in the multivesicular body of the rat epididymis are similar in morphology and cytochemical properties to the outer Golgi vesicles (that is to say, the transitional vesicles lying between the endoplasmic reticulum and the outer convex face of the Golgi complex and the vesicles at the ends of the Golgi stacks). Such vesicles and some of the vesicles in the multivesicular body were stained after prolonged fixation in osmium but other vesicular structures in the cell were not. The function of these vesicles in the multivesicular body (mvb) is obscure but it is speculated (Friend, 1969) that 'the mvb vesicles contain enzymes or other substances responsible for the acidification of the mvb'.

Plate 132

Fig. 1. Multivesicular bodies (M) found in monocytoid cells from a case of erythroleukaemia. ×35,000 (*Ghadially and Skinnider, unpublished electron micrograph*)

Fig. 2. Multivesicular bodies (M) found in a monocyte from the peripheral blood of a patient with hepatic cirrhosis. ×45,000 (*Ghadially and Skinnider, unpublished electron micrograph*)

Fig. 3. Pleomorphic multivesicular bodies (arrows) found in the colonic mucosa from a case of melanosis coli. ×32,000 (*Ghadially and Parry, unpublished electron micrograph*)

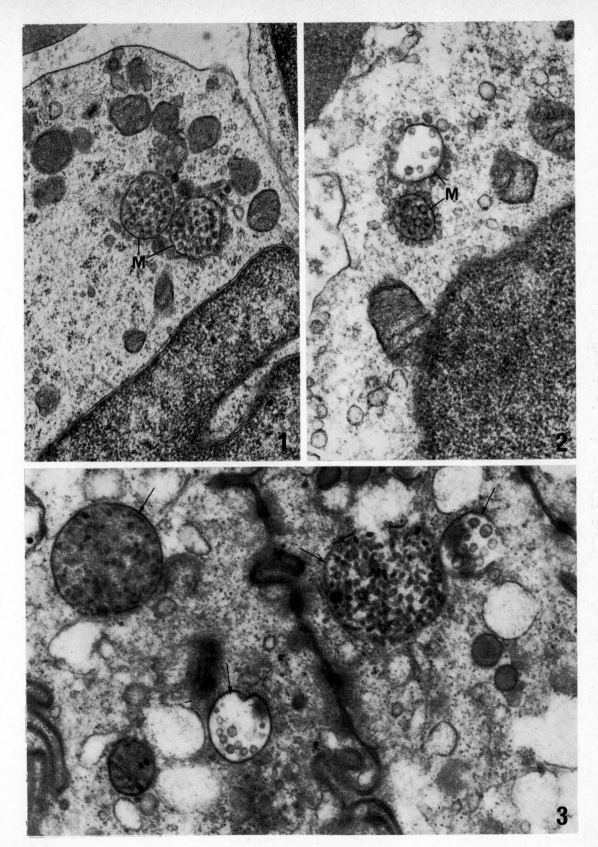

303

Another theory regarding the origin of the vesicles within the multivesicular body is that they arise by a process of invagination and budding from the wall of the limiting vacuole. It has also been speculated that endocytic vesicles carrying exogenous material may traverse the wall of the vacuole and find their way into multivesicular bodies (Novikoff *et al.*, 1964; Gordon *et al.*, 1965). Yet another concept is that a multivesicular body may form by autophagy of a cluster of vesicles (Ericsson, 1964; Kessel, 1966).

The various ideas mentioned above are not mutually exclusive and there is no compelling reason to believe that all multivesicular bodies arise in precisely the same manner or perform identical functions in all cell types.

In the great alveolar cells of the lung there is the situation where both the light and the dark varieties of multivesicular bodies are of common occurrence. These cells—which are at times also referred to as septal cells, type II epithelial cells or granular pneumocytes—are characterized by the presence of numerous single-membrane-bound bodies containing whorls or stacks of highly electron-dense membranes (*Plate 133*). These bodies, which are frequently referred to as cytosomes or multilamellar bodies, are now best referred to as myelinlc bodies (page 310). They are rich in phospholipids and give a positive reaction for acid phosphatase and other acid hydrolases (Balis and Conen, 1964; Hatasa and Nakamura, 1965; Goldfischer *et al.*, 1968; Kuhn, 1968; Corrin *et al.*, 1969; Vijeyaratnam and Corrin, 1972). It is also clear that the contents of these myelinoid bodies are discharged into the alveolar space and contribute to the surfactant layer which lowers surface tension and stabilizes the size of the alveolus. Although details of the intracellular mechanisms by which the surface-active lining layer precursors are synthesized are unclear, numerous investigators have shown that the myelinoid bodies evolve from multi-vesicular bodies (Campiche *et al.*, 1963; Hatasa and Nakamura, 1965; Balis *et al.*, 1966; Sorokin, 1966; Goldenberg *et al.*, 1967, 1969).

The probable sequence of events seems to be as follows. The light variety of multivesicular body is converted to the dense variety. Next a few osmiophilic membranes (myelinoid mem-branes) appear in the matrix of the dense multivesicular body. As the amount of membranous material increases the number of vesicles in the body diminishes until the fully mature myelinoid body packed with stacks or whorls of dense membranes (myelin figures) is formed. This then moves to the surface of the cell and its contents are discharged like any other merocrine secretion.

The precise manner in which the multivesicular bodies form in the great alveolar cells is not clear, but it is thought that vesicles containing the secretory material are pinched off from the rough endoplasmic reticulum and after their (probable) passage through the Golgi complex a cluster of vesicles is encompassed within a single limiting membrane, to form the multivesicular body.

Plate 133

Great alveolar cells from a newborn rat.

Fig. 1. Some of the stages of evolution of a myelinoid body (M) from light (L) and dark (D) multivesiculated bodies are seen in this electron micrograph. × 40,000

Fig. 2. A dark multivesicular body with vesicles (V) and dense membranes (M) is seen in company with another more mature form containing mainly laminated dense membranes. × 51,000

Fig. 3. Low power view showing a great alveolar cell with myelinoid bodies (M) and alveolar space (A) containing discharged secretory material (arrows). × 17,500

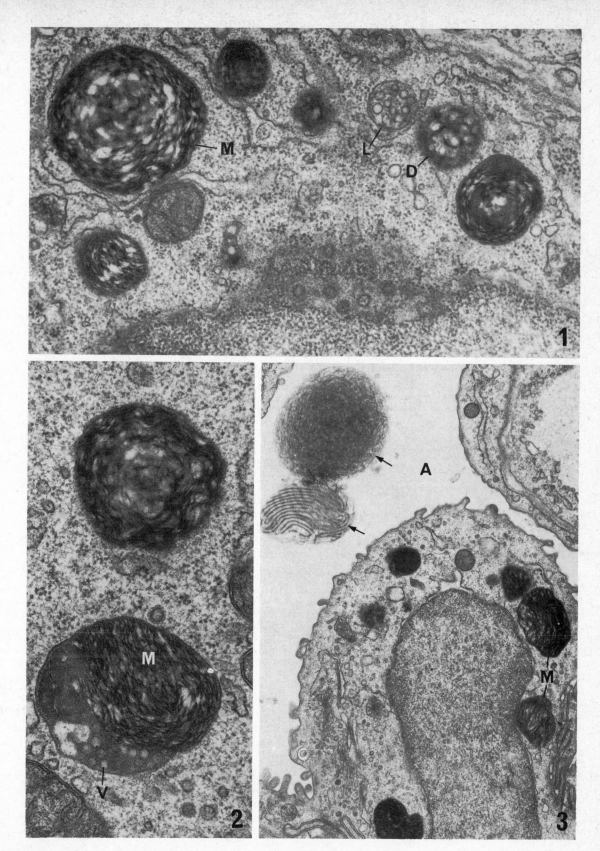

L

LIPOFUSCIN (RESIDUAL BODIES)

Although the golden yellow or brown pigment we now call lipofuscin has been known to light microscopists for over a century, its nature and manner of formation could not be truly appreciated until the lysosome concept had evolved. There is now ample evidence that the granules of lipofuscin and the identical or closely related pigments, haemofuscin and ceroid, represent residual bodies left behind in the cell after lysosomal activity. Ultrastructural studies have also revealed that although the major deposits of lipofuscin occur in the nervous system, heart and liver, there is hardly an organ or tissue where some lipofuscin-containing residual bodies do not occur (*Plates 134 and 135*).

The presence of pigment granules we now call lipofuscin was first noted by Hannover (1842) in nerve cells. The term 'lipofuscin' (meaning 'dusky fat') was coined later by Borst (1922). The abundance of this pigment in older individuals soon led workers to refer to it as the 'age pigment', 'wear and tear pigment' and 'womb to tomb pigment'. The term 'haemofuscin' was used by von Recklinghausen (1883) to distinguish the iron-free pigment granules in cases of haemochromatosis from those containing iron which were called 'haemosiderin'. The term 'ceroid' was used by Pappenheimer and Victor (1946) to describe the pigment in the motor neurons of vitamin-E-deficient rats and later extended to pigment deposits seen in various pathological situations. Histochemical evidence supports the view that lipofuscin, ceroid and haemofuscin are essentially the same material in different stages of oxidation (Lillie, 1965; Pearse, 1972). The variations in staining reaction and ultraviolet fluorescence observed in such pigment deposits are explainable on this basis. Porta and Hartroft (1969) succinctly express current feeling in this matter when they state, 'All the separate information gathered to date from investigations on the pigment related to ageing and to dietary factors favours their unification under lipofuscin pigment. To divide these closely related products into subentities seems unrealistic and only an accident of historic discoveries.'

Lipofuscin granules seem to be more abundant in humans than in other animals, but lipofuscin has been found in all vertebrates examined to date. It has also been found in gastropods (von Braunmuhl, 1957) and insects (Hodge, 1894). As early as 1886, Koneff had noted that the amount of lipofuscin in nerve cells increased with age. This was subsequently confirmed by many workers, for various species including man (Beams *et al.*, 1952; Sulkin and Kuntz, 1952; Sulkin, 1955; Wilcox, 1959; Brody, 1960; Samorajski *et al.*, 1965; Whiteford and Getty, 1966; Reichel *et al.*, 1968; Barden, 1969, 1970). Similar age-related increases of pigment also occur in the myocardium (Jayne, 1950; Strehler *et al.*, 1959; Munnell and Getty, 1968), liver (Bachmann, 1953), adrenal cortex and other organs (Planel and Guilhem, 1955; Samorajski and Ordy, 1967; Reichel, 1968).

In ultrathin sections these granules present as irregularly shaped bodies surrounded by a single membrane.

Plate 134

Fig. 1. Lipofuscin granules found in the myocardium of an elderly man. As pathology students well know, in the condition called brown atrophy of the heart such granules are abundant adjacent to the poles of the elongated nuclei of myocardial cells. This well known relationship of the pigment (P) to the nucleus (N) is demonstrated in this electron micrograph. × 18,500

Fig. 2. High power view of lipofuscin granules from the same specimen as *Fig. 1*. Note the characteristic dense granules, lipid droplets (L) and membrane surrounding the granules (arrows). × 45,000

Fig. 3. Lipofuscin granules found in an atrophic deltoid muscle of man. Note once again the presence of dense granular material and lipid droplets (L). × 23,000

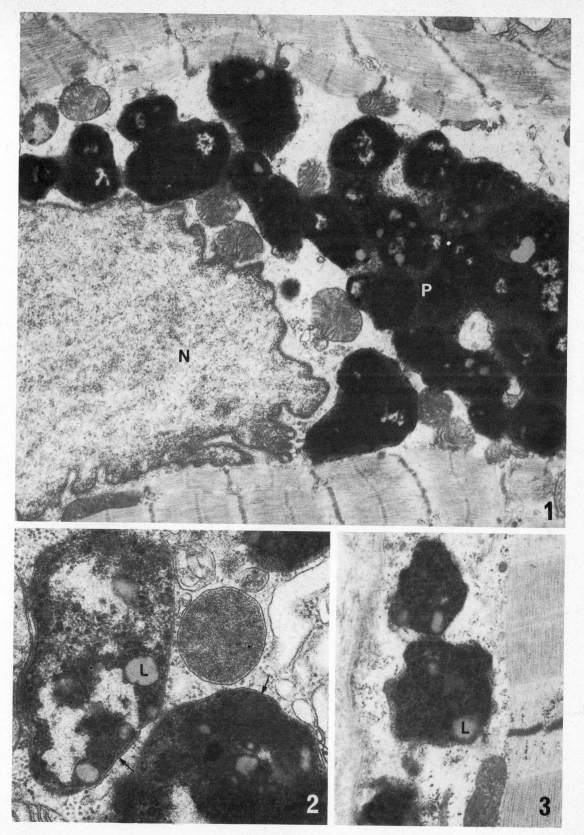

The contents are somewhat variable but in the main they consist of highly electron-dense material of a granular nature and usually also one or more medium-density or lucent lipidic droplets. On rare occasions recognizable remnants of cytoplasmic structures and/or electron-dense membranous material may be discerned in these lysosomal bodies.

The view that lipofuscin granules are lysosomal bodies is supported by many studies which have demonstrated the presence of acid phosphatase and other acid hydrolases such as esterases and cathepsins in them. This has been achieved by histochemical and cytochemical methods employing tissue sections and also by chemical analysis of isolated lipofuscin granules. By such techniques the lysosomal nature of lipofuscin granules has been confirmed in the liver (Essner and Novikoff, 1960; Goldfischer et al., 1966), heart (Bjorkerud, 1963; Jamieson and Palade, 1964; Goldfischer et al., 1966), mammary gland (Miyawaki, 1965), interstitial cells of the testis (Frank and Christensen, 1968) and neurons (Anderson and Song, 1962; Samorajski et al., 1964; Barden, 1969, 1970).

Both the ultrastructural appearance and the histochemical analysis of lipofuscin granules show that the pigment granule is not composed of a homogenous substance or a single chemical compound. According to the lysosome concept, one may look upon lipofuscin as a conglomerate of undigested residues derived by lysosomal hydrolysis and modification of sequestrated material prior to and after digestion. Such modifications include lipid peroxidation, polymerization and cross-linking of lipoproteins. (For references, see Barden, 1970.) The power of lysosomal hydrolases to degrade lipids (Mahadevan and Tappel, 1968a, b) is said to be limited, hence it is thought that they (lipids) are left behind and suffer stepwise oxidation producing lipofuscin. It has also been argued that the reason why such residues are left behind is that the lipids suffer oxidation at a very early stage and are hence not broken down by lysosomal enzymes.

The source of the material that is degraded in lysosomes and ultimately forms lipofuscin-containing residual bodies has not been extensively investigated, but a recent study (Travis and Travis, 1972) on rat myocardium shows that lipofuscin granules are formed here by the breakdown of mitochondria, glycogen and lipid within lysosomes. The fact that such residual bodies accumulate with age clearly shows that the power of many mammalian cells to excrete these bodies or their contents is limited or non-existent. It has been argued that such mounting accumulation of lipofuscin (which can at times constitute as much as one-third of the dry weight of the myocardium) may decrease the functional capacity of the organ (heart or brain) and may be a factor responsible for or involved in the ageing process. It remains for future work to determine whether the formation of these bodies can be suppressed or their elimination encouraged and whether this would be beneficial to the individual.

Plate 135

Fig. 1. These lipofuscin granules, composed of numerous dense granules and unusually large lipid droplets (L), were found in the liver tissue adjacent to a human hepatoma. The limiting membrane of these lysosomal bodies is discernible in some places (arrows). × 27,000 (*From Ghadially and Parry, 1966a*)

Fig. 2. Lipofuscin granules found in human gall-bladder epithelium. Here the lipid droplets (L) are small and numerous. × 26,000

Fig. 3. In these lipofuscin granules, found in a human synovial intimal cell, the electron-dense granular material is compacted and difficult to discern. Note once again the characteristic lipid droplets (L) and the enveloping membrane (arrows). × 60,000 (*From Ghadially and Roy, 1969*)

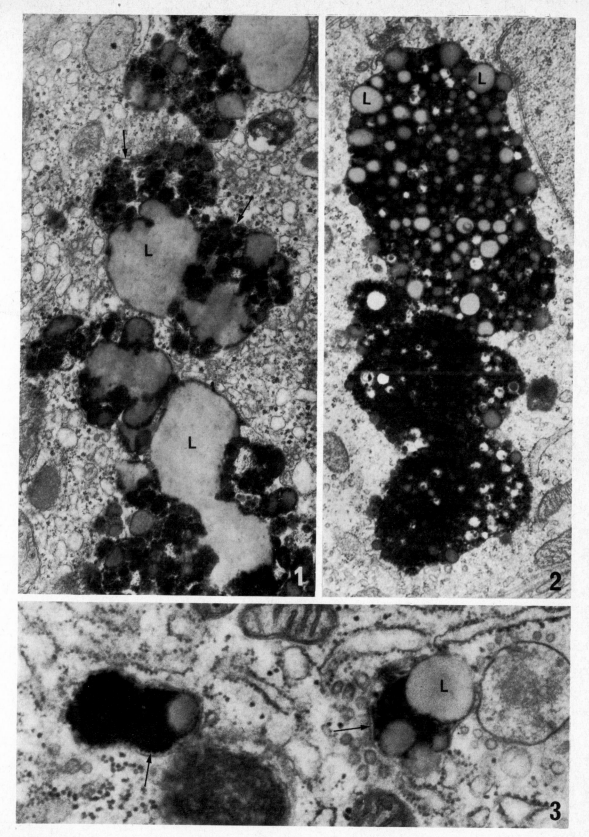

MYELIN FIGURES AND MYELINOID BODIES

The term 'myelin' was coined by Virchow (1854) to describe certain fatty substances obtainable from vegetable and animal materials (e.g. white matter of brain and egg yolk) which, when mixed with water, produced a laminated membranous structure. The term 'myelin' has subsequently been used mainly in connection with the medullary sheath of nerve fibres which, with the electron microscope, is seen to be an osmiophilic laminated membranous structure. Today the term 'myelinoid membranes' is used to describe markedly osmiophilic membranes, and the term 'myelin figures' is employed when such membranes show a stacked, reticulated or whorled arrangement. However, it should be remembered that the electron density realized in electron micrographs of myelin figures depends much on the tissue processing and photographic techniques employed so that at times the electron density may fall short of the expected ideal. Furthermore, the membranes comprising the myelin figure may not at times be too clearly visualized owing to obliquity of sectioning or other reasons.

Single-membrane-bound bodies containing myelin figures have frequently been encountered (see below) and acid phosphatase activity has been demonstrated in them. The term 'myeloid bodies' has been proposed to describe such lysosomal bodies (Hruban et al., 1965, 1972), but it seems more appropriate to use the term 'myelinoid bodies' since the word 'myeloid' means resembling or pertaining to the marrow.

Myelin figures are readily produced in tissues fixed in glutaraldehyde (Ericsson and Biberfeld, 1967), particularly if the fixation is prolonged for many hours or days. Since lipids are not fixed by glutaraldehyde, some (lipids) leach out of the cytomembranes. Mixtures of such liberated lipid with the aqueous environment produces membranous formations which are fixed by the osmium used as a post-fixative agent. These then present as myelin figures at electron microscopy. Such myelin figures may be found in extracellular sites and also within the cell, particularly common being myelin figures in the cytoplasmic matrix and mitochondria (*Plate 136, Figs.1–3*; see also *Plate 92*). The latter are likely to be mistaken for pathological or degenerative changes in the cell or mitochondrion.

Another interesting example of extracellular myelin figures or myelinoid membrane formation is found in the matrix of articular cartilage. The *in situ* necrosis of chondrocytes and the shedding of chondrocyte cell processes which normally occur in this tissue liberate much osmiophilic lipidic debris into the matrix (for references and details, see Ghadially and Roy, 1969). In man such material usually presents as electron-dense amorphous or granular material in the matrix, but in the rabbit small highly osmiophilic membranous formations (more often myelinoid membranes rather than the more complex myelin figures) are commonly produced (*Plate 136, Figs. 4 and 5*).

Virchow's observations on *in vitro* formation of myelin figures has been extended by some more recent studies. Such figures have been produced by Stoeckenius (1962) from brain phospholipid, by Revel et al. (1958) from egg lecithin and by Samuels et al. (1964) from a mixture of gangliosides, cholesterol, phospholipids, cerebrosides, amino acids and protein.

Plate 136

Figs. 1–3. Myelin figures produced in mitochondria and outside the cell by glutaraldehyde fixation. From a ganglion of the wrist. ×48,000; ×44,000; ×85,000 (*Ghadially and Mehta, unpublished electron micrographs*)

Fig. 4. Matrix of rabbit articular cartilage, showing lipidic debris which often presents as small highly osmiophilic membranous formations (arrows). ×48,000 (*From Ghadially, Meachim and Collins, 1965*)

Fig. 5. Matrix of human articular cartilage, showing lipid debris which usually presents as osmiophilic granular material. Membranous formations are, however, occasionally encountered. ×48,000 (*From Ghadially, Meachim and Collins, 1965*)

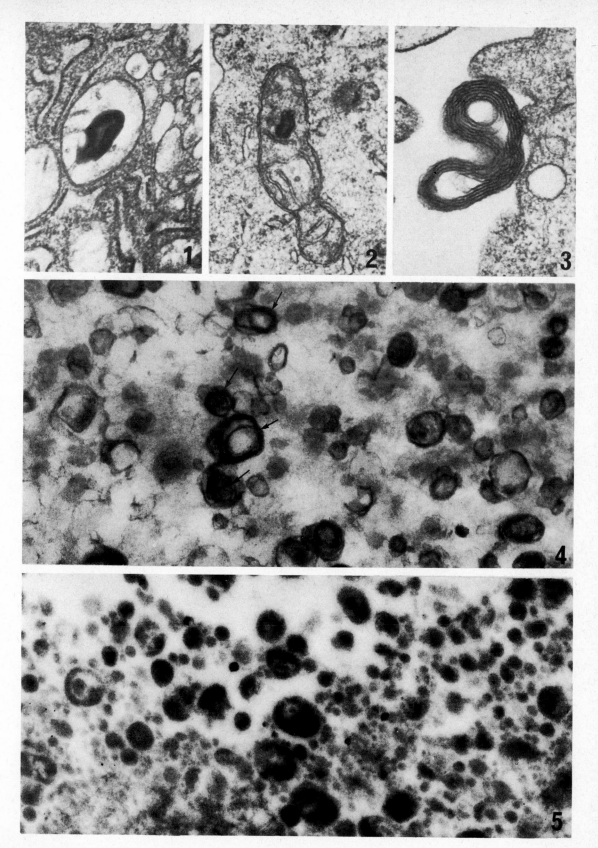

This mixture, based on the composition of myelinoid bodies found in Tay–Sachs disease (see below), produced myelin figures comparable to those found *in vivo* within lysosomes in this condition. Such experiments suggest that at least one of the ways in which myelin figures may be produced in lysosomes is by hydration of the lipidic component within these organelles. Thus one may speculate that lipid residues may present either as osmiophilic granules and droplets or, if hydrated, as myelin figures within the lysosome.

Myelinoid bodies are occasionally found in a wide variety of normal cells but in the great alveolar cells of the lung they are of common occurrence. Such bodies in this site, which are referred to as cytosomes or multilamellar bodies, represent the secretory granules normally produced by these cells (*Plate 133*). Myelinoid bodies are also occasionally seen in cells which engage in erythophagocytosis. Thus such osmiophilic membrane-containing lysosomes are at times found in Kupffer cells, in macrophages of the spleen and bone marrow and, as shown later, in synovial cells, from haemarthrotic joints (*Plate 140*). It is thought that in these instances the breakdown of the cholesterol-rich erythrocyte membrane within the phagolysosome is delayed and hence presents as osmiophilic membranous whorls.

Myelinoid bodies are pleomorphic structures which show infinite diversity of form. This is illustrated in *Plate 137* where myelinoid bodies from a herpesvirus-infected cell, a rat sarcoma, a human ovarian carcinoma and a synovial intimal cell after an intra-articular injection of egg yolk are depicted. In the last-mentioned instance it would appear that the myelinoid bodies represent phagosomes and phagolysosomes containing egg yolk.

Myelinoid bodies in great numbers are found in certain inborn errors of metabolism or storage diseases, which are now also referred to as 'inborn lysosomal diseases' or 'lysosomal storage diseases'. These bodies have been given various names such as 'lipid cytosomes', 'multi-membranous bodies', 'lamellar bodies', 'membranous cytoplasmic bodies' and 'zebra bodies'. All of these contain stacked, reticulated or whorled membranes. The last appellation (zebra bodies) is used to describe lysosomal bodies containing stacks of osmiophilic membranes, where adjacent membranes are closely apposed or fused, so that fairly wide alternating dense and light bands are produced. Myelinoid bodies of the zebra type and bodies containing whorled membranes have been seen in the neurons of cases of Tay–Sachs disease (Terry and Weiss, 1963) and also in some other (but not all) varieties of amaurotic idiocy (Menkes *et al.*, 1971). Acid phosphatase activity has been demonstrated in such bodies (Wallace *et al.*, 1964) and they have also at times been observed in various sites besides the brain in cases of Tay–Sachs disease (Hers and Van Hoof, 1969).

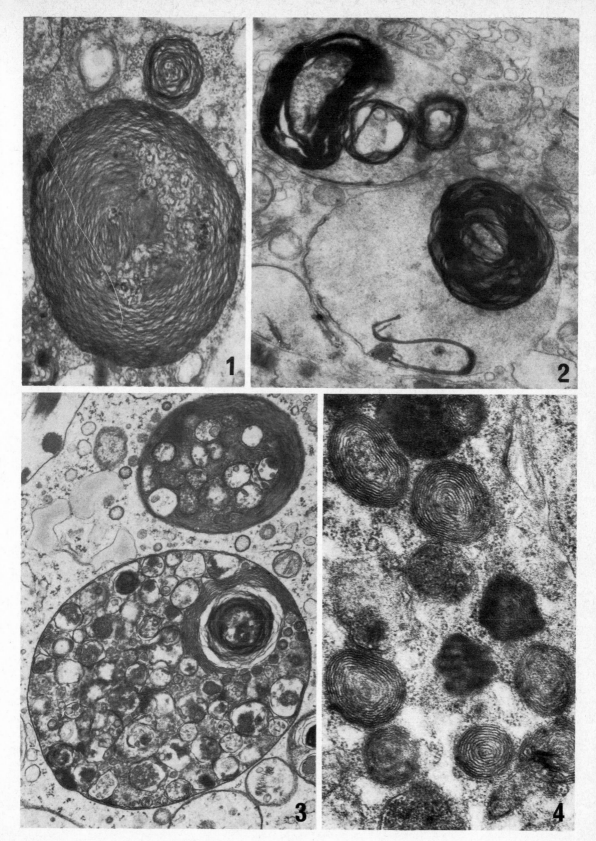

Membranous cytoplasmic bodies similar to those seen in man have also been noted in dogs with amaurotic idiocy (Diezel et al., 1967; Karbe, 1968). In certain types of Hurler's syndrome (pseudo-Hurler) mucopolysaccharide deposits occur in the liver, but myelinoid bodies are found in neurons (see review by Hers and Van Hoof, 1969). Recently zebra bodies have also been found in the neurons of a case of Fabry's disease (Grunnet and Spilsbury, 1973) (*Plate 138*).

In Fabry's disease, glycolipid deposits occur in the kidney epithelial cells and in blood vessels throughout the body. Myelinoid bodies have been described in this condition and acid phosphatase activity has been demonstrated in them (Rae et al., 1967; Tarnowski and Hashimoto, 1968). Niemann–Pick disease is characterized by sphingomyelin storage in the reticuloendothelial system and in various other sites. Myelinoid bodies containing mainly concentric laminated membranes have been described in this condition and acid phosphatase activity has been demonstrated in these bodies (Tanaka et al., 1963; Lynn and Terry, 1964; Wallace et al., 1965; Volk and Wallace, 1966; Lazarus et al., 1967; Luse, 1967).

In Gaucher's disease, however, the abnormal glucocerebroside accumulation in the reticulo-endothelial system (particularly the spleen) takes the form of microtubular material in single-membrane-bound bodies (De Marsh and Kautz, 1957; Salomon and Caroli, 1962; Jordan, 1964; Toujas et al., 1966). This is quite characteristic of the Gaucher cell. However, the neurons in some cases of this condition contain myelinoid bodies of the zebra type (Adachi et al., 1967).

It is now thought (Hers and Van Hoof, 1969; de Duve, 1970) that in most of the above-mentioned disorders there is a deficiency or absence of a specific lysosomal hydrolase. As a result of this, substances which need the deficient enzyme for their breakdown accumulate in the lysosome, which becomes overloaded with undigested material and increases considerably in size. However, enzymic defects outside the lysosome may be operative in some of these conditions, and these defects may lead to an accumulation of metabolite and its subsequent sequestration in the lysosome.

Myelinoid bodies have been produced in numerous cell types by a variety of drugs. An excellent review of these drug-induced myelinoid bodies has recently been published (Hruban et al., 1972) so a detailed list of references will not be presented. Drugs which have produced myelinoid bodies include triparanol, chloroquine, diazocholesterol, paraquat, clindamycin, erythromycin, 4,4-diethylaminoethoxyhexoestrol, chlorcyclizine, norchlorcyclizine and others.

Two main ideas have been put forward to explain the occurrence of myelin figures in lysosomes. The first theory is that any suitable lipidic residue may become hydrated and form myelin figures as evidenced by numerous *in vitro* studies. The second idea is that the myelin figures are, in some instances at least, incompletely digested cytomembranes. For example, it is thought that the cholesterol-rich erythrocyte membrane is difficult to digest, hence myelinoid bodies form in cells which phagocytose erythrocytes. Similarly, it is thought that some drug-induced myelinoid bodies are formed because the membranes contain bound drugs which makes them difficult to digest, or that the drugs selectively inhibit lysosomal enzymes.

Plate 138

Electron micrograph showing zebra bodies in a neuron from a case of Fabry's disease. × 34,000. (*From Grunnet and Spilsbury, 1973*)

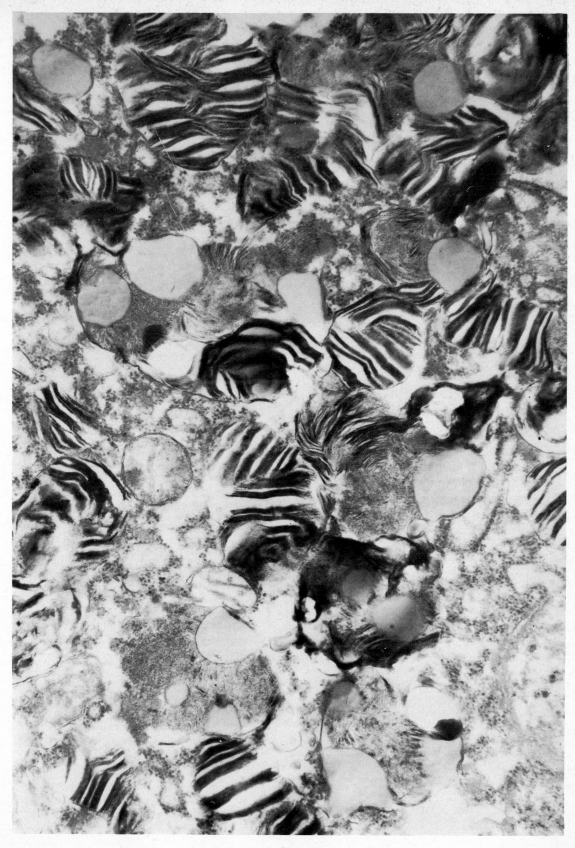

Splenic erythrophagocytosis was first described by Kolliker in 1849. It is now known that this is the mechanism by which aged and atypical erythrocytes are removed from the circulation by cells of the reticuloendothelial system, particularly the macrophages in the spleen and bone marrow. Similarly, erythrophagocytosis is also one of the processes by which erythrocytes are removed after haemorrhage (*Plate 139*). In both instances the ingested erythrocytes are broken down by lysosomal enzymes, but while in the former case most of the iron released forms ferritin and is reutilized, in the latter case much of the iron is converted to haemosiderin and stored for indefinite periods of time in residual bodies called siderosomes.

Phagocytosis of erythrocytes or their fragments (see below) is achieved by cell processes arising from the phagocytic cell which wrap around the erythrocyte. The erythrophagosome thus created does not contain acid phosphatase or other lysosomal enzymes but soon primary lysosomes from the phagocytic cell fuse with and discharge their contents into the phagosome and convert it to a phagolysosome where digestion of the ingested material occurs (Rifkind, 1965; Anton and Brandes, 1969; Aikawa and Sprinz, 1971). There is a certain similarity between erythrophagocytosis occurring in various sites, physiological and pathological states and in different species, but there are also interesting differences which remain to be investigated and understood.

One such difference relates to the fragmentation of the erythrocyte prior to ingestion by the phagocyte. (It should be noted that such fragments are membrane bound and contain haemoglobin. This phenomenon is quite distinct from lysis, where the haemoglobin escapes leaving behind a red cell ghost.) A review of the literature on erythrophagocytosis in the spleen, bone marrow and lymph nodes of man and experimental animals in physiological and pathological states shows that some observers believe that erythrocytes are fragmented prior to or during ingestion by the macrophage (Rous and Robertson, 1917; Rous, 1923; Crosby, 1959; Koyama *et al.*, 1964; Bessis, 1965; Wennberg and Weiss, 1968), while others hold that entire intact erythrocytes are ingested by the phagocytic cell (Smith, 1958; Simon and Pictet, 1964; Rifkind, 1965; Pictet *et al.*, 1969; Edwards and Simon, 1970; Simon and Burke, 1970; Aikawa and Sprinz, 1971). From available data one cannot clearly relate this difference to species variations or to physiological or pathological states, but it is abundantly clear from illustrations in the literature that both phenomena do occur.

Similar differences have also been noted in studies on the removal of shed blood. Thus, ultrastructural studies on haemorrhagic effusion in rats bearing the Novikoff ascites hepatoma have clearly shown that spherical or tear-drop-shaped membrane-bound fragments containing haemoglobin are cast off from the surface of erythrocytes and that such fragments and intact erythrocytes suffer phagocytosis by macrophages (Essner, 1960).

Plate 139

Erythrophagocytosis seen after injection of 1 ml of autologous blood into the rabbit knee joint.

Figs. 1 and 2. Phagocytosed erythrocytes in rabbit synovial cell (*Fig. 1*) and subsynovial macrophage (*Fig. 2*), showing erythrocytic segmentation. × 32,000; × 14,500 (*Fig. 1, from Roy and Ghadially, 1966; Fig. 2, from Ghadially and Roy, 1969*)

Figs. 3 and 4. Phagocytosed erythrocytes in rabbit synovial cell (*Fig. 3*) and subsynovial macrophage (*Fig. 4*), illustrating the formation of small surface projections (P) separated from the main erythrocyte mass by septa (S). It would appear that such fragments are later detached to form electron-dense bodies (D) containing whorled membranes. × 18,000; × 19,000 (*From Ghadially and Roy, 1969*)

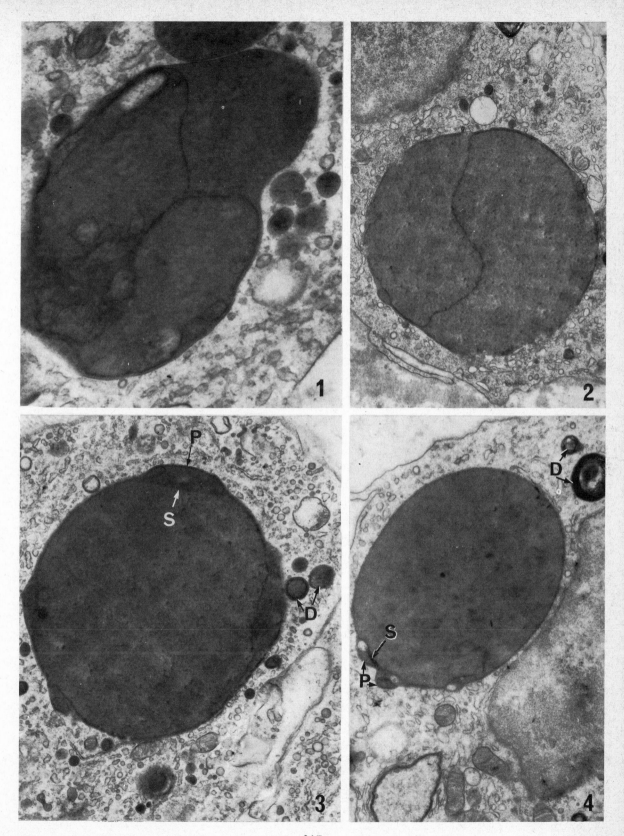

In traumatic haemarthrosis in man and experimentally produced haemarthrosis in the rabbit we found that entire erythrocytes were phagocytosed by synovial intimal cells and there was no evidence of fragmentation prior to ingestion (Roy and Ghadially, 1966, 1967, 1969; Ghadially and Roy, 1967b, 1969). However, a breaking up of the erythrocyte mass into smaller portions does occur within the phagocytic synovial cell. This is achieved in various ways, such as by the formation of septa which divide the erythrocyte or by the casting off of small fragments from the surface of the erythrocyte (*Plate 139*). Thus smaller sized phagosomes or phagolysosomes are derived from the main phagosomal mass where presumably a better contact between enzymes and substrates occurs.

In rat erythrocytes phagocytosed by splenic macrophages, Edwards and Simon (1970) report that canalization or 'tunnelization' of the erythrocyte occurs by deep invaginations of the limiting lysosomal membrane and that ferritin derived from the degraded erythrocyte escapes through the limiting membrane into the cytoplasm. Apparently no true siderosome formation or prolonged iron storage occurs, the ferritin being reutilized for building iron-containing compounds (Moore and Dubach, 1956; Edwards and Simon, 1970; Simon and Burke, 1970).

In haemarthrosis, canalization of the erythrocyte is seen only occasionally. The process of lysosomal digestion leads to the formation of two main types of residual bodies, one containing very electron-dense unicentric and multicentric myelin figures (lysosomal bodies containing myelin figures are referred as myelinoid bodies; see page 310) and another containing electron-dense iron-containing particles called siderosomes (page 320). Myelinoid bodies were rarely encountered by Edwards and Simon (1970) in rat splenic macrophages, but were abundant in the same situation in the rabbit (Simon and Burke, 1970). In the many human bone marrow specimens studied by us (Ghadially and Skinnider, unpublished observations), we have rarely seen good examples of myelinoid bodies in macrophages breaking down erythrocytes, yet, as already pointed out, such bodies are common in human synovial cells in haemarthrosis (*Plate 140*).

Since the power of lysosomal hydrolases to degrade lipids is limited and variable (Mahadevan and Tappel, 1968a, b) one may speculate that only in those circumstances where the lipid residue from the cholesterol-rich erythrocyte membrane persists in a suitably hydrated or altered form do myelin figures develop, while in other instances the lipid presents as osmiophilic droplets or electron-dense granules. Yet another possibility is that the cholesterol-rich erythrocyte membrane is not readily degraded in the lysosome and hence lingers awhile in the form of myelin figures. That such myelin figures within lysosomes do not persist indefinitely is evidenced by our observation that in animals examined some months after the injection of blood into the joint only residual bodies with electron-dense particles (siderosomes) are seen but myelinoid bodies are absent.

Plate 140

Fig. 1. Single-membrane-bound myelinoid body found in the synovial cell of a haemarthrotic rabbit knee joint. × 69,000 (*From Roy and Ghadially, 1966*)

Fig. 2. Unicentric (U) and multicentric (M) myelinoid bodies found in the synovial cell of a haemarthrotic rabbit knee joint. × 24,000 (*From Roy and Ghadially, 1966*)

Fig. 3. Myelinoid bodies essentially similar to those seen in the rabbit are also seen in this synovial intimal cell from a case of acute traumatic haemarthrosis in man. × 53,000 (*From Roy and Ghadially, 1967*)

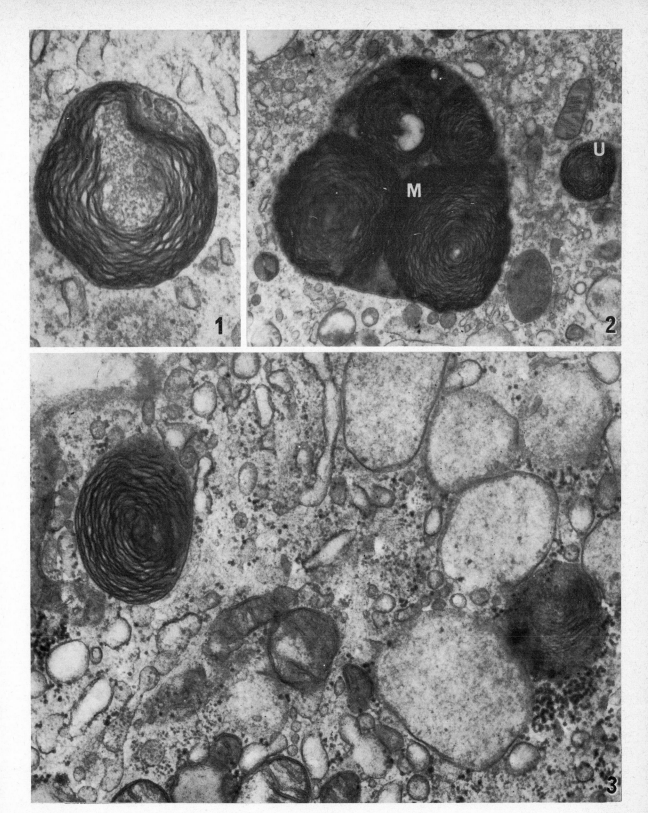

The term 'siderosome' was coined by Richter (1957) to describe single-membrane-bound bodies with aggregates of iron-containing electron-dense particles (50–60 Å diameter) within them. It is now clear that the Prussian-blue-positive haemosiderin granule of the light microscopist represents either a large siderosome or a clump of smaller siderosomes. Occasional siderosomes are normally found in the cells of the reticuloendothelial system but many more are encountered in diseases or experimental situations where an iron-overload is operative (e.g. pathological iron assimilation, blood transfusion, parenterally administered iron, etc.). In such states the paren-chymatous cells of various organs, particularly the liver also come to contain siderosomes. An example of this is illustrated in a later section of this chapter (*Plate 157*), where siderosomes formed in the liver of a rabbit which had received injections of iron dextran are depicted. In the same animal, siderosomes were also found in the chondrocytes of articular cartilage.

Siderosomes are also encountered in tissues after haemorrhage. For example, haemorrhage into a joint or injection of blood into a joint leads to the formation of siderosomes in both the cells of synovial membrane and articular cartilage* (*Plates 141–143*).

At one time it was thought that haemosiderin was deposited in mitochondria (Arnold, 1900; Gillman and Gillman, 1945) but it is now clear that, except in certain special instances (page 174). iron is not deposited in mitochondria and siderosomes do not form in this fashion. Current opinion regards the siderosome as a lysosomal body since acid phosphatase can be demonstrated in this structure (Novikoff *et al.*, 1956; Ericsson, 1965). The mature siderosome is, in fact, a residual body in which indigestible iron residues have been left behind after lysosomal enzyme activity has subsided.

There has been much confusion and controversy regarding the nature of the electron-dense particles in siderosomes. Some authors have called them 'ferritin' or 'ferritin aggregates', others have called them 'haemosiderin', while we (Ghadially and Roy, 1969) refer to them by the non-committal term 'electron-dense iron-containing particles'. The problem stems from differ-ences of opinion regarding the morphology of the ferritin molecule as seen with the electron microscope and the differences between haemosiderin and ferritin. About the latter, Richter (1958) stated that (1) 'the micelles of haemosiderin and ferritin are composed of the same sub-units' and (2) 'ferritin is a component of haemosiderin and at times a prominent one'. On the

*For details on siderosomes in articular cartilage see Ghadially *et al.* (1974).

Plate 141

Siderosomes in synovial cells from cases of acute traumatic haemarthrosis in man, and experimentally produced acute haemarthrosis in the rabbit.

Fig. 1. A collection of siderosomes of varied morphology is seen here. In some (A) the fine electron-dense particles are difficult to discern, but in others (B) the particles can easily be seen against a paler background. A siderosome containing a membranous structure is seen at C. ×37,000 (*From Ghadially and Roy, 1969*)

Fig. 2. A large siderosome (A), a few smaller siderosomes (B), and iron-containing electron-dense particles are seen scattered in the cytoplasm. The siderosomes are bounded by a single membrane. The appearance of a double membrane is due to linear regimentation of electron-dense particles along the periphery of the siderosome and is not a true second membrane. ×38,000 (*From Ghadially and Roy, 1969*)

Fig. 3. A large collection of nearly spherical siderosomes (S) is seen here. ×36,000 (*From Roy and Ghadially, 1969*)

Fig. 4. High power view of a siderosome, showing many electron-dense particles. ×96,000 (*From Ghadially and Roy, 1969*)

Fig. 5. High power view of siderosomes containing many electron-dense particles. Similar particles are also scattered throughout the cytoplasm. ×96,000 (*From Roy and Ghadially, 1969*)

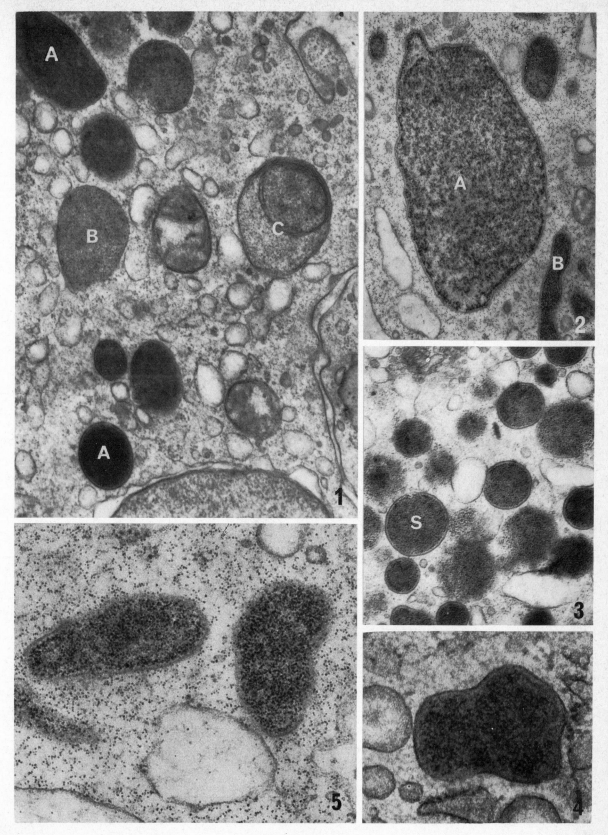

321

other hand, Shoden and Sturgeon (1961) have suggested that the haemosiderin granule is a relatively amorphous condensate of ferric hydroxide virtually free of protein, and that it probably arises by a process of degradation of the protein (apoferritin) matrix of ferritin.

Ferritin is a biochemically well-defined iron-containing protein which was isolated from the spleen on the basis of its water solubility by Laufberger (1934, 1937). By contrast, haemosiderin is insoluble in water and it is generally thought, on the basis of biochemical and histochemical studies, that it is probably not a single substance but varies in its composition depending upon the anatomical source, stage of maturation of the pigment and the iron preparations used to induce its formation. For example, besides iron, haemosiderin is thought to contain poly-saccharides, protein and lipid (e.g. Gedigk and Strauss, 1953). As Sturgeon and Shoden (1969) quite rightly point out, 'it is highly improbable that any of these substances other than iron constitutes an integral part of haemosiderin', and the different results obtained on chemical analysis could be attributable to the impossibility of obtaining 'pure' haemosiderin uncon-taminated by other cell components. Yet another explanation of the alleged heterogeneous nature of haemosiderin would be that haemosiderin granules are lysosomal bodies which, at least in the earlier stages of their evolution, may contain cytomembranes and other cytoplasmic material. Little wonder, then, that proteins and lipids are found when such granules are analysed or that with ageing and maturation of the pigment the iron concentration is found to increase.

Ultrastructural studies have shown that the ferritin molecule is roughly spherical in shape. It comprises a protein shell (apoferritin) of about 110 Å diameter with a centrally located 50 Å diameter core containing iron. The core as seen with the electron microscope is thought to consist of 4–6 subunits (called iron micelles) of about 27 Å in diameter (Farrant, 1954; Richter, 1959; Kerr and Muir, 1960; Bessis and Breton-Gorius, 1960; van Bruggen *et al.*, 1960). Although much has been made of such images and the so-called tetrads and hexads have been considered to be the characteristic 'signature' of ferritin, it is now evident that this appearance is almost certainly an artefact. Haydon (1969) has demonstrated that '(1) At a potential resolution of 5 Å near-focus electron micrographs of ferritin molecules show no substructure in the core and (2) by defocusing the microscope a computed amount, electron micrographs of the same ferritin molecule can be produced which show apparent core substructure similar to that shown in several patterns reported in the literature'. Such contentions are supported by x-ray diffraction studies (Harrison *et al.*, 1967) which show that iron micelles do exist in the ferritin core but they are randomly distributed and too small to be resolvable by currently available electron micro-scopes.

Such considerations and the fact that the electron-dense particles in siderosomes are often tightly packed and overlie each other so that it is difficult to resolve them (leave aside any sub-structure in them) have led us to use the non-committal term 'electron-dense iron-containing particles' to describe them.

Plate 142

Fig. 1. In this type B synovial cell two siderosomes (S) and innumerable electron-dense iron-containing particles are seen in the cytoplasmic matrix. From a rabbit knee joint after four once-weekly injections of autologous blood. × 43,000 (*From Roy and Ghadially, 1969*)

Fig. 2. The electron-dense iron-containing particles in the siderosomes seen in this synovial cell (type B) are highly compacted and difficult to discern. From a chronic haemarthrotic rabbit joint after 25 once-weekly injections of blood. × 40,000 (*From Roy and Ghadially, 1969*)

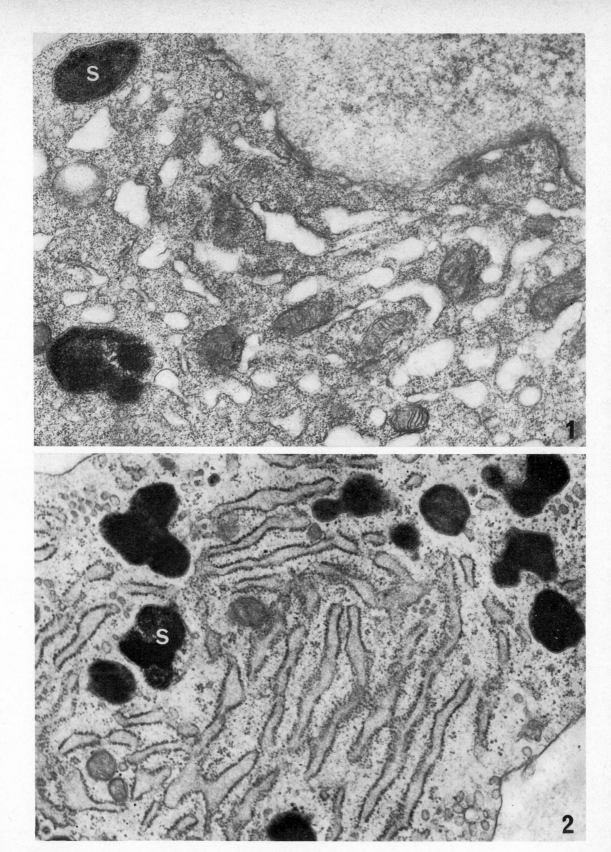

323

The chemical nature of haemosiderin is not unequivocally established, but recent electron probe x-ray analysis of siderosomes in haemarthrotic rabbit cartilage supports the idea that iron occurs in the siderosome as iron hydroxide and/or phosphate (Ghadially et al., 1974). Thus it would appear that lysosomal activity digests away most of the lipids and proteins derived from ingested erythrocytes or haemoglobin, leaving behind inorganic iron compound(s) in the siderosome. At this terminal stage of evolution the siderosome may be regarded as a variety of residual body. Such concepts are in keeping with what is seen in experimentally produced haemarthrosis (Roy and Ghadially, 1966, 1967, 1969; Ghadially and Roy, 1969). We found that in the early siderosomes produced in the synovial membrane soon after a single injection of blood into the joint space, the electron-dense iron-containing particles lay dispersed in a medium-density matrix, presumably protein in nature. With the passage of time the deposits became increasingly compact and electron opaque, and often their granular nature could not be discerned except at the periphery of such masses. This is even more evident in chronic haemarthrosis where quite large, highly electron-dense siderosomes develop with the passage of time.

The siderosomes seen in the synovial membrane in acute haemarthrosis vary in size but most of them are quite small and only occasionally is a large siderosome seen (*Plate 141*). These show a fairly uniform distribution of electron-dense iron-containing particles within them and there is no morphological ground for believing that the larger siderosome has arisen by the fusion of smaller ones. However, such a process of fusion is clearly evident in many of the very large siderosomes seen in chronic haemarthrosis. We (Roy and Ghadially, 1969) have coined the term 'compound siderosome' to describe these structures, where a conglomeration of partially fused siderosomes is seen (*Plate 143*). At times not only many siderosomes but also other organelles and inclusions are sequestrated in a large membrane-bound body which may be called a 'complex siderosome' (*Plate 143*).

Electron microscopic studies have helped clarify certain aspects of the staining reaction of haemosiderin seen with light microscopy. When tissues containing haemosiderin are subjected to the Prussian blue test, discrete blue granules, and at times also a diffuse blue hue, is seen in the cytoplasm. The latter type of staining has been ascribed in the past to a diffusion of Prussian blue from the granules or to differences in the diffusion of various constituents of haemosiderin (e.g. Lillie, 1954). Such hypotheses are now unnecessary, for electron microscopic studies provide a much more plausible explanation of this phenomenon. It is clear that at times numerous electron-dense iron-containing particles are found scattered in the cytopasm (*Plate 141, Fig. 5 and Plate 142, Fig. 1*). These are too small to be resolved by light microscopy but when present in sufficient numbers are likely to produce enough Prussian blue to give the cell a faint blue tint. Groups of small siderosomes, large siderosomes and compound and complex siderosomes are sizeable enough to produce the characteristic discrete blue granules or the larger blue masses seen in the Prussian blue test for haemosiderin.

Plate 143

Fig. 1. Compound siderosomes composed of several siderosomes, some of which are indicated as A, B, C, D and E. From synovial membrane of a rabbit after 24 once-weekly injections of blood into the joint. × 27,000 (*From Roy and Ghadially, 1969*)

Fig. 2. The complex siderosomes depicted here contain several siderosomes (S), lipid (L), mitochondria (M) and vesicles (V). From synovial membrane of a rabbit after six once-weekly injections of blood into the joint. × 37,000 (*From Roy and Ghadially, 1969*)

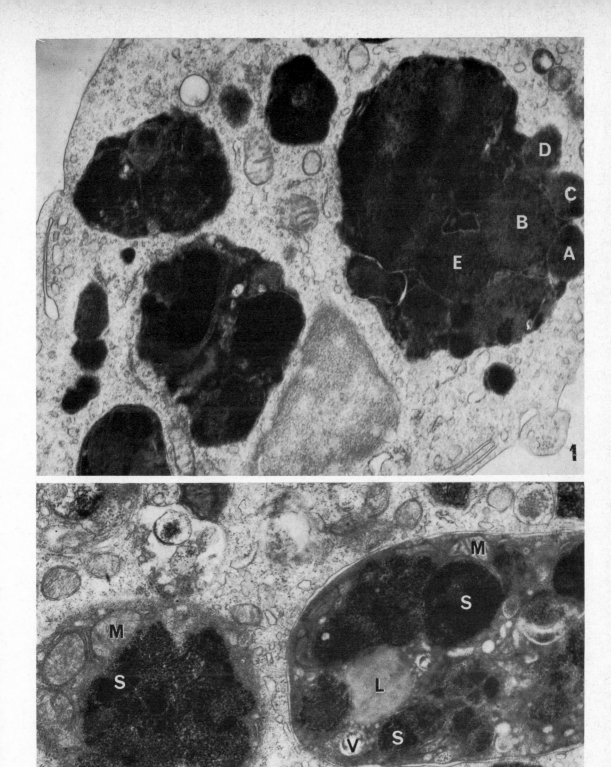

The ability of many mammalian cells to rid themselves of residual bodies seems to be strictly limited if not entirely non-existent. The mounting accumulation of residual bodies (lipofuscin) with age in various organs and the indefinite persistence of siderosomes (haemosiderin) after haemorrhage bear clear testimony to this fact. However, the cytolysosomes (autophagic vacuoles) and residual bodies (see below) that occur in erythrocytes are an exception. Appearances are seen which suggest that these cells can expel such bodies, and there is also evidence that they surrender them to the spleen during their passage through this organ.

Many and varied are the appearances of the contents of cytolysosomes seen in erythrocytes and reticulocytes (*Plates 144 and 145*). In some instances a portion of the haemoglobinized cytoplasm is seen sequestrated in a single-membrane-bound autophagic vacole. This no doubt represents an early stage of formation of one variety of cytolysosome (*Plate 145, Fig. 1*). Later stages of evolution are represented by bodies containing membranous structures, myelin figures and electron-dense material. Other cytolysosomes, particularly those seen in reticulocytes, at times contain recognizable organelle remnants derived from ribosomes, mitochondria and cytomembranes. This could be one of the ways in which the reticulocyte disposes of its organelles as it transforms into an erythrocyte.

It would appear that fully mature residual bodies, in which digestion of contents has been truly completed, rarely evolve from cytolysosomes that form in erythrocytes. Perhaps the enzyme content is not sufficiently potent or the cytolysosomes are expelled by the cell or removed by the spleen long before digestion is complete. The situation in the reticulocyte appears to be different, because siderosomes, which give a positive Prussian blue reaction and contain little else besides electron-dense iron-containing particles, are formed in these cells. Siderosomes found in erythrocytes are more likely to be those carried over from the normoblast or reticulocyte stage rather than new ones formed after the erythrocyte has matured.

Particularly intriguing are appearances which suggest that the contents of the autophagic vacuole are being or have been discharged. Such an appearance is depicted in *Plate 144, Fig. 2*, where a cytolysosome is seen to communicate with the exterior of the cell via a small opening. In other instances one sees 'holes' in erythrocytes (*Plate 145, Figs. 1 and 3*) which may appear empty or contain some residual lysosomal material and/or fibrillary proteinaceous precipitate identical in appearance to that seen outside the cell. Such appearances suggest that the contents of the cytolysosome have been discharged and the pit or vacuole created by this is now occupied by blood plasma.

Occasional erythrocytes containing cytolysosomes are found in normal individuals but many more are seen in patients with haematological disorders and in splenectomized individuals. We (Ghadially and Skinnider, unpublished observations) have seen them in the blood of various experimental animals, and they were found to be particularly frequent in the blood of some day-old rats we examined. Cytolysosomes have also been observed in the nucleated erythrocytes of amphibians (Tooze and Davies, 1965). Acid phosphatase activity has been demonstrated in the cytolysosome of human erythrocytes (Kent *et al.*, 1966; Schaeffer *et al.*, 1970).

Plate 144

From the peripheral blood of a splenectomized patient with hepatic cirrhosis (*Ghadially and Skinnider, unpublished electron micrographs*).

Fig. 1. Numerous pleomorphic cytolysosomes are seen in the cytoplasm of this erythrocyte. × 43,000
Fig. 2. Appearances seen here (arrow) suggest that a cytolysosome is about to discharge its contents. × 43,000

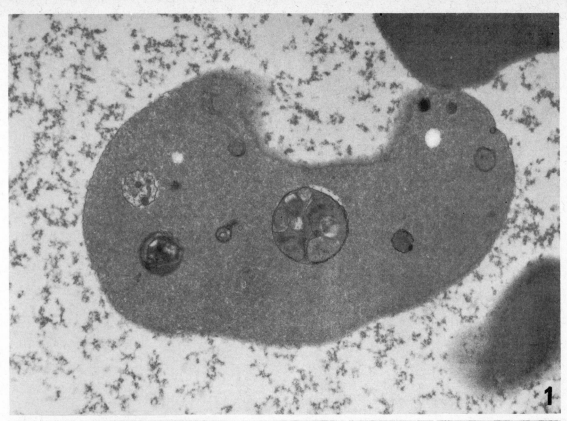

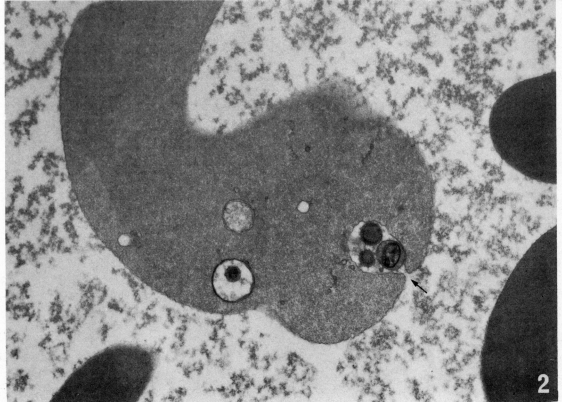

327

A detailed study of cytolysosomes in human erythrocytes and reticulocytes by Kent *et al.* (1966) has revealed many points of interest. According to them, 0·1–0·3 per cent of erythrocytes from normal individuals contain cytolysosomes. A tenfold increase in the percentage of erythrocytes containing cytolysosomes was noted in patients with haematological disorders and intact spleen, and an increase of similar magnitude was found in persons whose spleen had been removed after traumatic rupture and who had no haematological disorder.

The most profound increase, however, was noted in individuals whose spleen had been removed as a treatment of certain haematological disorders. Thus 16·3 per cent of the erythrocytes contained cytolysosomes in a post-splenectomized case of haemolytic anaemia, while the largest increase (36·5 per cent) was seen in a post-splenectomized case of haemoglobin C disease. These values were obtained by counting red blood cell profiles in ultrathin sections, so it stands to reason that the true incidence of cytolysosomes must be far greater than these figures.

The increase in cytolysosomes seen after splenectomy, both in normal individuals and in patients with haematological disorders, clearly shows that the spleen plays an important role in their removal and that in its absence cytolysosomes in erythrocytes are not eliminated efficiently. The situation here is reminiscent of the removal of siderotic granules (siderosomes) from erythrocytes. Siderocytes (erythrocytic cells containing siderosomes) are only rarely seen in normal blood but they are of common occurrence in post-splenectomized cases of haemolytic anaemia. The experiments of Crosby (1959) where [15]Cr-labelled siderocytes were transfused into normal and splenectomized subjects have shown that the number of detectable siderocytes diminishes rapidly in normal but not in splenectomized individuals. The loss, however, is in iron granules (siderosomes) and not cells, for the reduction in the number of Prussian-blue-positive siderocytes is not associated with a concurrent reduction of labelled donor cells. This demonstrates that the spleen can remove siderotic granules (siderosomes) without destroying the erythrocyte that contained them. The process by which this is achieved is referred to as 'pitting'. Crosby (1959) has defined the pitting function of the spleen as 'its ability to remove a solid particle from the cytoplasm of a red cell without destroying the cell itself much as a housewife plucks the stone from a cherry without crushing the fruit'.

The pitting function of the spleen, however, is not specific for siderosomes. In the absence of this organ various 'solid particles' such as Howell–Jolly bodies, Heinz bodies and malarial parasites are apt to be more numerous in the circulating erythrocytes. Thus, although the actual uptake of cytolysosomes by the spleen has not been demonstrated, it seems highly likely that the spleen is involved in their removal.

Plate 145

Fig. 1. A portion of erythrocyte cytoplasm, showing an early stage of cytolysosome formation (A) where a portion of the haemoglobinized cytoplasm appears sequestrated in a vacuole. The clear space (arrow) is probably a shrinkage artefact. Two other lucent vacuoles (B and C) are interpreted as cavities left behind after most of the lysosomal contents have been discharged. From a splenectomized case of thrombocytopenic purpura. × 85,000 (*Ghadially and Skinnider, unpublished electron micrograph*)

Fig. 2. Sequestrated haemoglobinized cytoplasm (H) and myelin figures (arrow) form the contents of this cytolysosome in an erythrocyte. From the same case as *Plate 114*. × 85,000 (*Ghadially and Skinnider, unpublished electron micrograph*)

Fig. 3. Transverse (T) and longitudinal (L) sections through pits left behind after discharge of lysosomal contents. From the same case as *Plate 144*. × 17,000 (*Ghadially and Skinnider, unpublished electron micrograph*)

Fig. 4. A cytolysosome (C) and a siderosome (S) are seen in this reticulocyte from a case of Hodgkin's disease with sideroblastic anaemia. × 50,000 (*Ghadially and Skinnider, unpublished electron micrograph*)

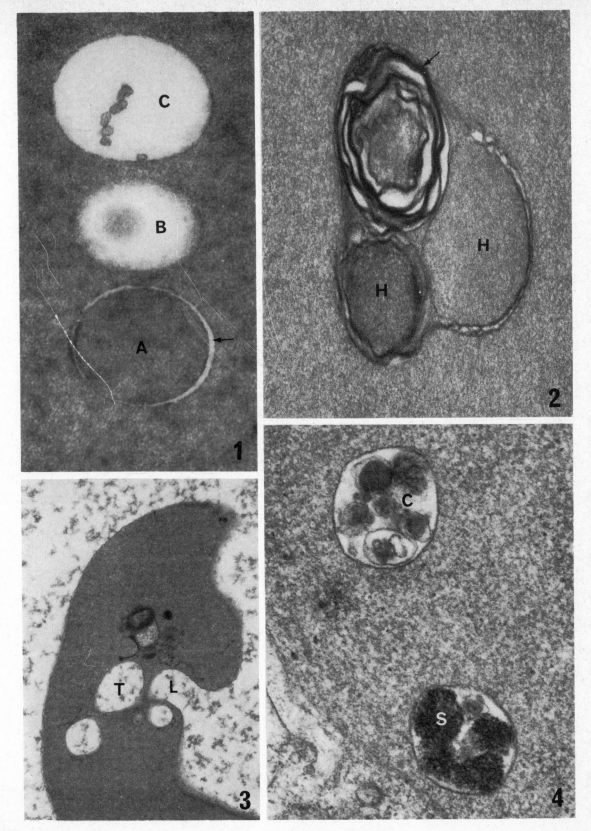

329

The morphological heterogeneity of the granules of the neutrophil leucocyte has long been recognized (Florey, 1962). At first, it was thought (Bessis and Thiery, 1961) that the various forms of granules represented different developmental stages of but a single granule type. Later work has shown this view to be incorrect, but there is still uncertainty as to how many different varieties of granules are present. Various lysosomal enzymes and also a variety of antibacterial substances such as lysozyme and phagocytin are present in these granules, but the distribution of these among the various types of granules is not established unequivocally.

It is now universally accepted that neutrophils of rabbit and man contain at least two distinct types of granules: a primary or azurophilic granule, and a secondary or specific granule (*Plate 146*) (Bainton and Farquhar, 1966, 1968; Wetzel *et al.*, 1967a, b; Dunn *et al.*, 1968). It is also clear that they are formed quite independently, at different periods of cell maturation. The primary granule is formed during the promyelocyte phase, while secondary granules are produced during later stages of neutrophil maturation (metamyelocyte, myelocyte and band form) after primary granule formation has virtually ceased. Recent ultrastructural, cytochemical and biochemical studies have indicated the existence of a tertiary granule which develops at a relatively late stage of neutrophil development (segmented forms) (Baggiolini *et al.*, 1969; Scott and Horn, 1970a).

Rabbit neutrophil (heterophil) polymorphs have been studied more extensively than any other. Here the three types of granules have been isolated and analysed. It has been shown that both primary and tertiary granules contain sulphated mucopolysaccharides and numerous acid hydrolases, including acid phosphatase, but myeloperoxidase is found only in the primary granules. There is evidence that the primary granules of human neutrophils also contain myeloperoxidase (Dunn *et al.*, 1968). Thus both the primary and tertiary granules are acceptable as primary lysosomes but the former are somewhat atypical because of their perioxidase content. The secondary granules of rabbits are known to contain alkaline phosphatase and various antibacterial substances. Thus secondary granules are not considered to be lysosomal in nature since they do not contain acid phosphatase or other typical lysosomal enzymes.

In the rabbit the primary granule presents as a single-membrane-bound electron-dense body approximately $0.8~\mu$ in diameter. The smaller $(0.3~\mu)$ primary granule of man may be round or elliptical, and as it matures a crystalloid develops in its interior.

Plate 146

Fig. 1. In this osmium-fixed immature neutrophil from human bone marrow the large dense primary granules (P) are easily distinguished from the smaller, less dense secondary granules (S). The presence of a well defined Golgi complex (G) and very small granules (arrows) of a density similar to the secondary granules suggests that the cell is at a stage of development where secondary granule production is in progress. × 27,000

Fig. 2. In this glutaraldehyde-fixed neutrophil from the peripheral blood of man, the secondary granules (S) are markedly extracted and appear electron lucent. A dense crystalloid (arrow) difficult to discern within the dense primary granules is present. × 28,000

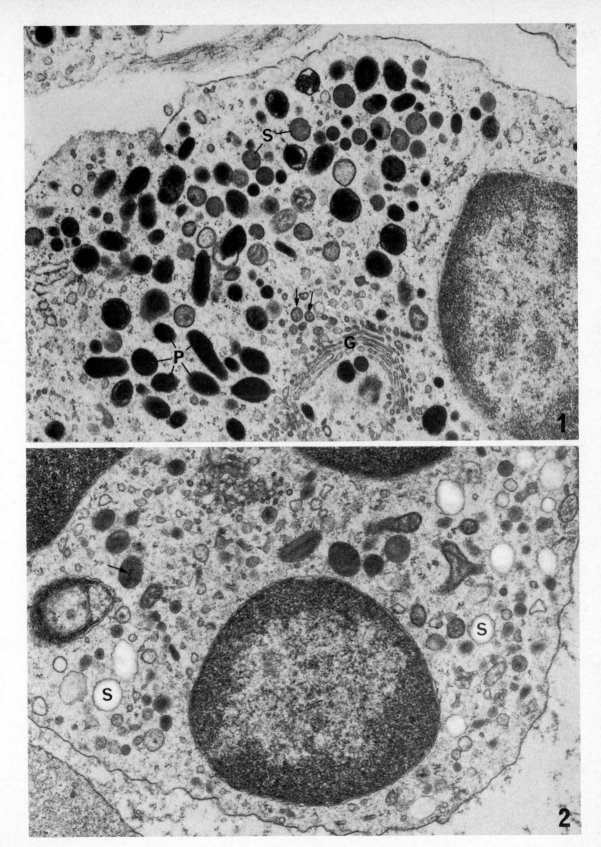

331

The secondary granules in both rabbit and man are less electron dense than the primary granules. In glutaraldehyde-fixed preparation of buffy coat from human blood the secondary granules are often slightly or markedly extracted. In such instances they present as electron-lucent granules with or without a denser periphery (*Plate 146*). The tertiary granules are small pleomorphic bodies seen mainly in mature circulating polymorphs. In man they are moderately to markedly electron dense and are said to vary in shape from round to quite elongated bacilliform bodies (*Plate 147*). The pleomorphism of this group suggests that a fourth type of granule may also exist in neutrophils (Daems, 1968).

The capacity of neutrophil leucocytes to phagocytose various materials such as bacteria, fungi, fibrin and also antigen–antibody complexes has been amply demonstrated (Riddle and Barnhart, 1964; Zucker-Franklin and Hirsch, 1964; Zucker-Franklin, 1968). It has already been noted that such material is taken in by a process of phagocytosis and comes to lie in a single-membrane-bound structure called a phagosome (page 296). Fusion of neutrophil granules with the wall of the phagosome and subsequent release of enzymes into the phagosome converts it into a phagolysosome, where the digestion of ingested material occurs. (Phagocytosis of bacteria by neutrophils is illustrated on *Plate 129*.) Ultrastructural studies show that all three types of granules fuse with the phagosome, and that this leads to a degranulation of the neutrophil. No new granules are formed after such an event.

It is thought that microtubules facilitate the association of neutrophil granules with the phagosome, for agents such as colchicine and vinblastine which are known to disrupt micro-tubules also interfere with the process of degranulation and phagolysosome formation, but phagocyte activity (i.e. phagosome formation) is unimpaired. On the other hand, cytochalasin B, which is thought to interfere with the action of contractile microfilaments, impairs phagocytosis and the uptake of bacteria—many of which remain adhered to the cell surface (for references, see Malawista *et al.*, 1971).

The manner in which the energy requirements for the phagocytic act and the killing of ingested organisms are met has been the subject of many studies (for references, see below). These indicate that the energy required for phagocytosis derives from glycolysis, but that the energy required for the events which follow is dependent upon oxidative metabolism and increased oxygen utilization. This marked increase in oxygen consumption is accompanied by oxidation of glucose via the hexose monophosphate shunt and hydrogen peroxide production, which is an important factor in the killing of certain organisms.

In certain inherited diseases, such as chronic granulomatous disease and Chediak–Higashi syndrome, there is a decreased ability to cope with some infections. There is no apparent abnormality of the immunological defence mechanism and it is thought that the defect resides in the neutrophil polymorph. In chronic granulomatous disease there is no impairment of phagocytosis, and according to most workers neither is there derangement of the fusion mechanism between granules and the phagosome, although according to Heyne *et al.* (1972) there may be 'a defect of the positive granule-taxis to the phagocytic vacuole'.

Plate 147

In this osmium-fixed polymorphonuclear neutrophil from peripheral blood of man, the primary and secondary granules cannot be confidently identified. It is worth noting that this is not infrequently the case. However, numerous bacilliform tertiary granules (arrows) are evident in this cell. These, together with the segmented nucleus, numerous glycogen particles (in circles) and an atrophic Golgi complex (G) represented by a few vesicles, are indicative of maturity in this leucocyte. Also seen is a lipid droplet (L). × 22,000

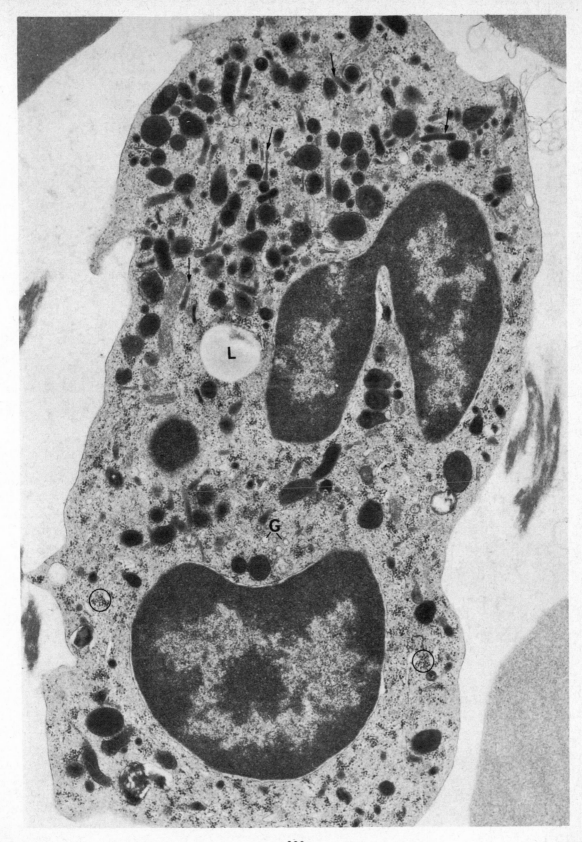

333

However, it has been shown that the neutrophils from these patients fail to show the burst of oxidative metabolism and hydrogen peroxide generation that follows the ingestion of particles by normal neutrophils. Several lines of investigation have indicated that it is this deficiency which is the bactericidal defect. Thus, for example, the neutrophils of these patients can kill fairly effectively organisms such as streptococci and pneumococci which generate hydrogen peroxide and thus contribute to their own destruction, but they are unable to cope with many Gram-negative pathogens and staphylococci that contain catalase which breaks down hydrogen peroxide. The many interesting aspects of phagocytic function and dysfunction and other defects such as myeloperoxidase deficiency are beyond the scope of this brief essay. For this information and support of statements made above the following papers and reviews should be consulted: Baehner and Nathan (1967, 1968), Holmes *et al.* (1966), MacFarlane *et al.* (1967), Quie *et al.* (1968), Klebanoff (1968, 1971), Klebanoff and White (1969), Elsbach *et al.* (1969), Spicer and Hardin (1969), Thompson *et al.* (1969), Lehrer (1971).

The Chediak–Higashi syndrome has been reported to occur in man, mink, mice and cattle (Beguez-Cesar, 1943; Higashi, 1954; Chediak, 1962; Kritzler *et al.*, 1964; Lutzner *et al.*, 1967; Padgett *et al.*, 1964; Padgett, 1967, 1968; Davis *et al.*, 11971). In all these species, large membrane-bound granules (acid-phosphatase-positive) occur in leucocytes and also in some other cell types. It is, however, worth noting that only a few granules in the neutrophils are so affected and that many others are of normal size. The significance and mechanism of production of the large granules in the neutrophil leucocytes have been interpreted in different ways by various workers. Thus they have been thought to be autophagic vacuoles, examples of toxic granulation, fused granules, or agglomerations of material liberated from normal granules and abnormally large granules produced by a failure of the mechanism which controls normal granule size. In mink neutrophils, Davis *et al.* (1971) found that pleomorphic primary granules, some smaller than normal and others larger than normal, were produced. However, the really large granules (megagranules) were produced by the fusion of primary granules. Secondary granules were not involved in the fusion process and appeared normal in size and number (*Plate 148*).

Certain prominent basophilic granules seen in neutrophils in various infections and other pathological states are often referred to as 'toxic' granules. Ultrastructural studies have not as yet clearly defined the nature of these granules. Spicer and Hardin (1969) have interpreted such granules seen after the injection of endotoxin as mucopolysaccharide-rich primary granules. Zucker-Franklin (1968) observed such granulation in phagocytosis experiments conducted with rheumatoid factor complexed with aggregated γ-globulin, and interpreted toxic granules as phagosomes and phagolysosomes.

The Döhle body which is also seen in a variety of infections and other disorders appears to be quite different from toxic granules. According to Cawley and Hayhoe (1972), the characteristic basophilia and pyroninophilia of these bodies is due to focal aggregates of rough endoplasmic reticulum in the neutrophil leucocyte.

Plate 148

Figs. 1 and 2. Neutrophils of mink with the homologue of the Chediak–Higashi trait of humans, showing large atypical granules (megagranules). One of these appears to be formed by the fusion of numerous large primary granules, as indicated by the arrows. The secondary granules (SG) are not involved in the fusion process and appear normal in size and number. $\times 23,000$; $\times 23,000$ (*From Davis, Spicer, Greene and Padgett, 1971*)

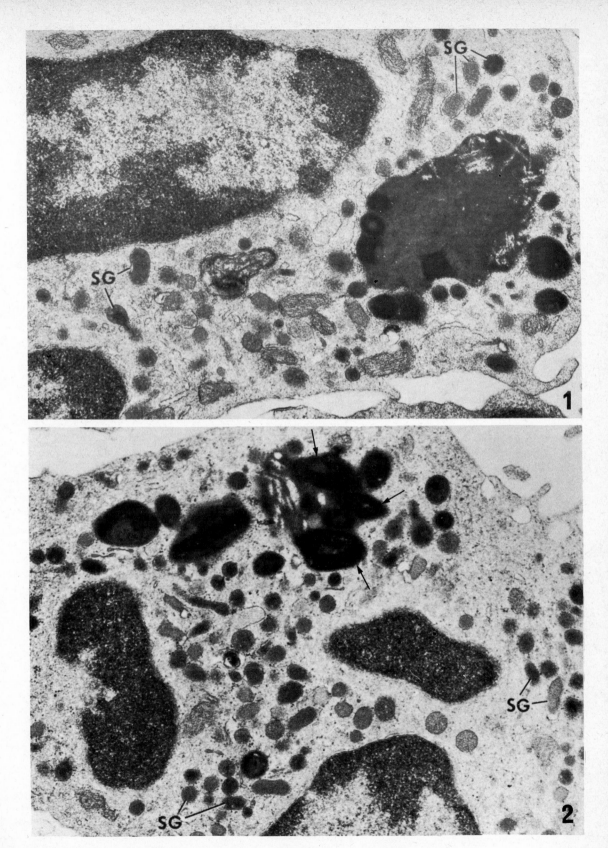

335

Despite numerous studies, the role of the eosinophil leucocyte in inflammation and allergic states is poorly understood. Since the eosinophilic granules of this leucocyte have now been shown to contain acid phosphatase (Ghidoni and Goldberg, 1966; Hudson, 1966) and also other hydrolases (Archer and Hirsch, 1963; Archer, 1963; Dunn et al., 1968), they are considered to be a variety of lysosome. Functionally, the ability of the eosinophil leucocyte to phagocytose foreign material has been demonstrated, as has the fusion of eosinophil granules with phagosomes to form secondary lysosomes. Electron microscopic studies show that eosinophils can phagocytose: (1) ferritin–antiferritin complexes (Sabesin, 1963); (2) zymosan particles (Zucker–Franklin and Hirsch, 1964); (3) mycoplasma (Zucker–Franklin et al., 1966); (4) E. coli (Cotran and Litt, 1969); (5) antigen–antibody complexes (Ishikawa et al., 1971); and (6) Candida albicans (Ishikawa et al., 1972).

The eosinophil granules of man, guinea-pig, rabbit, rat, mouse, cat, orang-utan, chimpanzee, sheep, cattle, horse and mink have been studied and numerous variations of internal structure have been described (for references, see Yamada and Sonoda, 1970).

In most mammalian species the precursors of the eosinophil granules (in the eosinophilic myelocyte) present as dense homogeneous rounded bodies, and there is evidence that they are produced either directly from the rough endoplasmic reticulum or by rough endoplasmic reticulum and Golgi complex in the manner that secretory granules are usually produced. As the cell matures, part of the granule content crystallizes, forming one or more plate-like structures which alter the form of the granule to an ellipsoid or discoid biconvex lens-like form. Details of the successive stages of maturation of the human eosinophil leucocyte and its granule have been described recently by Hardin and Spicer (1970).

According to Scott and Horn (1970b), not all granules of human eosinophil leucocytes mature in this fashion, for some immature granules are secreted by the eosinophil. A somewhat similar sentiment has been expressed by Barnhart and Riddle (1963), who found, with fluorescent antibody staining techniques, that profibrinolysin occurs in immature but not mature eosinophil granules of rabbit bone marrow. They therefore suggested that profibrinolysin was released during maturation. Unequivocal evidence of granule discharge by eosinophils has been seen by us (Skinnider and Ghadially 1974) in the bone marrow of a child thought to have chronic active hepatitis and in which there were episodes of disseminated intravascular coagulation. There was an increase in the population of eosinophils and many of them appeared to have discharged their granule content into the intercellular space which contained much fibrin (Plate 149). These observations support the idea that the eosinophil leucocyte may have a role in fibrinolysis.

Plate 149

An immature eosinophil from human marrow where crystalloid formation has commenced in only a few granules (C). Some of the granules are seen being discharged via deep channels (delineated by arrowheads) extending to the cell surface. Material presumed to be secretory product (P) and fibrin (F) is seen in the matrix. × 27,000 (*From Ghadially and Skinnider, (1974)*).

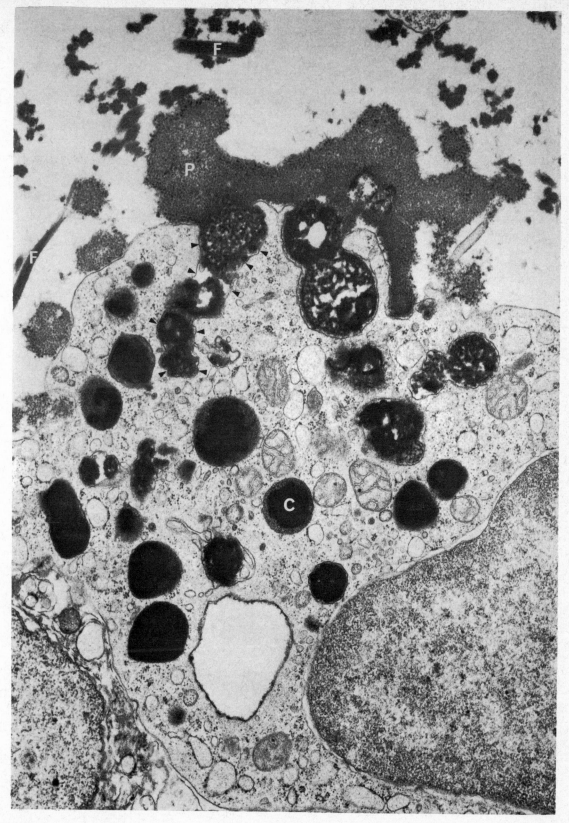

337

The dense core or plate of the mature granule has been examined by a number of workers and in some (but not all) species a crystalline structure has been demonstrated (Osako, 1959). In the mouse the crystalloid is described as a lamellated structure of alternating light and dense lines about 50 Å thick (Sheldon and Zetterquist, 1955). In the cat it is said to be a cylindrical structure composed of concentric lamellae (Bargmann and Knoop, 1958). In man and laboratory rodents, the crystal is described (Miller et al., 1966) as having a cubic lattice with a repeat of approximately 40 Å for man and 30 Å for rodents. Like many other protein crystals, in longitudinal section the crystal presents as a series of evenly spaced parallel dense lines, in oblique sections as a series of dense off-register dots, and in transverse sections as a square array of dots.

We (Ghadially and Parry, 1965b) have drawn attention to the fact that examination of electron micrographs of eosinophils published in the literature reveals two distinct appearances. In some eosinophils the granules have a dense core and pale crystalloid, while in others these densities are reversed (*Plate 150*). We have not as yet encountered an indubitable instance where both varieties of granules occurred in one eosinophil, but we have on a few occasions seen eosinophils, some containing one variety and some the other variety of granule in a single ultrathin section. The significance of this is not apparent from available data. That such appearances can be produced by different methods of handling the tissue is not doubted but this can hardly explain the phenomenon noted by us or by G. Kelenyi (personal communication) who has observed both varieties of granules in a single eosinophil.

Charcot–Leyden crystals and their association with focal accumulations of eosinophils have long been known to pathologists. They have been seen in the sputa of patients with bronchial asthma, pulmonary ascariasis and tropical eosinophilia. They have also been found in granulomas associated with tissue invasion by helminths, in the stools of patients with amoebic dysentery and indeed in many other instances where disintegrating eosinophils occur. They can also be produced *in vitro* by lysing eosinophils with a surface-active agent (Aerosol OT), and ultrastructural studies (El-Hashimi, 1971) show that these crystals are derived from the granule of the eosinophil leucocyte. The fact that Charcot–Leyden crystals occur in primates such as man and monkey, but not in a variety of other species studied, once more stresses species differences in these granules.

The chemical composition of the core and cortex of the eosinophil granule has not been fully elucidated. According to Miller et al. (1966), the available evidence suggests that the crystalline core comprises a specific peroxidase known to occur in the eosinophil granule, but Cotran and Litt (1969) believe that the peroxidase resides in the matrix rather than the crystalline core. The granule is also said to be rich in phospholipids and various lysosomal enzymes, such as cathepsin, ribonuclease, aryl sulphatase, β-glucuronidase and acid phosphatase. Antibacterial agents such as phagocytin and lysozyme were not found in eosinophil granule preparations by Archer and Hirsch (1963). The eosinophilia of the granules is said to be due to the presence of a high concentration of basic proteins. (For further references and details, see Miller et al., 1966; Hardin and Spicer, 1970; Scott and Horn, 1970b; Bainton and Farquhar, 1970.)

Plate 150

Fig. 1. The granules of this eosinophil leucocyte show an electron-dense crystalloid (C) set in a paler granular matrix (M). From human bone marrow fixed in osmium and stained with uranium and lead. × 34,000

Fig. 2. The granules of this eosinophil leucocyte show pale crystalloids (C) set in a granular matrix (M) (similar to the matrix of some of the crystalloids in *Fig. 1*) or a highly electron-dense matrix (D). From another specimen of human bone marrow prepared in the same way as *Fig. 1*. × 30,000

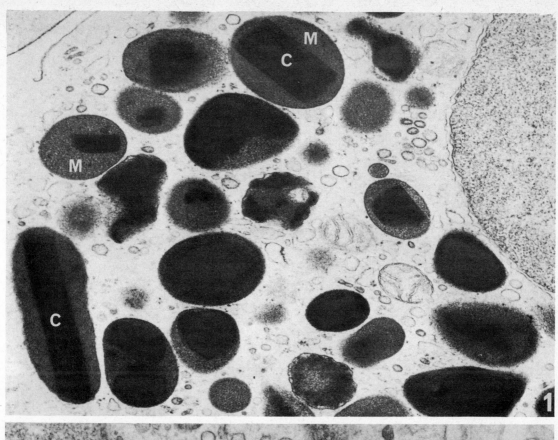

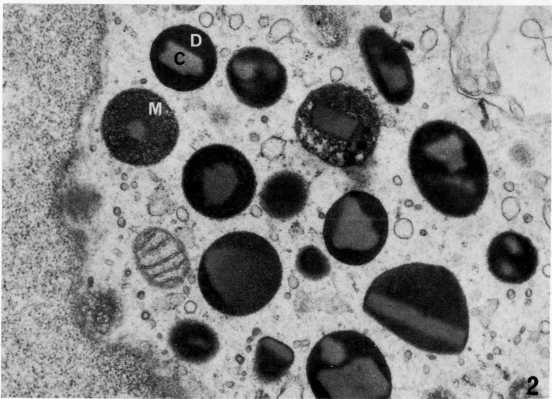

The abnormal brown or black pigmentation of the colonic mucosa, which is now called melanosis coli, was first described by Cruveilhier in 1829. The term 'melanosis coli' was first used by Virchow (1857). Melanosis coli is dismissed rather briefly as a curiosity in most standard works on medicine and pathology for, although the condition is tinctorially spectacular, it is not thought to produce severe or specific symptomatology on its own. Symptoms which may be manifest are attributed to the accompanying conditions and these range from 'idiopathic' constipation to carcinoma of the colon.

Much interest has, however, existed for a long time regarding the nature of the pigment, the aetiology of the condition and its alleged association with carcinoma of the colon. Numerous excellent clinical, pathological, histochemical and experimental studies have been reported (McFarland, 1917; Stewart and Hickman, 1931; Bockus et al., 1933; Roden, 1940; Speare, 1951; Cabanne and Couderc, 1963), and the ultrastructure of the pigment granules and the colon (Plates 151 and 152) in this condition has been reported and reviewed by us (Ghadially and Parry, 1966b, 1967).

Many of the earlier theories regarding the causation of melanosis coli have long been abandoned. For instance, the view that ingestion of heavy metals, with their deposition in the colon, was responsible for the pigmentation has not been supported by chemical analyses of affected tissue, and the belief that the colonic pigment may be of haematogenous origin as suggested by Virchow was discarded when attempts to produce the condition experimentally by introducing blood into the colon of animals failed. The more recent ideas regarding the aetiology of this condition centre around two factors: firstly, disturbance of bowel function resulting in chronic constipation, and, secondly, the chronic ingestion of cathartics of the anthracene group such as cascara, senna, aloes and rhubarb. The role of such purgatives (particularly cascara) in the production of this condition has been unequivocally demonstrated by experimental studies both in monkey and man (Bockus et al., 1933; Roden, 1940; Speare, 1951), for, by sigmoidoscopy and biopsy, the colonic pigment has been observed to wax and wane with cycles of administration and withdrawal of the drug.

The theory that the pigment might be melanin or a melanin-like substance has been popular for a long time. McFarland (1917) classified the pigment as intermediate between true melanin and the wear and tear pigment, lipofuscin. Cabanne and Couderc (1963) believe that both lipofuscin and malanin occur in the pigment granules of melanosis coli. The histochemical studies

---

Plate 151

Fig. 1. Low power view of colonic mucosa from a case of melanosis coli, showing numerous single-membrane-bound dense bodies (D) lying between the nucleus (N) and some mucus droplets (M). Besides electron-dense particles and granules, these bodies also contain some membranous structures. They are thus interpreted as being derived from autophagic vacuoles (cytolysosomes). × 12,500 (From Ghadially and Parry, 1966b)

Fig. 2. High power view of two cytolysosomes found in a colonic epithelial cell; one (A) contains numerous vesicles and a mitochondrion, while the other (B) contains endoplasmic reticulum, mitochondria and glycogen. From the same case as Fig. 1. See also Plate 160, which shows glycogen-containing cytolysosomes found in submucosal cells of the same patient. × 24,000 (From Ghadially and Parry, 1966b)

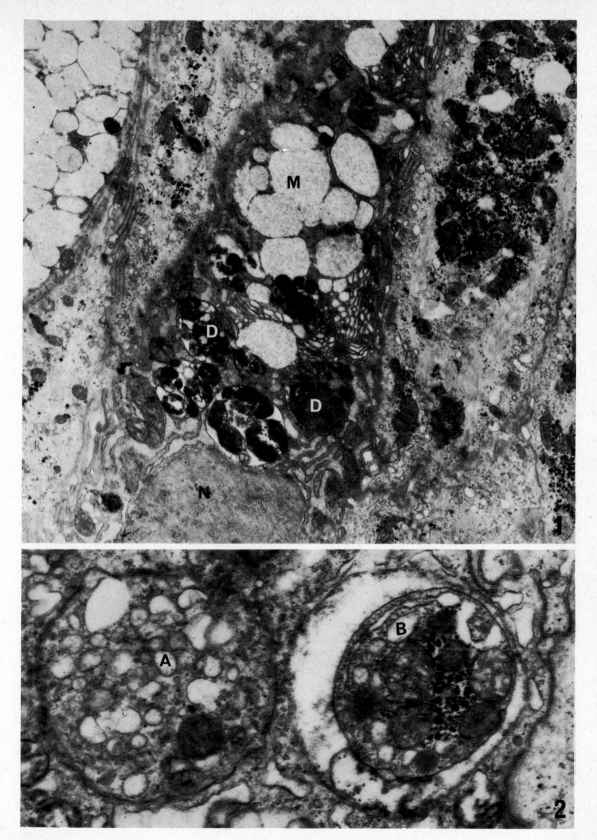

conducted by us (Ghadially and Parry, 1966b) also showed that the pigment gives many of the reactions for both lipofuscin and melanin. In our hands, Lillie's Nile blue sulphate reaction, however, supports the idea that the pigment is lipofuscin.

A strong argument against the pigment being melanin is that no melanocytes are found in this region. If one accepts the now well proven fact that melanin is synthesized in melanocytes and melanosomes which contain the enzyme tyrosinase, then it is clear that melanin derived by enzymic oxidation, as found in the skin or the eye, cannot be produced in sites where these cells are absent. Nevertheless, it is known that oxidation of many cyclic compounds such as phenol, pyrogallol, indole and skatole may produce melanin-like compounds without the intervention of melanocytes (Thomson, 1962). Thus, while one can exclude the occurrence of what might be called 'normal' melanin derived from the enzymatic oxidation of tyrosine, one cannot rule out the possibility of melanin-like pigment derived from other sources in other ways.

Our (Ghadially and Parry, 1966b) ultrastructural studies, however, clearly showed that the pigment granules in melanosis coli contain lipofuscin, since many lysosomes and residual bodies were found in the colonic tissue. Cytolysosomes containing mitochondria, endoplasmic reticulum and glycogen were seen in the mucosal cells (*Plate 151*), even though in the past light microscopists have repeatedly reported that no pigment is seen in the mucosa but only in the macrophages in the submucosa. However, it is true that most of the pigment granules do lie in this region (submucosa), for the electron microscope shows huge phagocytic cells filled with innumerable single-membrane-bound bodies with electron-dense, granular and amorphous material and also occasionally lipid droplets so characteristic of lipofuscin (*Plate 152*). Such bodies are akin to residual bodies containing lipofuscin known to be derived by lysosomal activity (page 306).

It has already been noted that cytolysosomes are commonly produced as a result of organelle injury by many drugs and other noxious influences (page 300). It would therefore appear that melanosis coli is a condition produced by the damaging effect of some constituent in the anthracene group of purgatives, which leads to the formation of cytolysosomes and lipofuscin-containing residual bodies. Whether such bodies also contain some pigmented material produced in the gut or present in the purgative, which is phagocytosed by cells, remains a matter of conjecture.

Plate 152

Fig. 1. Typical pigment-bearing macrophages found in the colonic submucosa from a case of melanosis coli. It will be noted that with the electron microscope the pigment granules have the morphology of lipofuscin-containing residual bodies. × 5,000 (*From Ghadially and Parry, 1966b*)

Fig. 2. High power view of some of the residual bodies shown in *Fig. 1*. Note the presence of electron-dense particles and granules and also the occasional medium-density lipid droplets (L) so characteristic of lipofuscin. Compare with other lipofuscin-containing residual bodies shown in *Plates 134 and 135*. × 21,000 (*From Ghadially and Parry, 1966b*)

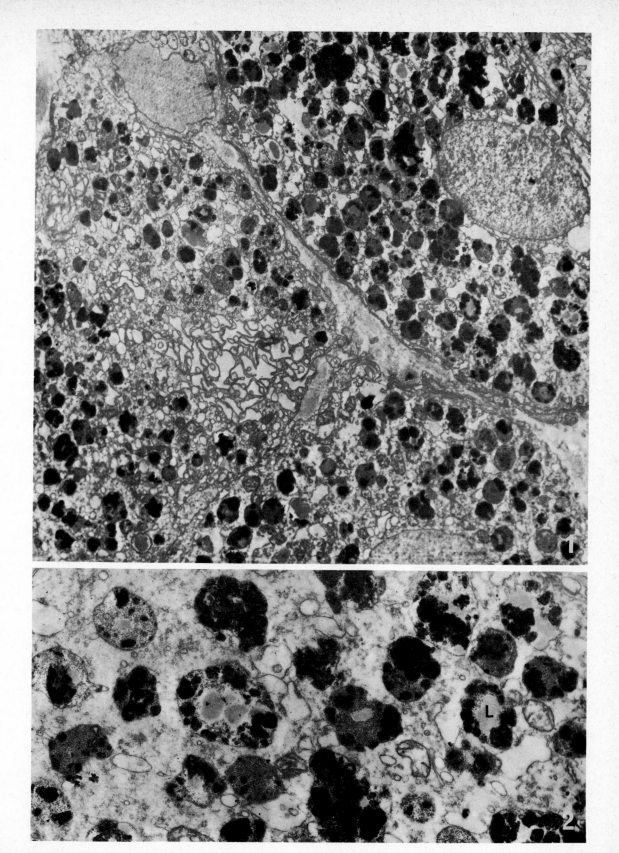

343

Numerous studies attest to the fact that lysosomes and their enzymes play an important role in inflammatory processess (de Duve and Wattiaux, 1966; Weissmann, 1966, 1967; Houck, 1968; Fell, 1969). It would appear that some of the morphological changes seen in chronic inflammation are due to the release of hydrolytic enzymes from lysosomes that develop in the cells of the inflamed tissues and/or from the neutrophils and macrophages which invade the tissue. In order to illustrate this point the following discussion will be limited to one well known and much studied example of chronic inflammation, namely rheumatoid arthritis. A striking increase in the number of lysosomes (*Plates 128, 153 and 154*) has been observed in the synovial membrane in rheumatoid arthritis by many workers (Barland *et al.*, 1964; Wyllie *et al.*, 1966; Norton and Ziff, 1966; Ghadially and Roy, 1967a, 1969), but it must be noted that this change is not specific and that modest increases in lysosomes are common enough in many pathological synovial membranes.

The manner in which the initial increase in lysosomes occurs is not clear. One theory is that the lysosomes are derived from phagocytosis of the interaction product of γ-globulin and the rheumatoid factor (Hollander *et al.*, 1965; Robinson, 1966). On the other hand, Hamerman (1966) has suggested that phagocytosis of bacterial or cell fragments may be the exciting factor. It is also possible that the noxious aetiological agent, whatever it might be, primarily damages cell organelles and leads to the formation of an excessive number of cytolysosomes. Our morphological studies reveal that fibrin, cell fragments and erythrocytes are avidly phagocytosed by synovial cells (*Plate 154*). At times electron-dense iron-containing particles are also formed in these lysosomes and cytoplasmic matrix. Such particles have been regarded as ferritin by other workers (Muirden, 1966; Muirden and Senator, 1968). Acid phosphatase has been demonstrated in the lysosomes of synovial cells, and also of leucocytes occurring in the synovial fluid from cases of rheumatoid arthritis (*Plate 128*) (Barland *et al.*, 1964; Coimbra and Lopes-Vaz, 1967).

Results of biochemical studies are in keeping with morphological observations, for an increase in the amount of lysosomal enzymes has been demonstrated in the synovial membrane (Luscombe, 1963; Hendry and Carr, 1963) and in the synovial fluid (Jacox and Feldmahn, 1955; Lehman *et al.*, 1964; Caygill and Pitkeathly, 1966). The bulk of the hydrolytic enzymes are probably derived from the synovial cell lysosome and not from the lysosomes of polymorphonuclear leucocytes, as there is no concurrent increase in the amount of alkaline phosphatase (Lehman *et al.*, 1964), an enzyme found in the secondary granules of this leucocyte.

Thus biochemical findings clearly show that hydrolytic enzymes are liberated from lysosomes, and many theories have been proposed to explain this phenomenon. Regarding the rupture of lysosomes in other situations, de Duve (1963) has suggested that cellular over-feeding, especially with non-consumable diets, may be responsible and he has also suggested that newly formed

---

Plate 153

Synovial intimal cells from cases of rheumatoid arthritis. (*From Ghadially and Roy, 1967a*)

Fig. 1. Type A synovial cell containing numerous lysosomes (L). × 34,000

Fig. 2. The lysosome containing membranous formations may be interpreted as a cytolysosome (C) for there is little to suggest that it is a phagolysosome derived from an ingested cell fragment. Other lysosomes containing medium-density material are present. The limiting membrane of one of these organelles is ruptured and the contents appear to have extruded into the cytoplasm (arrow). Whether this is an artefact of tissue collection or a meaningful *in vivo* event is debatable. × 30,000

Fig. 3. Lysosomal pleomorphism is depicted in this electron micrograph. × 32,000

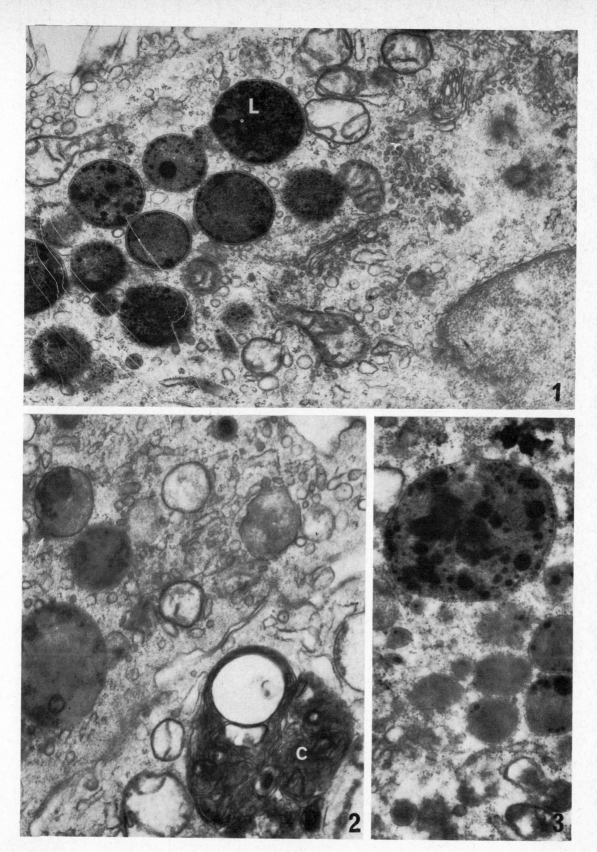

345

lysosomes may be unstable and rupture easily. An extension of this concept was proposed by Page Thomas (1969) who coined the term 'intraphagosomal dyslysis' to describe this phenomenon. Here it is visualized that there is a relative lack of lysosomal enzymes, in the presence of an appropriate substrate (i.e. basically digestible) due to excessive phagocytosis, and that such a situation leads to an increased production of primary lysosomes (via a feedback mechanism), some of which discharge their contents extracellularly. Besides the above-mentioned mechanisms there is also the obvious one whereby lysosomal enzymes are liberated when synovial cells die and suffer autolysis.

Whatever the mechanisms involved may be, it is clear that a release of lysosomal enzymes does occur and it is not difficult to visualize that this can lead to tissue damage and inflammation; indeed it has been shown that inflammation of subcutaneous tissues or joints can be produced by injections of purified extracts of leucocyte lysosomes (Weissmann, 1966). The inflammation and cell damage engendered by the release of hydrolytic enzymes may in turn lead to further phagocytic activity by the synovial cells and the production of more lysosomes. One could speculate that ultimately a situation might well be reached in which the joint tissues proceed to destroy themselves without any further assistance from the noxious agent which initiated the process.

It is interesting to note that agents of value in the treatment of joint diseases, such as glucocorticoids, chloroquine, gold salts and colchicine, are said to stabilize lysosomal membranes while agents which labilize lysosomal membranes, such as streptolysin S and filipin, produce inflammation, arthritis and destruction of cartilage when injected into the joint (Weissmann and Thomas, 1964; Weissmann et al., 1965; Pras and Weissmann, 1966).

The idea that lysosomal dysfunction and release of hydrolytic enzymes may be operative in rheumatoid arthritis is also supported by the work of Page Thomas (1969). He has shown that intra-articular injections of dyes such as Congo red which inhibit lysosomal hydrolases, or the injection of polysaccharides such as chitin which presumably do not suffer rapid degradation in synovial lysosomes, lead to a morphological picture (light microscopic studies) reminiscent of rheumatoid arthritis. Such changes include synovial hyperplasia, villus formation, focal round cell aggregation and plasma cell infiltration.

Plate 154

This electron micrograph illustrates the manner in which synovial cells phagocytose fibrinoid material and cellular detritus from the joint space. Fibrinoid material can be seen lying in the joint space at A. This material can also be seen trapped between the cell wall and a filopodium at B. Furthermore, morphologically similar material can be demonstrated in single-membrane-bound structures (phagosomes and phagolysosomes) within the cell (C). These appearances are compatible with the idea that the fibrinoid material is being phagocytosed by the synovial cell to form phagosomes. Phagosomes are known to acquire hydrolytic enzymes by fusing with primary lysosomes arising from the Golgi complex and thus become converted into phagolysosomes. It is interesting, therefore, to observe that many small vesicles, probably arising from the Golgi complex (G), are seen adjacent to or in contact with (arrows) the phagosomes and phagolysosomes. An early stage of phagocytosis of a cell fragment is also probably depicted in this picture. In the joint space is seen a cell fragment (identified as such by micropinocytotic vesicles (P) along its plasma membrane, intracytoplasmic filaments (F), lipid droplet (L) and electron-dense bodies (D), (probably lysosomal in nature) ensheathed by a somewhat complex array of synovial cell filopodia. ×43,000 (*From Ghadially and Roy, 1967a*)

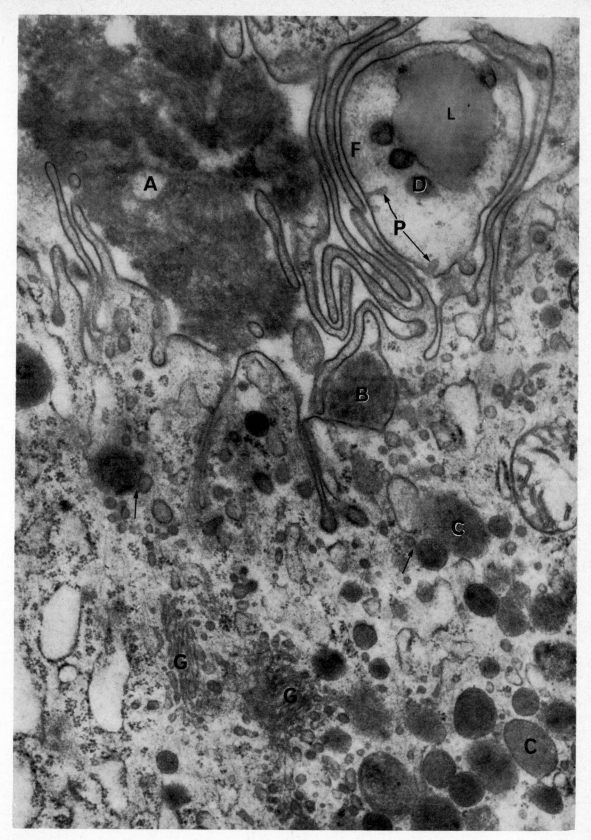

347

LYSOSOMES IN THE LIVER OF THE TUMOUR-BEARING HOST

A marked increase in numbers and also to some extent in the size of peribiliary dense bodies, occurs in rats bearing a variety of tumours (*Plate 155*). This phenomenon, noted by us (Ghadially and Parry, 1965a) during ultrastructural studies on the liver of rats bearing carcinogen-induced subcutaneous sarcomas in their flank, has since been extended by us and others to other tumour–host systems. It should be noted that such changes occur in the liver free of metastatic growth. Before this interesting phenomenon is discussed it is worth recalling some aspects of tumour–host relationships.

Many striking morphological and biochemical changes occur in animals bearing tumours. One such constant phenomenon is an increase in liver weight (Medigreceanu, 1910; Abels *et al.*, 1942; Annau *et al.*, 1951), associated with a decreased liver catalase activity (Greenstein, 1954). This increase in liver weight is particularly remarkable, for it occurs in an animal that is wasting away to satisfy the metabolic needs of the growing tumour (see the review by Wiseman and Ghadially, 1958). It is now clear that the increase in liver weight is due to an increase in liver nitrogen (Yeakel, 1948; Sherman *et al.*, 1950; Yeakel and Tobias, 1951) as well as in liver water content (McEwan and Haven, 1941). Thus, protein is diverted not only to the growing tumour mass but also to the liver of the cachectic host.

Despite these changes, light microscopic examination of routine histological preparations of the liver reveals either a normal-looking organ or one that shows only some cloudy swelling and occasional focal necrosis. However, ultrastructural studies have shown various changes in the liver of the tumour-bearing host. These include dilatation and vesiculation of the endoplasmic reticulum, mitochondrial swelling, reduction of liver glycogen, decrease in the number of micro-bodies (see also page 375) and an increase in hepatocellular lysosomes of the peribiliary dense body variety. No overt increase in cytolysosomes was seen by us in the liver except during the terminal stages of the life of the tumour-bearing host (Ghadially and Parry, 1965a; Parry and Ghadially, 1966). The increase in hepatocellular lysosomes can be quite marked; at times as many as 40–120 peribiliary dense bodies may be seen around a single bile canaliculus. This change has been quantified by Parry (1969) and shown to be statistically significant. He found that the mean number of lysosomes per bile canalicular section was 1·8 in the normal state, 4·4 in an animal bearing a 6 g tumour, and 9·8 in an animal with a 293 g tumour.

An increase in hepatocellular lysosomes or lysosomal enzymes has been observed in: (1) rats bearing 9:10-dimethyl-1:2-benzanthracene-induced sarcoma (Ghadially and Parry, 1965); (2) rats bearing a variety of transplanted tumours such as squamous cell carcinoma of the skin, mammary carcinoma, hepatoma and sarcomas (Parry and Ghadially, 1967; Rogers *et al.*, 1967; Butterworth, 1970; Shamberger *et al.*, 1971); and (3) patients with hepatoma (Ghadially and Parry, 1966a), Hodgkin's disease (*Plate 156*) and renal and gastric carcinoma (Schersten *et al.*, 1969; Stein *et al.*, 1971).

Plate 155

Fig. 1. Numerous lysosomes are seen in this hepatocyte of a rat bearing a carcinogen-induced subcutaneous sarcoma. × 30,000 (*From Parry, 1969*)

Fig. 2. Liver of rat bearing a carcinogen-induced sarcoma, showing a collection of lysosomes and other organelles. Tissue was fixed in glutaraldehyde and treated according to the method of Holt and Hicks (1961). The intensely electron-dense material deposited mainly on or close to the lysosomal membranes (arrows) is lead phosphate resulting from acid phosphatase activity in these organelles. × 40,000 (*From Ghadially and Parry, 1965a*)

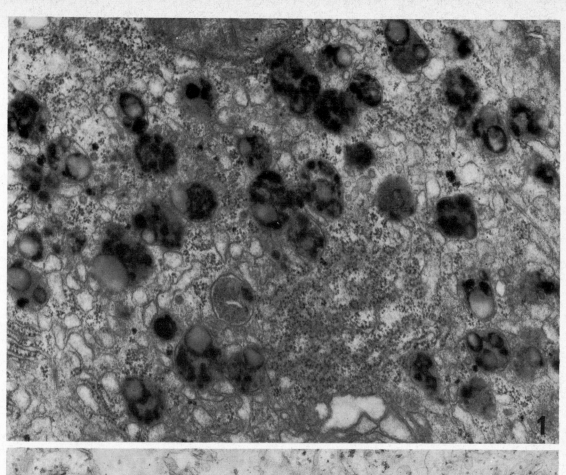

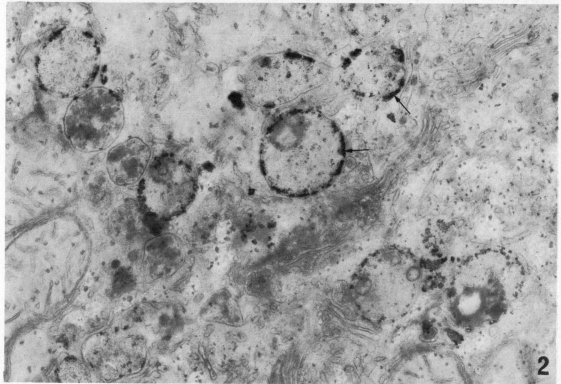

Furthermore, we (Parry and Ghadially, 1969) have demonstrated that necrotic tumour tissue does not produce this effect, but injections of toxohormone, a much-studied polypeptide that can be extracted from a variety of tumours of experimental animals and man, does produce a statistically significant increase in the lysosome population (Parry and Ghadially, 1970).

Contrary to the above-mentioned findings is the report by Khandekar *et al.* (1972), who studied the liver of rats bearing Walker carcinoma and failed to find an increase in lysosomes but noted a hypertrophy of the smooth endoplasmic reticulum. The Walker carcinoma is one of the fastest growing transplantable tumours and almost invariably shows much necrosis, so the absence of a detectable increase in hepatocellular lysosomes may have been dependent upon a paucity of viable tumour tissue. In mice bearing Ehrlich ascites tumours also, no increase in hepatocellular lysosomes has been noted (Tsukada *et al.*, 1966; Lee and Aleyassine, 1971). This may be due to the type of tumour used, to species differences and to the difficulty of confidently distinguishing peribiliary dense bodies in this animal.

The significance of the increase in the hepatocellular lysosomes noted in tumour-bearing rats is not too clear. A possible explanation would be that toxohormone (and perhaps also other toxic substances produced by viable tumour tissue) is taken into the hepatocytes by a process of endocytosis and is then sequestrated into the peribiliary dense bodies, as are metals and detergents. Thus, this phenomenon could be looked upon as a detoxicating mechanism of survival value to the tumour-bearing animal.

The precise cause of death of animals bearing tumours is not known. In the absence of haemorrhage or gross involvement of vital organs by tumour metastasis, it seems likely that death results from some biochemical disturbance. This idea is neither new nor novel and has been mooted by many workers (see review by Wiseman and Ghadially, 1958). Furthermore, it is known that some remarkable changes occur in the tumour-bearing rat just prior to its death. During this terminal stage in the life of the animal, when most of the normal tissues are markedly wasted, even the rate of growth of the tumour becomes retarded and the liver shows a sudden marked weight loss (McEwen and Haven, 1941). At this stage the light microscope shows degenerative changes and sizeable areas of hepatic necrosis. With the electron microscope the most salient feature is a swelling and rupture of many hepatocellular lysosomes, and also the presence of numerous cytolysosomes (Parry and Ghadially, 1966). The appearances seen are in fact consistent with the 'suicide bag' hypothesis of de Duve whereby it is proposed that rupture of lysosomes or seepage of lysosomal enzymes could occur and the released acid hydrolases would then damage or kill the cell. Although in this instance one cannot be certain from static pictures alone whether cell death precedes or follows the rupture of lysosomes, there are now many situations in which tissue damage and cell death are thought to be mediated in this fashion (for examples see pages 346 and 352).

Plate 156

Hepatocytes from a patient with Hodgkin's disease, showing a large number of lysosomes. × 10,000 (*Ghadially, Ailsby and Larsen, unpublished electron micrograph*)

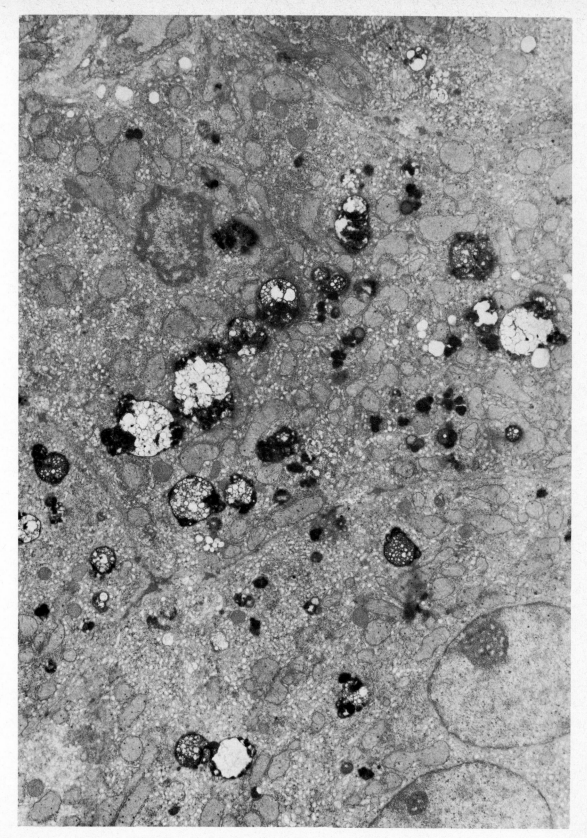

Numerous studies now attest to the fact that lysosomes in various tissues come to contain metals such as iron (*Plate 157*), copper, silver, lead, mercury, gold and thorium when compounds of these metals are administered to experimental animals (Kent *et al.*, 1963a, b, 1965; Koenig, 1963; Taylor, 1965; Ganote *et al.*, 1966; Ericcson, 1969; Wessel *et al.*, 1969; Southwick and Bensch, 1971; Oryschak and Ghadially, 1974). Needless to say this is not the only site where metals can accumulate, but in various tissues lysosomes are the most common site of accumulation of a variety of metals and there is evidence that this may be of pathological import.

The accumulation of metals in lysosomes is also seen in some human diseases. For example, in Wilson's disease where there is an inherited disorder of copper metabolism, copper accumulates in the hepatocellular lysosomes (Goldfischer and Moskal, 1966), while in haemochromatosis iron deposits occur in hepatocellular lysosomes (Novikoff and Essner, 1960; Kent *et al.*, 1963a, b). Similarly, in human and experimentally produced chronic haemarthrosis, synovial membrane and articular cartilage come to contain numerous iron-loaded lysosomes (siderosomes). (For a review and references, see Ghadially and Roy, 1969.) In all the above-mentioned instances, varying degrees of cell necrosis and/or fibrosis are seen, and it has long been debated to what extent, if any, the metallic deposits in the tissue are responsible for such pathological changes. Against such an idea it has been pointed out that: (1) the normal fetal and newborn liver can tolerate concentrations of copper comparable to those seen in Wilson's disease and that large amounts of copper may be present with normal liver function; (2) in haemochromatosis the cirrhosis can antedate the iron deposits, and there is evidence that nutritional deficiences are also operative which may be responsible for the cirrhosis; and (3) the studies of Kent *et al.* (1963a, b) have shown that substantial quantities of iron are not taken up by hepatocytes unless these cells are first damaged by hepatotoxic agents.

Nevertheless, there is now a growing body of evidence which suggests that metallic deposits in lysosomes are not innocuous and that they can contribute to the pathological changes that occur. It is thought that if lysosomes are overloaded with undigestible materials or substances which inhibit enzyme activity so that their normal function is impaired, rupture of lysosomes or seepage of enzymes may occur, leading to cell damage and necrosis.

Thus, *in vitro* studies on isolated lysosomes show that the activity of acid phosphatase and β-glucuronidase is inhibited by copper and that a high concentration of iron or copper can produce a marked leakage of enzymes from lysosomes (Schaffner *et al.*, 1962; Koenig and Jibril, 1962). Similarly, Allison *et al.* (1966) have shown that when lung macrophages take up silica or asbestos, the lysosomal membrane becomes unstable and hydrolytic enzymes are released into the cell with resultant injury or cell death. Such an event releases the silica particles which are taken up once more by another cell, and it seems feasible that such a self-perpetuating mechanism could lead to necrosis and fibrosis as seen in silicosis.

Finally, it is worth pointing out that certain non-metallic (but also indigestible) materials can also lead to a release of hydrolytic enzymes. For example, when the detergent Triton WR-1339 is injected into rats, the hepatocellular lysosomes become loaded with this material and there is a marked increase in the acid phosphatase content of the bile, no doubt released from the lysosomes.

Plate 157

Iron-loaded electron-dense lysosomes found in the liver of a rabbit that had received injections of iron dextran. × 48,000

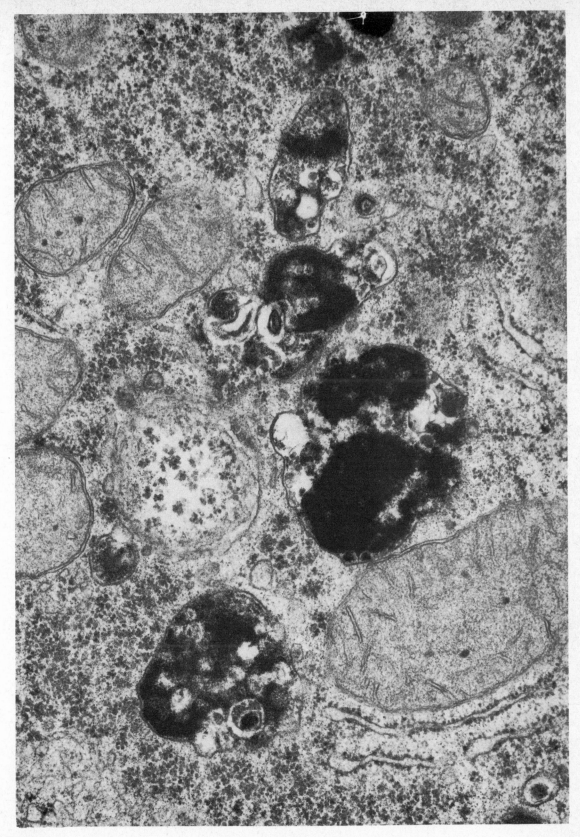

COLLAGEN IN LYSOSOMES

It is now generally accepted that collagen is formed extracellularly by polymerization of tropo-collagen molecules secreted by fibroblastic cells, but the manner in which collagen is resorbed or removed is less well established. In most tissues collagen appears to be quite stable and provides little opportunity for studying its turnover. This phenomenon may be studied more readily in situations where substantial amounts of collagen are degraded and removed over a short period of time. Such situations include the resorption and remodelling of tissues which occurs during: (1) morphogenesis and metamorphosis (Weber, 1963; Gross, 1964; Usuku and Gross, 1965; Woessner, 1968); (2) wound healing (Grillo and Gross, 1967; Ross and Odland, 1968; Williams, 1970; and (3) post-partum involution of the uterus (Deno, 1936; Harkness and Moralee, 1956; Maibenco, 1960; Lobel and Deane, 1962; Woessner, 1962, 1965; Luse and Hutton, 1964; Schwarz and Guldner, 1967; Parakkel, 1968).

Many biochemical studies have shown a marked increase in acid hydrolases in tissues under-going resorption and remodelling (Harkness and Morales, 1956; Lobel and Deane, 1962; Weber, 1963; Goodall, 1965; Woessner, 1965, 1968) but early attempts to demonstrate collagen-ase in such systems were unsuccessful. However, Gross and his colleagues (Gross et al., 1963; Gross, 1964; Grillo and Gross, 1967) have now succeeded in demonstrating a collagenase in regressing tissue which at physiological temperatures and neutral pH (hence non-lysosomal) is capable of lysing a reconstituted collagen gel.

Animal collagenase, unlike bacterial collagenase, appears to be incapable of completely degrading collagen, and Woessner (1968) has proposed that the collagen fibres are first frag-mented by the collagenase (non-lysosomal) and then picked up by phagocytic cells where they suffer further degradation within lysosomes.

Electron microscopic studies on the involuting rat and mouse uterus support such a concept, for cells with numerous single-membrane-bound vacuoles, containing collagen fibres are found (*Plate 158*). While some of these may be no more than invaginations of the plasma membrane surrounding collagen fibres lying in the matrix, others have to be regarded as phagosomes and phagolysosomes since disintegrating collagen and acid phosphatase activity have been demon-strated in these structures and in the dense bodies that evolve from them (Parakkal, 1968).

Some doubt exists as to the nature and origin of the phagocytic cell involved in the removal of collagen in the involuting uterus. Luse and Hutton (1964) concluded that it was the fibroblast which was responsible, while Schwarz and Guldner (1967) interpreted these cells as histiocytes and Parakkal (1968) called them macrophages. Often these cells are well endowed with rough endoplasmic reticulum and Golgi complex. Such features are more characteristic of fibroblasts than macrophages. However, it is the resting or not too active macrophage which shows a paucity of these organelles. Stimulated macrophages in culture (Cohn et al., 1966a, b; Sutton and Weiss, 1966) and wound healing (Ross and Odland, 1968) show a hypertrophy of these organelles, which would be necessary for the synthesis of hydrolytic enzymes and primary lysosomes.

Plate 158

Figs. 1 and 2. Macrophages from involuting rat uterus three days after delivery, showing vacuoles containing collagen fibres cut in various planes. In this preparation the fibres (C) in the matrix and vacuoles are intensely stained by phos-photungstic acid. ×20,000; ×22,000

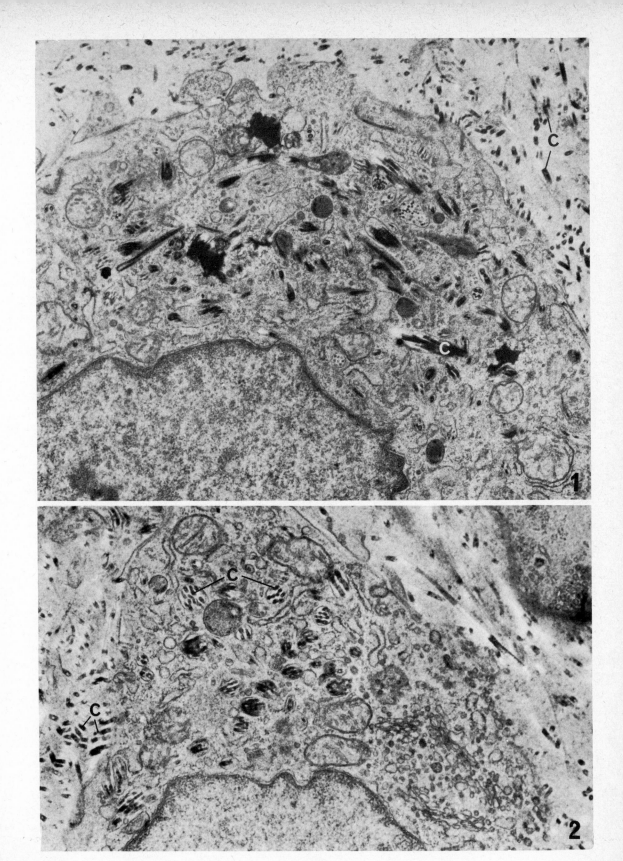

GLYOGEN IN LYSOSOMES

Accumulation of glycogen in lysosomes has been noted in various conditions, but the most marked example of this is seen in Pompe's disease (glycogenosis type II). In this genetic disorder there is a deficiency of lysosomal acid α-glucosidase (acid maltase) and large amounts of glycogen accumulate in single-membrane-bound bodies (Hers, 1963; Baudhuin *et al.*, 1964; Cardiff, 1966; Hug and Schubert, 1967; Hers and Van Hoof, 1969), which are regarded as lysosomes because acid phosphatase activity has been demonstrated in them (Garancis, 1968). Such bodies occur mainly in the liver and kidney but are also found in various other organs (Witzleben, 1969). Excessive deposits of glycogen occur in muscle but much of this is outside the lysosomes. It has been suggested that this is probably due to lysosomal rupture by mechanical pressure from muscle contraction. This could also account for the destruction of myocardium and skeletal muscle seen in Pompe's disease since acid hydrolases would also be released (Hers and Van Hoof, 1969). This disease is also said to occur in cats, and glycogen-laden lysosomes have been described in the central nervous system of this animal (Sandstrom *et al.*, 1969).

It is worth noting that single-membrane-bound structures containing glycogen have been seen in muscle tissues on several occasions, and not only in Pompe's disease. We have noted occasional membrane-bound structures containing glycogen in biopsies of human myocardium and skeletal muscle (*Plate 159, Figs. 1 and 2*). Engel (1969) states that 'occasional glycogen sequestration in simple membrane-bound sacs can be seen in any myopathy while the presence of glycogen in ordinary autophagic vacuoles with heterogeneous contents occurs in chloroquine myopathy, polymyositis and other chronic myopathies'. His studies show that acid phosphatase activity can be demonstrated in some but not all single-membrane-bound structures containing glycogen.

Autophagic vacuoles (cytolysosomes) containing glycogen have been found in many cell types. Even so, it must be conceded that this is rather a rare phenomenon. We have found cytolysosomes containing glycogen in: (1) erythrocytic cells from cases of erythroleukaemia (*Plate 159, Fig. 3*); (2) a carcinogen-induced subcutaneous sarcoma of the rat (*Plate 159, Fig. 4*); (3) a normal cow hepatocyte (*Plate 159, Fig. 5*); (4) cells in the mucosa and submucosa in melanosis coli (*Plate 160, Figs. 1 and 2*); and (5) in the liver of rats treated with toxohormone (Parry and Ghadially, 1970). In most of these examples, the amount of glycogen found in the lysosome is quite small and one might contend that such inclusions of glycogen in cytolysosomes are fortuitous.

On rare occasions a few glycogen particles have been seen in some lysosomes of apparently normal adult rat liver, but lysosomes containing much glycogen are not hard to find in the livers of newborn mice and rats (Jézéquel *et al.*, 1965; Phillips and Unakar, 1967).

Plate 159

Figs. 1 and 2. Membrane-bound collections of glycogen found in human myocardium. Whether these structures are lysosomes or not is debatable. From the same case as *Plate 42*. × 30,000; × 30,000

Fig. 3. Mature erythrocyte with monoparticulate glycogen in cytoplasm (arrow) and numerous cytolysosomes (C), some containing glycogen deposits. × 130,000 (*From Skinnider and Ghadially, 1973*)

Fig. 4. Glycogen-containing cytolysosomes found in a tumour cell. From a subcutaneous sarcoma of the rat, produced by 9:10-dimethyl-1:2-benzanthracene. × 28,000 (*Parry and Ghadially, unpublished electron micrograph*)

Fig. 5. Cytolysosome containing glycogen rosettes found in a normal cow hepatocyte. × 72,000 (*Ghadially and Ailsby, unpublished electron micrograph*)

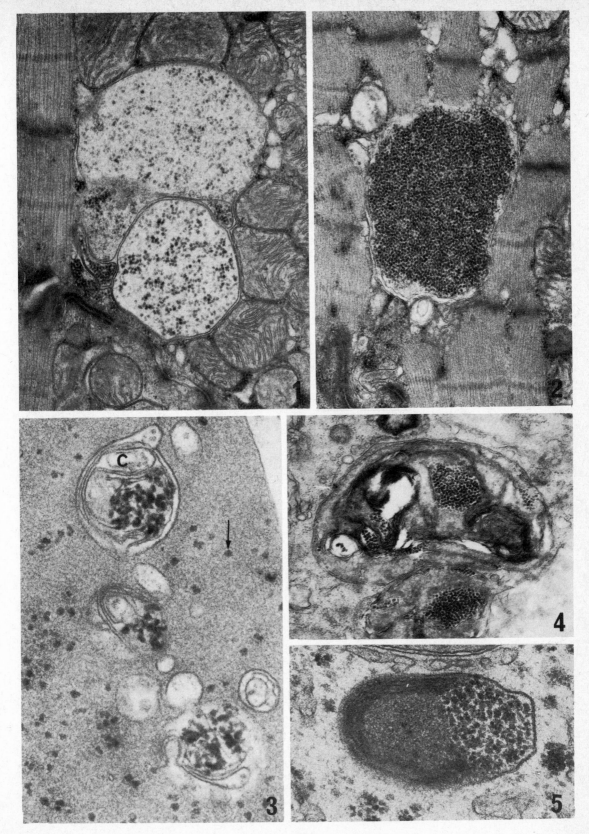

Glycogen-laden lysosomes have not been reported to occur in experimental animals after the administration of barbiturates, and our Ghadially and Bhatnagar, unpublished observations) experience is in keeping with this. However, in one hamster that had been so treated numerous massively enlarged glycogen-containing lysosomes were noted (*Plate 160*). Some of the lysosomes seemed to contain only glycogen but others contained small amounts of membranous and osmiophilic material also. The appearances seen here are in every way similar to those found in Pompe's disease but the significance of this finding is hard to assess on the limited data available. Glycogen-containing lysosomes have also been found in the kidney tubular cells of diabetic spiny mice (*Acomys cahirinus*) and in rats made hyperglycaemic by the administration of streptozotocin (Junod *et al.*, 1969; Orci *et al.*, 1970; Orci and Stauffacher, 1971). Here also some 'pure' glycogen-containing lysosomes were seen but others contained lipid and membranous structures as well as glycogen.

The functional basis of the accumulation of glycogen in lysosomes is not established unequivocally except in the case of Pompe's disease. Here it is clear that a genetic defect leading to the absence of a single lysosomal enzyme (acid maltase), necessary for the breakdown of glycogen to glucose, produces accumulations of glycogen in lysosomes. Although the lysosomal pathway for glycogen breakdown is said to be a minor one compared to phosphorylytic degradation, and the latter system is normal in patients with Pompe's disease, it is not difficult to visualize how, over a period of time, massive lysosomes containing glycogen develop.

Regarding the occurrence of glycogen-containing lysosomes in newborn animals, it is thought that there might be a transient enzyme deficiency in the lysosome during the neonatal period or that a relative deficiency develops due to a rapid increase of glycogen metabolism at this stage of life (Jézéquel *et al.*, 1965; Phillips and Unakar, 1967). In diabetic animals there is an excess of cytoplasmic glycogen in the kidney tubules; therefore a relative enzyme deficiency could develop due to the excessive amounts of substrate taken in by the lysosomes. On the other hand, one could speculate that there might be a primary diabetes-induced enzyme defect produced in these animals (Orci and Stauffacher, 1971). In this connection it may be noted that hyperglycaemia occurs in these animals and it has been found that the presence of glucose is known to diminish the activity α-1,4-glucosidase.

Plate 160

Figs. 1 and 2. Cytolysosomes containing glycogen found in an unidentified cell in the submucosa of a case of melanosis coli. *See also Plate 151, Fig. 2.* × 34,000; × 34,000 (*Ghadially and Parry, unpublished electron micrographs*)

Fig. 3. Lysosomes containing glycogen found in the hepatocyte of a hamster that had received phenobarbitone. × 36,000. (*Ghadially and Bhatnagar, unpublished electron micrograph*)

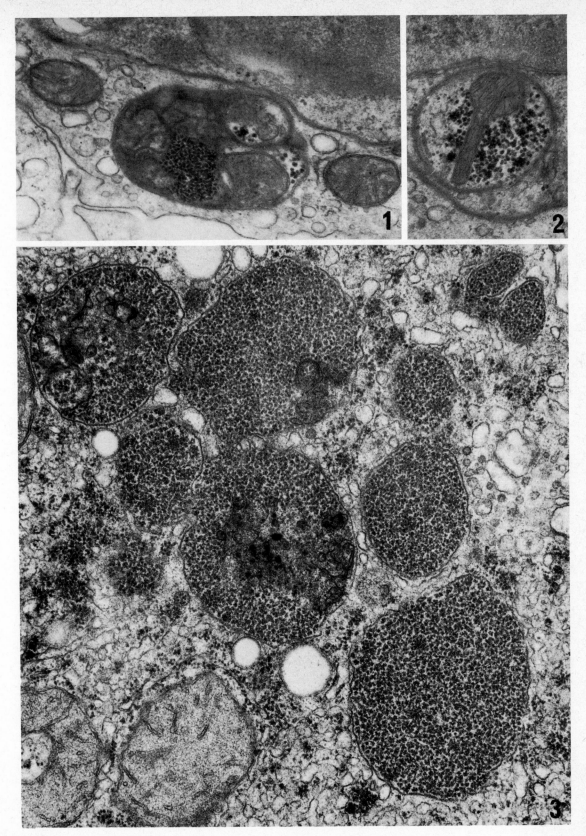

REFERENCES

Abels, J. C., Rekers, P. E., Binkley, G. E., Pack, G. T. and Rhoads, C. P. (1942). 'Metabolic studies in patients with cancer of the gastro-intestinal tract. II. Hepatic dysfunction.' *Ann. intern. Med.* **16**, 221

Adachi, M., Wallace, B. J., Schneck, L. and Volk, B. W. (1967). 'Fine structure of central nervous system in early infantile Gaucher's disease.' *Archs Path.* **83**, 513

Aikawa, M. and Sprinz, H. (1971). 'Erythrophagocytosis in the bone marrow of canary infected with malaria. Electron microscope observations.' *Lab. Invest.* **24**, 45

Allison, A. C., Harington, J. S. and Birbeck, M. (1966). 'An examination of the cytotoxic effects of silica on macrophages.' *J. exp. Med.* **124**, 141

Anderson, P. J. and Song, S. K. (1962). 'Acid phosphatase in the nervous system.' *J. Neuropath. exp. Neurol.* **21**, 263

Annau, E., Manginelli, A. and Roth, A. (1951). 'Increased weight and mitotic activity in the liver of tumor-bearing rats and mice.' *Cancer Res.* **11**, 304

Anton, E. and Brandes, D. (1968). 'Lysosomes in mice mammary tumors treated with cyclophosphamide.' *Cancer* **21**, 483

— — (1969). 'Role of lysosomes in cellular lytic processes. IV. Ultrastructural and histochemical changes in lymphoid tissue of thymectomized mice with wasting disease.' *J. Ultrastruct. Res.* **26**, 69

Archer, R. K. (1963). *The Eosinophilic Leucocyte.* Oxford: Blackwell Scientific

Archer, G. T. and Hirsch, J. G. (1963). 'Isolation of granules from eosinophil leukocytes and study of their enzyme content.' *J. exp. Med.* **118**, 277

Arnold, J. (1900). 'Uber Siderosis und siderofere Zellen, zugleich ein Beitrag zur "Granulalehre".' *Virchows Arch. path. Anat. Physiol.* **161**, 284

Bachmann, K. D. (1953). 'Uber das Lipofuscin der Leber.' *Virchows Arch. path. Anat. Physiol.* **323**, 133

Baehner, R. L. and Nathan, D. G. (1967). 'Leukocyte oxidase. Defective activity in chronic granulomatous disease.' *Science* **155**, 835

— — (1968). 'Quantitative nitroblue tetrazolium test in chronic granulomatous disease.' *New Engl. J. Med.* **278**, 971

Baggiolini, M. Hirsch, J. G. and De Duve, C. (1969). 'Resolution of granules from rabbit heterophil leukocytes into distinct populations by zonal sedimentation.' *J. Cell Biol.* **40**, 529

Bainton, D. F. and Farquhar, M. G. (1966). 'Origin of granules in polymorphonuclear leukocytes. Two types derived from opposite faces of the Golgi complex in developing granulocytes.' *J. Cell Biol.* **28**, 277

— — (1968). 'Differences in enzyme content of azurophil and specific granules of polymorphonuclear leukocytes. I. Histochemical staining of bone marrow smears.' *J. Cell Biol.* **39**, 286

— — (1970). 'Segregation and packaging of granule enzymes in eosinophilic leukocytes.' *J. Cell Biol.* **45**, 54

Balis, J. U. and Conen, P. E. (1964). 'The role of alveolar inclusion bodies in the developing lung.' *Lab. Invest.* **13**, 1215

— Delivoria, M. and Cohen, P. E. (1966). 'Maturation of postnatal human lung and the idiopathic respiratory distress syndrome.' *Lab. Invest.* **15**, 1530

Barden, H. (1969). 'The histochemical relationship of neuromelanin and lipofuscin.' *J. Neuropath. exp. Neurol.* **28**, 419

— (1970). 'Relationship of Golgi thiaminepyrophosphatase and lysosomal acid phosphatase to neuromelanin and lipofuscin in cerebral neurons of the aging Rhesus monkey.' *J. Neuropath. Exp. Neurol.* **29**, 225

Bargmann, W. and Knoop, A. (1958). 'Uber das granulum des eosinophilen.' *Z. Zellforsch. mikrosk. Anat.* **48**, 130

Barland, P., Novikoff, A. B. and Hamerman, D. (1964). 'Fine structure and cytochemistry of the rheumatoid synovial membrane, with special reference to lysosomes.' *Am. J. Path.* **44**, 853

Barnhart, M. I. and Riddle, J. M. (1963). 'Cellular localization of profibrinolysin (plasminogen).' *Blood* **21**, 306

Baudhuin, P., Hers, H. G. and Loeb, H. (1964). 'An electron microscopic and biochemical study of type II glycogenosis.' *Lab. Invest.* **13**, 1139

Beams, H. W., van Breeman, V., Newfang, D. M. and Evans, T. (1952). 'A correlated study of spinal ganglion cells and associated nerve fibers with the light and electron microscopes.' *J. comp. Neurol.* **96**, 249

Beguez-Cesar, A. (1943). 'Neutropenia cronica maligna familiar congranulaciones antipicas de los leucocitosi.' *Boln Soc. cuba. Pediat.* **15**, 900

Bessis, M. (1965). 'Cellular mechanisms for the destruction of erythrocytes.' *Semin. Hemat.* **2**, 59

— and Breton-Gorius, J. (1960). 'Aspects de la molecule de ferritine et d'apoferritine au microscope électronique.' *C.r. Acad. Sci., Paris* **250**, 1360

— and Thiery, J. P. (1961). 'Electron microscopy of human white blood cells and their stem cells.' *Int. Rev. Cytol.* **12**, 199

Biberfeld, P., Ericsson, J. L. E., Perlmann, P. and Raftell, M. (1966). 'Ultrastructural features of *in vitro* propagated rat liver cells.' *Z. Zellforsch. mikrosk. Anat.* **71**, 153

Bjorkerud, S. (1963). 'The isolation of lipofuscin granules from bovine cardiac muscle, with observations on the properties of the isolated granules on the light and electron microscopic levels.' *J. Ultrastruct. Res.* Suppl. 5

Bockus, H. L., Willard, J. H. and Bank, J. (1933). 'Melanosis coli. The etiologic significance of the anthracene laxatives: a report of forty-one cases.' *J. Am. med. Ass.* **101**, 1

Borst, M. (1922). *Pathologische Histologie.* Leipzig: Vogel

Brody, H. J. (1960). 'The deposition of aging pigment in the human cerebral cortex.' *J. Geront.* **15**, 258

Butterworth, S. T. G. (1970). 'Changes in liver lysosomes and cell functions close to an invasive tumour.' *J. Path.* **101**, 227

Cabanne, F. and Couderc, P. (1963). 'Melanose colique generalisée idiopathique. Etude anatomo-clinique et histochimique d'une observation.' *Annls Anat. path.* **8**, 609

Campiche, M. A., Gautier, A., Hernandez, E. I. and Reymond, A. (1963). 'An electron microscope study of the fetal development of human lung.' *Pediatrics* **32**, 976

360

Cardiff, R. D. (1966). 'A histochemical and electron microscopic study of skeletal muscle in a case of Pompe's disease (glycogenosis II).' *Pediatrics* **37**, 249

Cawley, J. C. and Hayhoe, F. G. J. (1972). 'The inclusions of the May–Hegglin anomaly and Dohle bodies of infection: an ultrastructural comparison.' *Br. J. Haematol.* **22**, 491

Caygill, J. C. and Pitkeathly, D. A. (1966). 'A study of beta-acetylglucosaminase and acid phosphatase in pathological joint fluids.' *Ann. rheum. Dis.* **25**, 137

Chediak, M. (1962). 'Nouvelle anomalie leucocytaire de caractère constitutionnel et familial.' *Nouv. Revue franc. Hematol.* **7**, 362

Cohn, Z. A. and Fedorko, M. E. (1969). 'The formation and fate of lysosomes.' In *Lysosomes in Biology and Pathology*, Vol. 1, p 43. Ed. by J. T. Dingle and H. B. Fell. Amsterdam and London: North Holland Publ.

— Hirsch, J. G. and Fedorko, M. E. (1966a). 'The *in vitro* differentiation of mononuclear phagocytes. IV. The ultrastructure of macrophage differentiation in the peritoneal cavity and in culture.' *J. exp. Med.* **123**, 747

— Fedorko, M. E. and Hirsch, J. G. (1966b). 'The *in vitro* differentiation of mononuclear phagocytes. V. The formation of macrophage lysosomes.' *J. exp. Med.* **123**, 757

Coimbra, A. and Lopes-Vaz, A. (1967). 'Acid phosphatase positive cytoplasmic bodies in leucocytes of rheumatoid synovial fluid.' *Arthritis Rheum.* **10**, 337

Corrin, B., Clark, A. E. and Spencer, H. (1969). 'Ultrastructural localization of acid phosphatase in the rat lung.' *J. Anat.* **104**, 65

Cotran, R. S. and Litt, M. (1969). 'The entry of granule-associated peroxidase into the phagocytic vacuoles of eosinophils.' *J. exp. Med.* **129**, 1291

Crosby, W. H. (1959). 'Normal functions of the spleen relative to red blood cells: a review.' *Blood* **14**, 399

Cruveilhier, J. (1829). *Anatomie Pathologique du Corps Humain*, **19**, 1; 18, 29. Paris: Baillière

Daems, W. T. (1968). 'On the fine structure of human neutrophilic leukocyte granules.' (letter to the editor) *J. Ultrastruct. Res.* **24**, 343

— Wisse, E. and Brederoo, P. (1969). 'Electron microscopy of the vacuolar apparatus.' In *Lysosomes in Biology and Pathology*, Vol. 1, p. 64. Ed. by J. T. Dingle and H. B. Fell. Amsterdam and London: North Holland Publ.

Davis, W. C., Spicer, S. S., Greene, W. B. and Padgett, G. A. (1971). 'Ultrastructure of bone marrow granulocytes in normal mink and mink with the homolog of the Chediak–Higashi trait of humans. I. Origin of the abnormal granules present in the neutrophils of mink with the C–HS trait.' *Lab. Invest.* **24**, 303

de Duve, C. (1963). 'The lysosome concept.' In Ciba Foundation Symposium on *Lysosomes*, p. 1. Ed. by A. V. S. de Reuck and M. P. Cameron. Edinburgh and London: Churchill Livingstone

— (1969). 'The lysosome in retrospect.' In *Lysosomes in Biology and Pathology*, Vol. 1, p. 3. Ed. by J. T. Dingle and H. B. Fell. Amsterdam and London: North Holland Publ.

— (1970). 'The role of lysosomes in cellular pathology.' *Triangle* **9**, 200

— and Wattiaux, R. (1966). 'Functions of lysosomes.' *A. Rev. Physiol.* **28**, 435

— Pressman, B. C., Gianetto, R., Wattiaux, R. and Appelmans, F. (1955). 6. Tissue fractionation studies. 'Intracellular distribution patterns of enzymes in rat liver tissue.' *Biochem. J.* **60**, 604

de Marsh, Q. B. and Kautz, J. (1957). 'The submicroscopic morphology of Gaucher cells.' *Blood* **12**, 324

Deno, R. A. (1936). 'Uterine macrophages in the mouse and their relation to involution.' *Anat. Rec.* **60**, 433

Diezel, P. B., Rossner, J. A., Koppang, N., Ritzhaupt, P. and Bartling, D. (1967). 'Juvenile form of amaurotic family idiocy. A contribution to the morphological, histochemical and electron microscopic aspects.' In *Inborn Diseases of Sphingolipid Metabolism*, p. 23. Ed. by S. M. Aronson and B. W. Volk. New York: Academic Press

Djaczenko, W., Filadoro, F. and Pezzi, R. (1969). 'On the presence of multivesicular bodies in *Leishmania donovani*.' *Experientia* **25**, 666

Dunn, W. B., Hardin, J. H. and Spicer, S. S. (1968). 'Ultrastructural localization of myeloperoxidase in human neutrophil and rabbit heterophil and eosinophil leukocytes.' *Blood* **32**, 935

Edwards, V. D. and Simon, G. T. (1970). 'Ultrastructural aspects of red cell destruction in the normal rat spleen.' *J. Ultrastruct. Res.* **33**, 187

El-Hashimi, W. (1971). 'Charcot–Leyden crystals. Formation from primate and lack of formation from nonprimate eosinophils.' *Am. J. Path.* **65**, 311

Elsbach, P., Zucker-Franklin, D. and Sansaricq, C. (1969). 'Increased lecithin synthesis during phagocytosis by normal leukocytes and by leukocytes of a patient with chronic granulomatous disease.' *New Engl. J. Med.* **280**, 1319

Engel, A. G. (1969). 'Acid maltase deficiency in adult life. Morphologic and biochemical data in 3 cases of a syndrome simulating other myopathies.' In *Muscle Diseases*. Excerpta Medica Int. Congr. Series No. 199

Ericsson, J. L. E. (1964). 'Absorption and decomposition of homologous hemoglobin in renal proximal tubular cells.' *Acta path. microbiol. scand.* **168** (Suppl.), 1

— (1965). 'Transport and digestion of hemoglobin in the proximal tubules. II. Electron microscopy.' *Lab. Invest.* **14**, 16

— (1969). 'Mechanism of cellular autophagy.' In *Lysosomes in Biology and Pathology*, Vol. 2, p. 345. Ed. by J. T. Dingle and H. B. Fell. Amsterdam and London: North Holland Publ.

— and Biberfeld, P. (1967). 'Studies on aldehyde fixation. Fixation rates and their relation to fine structure and some histochemical reactions in liver.' *Lab. Invest.* **17**, 281

Essner, E. (1960). 'An electron microscopic study of erythrophagocytosis.' *J. biophys. biochem. Cytol.* **7**, 329

— and Novikoff, A. B. (1960). 'Human hepatocellular pigments and lysosomes.' *J. Ultrastruct. Res.* **3**, 374

Farquhar, M. G. and Palade, G. E. (1962). 'Functional evidence for the existence of a third cell type in the renal glomerulus.' *J. Cell Biol.* **13**, 55

Farrant, J. L. (1954). 'An electron microscopic study of ferritin.' *Biochim. biophys. acta* **13**, 569

Fedorko, M. E. (1968). 'Effect of Chloroquine on morphology of leukocytes and pancreatic exocrine cells from the rat.' *Lab. Invest.* **18**, 27

Fell, H. B. (1969). 'Heberden Oration, 1968. Role of biological membranes in some skeletal reactions.' *Ann. rheum. Dis.* **28**, 213

Florey, H. W. (Ed.) (1962). 'Inflammation.' In *General Pathology,* 3rd edn., p. 68, Philadelphia, Pa: W. B. Saunders

Frank, A. L. and Christensen, A. K. (1968). 'Localization of acid phosphatase in lipofuscin granules and possible autophagic vacuoles in interstitial cells of the guinea pig testis.' *J. Cell Biol.* **36**, 1

Friend, D. S. (1969). 'Cytochemical staining of multivesicular body and Golgi vesicles.' *J. Cell Biol.* **41**, 269

—— and Farquhar, M. G. (1967). 'Functions of coated vesicles during protein absorption in the rat vas deferens.' *J. Cell Biol.* **35**, 357

—— and Murray, M. J. (1965). 'Osmium impregnation of the Golgi apparatus.' *Am. J. Anat.* **117**, 135

Ganote, C. E., Beaver, D. L. and Moses, H. L. (1966). 'Renal gold inclusions.' *Archs Path.* **81**, 429

Garancis, J. C. (1968). 'Type II glycogenosis. Biochemical and electron microscopic study.' *Am. J. Med.* **44**, 289

Gedigk, P. and Strauss, G. (1953). 'Zur Histochemie des Hamosiderins.' *Virchows Arch. path. Anat. Physiol.* **324**, 373

Ghadially, F. N. and Parry, E. W. (1965a). 'Ultrastructure of the liver of the tumor-bearing host.' *Cancer* **18**, 485

—— (1965b). 'Probable significance of some morphological variations in the eosinophil granule revealed by the electron microscope.' *Nature, Lond.* **206**, 632

—— (1966a). 'Ultrastructure of a human hepatocellular carcinoma and surrounding non-neoplastic liver.' *Cancer* **19**, 1989

—— (1966b). 'An electron-microscope and histochemical study of melanosis coli.' *J. path. Bact.* **92**, 313

—— (1967). 'Melanosis coli.' *Curr. Med. Drugs* **8**, 13

—— and Roy, S. (1967a). 'Ultrastructure of synovial membrane in rheumatoid arthritis.' *Ann. rheum. Dis.* **26**, 426

—— (1967b). 'Phagocytosis by synovial cells.' *Nature, Lond.* **213**, 1041

—— (1969). *Ultrastructure of Synovial Joints in Health and Disease.* London: Butterworths

— Meachim, G. and Collins, D. H. (1965). 'Extracellular lipid in matrix of human articular cartilage.' *Ann. rheum. Dis.* **24**, 136

— Oryschak, A. F., Ailsby, R. L. and Mehta, P. N. (1974). 'Electron probe x-ray analysis of siderosomes in haemarthrotic articular cartilage.' *Virchows Arch. Abt. B. Zellpath.* **16**, 43

Ghidoni, J. J. and Goldberg, A. F. (1966). 'Light and electron microscopic localization of acid phosphatase activity in human eosinophils.' *Am. J. clin. path.* **45**, 402

Gillman, J. and Gillman, T. (1945). 'Structure of the liver in pellagra.' *Arch Path.* **40**, 239

Goldenberg, V. E., Buckingham, S. and Sommers, S. C. (1967). 'Pulmonary alveolar lesions in vagotomized rats.' *Lab. Invest.* **16**, 693

—— (1969). 'Pilocarpine stimulation of granular pneumocyte secretion.' *Lab. Invest.* **20**, 147

Goldfischer, S. and Moskal, J. (1966). 'Electron probe microanalysis of liver in Wilson's disease. Simultaneous assay for copper and for lead deposited by acid phosphatase activity in lysosomes.' *Am. J. Path.* **48**, 305

— Villaverde, H. and Forschirm, R. (1966). 'The demonstration of acid hydrolase, thermostable reduced diphospho-pyridine neucleotide tetrazolium reductase and peroxidase activities in human lipofuscin pigment granules.' *J. Histo-chem. Cytochem.* **14**, 641

— Kikkawa, Y. and Hoffman, L. (1968). 'The demonstration of acid hydrolase activities in the inclusion bodies of type II alveolar cells and other lysosomes in the rabbit lung.' *J. Histochem. Cytochem.* **16**, 102

Goodall, F. R. (1965). 'Degradative enzymes in the uterine myometrium of rabbits under different hormonal conditions.' *Archs Biochem. Biophys.* **112**, 403

Gordon, G. B., Miller, L. R. and Bensch, K. G. (1965). 'Studies on the intracellular digestive process in mammalian tissue culture cells.' *J. Cell Biol.* **25**, 41

Greenstein, J. P. (1954). *Biochemistry of Cancer,* p. 507. New York: Academic Press

Grillo, H. C. and Gross, J. (1967). 'Collagenolytic activity during mammalian wound repair.' *Devl Biol.* **15**, 300

Gross, J. (1964). 'Studies on the biology of connective tissues. Remodelling of collagen in metamorphosis.' *Medicine, Baltimore* **43**, 291

— Lapiere, C. M. and Lanzer, M. L. (1963). 'Organization and disorganization of extracellular substances: the collagen system.' In *Cytodifferentiation and Macromolecular Synthesis,* p. 175. Ed. by M. Locke. New York: Academic Press

Grunnet, M. L. and Spilsbury, P. R. (1973). 'The central nervous system in Fabry's disease. An ultrastructural study.' *Archs Neurol., Chicago* **28**, 231

Hamerman, D. (1966). 'New thoughts on the pathogenesis of rheumatoid arthritis.' *Am. J. Med.* **40**, 1

Hannover, A. (1842). *Videnskapasselskapets Naturv og Math. Afh. Copenhagen* **10**, 1

Hardin, J. H. and Spicer, S. S. (1970). 'An ultrastructural study of human eosinophil granules: maturational stages and pyroantimonate reactive cation.' *Am. J. Anat.* **128**, 283

Harkness, R. D. and Moralee, B. E. (1956). 'The time-course and route of loss of collagen from the rat's uterus during post-partum involution.' *J. Physiol.* **132**, 502

Harrison, P. M., Fischbach, F. A., Hoy, T. G. and Haggis, G. H. (1967). 'Ferric oxyhydroxide core of ferritin.' *Nature, Lond.* **216**, 1188

Hatasa, K. and Nakamura, T. (1965). 'Electron microscopic observations of lung alveolar epithelial cells of normal young mice, with special reference to formation and secretion of osmiophilic lamellar bodies.' *Z. Zellforsch. mikrosk. Anat.* **68**, 266

Haydon, G. B. (1969). 'Visualization of substructure in ferritin molecules: an artifact.' *J. Microscopy* **89**, 251

Hendry, N. G. C. and Carr, A. J. (1963). 'Glycosidase abnormality in synovial membrane in joint disease.' *Nature, Lond.* **199**, 392

Hers, H. G. (1963). 'A glucosidase deficiency in generalized glycogen storage disease (Pompe's disease).' *J. Biochem.* **86**, 11

— and Van Hoof, F. (1969). 'Genetic abnormalities of lysosomes.' In *Lysosomes in Biology and Pathology,* Vol. II, p. 19. Ed. by J. T. Dingle and H. B. Fell. Amsterdam: North Holland Publ.

Heyne, K., Kemmer, C. and Rudolph, S. (1972). 'Beitrag zur ultrastruktur Phagozytierender granulozyten bei progressiver Septischer granulomatose des Kindes.' *Pathologia Microbiol.* **38**, 133

Higashi, O. (1954). 'Congenital gigantism of peroxidase granules.' *Tohoku J. exp. Med.* **59**, 315

Hodge, C. F. (1894). 'Changes in ganglion cells from birth to senile death. Observations on man and honey-bee.' *J. Physiol.* **17**, 129

Hollander, J. L., McCarty, D. J., Astorga, G. and Castro-Murillo, E. (1965). 'Studies on the pathogenesis of rheumatoid joint inflammation. I. The R.A. cells and a working hypothesis.' *Ann. intern. Med.* **62**, 271

Holmes, B., Quie, P. G., Windhorst, D. B. and Good, R. A. (1966). 'Fatal granulomatous disease of childhood. An inborn abnormality of phagocytic function.' *Lancet* **1**, 1225

Holt, S. J. and Hicks, R. M. (1961). 'The localisation of acid phosphatase in rat liver cells as revealed by combined cytochemical staining and electron microscopy.' *J. Biophys. Biochem. Cytol.* **11**, 47

Holtzman, E. and Dominitz, R. (1968). 'Cytochemical studies of lysosomes, Golgi apparatus and endoplasmic reticulum in secretion and protein uptake by adrenal medulla cells of the rat.' *J. Histochem. Cytochem.* **16**, 320

Houck, J. C. (1968). 'A personal overview of inflammation.' *Biochem. Pharmac. Suppl.* 1, No. 17, p. 1

Hruban, Z., Swift, H. and Slesers, A. (1965). 'Effect of triparanol and diethanolamine on the fine structure of hepatocytes and pancreatic acinar cells.' *Lab. Invest.* **14**, 1652

— Slesers, A. and Hopkins, E. (1972). 'Drug-induced and naturally occurring myeloid bodies.' *Lab. Invest.* **27**, 62

Hudson, G. (1966). 'Eosinophil granules and phosphotungstic acid: an electron microscope study of guinea-pig bone marrow.' *Expl Cell Res.* **41**, 265

Hug, G. and Schubert, W. K. (1967). 'Glycogenosis type II.' *Archs Path.* **84**, 141

Ishikawa, T., Evans, R., Wicher, K. and Arbesman, C. E. (1971). '*In vitro* and *in vivo* adhesion of antigen–antibody complexes to eosinophils.' *Fedn Proc.* **30**, 2788 (Abstract)

— Yu, M. C. and Arbesman, C. E. (1972). 'Electron microscopic demonstration of phagocytosis of *Candida albicans* by human eosinophilic leukocytes.' *J. Allergy Clin. Immun.* **50**, 183

Jacox, R. F. and Feldmahn, A. (1955). 'Variations of beta-glucuronidase concentrations in abnormal human synovial fluid.' *J. clin. Invest.* **34**, 263

Jamieson, J. D. and Palade, G. E. (1964). 'Specific granules in atrial muscle cells.' *J. Cell Biol.* **23**, 151

Jayne, E. P. (1950). 'Cytochemical studies of age pigments in the human heart.' *J. Geront.* **5**, 319

Jézéquel, A. M., Arakawa, K. and Steiner, J. W. (1965). 'The fine structure of the normal, neonatal mouse liver.' *Lab. Invest.* **14**, 1894

Jordan, S. W. (1964). 'Electron microscopy of Gaucher cells.' *Expl Molec. Path.* **3**, 76

Junod, A., Lambert, A. E., Stauffacher, W. and Renold, A. E. (1969). 'Diabetogenic action of streptozotocin: relationship of dose to metabolic response.' *J. clin. Invest.* **48**, 2129

Karbe, E. (1968). 'Amaurotische Idiotie bei Hund und Mensch.' *Bull. schweiz. Akad. med. Wiss.* **24**, 95

Kent, G., Minick, O. T., Volini, F. I., Orfei, E. and de la Huerga, J. (1963a). 'Iron storage in N-2-fluorenylacetamide-induced hepatic injury. Electron microscopic observations following the injection of iron-dextran.' *Lab. Invest.* **12**, 1102

— Volini, F. I., Orfei, E., Minick, O. T. and de la Huerga, J. (1963b). 'Effect of hepatic injuries upon iron storage in the liver.' *Lab. Invest.* **12**, 1094

— Minick, O. T., Orfei, E., Volini, F. I. and Madera-Orsini, F. (1965). 'The movement of iron-laden lysosomes in rat liver cells during mitosis.' *Am. J. Path.* **46**, 803

—— Volini, F. E. and Orfei, E. (1966). 'Autophagic vacuoles in human red cells.' *Am. J. Path.* **48**, 831

Kerr, D. N. and Muir, A. R. (1960). 'A demonstration of the structure and disposition of ferritin in the human liver cell.' *J. Ultrastruct. Res.* **3**, 313

Kessel, R. G. (1966). 'Electron microscope studies on the origin and maturation of yolk in oocytes of the tunicate *Ciona intestinalis*.' *Z. Zellforsch. mikrosk. Anat.* **71**, 525

Khandekar, J. D., Dardachti, D., Garg, B. D., Tuchweber, B. and Kovacs, K. (1972). 'Hepatic fine structural changes and microsomal hypofunction in Walker tumor-bearing rats.' *Cancer* **29**, 738

Klebanoff, S. J. (1968). 'Myeloperoxidase–halide–hydrogen peroxide antibacterial system.' *J. Bact.* **95**, 2131

— (1971). 'Neutrophils and host defense.' *Calif. Med.* **114**, 47

— and White, L. R. (1969). 'Iodination defect in the leukocytes of a patient with chronic granulomatous disease of childhood.' *New Engl. J. Med.* **280**, 460

Koenig, H. (1963). 'Intravital staining of lysosomes by basic dyes and metallic ions.' *J. Histochem. Cytochem.* **11**, 120

— and Jebril, A. (1962). 'Acidic glycolipids and the role of ionic bonds in the structure-linked latency of lysosomal hydrolases.' *Biochim. biophys. acta* **65**, 543

Kolliker, A. (1849). In *Todd's Cyclopaedia of Anatomy and Physiology,* Vol. IV, p. 771. London: Longman Brown, Green, Longman and Roberts

Koneff, H. (1886). 'Bertrage zur Kenntniss der Nervenzellen in den peripheren Ganglien.' *Mitt. naturf. Ges. Bern* **44**, 13

Koyama, S., Sadako, A. and Deguchi, K. (1964). 'Electron microscopic observations of the splenic red pulp with special reference to the pitting function.' *Mie med. J.* **14**, 143

Kritzler, R. A., Terner, J. Y., Lindenbaum, J., Magidson, J., Williams, R., Preisig, R. and Phillips, G. B. (1964). 'Chediak–Higashi syndrome. Cytologic and serum lipid observations in a case and family.' *Am. J. Med.* **36**, 583

Kuhn, C. (1968). 'Cytochemistry of pulmonary alveolar epithelial cells.' *Am. J. Path.* **53**, 809

Laufberger, V. (1934). 'O výměně železa.' *Biol. Listy* **19**, 73

— (1937). 'Sur la cristallisation de la ferritine.' *Bull. Soc. Chim. biol.* **19**, 1575

Lazarus, S. S., Vethamany, V. G., Schneck, L. and Volk, B. W. (1967). 'Fine structure and histochemistry of peripheral blood cells in Niemann–Pick disease.' *Lab. Invest.* **17**, 155

Lee, S. H. and Aleyassine, H. (1971). 'Morphologic changes in the liver of mice bearing Ehrlich ascites tumor.' *Lab. Invest.* **24**, 513

Lehman, M. A., Kream, J. and Brogna, D. (1964). 'Acid and alkaline phosphatase activity in serum and synovial fluid of patients with arthritis.' *J. Bone Jt Surg.* **46A**, 1732

Lehrer, R. I. (1971). 'The role of phagocyte function in resistance to infection.' *Calif. Med.* **114**, 17

Lillie, R. D. (1954). *Histopathologic Technic and Practical Histochemistry*, p. 243. New York: Blakiston

— (1965). *Histopathologic Technic and Practical Histochemistry*, 3rd edn. New York: McGraw–Hill

Lobel, B. L. and Deane, H. W. (1962). 'Enzymic activity associated with postpartum involution of the uterus and with its regression after hormone withdrawal in the rat.' *Endocrinology* **70**, 576

Locke, M. and Collins, J. V. (1967). 'Protein uptake in multivesicular bodies in the molt–intermolt cycle of an insect.' *Science* **155**, 467

Luscombe, M. (1963). 'Acid phosphatase and catheptic activity in rheumatoid synovial tissue.' *Nature, Lond.* **197**, 1010

Luse, S. (1967). 'The fine structure of the brain and other organs in Niemann–Pick disease.' In *Inborn Disorders of Sphingolipid Metabolism*, p. 93. Ed. by S. M. Aronson and B. W. Volk. New York: Academic Press

— and Hutton, R. (1964). 'An electron microscopic study of the fate of collagen in the post-partum rat uterus.' *Anat. Rec.* **148**, 308

Lutzner, M. A., Lowrie, C. T. and Jordon, H. W. (1967). 'Giant granules in leukocytes of the beige mouse.' *J. Hered.* **58**, 299

Lynn, R. and Terry, R. D. (1964). 'Lipid histochemistry and electron microscopy in adult Niemann–Pick disease.' *Am. J. Med.* **37**, 987

McEwen, H. D. and Haven, F. L. (1941). 'The effect of carcinosarcoma 256 on the water content of the liver.' *Cancer Res.* **1**, 148

McFarland, W. L. (1917). 'Pigmentation of the hind-gut. A pathologic and experimental study.' *J. Am. med. Ass.* **69**, 1946

MacFarlane, P. S., Speirs, A. L. and Sommerville, R. G. (1967). 'Fatal granulomatous disease of childhood and benign lymphocytic infiltration of skin (congenital dysphagocytosis).' *Lancet* **1**, 408

Mahadevan, S. and Tappel, A. L. (1968a). 'Lysosomal lipases of rat liver and kidney.' *J. biol. Chem.* **243**, 2849

— — (1968b). 'Hydrolysis of higher fatty acid esters of *p*-nitrophenol by rat liver and kidney lysosomes.' *Archs Biochem. Biophys.* **126**, 945

Maibenco, H. G. (1960). 'Connective tissue changes in post-partum uterine involution in the albino rat.' *Anat. Rec.* **136**, 59

Malawista, S. E., Gee, J. B. L. and Bensch, K. G. (1971). 'Cytochalasin B reversibly inhibits phagocytosis: functional, metabolic and ultrastructural effects in human blood leukocytes and rabbit alveolar macrophages.' *Yale J. Biol. Med.* **44**, 286

Medigreceanu, F. (1910). 'On the relative sizes of the organs of rats and mice bearing malignant new growths.' *Proc. R. Soc. B.* **82**, 286

Meller, K. and Breipohl, W. (1971). 'Elektronenmikroskopische und histoautoradiographische Befunde zur Puromycinwirkung auf ausreifende Plexus chorioideus-zellen *in vitro*.' *Z. Zellforsch. mikrosk. Anat.* **118**, 428

Menkes, J. H., O'Brien, J. S., Okada, S., Grippo, J., Andrews, J. M. and Cancilla, P. A. (1971). 'Juvenile G_{M2} gangliosidosis.' *Archs Neurol., Chicago* **25**, 14

Miller, F., de Harven, E. and Palade, G. E. (1966). 'The structure of eosinophil leukocyte granules in rodents and in man.' *J. Cell Biol.* **31**, 349

Miyawaki, H. (1965). 'Histochemistry and electron microscopy of iron-containing granules, lysosomes and lipofuscin in mouse mammary glands.' *J. natn Cancer Inst.* **34**, 601

Moe, H., Rostgaard, J. and Behnke, O. (1965). 'On the morphology and origin of virgin lysosomes in the intestinal epithelium of the rat.' *J. Ultrastruct. Res.* **12**, 396

Moore, C. V. and Dubach, R. J. (1956). 'Metabolism and requirements of iron in the human.' *J. Am. med. Ass.* **162**. 197

Muirden, K. D. (1966). 'Ferritin in synovial cells in patients with rheumatoid arthritis.' *Ann. rheum. Dis.* **25**, 387

— and Senator, G. B. (1968). 'Iron in the synovial membrane in rheumatoid arthritis and other joint diseases.' *Ann. rheum. Dis.* **27**, 38

Munnell, J. F. and Getty, R. (1968). 'Rate of accumulation of cardiac lipofuscin in the aging canine.' *J. Geront.* **23**, 154

Norton, W. L. and Ziff, M. (1966). 'Electron microscopic observations on the rheumatoid synovial membrane.' *Arthritis Rheum.* **9**, 589

Novikoff, A. B. (1961). 'Lysosomes and related particles.' In *The Cell*, Vol. 2, p. 423, Ed. by J. Brachet and A. E. Mirsky. New York and London: Academic Press

— and Essner, E. (1960). 'The liver cell: some new approaches to its study.' *Am. J. Med.* **29**, 102

— Beaufay, H. and de Duve, C. (1956). 'Electron microscopy of lysosome-rich fractions from rat liver.' *J. biophys. biochem. Cytol.* **2**, 179

— Essner, E. and Quintana, N. (1964). 'Golgi apparatus and lysosomes.' *Fedn Proc.* **23**, 1010

Orci, L. and Stauffacher, W. (1971). 'Glycogenosomes in renal tubular cells of diabetic animals.' *J. Ultrastruct. Res.* **36**, 499

— — Amherdt, M., Pictet, R., Renold, A. E. and Rouiller, Ch. (1970). 'The kidney of spiny mice *(Acomys cahirinus)*: electron microscopy of glomerular changes associated with ageing and tubular glycogen accumulation during hyperglycemia.' *Diabetologia* **6**, 343

Osako, R. (1959). 'An electron microscopic observation on the specific granules of eosinophil leukocytes of vertebrates.' *Acta haemat. Jap.* **22**, 134

Oryschak, A. F. and Ghadially, F. N. (1974). 'Aurosomes in rabbit articular cartilage.' *Virchows Arch. Abt. B. Zellpath.* **17**, 159

Padgett, G. A. (1967). 'Neutrophilic function in animals with the Chediak–Higashi syndrome.' *Blood* **29**, 906

— (1968). 'The Chediak–Higashi syndrome.' *Adv. vet. Sci.* **12**, 239

— Leader, R. W., Gorham, J. R. and O'Mary, C. C. (1964). 'The familial occurrence of the Chediak–Higashi syndrome in mink and cattle.' *Genetics* **49**, 505

Page Thomas, D. P. (1969). 'Lysosomal enzymes in experimental and rheumatoid arthritis.' In *Lysosomes in Biology and Pathology,* Vol. 2, p. 87. Ed. by J. T. Dingle and H. B. Fell. Amsterdam and London: North Holland Publ.

Pappenheimer, A. M. and Victor, J. (1946). '"Ceroid" pigment in human tissues.' *Am. J. Path.* **22**, 395

Parakkal, P. F. (1968). 'Involvement of macrophages in collagen resorption.' *Brief Notes* Publication No. 365, *J. Cell Biol.* **41**, 345

Parry, E. W. (1969). 'A quantitative method for assessment of hepatocellular lysosomes—its application to normal and tumour-bearing animals.' *J. Path.* **97**, 155

— and Ghadially, F. N. (1965). 'Ultrastructure of carcinogen-induced rat sarcoma.' *Cancer* **18**, 1026

— — (1966). 'Ultrastructural changes in the liver of tumor-bearing rats during the terminal stages of life.' *Cancer* **19**, 821

— — (1967). 'Ultrastructure of the livers of rats bearing transplanted tumours.' *J. Path. Bact.* **93**, 295

— — (1969). 'Effects of necrotic tumor on hepatic cells in the rat.' *Cancer* **23**, 475

— — (1970). 'The effects of toxohormone on the ultrastructure of rat hepatocytes.' *J. Path.* **100**, 161

Pearse, A. G. E. (1972). *Histochemistry: Theoretical and Applied,* 3rd edn. Edinburgh and London: Churchill Livingstone

Phillips, M. J., Unakar, N. J., Doornewaard, G. and Steiner, J. W. (1967). 'Glycogen depletion in the newborn rat liver: 'an electron microscopic and electron histochemical study.' *J. Ultrastruct. Res.* **18**, 142

Pictet, R., Orci, L., Forssmann, W. G. and Girardier, L. (1969). 'An electron microscope study of the perfusion-fixed spleen. II. Nurse cells and erythrophagocytosis.' *Z. Zellforsch. mikrosk. Anat.* **96**, 400

Planel, H. and Guilhem, A. (1955). 'Contribution à l'étude histochimique des pigments de la glande surrénale du cobaye en fonction de l'âge.' *C.r. Soc. Biol.* **149**, 1504

Porta, E. A. and Hartroft, W. S. (1969). 'Lipid pigments in relation of aging and dietary factors (lipofuscins)'. In *Pigments in Pathology.* Ed. by M. Wolman. New York and London: Academic Press

Pras, M. and Weissmann, G. (1966). 'Filipin-induced arthritis.' *Arthritis Rheum.* **9**, 533 (abstr.)

Quie, P. G., Kaplan, E. L., Page, A. R., Gruskay, F. L. and Malawista, S. E. (1968). 'Defective polymorphonuclear-leukocyte function and chronic granulomatous disease in two female children.' *New Engl. J. Med.* **278**, 976

Rae, A. I., Lee, J. C. and Hopper, J. (1967). 'Clinical and electron microscopic studies of a case of glycolipid lipoidosis (Fabry's disease)'. *J. clin. Path.* **20**, 21

Rebhun, L. I. (1960). 'Aster associated particles in the cleavage of marine invertebrate eggs.' *Ann. N.Y. Acad. Sci.* **90**, 357

Reichel, W. (1968). 'Lipofuscin pigment accumulation and distribution in five rat organs as a function of age.' *J. Gerontol.* **23**, 145

— Hollander, J., Clark, J. and Strehler, B. L. (1968). 'Lipofuscin pigment accumulation as a function of age and distribution in rodent brain.' *J. Gerontol.* **23**, 71

Revel, J. P., Ito, S. and Fawcett, D. W. (1958). 'Electron micrographs of myelin figures of phospholipid simulating intracellular membranes.' *J. biophys. biochem. Cytol.* **4**, 495

Richter, G. W. (1957). 'A study of hemosiderosis with the aid of electron microscopy.' *J. exp. Med.* **106**, 203

— (1958). 'Electron microscopy of hemosiderin. Presence of ferritin and occurrence of crystalline lattices in hemosiderin deposits.' *J. biophys. biochem. Cytol.* **4**, 55

— (1959). 'The cellular transformation of injected colloidal iron complexes into ferritin and hemosiderin in experimental animals.' *J. Expl Med.* **109**, 197

Riddle, J. M. and Barnhart, M. I. (1964). 'Ultrastructural study of fibrin dissolution via emigrated polymorphonuclear neutrophils.' *Am. J. Path.* **45**, 805

Rifkind, R. A. (1965). 'Heinz body anemia: an ultrastructural study. II. Red cell sequestration and destruction.' *Blood* **26**, 433

Robbins, E., Marcus, P. I. and Gonatas, N. K. (1964). 'Dynamics of acridine orange cell interaction. II. Dye-induced ultrastructural changes in multivesicular bodies (acridine orange particles).' *J. Cell Biol.* **21**, 49

Robinson, W. D. (1966). 'The etiology of rheumatoid arthritis.' In *Arthritis and Allied Conditions. A Textbook of Rheumatology,* p. 181. Ed. by J. L. Hollander. London: Kimpton

Roden, D. (1940). 'Melanosis coli. A pathological study: its experimental production in monkeys.' *Ir. J. med. Sci.* (Sept.) 654

Rogers, L. A., Morris, H. P. and Fouts, J. R. (1967). 'The effect of phenobarbital on drug metabolic enzyme activity, ultrastructure and growth of a "minimal deviation" hepatoma (Morris 7800).' *J. Pharmac. exp. Ther.* **157**, 227

Rosenbluth, J. and Wissig, S. L. (1964). 'The distribution of exogenous ferritin in toad spinal ganglia and the mechanism of its uptake by neurons.' *J. Cell Biol.* **23**, 307

Ross, R. and Odland, G. (1968). 'Human wound repair. II. Inflammatory cells, epithelial-mesenchymal interrelations, and fibrogenesis.' *J. Cell. Biol.* **39**, 152

Rouiller, C. (1954). 'Les canalicules biliaires. Etude au microscope electronique.' *C.r. Soc. Biol.* **148**, 2008

Rous, P. (1923). 'Destruction of the red blood corpuscles in health and disease.' *Physiol. Rev.* **3**, 75

— and Robertson, O. H. (1917). 'The normal fate of erythrocytes. I. The findings in healthy animals.' *J. exp. Med.* **25**, 651

Roy, S. and Ghadially, F. N. (1966). 'Pathology of experimental haemarthrosis.' *Ann. rheum. Dis.* **25**, 402

— — (1967). 'Ultrastructure of synovial membrane in human haemarthrosis.' *J. Bone Jt Surg.* **49A**, 1636

— — (1969). 'Synovial membrane in experimentally produced chronic haemarthrosis.' *Ann. rheum. Dis.* **28**, 402

Sabesin, S. M. (1963). 'A function of the eosinophil: phagocytosis of antigen–antibody complexes.' *Proc. Soc. exp. Biol. Med.* **112**, 667

Salomon, J. C. and Caroli, J. (1962). 'Apropos of a case of Gaucher's disease: study by electron microscopy of a fragment of hepatic tissue.' *Rev. Intern. Hepatol.* **12**, 281

365

Samorajski, T. and Ordy, J. M. (1967). 'The histochemistry and ultrastructure of lipid pigment in the adrenal glands of aging mice.' *J. Gerontol.* **22**, 253

—— and Keefe, J. R. (1965). 'The fine structure of lipofuscin age pigment in the nervous system of aged mice.' *J. Cell Biol.* **26**, 779

———— (1965). 'The fine structure of lipofuscin age pigment in the nervous system of aged mice.' *J. Cell Biol.* **26**, 779

Samuels, S., Gonatas, N. K. and Weiss, M. (1964). 'Chemical and ultrastructural comparison of synthetic and pathologic membrane system.' *J. Cell Biol.* **21**, 148

Sandstrom, B., Westman, J. and Ockerman, P. A. (1969). 'Glycogenosis of the central nervous system in the cat.' *Acta Neuropath.* **14**, 194

Schaeffer, K., Brinkley, B. R., Young, J. E., Oliver, S. S., Chang, J. P. and Guillen, W. M. (1970). 'The occurrence of lysosome-like structures in sickling erythrocytes.' *Lab. Invest.* **23**, 297

Schaffner, F., Sternlieb, I., Barka, T. and Popper, H. (1962). 'Hepatocellular changes in Wilson's disease. Histochemical and electron microscopic studies.' *Am. J. Path.* **41**, 315

Schersten, T., Wahlqvist, L. and Johansson, L. G. (1969). 'Lysosomal enzyme activity in liver tissue from patients with renal carcinoma.' *Cancer* **23**, 608

Schwarz, W. and Guldner, F. H. (1967). 'Elektronenmikroskopische. Untersuchungen des Kollagenabbaus im Uterus der Ratte nach de Schwangerschaft.' *Z. Zellforsch. mikrosk. Anat.* **83**, 416

Scott, R. E. and Horn, R. G. (1970a). 'Ultrastructural aspects of neutrophil granulocyte development in humans.' *Lab. Invest.* **23**, 202

—— (1970b). 'Fine structural features of eisinophil granulocyte development in human bone marrow. Evidence for granule secretion.' *J. Ultrastruct. Res.* **33**, 16

Sedar, A. W. (1966). 'Transport of exogenous peroxidase across the epididymal epithelium.' In *Proceedings of the 6th International Congress for Electron Microscopy*, Vol. 2, p. 591. Ed. by Kyoto R. Uyeda. Tokyo: Maruzen

Shamberger, R. J., Hozumi, M. and Morris, H. P. (1971). 'Lysosomal and nonlysosomal enzyme activities of Morris hepatomas.' *Cancer Res.* **31**, 1632

Sheldon, H. and Zetterquist, H. (1955). 'Internal ultrastructure in granules of white blood cells of the mouse.' *Bull. Johns Hopkins Hosp.* **96**, 135

Sherman, C. D., Jr., Morton, J. J. and Mider, G. B. (1950). 'Potential sources of tumour nitrogen.' *Cancer Res.* **10**, 374

Shoden, A. and Sturgeon, P. (1961). 'Formation of haemosiderin and its relation to ferritin.' *Nature, Lond.* **189**, 846

Simon, G. T. and Burke, J. S. (1970). 'Electron microscopy of the spleen. III. Erythro-leukophagocytosis.' *Am. J. Path.* **58**, 451

—— and Pictet, R. (1964). 'Etude au microscope electronique des sinus spleniques et des cordons de Billroth chez le rat.' *Acta anat.* **57**, 163

Skinnider, L. F. and Ghadially, F. N. (1973). 'Glycogen in erythroid cells.' *Archs Path.* **95**, 139

—— and Ghadially, F. N. (1974). 'Secretion of granule content by eosinophils.' *Archs. Path.* **98**, 58

Smith, F. (1958). 'Erythrophagocytosis in human lymph-glands.' *J. Path. Bact.* **76**, 383

Smith, R. E. and Farquhar, M. G. (1966). 'Lysosome function in the regulation of the secretory process in cells of the anterior pituitary gland.' *J. Cell Biol.* **31**, 319

Sorensen, G. D. (1961). 'Electron microscopic observations of viral particles within myeloma cells of man.' *Expl Cell Res.* **25**, 219

Sorokin, S. P. (1966). 'A morphologic and cytochemical study on the great alveolar cell.' *J. Histochem. Cytochem.* **14**, 884

Southwick, W. O. and Bensch, K. G. (1971). 'Phagocytosis of colloidal gold by cells of synovial membrane.' *J. Bone Jt Surg.* **53A**, 729

Speare, G. S. (1951). 'Melanosis coli. Experimental observations on its production and elimination in twenty-three cases.' *Am. J. Surg.* **82**, 631

Spicer, S. S. and Hardin, J. H. (1969). 'Ultrastructure, cytochemistry and function of neutrophil leukocyte granules. A review.' *Lab. Invest.* **20**, 488

Spors, S. (1971). 'Elektronenmikroskopische Untersuchungen der Membran-Phosphatasen und der Lysosomen im proximalen Tubulus der Rattenniere nach Folsauregabe.' *Virchows Arch. Abt. B. Zellpath.* **9**, 198

Stein, U., Heismeyer, H., Zimmermann, W. and Lesch, R. (1971). 'Cathepsin D and acid carboxypeptidase activities of human liver tissue from subjects with different liver dieases.' The 6th Meeting Europ. Assoc. for the Study of the Liver, London.(Abstr.) Quoted by Schersten, T. and Lundholm, I. I. (1972) 'Lysosomal enzyme activity in muscle tissue from patients with malignant tumor.' *Cancer* **30**, 1246

Stewart, M. J. and Hickman, E. M. (1931). 'Observations on melanosis coli.' *J. Path. Bact.* **34**, 61

Stoeckenius, W. (1962). 'The molecular structure of lipid-water systems and cell membrane models studied with the electron microscope.' In *The Interpretation of Ultrastructure*, p. 349. Ed. by R. J. C. Harris. New York: Academic Press

Straus, W. (1958). 'Colorimetric analysis with N,N-dimethyl-*p*-phenylenediamine of the uptake of intravenously injected horse-radish peroxidase by various tissues of the rat.' *J. biophys. biochem. Cytol.* **4**, 541

—— (1964). 'Cytochemical observations on the relationship between lysosomes and phagosomes in kidney and liver by combined staining for acid phosphatase and intravenously injected horse-radish peroxidase.' *J. Cell Biol.* **20**, 497

Strehler, B. L., Mark, D. D., Mildvan, A. S. and Gee, M. V. (1959). 'Rate and magnitude of age pigment accumulation in the human myocardium.' *J. Gerent.* **14**, 430

Sturgeon, P. and Shoden, A. (1969). 'Hemosiderin and ferritin.' In *Pigments of Pathology*. Ed. by M. Wolman. New York and London: Academic Press

Sulkin, N. M. (1955). 'The properties and distribution of P.A.S. positive substances in the nervous system of the senile dog.' *J. Geront.* **10**, 135

—— and Kuntz, A. (1952). 'Histochemical alterations in autonomic ganglion cells associated with aging.' *J. Geront.* **7**, 533

366

Sutton, J. S. and Weiss, L. (1966). 'Transformation of monocytes in tissue culture into macrophages, epithelioid cells, and multinucleated giant cells. An electron microscope study.' *J. Cell Biol.* **28**, 303

Tanaka, Y., Brecher, G. and Fredrickson, D. S. (1963). 'Cellules de la maladie de Nieman–Pick et du quelques autres lipoidoses.' *Nouv. Revue franc. Hematol.* **3**, 5

Tappel, A. L. (1969). 'Lysosomal enzymes and other components.' In *Lysosomes in Biology and Pathology,* Vol. 2, p. 207. Ed. by J. T. Dingle and H. B. Fell. Amsterdam and London: North Holland Publ.

Tarnowski, W. M. and Hashimoto, K. (1968). 'Lysosomes in Fabry's disease.' *Acta derm.-vener.* **48**, 143

Taylor, N. S. (1965). 'Histochemical studies of nephrotoxicity with sublethal doses of mercury in rats.' *Am. J. Path,* **46**. 1

Terry, R. D. and Weiss, M. (1963). 'Studies in Tay–Sachs disease. II. Ultrastructure of the cerebrum.' *J. Neuropath. exp. Neurol.* **22**, 18

Thompson, E. N., Chandra, R. K., Cope, W. A. and Soothill, J. F. (1969). 'Leucocyte abnormality in both parents of a patient with chronic granulomatous disease.' *Lancet* **1**, 799

Thomson, R. H. (1962). 'Some naturally occurring black pigments.' In *Recent Progress in the Chemistry of Natural and Synthetic Colouring Matters and Related Fields,* p. 99. Ed. by T. G. Gore, B. S. Joshi, S. V. Sunthankar and B. D. Tilak. New York and London: Academic Press

Tooze, J. and Davies, H. G. (1965). 'Cytolysosomes in amphibian erythrocytes.' *J. Cell Biol.* **24**, 146

Toujas, L., Juif, J. G., Cussac, Y., Porte, A. and Platt, E. (1966). 'Sur les modifications ultrastructurales du foie dans un cas de maladie de Gaucher.' *Ann. Anat. Path.* **11**, 101

Travis, D. F. and Travis, A. (1972). 'Ultrastructural changes in the left ventricular rat myocardial cells with age.' *J. Ultrastruct. Res.* **39**, 124

Tsukada, H., Fujiwara, S., Mochizuki, Y., Shibuya, M. and Kaneko, A. (1966). 'Malignancy of Ehrlich ascites tumor and changes in the liver of the tumor-bearing mice.' *Tumor Res.* **1**, 41

Usuku, G. and Gross, J. (1965). 'Morphologic studies of connective tissue resorption in tail fin of metamorphosing bullfrog tadpole.' *Devl Biol.* **11**, 352

van Bruggen, E. F. J., Wiebenga, E. H. and Gruber, M. (1960). 'Electron micrographs of ferritin and apoferritin molecules.' *J. molec. Biol.* **2**, 81

Vasquez, C., Pavlovsky, A. and Bernhard, W. (1963). 'Lésions nucleaires et inclusions cytoplasmiques particulieres dans deux cas de lymphoreticulo-sarcomes humains.' *C. R. Acad. Sci., Paris* **256**, 2261

Vijeyaratnam, G. S. and Corrin, B. (1972). 'Pulmonary histiocytosis simulating desquamative interstitial pneumonia in rats receiving oral iprindole.' *J. Path.* **108**, 105

Virchow, R. (1857). 'II. Die pathologischen Pigmente.' *Arch. path. Anat.* **1**, 379

Geweben.' *Virchows Arch.* **6**, 562

Virchow, R. (1857). *Arch. path. Anat.* **1**, 379

Volk, B. W. and Wallace, B. J. (1966). 'The liver in lipidosis. An electron microscopic and histochemical study.' *Am. J. Path.* **49**, 203

von Braunmuhl, A. (1957). In *Handbuch der Speziellen Pathologischen Anatomie und Histologie,* Vol. 13, Part 1, 357. Ed. by O. Lubarsch, F. Henke and R. Rossle. Berlin: Springer

von Recklinghausen, F. (1883). *Handbuch der allgem Pathologie des Kreislanfs und der Ernahrung,* Deut. Chir II and III. (Quoted by Porta, E. A. and Hartroft, W. S. (1969) in *Pigments in Pathology,* ed. by M. Wolman. New York and London: Academic Press)

Wallace, B. J., Volk, B. W. and Lazarus, S. S. (1964). 'Fine structural localization of acid phosphatase activity in neurons of Tay–Sachs disease.' *J. Neuropath. exp. Neurol.* **23**, 676

— Schneck, L., Kaplan, H. and Volk, B. W. (1965). 'Fine structure of the cerebellum of children with lipidoses.' *Archs Path.* **80**, 466

Wattiaux, R. (1969). *'Biochemistry and function of lysosomes.'* In *Handbook of Molecular Cytology.* Ed. by A. Lima-de-Faria. Amsterdam and London: North Holland Publ.

Weber, R. (1963). 'Behaviour and properties of acid hydrolases in regressing tails of tadpoles during spontaneous and induced metamorphosis in vitro.' In Ciba Foundation Symposium on *Lysosomes,* p. 282. Ed. by A. V. R. de Reuck and M. P. Cameron. Edinburgh and London: Churchill Livingstone

Weissmann, G. (1966). 'Lysosomes and joint disease.' *Arthritis Rheum.* **9**, 834

— (1967). 'The role of lysosomes in inflammation and disease.' *A. Rev. Med.* **18**, 97

— and Thomas, L. (1964). 'Effects of corticosteroids on connective tissue and lysosomes.' *Recent Prog. Horm. Res.* **20**, 215

— Becker, B., Wiedermann, G. and Bernheimer, A. W. (1965). 'Studies on lysosomes. VII. Acute and chronic arthritis produced by intra-articular injections of streptolysin S in rabbits.' *Am. J. Path.* **46**, 129

Wennberg, E. and Weiss, L. (1968). 'Splenic erythroclasia: an electron microscopic study of hemoglobin H disease.' *Blood* **31**, 778

Wessel, W., Georgsson, G. and Segschneider, I. (1969). 'Elektronenmikroskopische Untersuchungen uber Weg und Wirkung hochdosierten Sublimats nach Injektion in die Arteria renalis.' *Virchows Arch. Abt. B. Zellpath.* **3**, 88

Wetzel, B. K., Horn, R. G. and Spicer, S. S. (1967a). 'Fine structural studies on the development of heterophil, eosinophil, and basophil granulocytes in rabbits.' *Lab. Invest.* **16**, 349

— Spicer, S. S. and Horn, R. G. (1967b). 'Fine structural localization of acid and alkaline phosphatases in cells of rabbit blood and bone marrow.' *J. Histochem. Cytochem.* **15**, 311

Whiteford, R. and Getty, R. (1966). 'Distribution of lipofuscin in the canine and porcine brain as related to aging.' *J. Geront.* **21**, 31

Wilcox, H. H. (1959). 'Structural changes in the nervous system related to the process of aging P16.' In *The Process of Aging in the Nervous System.* Ed. by J. E. Birren, H. A. Inus and W. F. Windle. Springfield, Ill: Charles C Thomas

Williams, G. (1970). 'The late phases of wound healing: histological and ultrastructural studies of collagen and elastic-tissue formation.' *J. Path.* **102**, 61

Wiseman, G. and Ghadially, F. N. (1958). 'A biochemical concept of tumour growth, infiltration and cachexia.' *Br. med. J.* **2**, 18

Witzleben, C. L. (1969). 'Renal cortical tubular glycogen localization in glycogenosis type II (Pompe's disease).' *Lab. Invest.* **20**, 424

Woessner, J. F., Jr. (1962). 'Catabolism of collagen and non-collagen protein in the rat uterus during post-partum involution.' *Biochemistry* **83**, 304

— (1965). 'Uterine involution and collagen breakdown.' In *Structure and Function of Connective and Skeletal Tissues*, p. 442. Ed. by S. Fitton Jackson, R. D. Harkness, S. M. Partridge and G. R. Tristram. London: Butterworths

— (1968). 'Biological mechanisms of collagen resorption.' In *Treatise on Collagen, Part B. Biology of Collagen*, Vol. 2, p. 253. Ed. by B. S. Gould. New York: Academic Press.

Wyllie, J. C., Haust, M. D. and More, R. H. (1966). 'The fine structure of synovial lining cells in rheumatoid arthritis.' *Lab. Invest.* **15**, 519

Yamada, Y. and Sonoda, M. (1970). 'Eosinophils of ovine peripheral blood in electron microscopy.' *Jap. J. vet. Res.* **18**, 117

Yeakel, E. H. (1948). 'Increased weight of the liver in Wistar albino rats with induced and transplanted tumours.' *Cancer Res.* **8**, 392

— and Tobias, G. L. (1951). 'Liver nitrogen in tumor-bearing rats.' *Cancer Res.* **11**, 830

Zucker-Franklin, D. (1968). 'Electron microscopic studies of human granulocytes. Structural variations related to function.' *Semin. Hemat.* **5**, 109

— and Hirsch, J. G. (1964). 'Electron microscope studies on the degranulation of rabbit peritoneal leukocytes during phagocytosis.' *J. exp. Med.* **120**, 569

Zucker-Franklin, D., Davidson, M. and Thomas, L. (1966). 'The interaction of mycoplasmas with mammalian cells. *J. exp. Med.* **124**, 521

CHAPTER VIII

Microbodies (Peroxisomes)

INTRODUCTION

The term 'microbody' was coined by Rhodin (1954, 1956) to describe certain single-membrane-bound organelles containing a fine granular matrix found in the proximal tubular cells of the mouse kidney. Morphologically similar bodies but with a dense crystalloid set in the granular matrix were subsequently found in rat hepatocytes (Gansler and Rouiller, 1956; Rouiller and Bernhard, 1956). Later biochemical studies (de Duve, 1965; de Duve and Baudhuin, 1966; de Duve, 1969a, b) on isolated microbodies showed that they contain several oxidases such as urate oxidase, D-amino acid oxidase and α-hydroxy acid oxidase which generate hydrogen peroxide and also catalase which destroys hydrogen peroxide. Because of their involvement in hydrogen peroxide metabolism the term 'peroxisome' was coined by de Duve (1965) to describe them. Similarly, the presence of urate oxidase (uricase) within the crystalloid of the hepatic microbodies of some species led Afzelius (1965) to suggest that such microbodies be called 'uricosomes'. This term has not gained much popularity. The term 'peroxisome' is often used as well as the term 'microbody' coined by Rhodin.

Microbodies found in the liver and kidney are usually round or oval organelles about 0·5 μ in diameter. However, there are many interesting morphological differences discernible in microbodies from various sites and species (page 372). Initially, it appeared that microbodies were confined to a few plant cells and protozoa and to the hepatic and renal tubular epithelial cells of vertebrates. On the basis of this observation and their enzyme content it was speculated that microbodies were perhaps vestigial organelles representing a phylogenetically primitive oxidative pathway. However, the development of a cytochemical method for staining microbodies at the ultrastructural level (Fahimi, 1968; Hirai, 1968: Novikoff and Goldfischer, 1968) and also further morphological and biochemical studies have now shown that catalase-containing organelles acceptable as microbodies are found in quite a few other vertebrate cells. Such studies have also shown that all microbodies contain catalase (in rat hepatic microbodies up to 40 per cent of the microbody protein is catalase) but the hydrogen-peroxide-producing oxidases differ in number and specificity in microbodies found in various sites (de Duve, 1969a, b). Thus, catalase has become the marker for the identification of microbodies as has acid phosphatase for lysosomes.

The significance and function of microbodies in mammalian cells is poorly understood but various possibilities have been considered. It is thought that they might: (1) be involved in

N

glyconeogenesis; (2) provide an ancillary site for carbohydrate oxidation; (3) participate in the oxidation of reduced nicotinamide adenine dinucleotide; (4) play a part in lipid metabolism; and (5) protect cells against oxygen toxicity.

STRUCTURE, FUNCTION AND VARIATIONS

As pointed out in the introduction, initial work on microbodies created the impression that microbodies in vertebrates were present only in hepatic and renal tubular epithelial cells, but it was recognized that they were found also in some plant cells and protozoa. Later studies have established that microbodies are much more widely distributed.

Microbodies have now been found in: (1) algae, yeasts, plant cells and protozoa (Frederick and Newcomb, 1959, 1969; de Duve and Baudhuin, 1966; Frederick *et al.*, 1968; Muller *et al.*, 1968; Tolbert *et al.*, 1968; de Duve, 1969a, b; Muller, 1969; Tolbert and Yamazaki, 1969; Vigil, 1969, 1970; Matsushima, 1971; Clandinin, 1972); (2) fat body of an insect (Locke and McMahon, 1971); (3) hepatocytes and renal tubular epithelial cells of a large number of vertebrates including mammals (for references, see below); (4) brown adipose tissue of the rat (Ahlabo and Barnard, 1971); (5) rat adrenals (Beard, 1972); (6) Clara cells and great alveolar cells of a variety of primates and rodents (Petrik, 1971; Schneeberger, 1972a, b); (7) interstitial cells (Leydig cells) of rodent testes (Reddy and Svoboda, 1972); (8) absorptive cells of mammalian small intestine (Novikoff and Novikoff, 1972); and (9) the parenchymal cells of various exocrine glands of the rat such as pancreas, parotid, submandibular, lacrimal, nasal mucosal and von Ebner's glands (Hand, 1973).

The morphology of microbodies from hepatocytes and renal tubular epithelial cells has been studied extensively (Gansler and Rouiller, 1956; Rouiller and Bernhard, 1956; Rhodin, 1958; Ashford and Porter, 1962; Novikoff and Shin, 1964; Afzelius, 1965; Ericsson and Trump, 1966; Svoboda *et al.*, 1967; Tsukada *et al.*, 1968; Tisher *et al.*, 1968; Beard and Novikoff, 1969) and their enzyme content has also been the subject of many reports (Beaufay *et al.*, 1964; Afzelius, 1965; Allen and Beard, 1965; Baudhuin *et al.*, 1965a, b; Schnitka, 1966; Tsukada *et al.*, 1966).

These studies show that microbodies are round, oval or elongated structures bounded by a single membrane and that they contain a granular matrix. However, some microbodies have a nucleoid while others do not (*Plate 161*). If the nucleoid is present it may be either amorphous or crystalline. Rat hepatocyte microbodies contain catalase, urate oxidase, D-amino acid oxidase and α-hydroxy acid oxidase. The catalase and D-amino acid oxidase reside in the matrix while the urate oxidase is located in the crystalline cores or nucleoids. In rat kidney microbodies, catalase, D-amino acid oxidase, and L-amino- and L-α-hydroxy acid oxidase have been demonstrated, but urate oxidase is absent.

A positive correlation between the presence of urate oxidase and nucleoids (particularly nucleoids with a crystalline structure) has now been reported for hepatic and renal microbodies of a large number and variety of vertebrates (Afzelius, 1965; de la Inglesia *et al.*, 1966; Schnitka, 1966; Hruban and Rechcigl, 1967). Thus the liver of man and birds does not possess urate oxidase

---

Plate 161

Fig. 1. Hepatic microbody from a rat, showing granular matrix (M) and a crystalline nucleoid (N). × 90,000
Fig. 2. Hepatic microbody from a hamster, showing rod-like and curved nucleoids (N) × 50,000
Fig. 3. Microbodies (M) from human liver. Note the absence of nucleoids. × 27,000
Fig. 4. Microbodies (M) from the liver of a canary. Note their smaller size, denser matrix and the absence of nucleoids. × 29,000

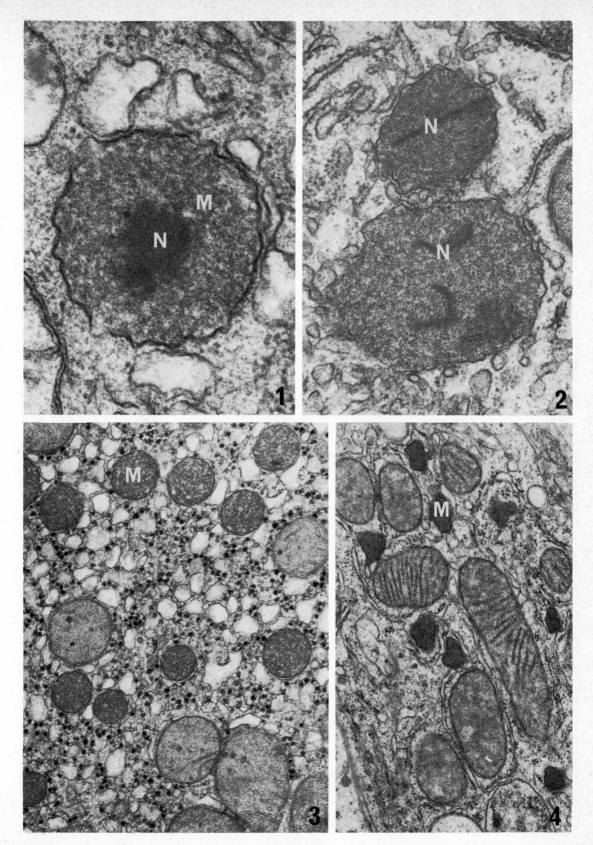

activity and the hepatic microbodies lack nucleoids. However, some exceptions to such generalizations do seem to exist. For example, the kidney tissue of man, rat and Rhesus monkey (*Macaca mulatta*) lacks urate oxidase activity, but amorphous nucleoids have been found in the renal microbodies of man, amorphous and crystalline nucleoids have been described in the renal microbodies of the rat and crystalline nucleoids have been shown in Rhesus kidney microbodies (Tisher *et al.*, 1968). Nucleoids have not been noted in microbodies found in other sites such as brown adipose tissue, adrenals, alveolar epithelial cells and interstitial cells of the testis.

Many interesting species-related and other differences in the nucleoids of microbodies have been noted (*Plates 161 and 162*). Thus the nucleoids of the microbodies of rat hepatocytes are rounded or compact bodies while in the hamster they present in ultrathin sections as one or more rod-like or filamentous structures which are sometimes curved upon themselves or angulated. Their three-dimensional form probably resembles a thin plate or a folded sheet. In bovine microbodies a linear density or marginal plate apposed against the membrane covering the microbody has been described, and this is thought to represent a filamentous nucleoid. We (Ghadially and Ailsby, unpublished observations) have seen such a plate or plates in hepatic and renal microbodies of the cow (*Plate 162*) and rabbit. Hepatic microbodies of Rhesus monkey generally do not contain a nucleoid but a rare microbody with a small nucleoid is seen. However, in the squirrel monkey, microbodies with irregular, linear or angular nucleoids occur (Wattiaux-DeConinck *et al.*, 1965; Svoboda *et al.*, 1967). Although the hepatic microbodies of normal man do not contain a nucleoid, Biempica (1966) found that in a complex disease state the microbodies developed a crystalline nucleoid.

Newly formed microbodies lack a nucleoid because this structure is developed at a later stage of maturation of the microbody. Thus in the hepatocytes of fetal rats only rarely do microbodies contain nucleoids and the matrix is not as dense as in the adult rat (Tsukada *et al.*, 1968). Similarly, most of the abundant newly formed microbodies in the regenerating rat liver also lack a nucleoid (Svoboda *et al.*, 1967).

It would appear that the number and size of microbodies show many variations. Hepatic microbodies from various species range in size from 0·1 to 1 μ, but most measure approximately 0·5 μ in diameter. In the great alveolar cells, microbodies are much smaller and measure between 0·1 and 0·2 μ in diameter. The ratio of microbodies to mitochondria is said to be approximately 1 to 4 in hepatocytes and between 1 to 1 and 1 to 2 in the great alveolar cells. (Schneeberger, 1972a).

Plate 162

Fig. 1. Microbodies from a cow hepatocyte, showing linear densities which probably represent a transverse section through a marginal plate (P). Also seen are structures resembling conventional nucleoids but they are more likely to be tangential (T) sections through the marginal plate. × 37,000

Fig. 2. Microbodies from a renal tubular epithelial cell of a cow. Multiple marginal plates (P) can be seen in these microbodies, as are crystalline bodies in the matrix. The latter probably represent tangential (T) sections through a marginal plate. × 40,000

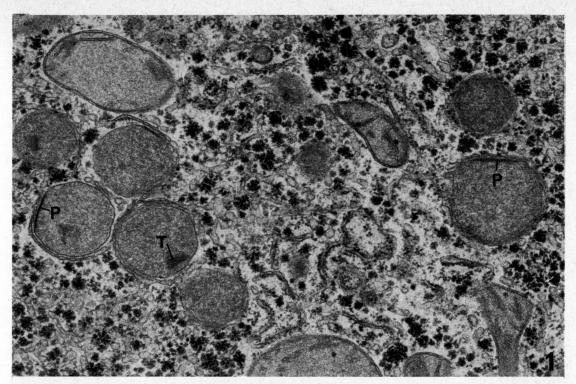

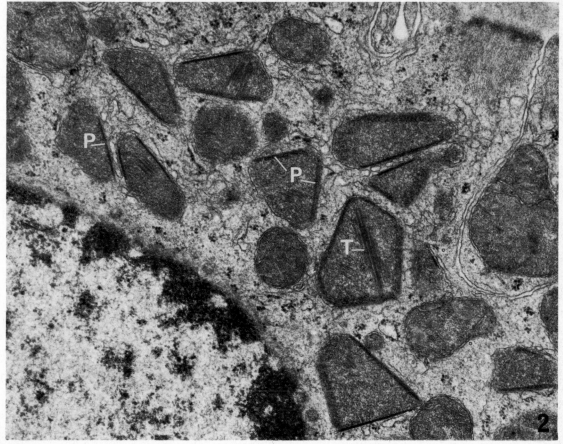

The site of origin and the manner in which microbodies are produced remain speculative. There is said to be a turnover of microbodies (Poole et al., 1969) but how these organelles regress is not clear either. Suggested mechanisms for the removal of microbodies include: (1) transformation or incorporation into lysosomes; and (2) dissolution of the organelle into the surrounding cytoplasm (Svoboda et al., 1967). The idea that microbodies may arise from or develop into mitochondria (Gansler and Rouiller, 1956; Rouiller and Bernhard, 1956; Engfeldt et al., 1958) has been abandoned by most workers, although there are some who still support such concepts (Pavel et al., 1971). A possible origin of microbodies from the following structures has been proposed: (1) smooth endoplasmic reticulum (Hagiwara et al., 1961; Hruban et al., 1963, 1965; Novikoff and Shin, 1964; Essner, 1966; Svoboda and Azarnoff, 1966; Tsukada et al., 1966; Svoboda et al., 1967); (2) Golgi complex and multivesicular bodies (Rouiller and Bernhard, 1956; Rouiller and Jezequel, 1963; Bruni and Porter, 1965; Ericsson and Glinsmann, 1966; Dvorak and Mazanec, 1967); and (3) rough endoplasmic reticulum (Essner and Masin, 1967; Tsukada et al., 1968; Mochizuki, 1968).

Regarding hepatic microbodies there was, until recently, general agreement that the necessary enzymes were produced by the ribosomes on the rough endoplasmic reticulum and that the material was then sequestrated in diverticula arising from the endoplasmic reticulum or travelled to the Golgi complex where it was parcelled off to form microbodies. Recent cytochemical studies have, however, cast a doubt on this thesis and it is now suggested by Wood and Legg (1970) that 'new microbodies may arise from pre-existing microbodies and that catalase after formation on the ribosomes of the rough endoplasmic reticulum, may be transferred directly into microbodies without passing through the cisternae of either the endoplasmic reticulum or Golgi apparatus'. Similar sentiments are expressed by Schneeberger (1972a), who found that in the great alveolar cells of the lung there is a threefold increase in the number of microbodies immediately before birth, and that microbodies at all stages of development are found in close proximity to the rough endoplasmic reticulum. However, physical connections between the two were not demonstrable and she states, 'It appeared that peroxisomes were formed de novo within the cytoplasm'.

The role of microbodies in cell physiology is poorly understood. (Various suggestions on this point are summarized on page 369.) They do not appear to be very responsive to altered states engendered by disease or experimental procedures. However, in a few instances, alterations in the population density and morphology of these bodies are known to occur.

A rapid and sustained increase in hepatic or hepatic and renal microbodies can be produced in some species by feeding clofibrate (ethyl chlorophenoxyisobutyrate). Such an increase may also be accompanied by an alteration in the size and shape of microbodies (Plate 163; Plate 164, Figs. 1 and 2). This includes the formation of elongate and bipartite microbodies, and the appearance of tail-like or strap-like protuberances from them (Hess et al., 1965; Svoboda et al., 1967; Hartman and Tousimis, 1969). Clofibrate is a hypolipidaemic agent which lowers serum

---

Plate 163

The marked increase in the number of microbodies produced in rat hepatocytes by feeding clofibrate is illustrated in this electron micrograph. Only a few of the microbodies contain a nucleoid (N) but some (arrow) contain multiple small nucleoids. ×15,500

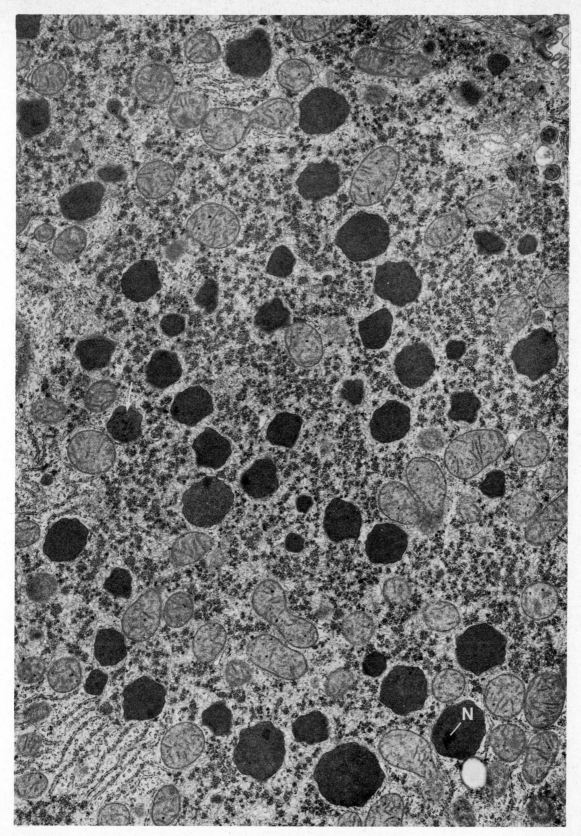

cholesterol and triglycerides in man, but hypolipidaemia in itself does not appear to be responsible for the increase, since many other hypolipidaemic agents do not produce this change. The response is also sex and species specific. For example, in the male rat, hepatic and renal microbodies are increased in number after clofibrate feeding but this is not so in the female. An increase in hepatic microbodies after clofibrate is seen in mice, dogs and hamsters but not in the guinea-pig, rabbit and squirrel-monkey (Svoboda et al., 1967).

Reports on other drugs which have altered microbody population and/or morphology include: (1) alterations of microbody population after ethionine; (2) increase in number and size after salicylates; (3) increase in number and changes in matrix after thioacetamide; (4) enlargement of crystalloid core after azaserine and terephthalanilides; and (5) extrusion of nucleoid after hexahydrosalicylic acid and sodium tungstate (for references, see Svoboda et al., 1967). Alterations in microbodies have not been reported after phenobarbitone administration and our experience is in keeping with this. However, in a hamster treated with this drug we (Ghadially and Bhatnagar, unpublished observations) found some large microbodies (*Plate 164, Fig. 3*) and some microbodies containing glycogen (*Plate 121, Fig. 1*). The glycogen lay either free in the microbody matrix or within a vacuole containing electron-lucent material. In one instance an appearance which could be interpreted as a glycogen-containing vacuole entering a microbody was seen. In hepatomas there is usually a reduction in the number of microbodies. It is said that the number of microbodies present is inversely proportional to the growth rate of the tumour (Dalton, 1964).

Perhaps the most constant and frequently studied biochemical change known to occur in animals bearing a variety of tumours is the reduction of liver catalase activity (Greenstein, 1954) and it would appear that there is also a decrease in the number of microbodies in the hepatocytes (Ghadially and Parry, 1965; Mochizuki, 1968). Since 80 per cent of the liver catalase activity is believed to be localized in microbodies and about 40 per cent of microbody protein can be ascribed to catalase (Beaufay et al., 1964; Fugiwara, 1964; de Duve and Baudhuin, 1966), a reduction of microbodies in the liver of the tumour-bearing host may be expected. The mechanism and specificity of catalase depression in the liver of the tumour-bearing host have been the subject of much dispute but there is now overwhelming evidence that this change and the remarkable increase in hepatocellular lysosomes that occurs in the tumour-bearing animal is engendered by a toxic polypeptide (toxohormone) produced by viable tumour tissue (for references to the considerable literature on the subject, see Kampschmidt, 1965; Nakahara, 1967; Parry and Ghadially, 1970).

Plate 164

Fig. 1. The marked increase in the number of microbodies produced in renal tubular epithelial cells of the rat by feeding clofibrate is illustrated in this electron micrograph. Many microbodies (arrows) show multiple nucleoids. × 16,000 (*Ghadially and Ailsby, unpublished electron micrograph*)

Fig. 2. High power view of two of the microbodies shown in *Fig. 1.* × 51,000 (*Ghadially and Ailsby, unpublished electron micrograph*)

Fig. 3. An unusually large microbody (approximately 2·4 μ long) found in the liver of a hamster that had received phenobarbitone. × 40,000 (*Ghadially and Bhatnagar, unpublished electron micrograph*)

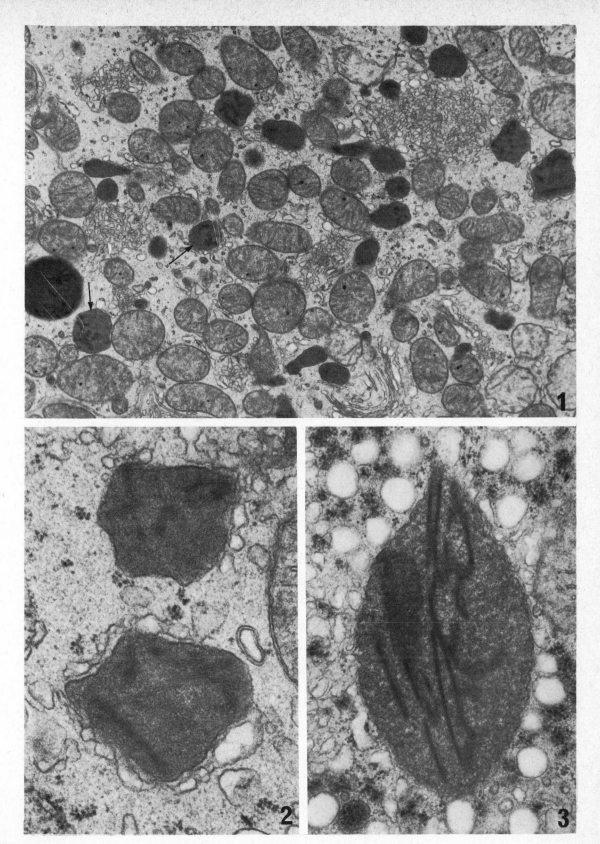

377

Afzelius, B. (1965). 'The occurrence and structure of microbodies. A comparative study.' *J. Cell Biol.* **26**, 835

Ahlabo, I. and Barnard, T. (1971). 'Observations of peroxisomes in brown adipose tissue of the rat.' *J. Histochem. Cytochem.* **19**, 670

Allen, J. and Beard, M. (1965). 'Alpha-hydroxy acid oxidase: localization in renal microbodies.' *Science* **149**, 1507

Ashford, T. P. and Porter, K. R. (1962). 'Cytoplasmic components in hepatic cell lysosomes.' *J. cell. Biol. Cytol.* **12**, 198

Baudhuin, P., Beaufay, H. and de Duve, C. (1965a). 'Combined biochemical and morphological study of particulate fractions from rat liver; analysis of preparations enriched in lysosomes or in particles containing urate oxidase, D-amino acid oxidase, and catalase.' *J. Cell Biol.* **26**, 219

— Muller, M., Poole, B. and de Duve, C. (1965b). 'Non-mitochondrial oxidizing particles (microbodies) in rat liver and kidney and in *Tetrahymena pyriformis*.' *Biochem. Biophys. Res. Commun.* **20**, 53

Beard, M. E. (1972). 'Identification of peroxisomes in the rat adrenal cortex.' *J. Histochem. Cytochem.* **20**, 173

— and Novikoff, A. B. (1969). 'Distribution of peroxisomes (microbodies) in the nephron of the rat. A cytochemical study.' *J. Cell Biol.* **42**, 501

Beaufay, H., Jacques, P., Baudhuin, P., Sellinger, O. Z., Berthet, J. and de Duve, C. (1964). 'Tissue fractionation studies. 18. Resolution of mitochondrial fractions from rat liver into three distinct populations of cytoplasmic particles by means of density equilibration in various gradients.' *Biochem. J.* **92**, 184

Biempica, L. (1966). 'Human hepatic microbodies with crystalloid cores.' *J. Cell Biol.* **29**, 383

Bruni, C. and Porter, K. R. (1965). 'The fine structure of the parenchymal cell of the normal rat liver. I. General Obervations.' *Am. J. Path.* **46**, 691

Clandinin, M. T. (1972). 'Some ultrastructural observations of cotyledonary tissue and microbodies from *Pisum sarivum*.' *Experientia* **28**, 237

Dalton, A. J. (1964). 'An electron microscopical study of a series of chemically induced hepatomas.' In *Cellular Control Mechanisms and Cancer*, p. 211. Ed. by P. Emmelot and O. Muhlbock. New York: American Elsevier

de Duve, C. (1965). 'Functions of microbodies (peroxisomes).' *J. Cell Biol.* **27**, 25A

— (1969a). 'The peroxisome: a new cytoplasmic organelle.' *Proc. R. Soc. (Biol).* **173**, 71

— (1969b). 'Evolution of the peroxisome.' *Ann. N.Y. Acad. Sci.* **168**, 369

— and Baudhuin, P. (1966). 'Peroxisomes (microbodies and related particles).' *Physiol. Rev.* **46**, 323

de la Inglesia, F. A., Porta, E. A. and Hartcroft, W. S. (1966). 'Histochemical urate oxidase activity and microbodies in non-human primate liver.' *J. Histochem. Cytochem.* **14**, 685

Dvorak, M. and Mazanec, K. (1967). 'Differenzierung der Feinstruktur der Leberzelle in der fruhen Postnatalen Periode.' *Z. Zellforsch. mikrosk. Anat.* **80**, 370

Engfeldt, B., Gardell, S., Hellstrom, J., Ivemark, B., Rhodin, J. and Strandh, J. (1958). 'Effect of experimentally induced hyperparathyroidism on renal function and structure.' *Acta endocr.* **29**, 15

Ericsson, J. L. E. and Glinsmann, W. H. (1966). 'Observations on the subcellular organization of hepatic parenchymal cells. I. Golgi apparatus, cytosomes, and cytosegresomes in normal cells.' *Lab. Invest.* **15**, 750

— and Trump, B. F. (1966). 'Electron microscopic studies of the epithelium of the proximal tubule of the rat kidney. III. Microbodies, multivesicular bodies, and the Golgi apparatus.' *Lab. Invest.* **15**, 1610

Essner, E. (1966). 'Endoplasmic reticulum and the origin of microbodies in fetal liver.' *Fedn Proc.* **25**, 361

— and Masin, E. J. (1967). 'Endoplasmic reticulum and the origin of microbodies in fetal mouse liver.' *Lab. Invest.* **17**, 71

Fahimi, H. D. (1968). 'Cytochemical localization of peroxidase activity in rat hepatic microbodies (peroxisomes).' *J. Histochem. Cytochem.* **16**, 547

Frederick, S. E. and Newcomb, E. H. (1959). 'Microbody-like organelles in leaf cells.' *Science* **163**, 1353

— — (1969). 'Cytochemical localization of catalase in leaf microbodies (peroxisomes).' *J. Cell Biol.* **43**, 343

— — Vigil, E. L. and Wergin, W. P. (1968). 'Fine-structural characterization of plant microbodies.' *Planta med.* **81**, 229

Fujiwara, F. (1964). 'Influences of fractionation media on the release of enzymes in light-mitochondrial fraction in rat and mouse liver cells, with special reference to uricase-containing particles.' *Sapporo med. J.* **26**, 102

Gansler, H. and Rouiller, C. (1956). 'Modifications physiologiques et pathologiques du chondriome. Etude au microscope electronique.' *Schweiz. Z. Path. Bakt.* **19**, 217

Ghadially, F. N. and Parry, E. W. (1965). 'Ultrastructure of the liver of the tumor-bearing host.' *Cancer* **18**, 485

Greenstein, J. P. (1954). *Biochemistry of Cancer.* New York: Academic Press

Hagiwara, A., Suzuki, T. and Takaki, F. (1961). 'Electron microscopic cyto-histopathology (VIII). Electron microscopic studies of the liver. (2) Studies on the origin of so-called "microbodies" as a precursor of rat liver mitochondria, and their relations to the secretion granules of the bile.' *Jikei med.* **8**, 51

Hand, A. R. (1973). 'Morphologic and cytochemical identification of peroxisomes in the rat parotid and other exocrine glands.' *J. Histochem. Cytochem.* **21**, 131

Hartman, H. A. and Tousimis, A. J. (1969). 'Rat hepatocyte peroxisomes: ultrastructural alterations following cessation of chronic dietary clofibrate administration.' *Experientia* **25**, 1248

Hess, R., Staubli, W. and Riess, W. (1965). 'Nature of the hepatomegalic effect produced by ethyl-chlorophenoxyisobutyrate in the rat.' *Nature, Lond.* **208**, 856

Hirai, K. (1968). 'Specific affinity of oxidized amine dye (radical intermediates) for heme enzymes: study in microscopy and spectrophotometry.' *Acta histochem. cytochem.* **1**, 43

Hruban, Z. and Rechcigl, M., Jr. (1967). 'Comparative ultrastructure of microbodies.' *Fedn Proc.* **26**, 513

— Swift, H. and Wissler, R. J. (1963). 'Alterations in the fine structure of hepatocytes produced by β-3-thienylalanine.' *J. Ultrastruct. Res.* **8**, 236

— — and Slesers, A. (1965). 'Effect of azaserine on the fine structure of the liver and pancreatic acinar cells.' *Cancer Res.* **25,** 708

Kampschmidt, R. F. (1965). 'Mechanism of liver catalase depression in tumor-bearing animals: a review.' *Cancer Res.* **25,** 34

Locke, M. and McMahon, J. T. (1971). 'The origin and fate of microbodies in the fat body of an insect.' *J. Cell Biol.* **48,** 61

Matsushima, H. (1971). 'The microbody with a crystalloid core in tobacco cultured cell clone XD-6S. I. Cytochemical studies on the microbody.' *J. Electron Microsc.* **20,** 120

Mochizuki, Y. (1968). 'An electron microscope study on hepatocyte microbodies of mice bearing Ehrlich ascites tumor.' *Tumor Res.* **3,** 1

Muller, M. (1969). 'Peroxisomes of protozoa.' *Ann. N.Y. Acad. Sci.* **168,** 292

— Hogg, J. F. and de Duve, C. H. (1968). 'Distribution of tricarboxylic acid cycle enzymes and glyozylate cycle enzymes between mitochondria and peroxisomes in *Tetrahymena pyriformis.' J. Biol. Chem.* **243,** 5385

Nakahara, W. (1967). 'Toxohormone.' In *Methods in Cancer Research,* Vol. 2, p. 203. Ed. by H. Busch. New York: Academic Press

Novikoff, A. B. and Goldfischer, S. (1968). 'Visualization of microbodies for light and electron microscopy.' *J. Histochem. Cytochem.* **16,** 507

— and Shin, W. Y. (1964). 'The endoplasmic reticulum in the Golgi zone and its relations to microbodies, Golgi apparatus and autophagic vacuoles in rat liver cells.' *J. Microscopie* **3,** 187

Novikoff, P. M. and Novikoff, A. B. (1972). 'Peroxisomes in absorptive cells of mammalian small intestine.' *J. Cell Biol.* **53,** 532

Parry, E. W. and Ghadially, F. N. (1970). 'The effects of toxohormone on the ultrastructure of rat hepatocytes.' *J. Path.* **100,** 161

Pavel, I., Bonaparte, H. and Petrovici, A. (1971). 'Involution of liver mitochondria in viral hepatitis.' *Archs Path.* **91,** 294

Petrik, P. (1971). 'Fine structural identification of peroxisomes in mouse and rat bronchiolar and alveolar epithelium.' *J. Histochem. Cytochem.* **19,** 339

Poole, B., Leighton, F. and de Duve, C. (1969). 'The synthesis and turnover of rat liver peroxisomes. II. Turnover of peroxisome proteins.' *J. Cell Biol.* **41,** 536

Reddy, J. and Svoboda, D. (1972). 'Microbodies (peroxisomes) in the interstitial cells of rodent testes.' *Lab. Invest.* **26,** 657

Rhodin, J. (1954). 'Correlation of ultrastructural organization and function in normal and experimentally changed proximal convoluted tubule cells of the mouse kidney.' Thesis, Karolinska Institute, Stockholm, Aktiebolaget Godvil

— (1956). 'Further studies on the nephron ultrastructure in mouse. Terminal part of proximal convolution.' In *Proceedings Stockholm Conference Electron Microscopy.* Ed. by Almqvist A. Wiksell. Stockholm

— (1958). 'Electron microscopy of the kidney.' *Am. J. Med.* **24,** 661

Rouiller, C. and Bernhard, W. (1956). 'Microbodies and the problem of mitochondrial regeneration in liver cells.' *J. biophys. biochem. Cytol.* **2,** Suppl. 4, 355

— and Jezequel, A. (1963). 'Electron microscopy of the liver.' In *The Liver: Morphology, Biochemistry, Physiology,* Vol. 1, p. 195. Ed. by C. Rouiller. New York: Academic Press

Schneeberger, E. E. (1972a). 'Development of peroxisomes in granular pneumocytes during pre- and postnatal growth.' *Lab. Invest.* **27,** 581

— (1972b). 'A comparative cytochemical study of microbodies (peroxisomes) in great alveolar cells of rodents, rabbit and monkey.' *J. Histochem. Cytochem.* **20,** 180

Schnitka, T. K. (1966). 'Comparative ultrastructure of hepatic microbodies in some mammals and birds in relation to species differences in uricase activity.' *J. Ultrastruct. Res.* **16,** 598

Svoboda, D. J. and Azarnoff, D. L. (1966). 'Response of hepatic microbodies to a hypolipidemic agent, ethyl chlorophenoxyisobutyrate (CPIB).' *J. Cell Biol.* **30,** 442

— Grady, H. and Azarnoff, D. (1967). 'Microbodies in experimentally altered cells.' *J. Cell Biol.* **35,** 127

Tisher, C. C., Finkel, R. M., Rosen, S. and Kendig, E. M. (1968). 'Renal microbodies in the Rhesus monkey.' *Lab. Invest.* **19,** 1

Tolbert, N. E. and Yamazaki, R. K. (1969). 'Leaf peroxisomes and their relation to photorespiration and photosynthesis.' *Ann. N.Y. Acad. Sci.* **168,** 325

— Oeser, A., Kisaki, T., Hageman, R. H. and Yamazaki, R. K. (1968). 'Peroxisomes from spinach leaves containing enzymes related to glycolate metabolism.' *J. Biol. Chem.* **243,** 5179

Tsukada, H., Mochizuki, Y. and Fujiwara, S. (1966). 'The nucleoids of rat liver cell microbodies. Fine structure and enzymes.' *J. Cell Biol.* **28,** 449

— — and Konishi, T. (1968). 'Morphogenesis and development of microbodies of hepatocytes of rats during pre- and postnatal growth.' *J. Cell Biol.* **37,** 231

Vigil, E. L. (1969). 'Intracellular localization of catalase (peroxidatic) activity in plant microbodies'. *J. Histochem. Cytochem.* **17,** 425

— (1970). 'Cytochemical and developmental changes in microbodies (glyxysomes) and related organelles of castor bean endosperm.' *J. Cell Biol.* **46,** 435

Wattiaux-de Coninck, S., Rutgeerts, M. and Wattiaux, J. (1965). 'Lysosomes in rat-kidney tissue.' *Biochim. biophys. acta* **105,** 446

Wood, R. L. and Legg, P. G. (1970). 'Peroxidase activity in rat liver microbodies after amino-triazole inhibition.' *J. Cell Biol.* **45,** 576

CHAPTER IX

Melanosomes

INTRODUCTION

A melanosome may be defined as the specific organelle of the melanocyte in which melanin is synthesized. The end-product of its action is the melanin granule (now called stage IV melanosome), into which it is ultimately transformed. Melanosomes are produced by melanocytes, and melanosomes in early stages of development are found only in these cells. Later stages of development are found both in melanocytes and other cells such as the basal and prickle cells of the epidermis (keratinocytes) and phagocytic cells in the dermis (melanophages). Masson (1948) recognized two types of melanocytes: continent and incontinent. An example of continent melanocytes is found in the pigment epithelium of the eye where these cells retain the synthesized melanin throughout their life. The incontinent melanocytes of the epidermis and hair follicles discharge their melanin (melanosomes) into epithelial cells by a process which Masson called 'cytocrine activity'.

In the past there was much confusion regarding the nomenclature of melanin-containing cells, and it was widely held that a variety of cells, such as the basal cells of the epidermis and also various mesenchymal cells, could all synthesize melanin. This confusion was reflected also in the concepts and nomenclature of malignant melanomas, which were called melanocarcinomas or melanosarcomas; and the benign melanoma (naevus) was generally thought to arise from the basal cells of the epidermis. Innumerable later studies have, however, clearly established the melanocyte as a specific cell type, and its origin from the neural crest has also been long established (Rawles, 1947, 1948).

In this era, however, melanocytes were often referred to as melanoblasts, and melanophages as melanophores. At the Third International Pigment Cell Conference it was decided (Gordon, 1953) to call the mature melanin-producing and melanin-containing cell a melanocyte and to reserve the term melanoblast for the embryonic precursor capable of transforming into a melanocyte. It was also pointed out that the term 'melanophore' had long been used to describe certain pigment-effector cells of lower vertebrates (now thought to be a variety of melanocyte in which dispersion or aggregation of pigment leads to rapid skin colour changes) and the principle of priority in scientific nomenclature dictated that this term should not be used to describe the functionally and morphologically different melanophages of man and higher vertebrates, which contained phagocytosed melanin.

The melanocyte is now recognized as the basic pigment cell not only of human melanomas but of melanomas of all vertebrates. This view, first advocated by Gordon (1948) from the study of piscine melanomas produced by genetic methods in *Platypoecilus* x *Xiphophorus* hybrids (Gordon 1937; Grand *et al.*, 1941), was also found to be so for the *Lebistes* x *Mollienesia* hybrid (Ghadially and Gordon, 1957)* and the abundant melanotic tumours that arise in hamster skin painted with carcinogens (Ghadially and Barker, 1960; Illman and Ghadially, 1960; Ghadially and Illman, 1964, 1966).

The discovery of the melanosome by Seiji *et al.* in 1961 marks the last step in establishing unequivocally the melanocyte as a race of cells quite distinct and different from others. This advance led to a reconsideration of the nomenclature of pigment cells, and at the Sixth International Pigment Cell Conference the melanocyte was defined as 'A cell which synthesizes a specialized melanin-containing organelle, the melanosome' (Fitzpatrick *et al.*, 1966).

* According to the Rosen and Bailey (1963) classification, fishes of the genera *Lebistes* and *Mollienesia* are now classified under the genus *Poecilia*. The genus *Platypoecilus* has been absorbed into the genus *Xiphophorus*. (For colour illustrations and descriptions of these fishes, see Ghadially, 1969).

382

The concept that melanin synthesis occurs in a specialized organelle of the melanocyte called the melanosome was first proposed by Seiji *et al.* (1961). It is now clear that this organelle contains tyrosinase, an enzyme which is involved in the oxidation of the colourless amino acid, tyrosine, to the pigmented polymers we call the melanins (eumelanins are brownish-black, phaeomelanins are yellowish-red). Dopa (3,4-dihydroxyphenylalanine) is an intermediate compound formed during the first stage of this oxidative reaction. Thus, when either dopa or tyrosine is presented to cells containing tyrosinase, they show increased pigmentation. This is the basis of the dopa reaction (Bloch, 1927) and the tyrosinase reaction (Fitzpatrick *et al.*, 1950); both reveal the presence of the only known enzyme involved in melanin synthesis, namely tyrosinase.

The latest classification of melanosomes (Fitzpatrick *et al.*, 1971) recognizes four stages of melanosome development. The first or earliest stage of development contains no melanin. The last stage is the fully mature melanin granule where the internal structure of the melanosome is totally masked or destroyed by melanin deposition (*Plates 165 and 166*). The earlier stages possess an active tyrosinase system; the last stage does not. The ontogeny of melanosomes has been the subject of excellent reviews (Toda *et al.*, 1968; Fitzpatrick *et al.*, 1971). It is now generally held that tyrosinase is synthesized by the ribosomes of the rough endoplasmic reticulum and transported via this organelle to the Golgi complex where it is parcelled off into small vesicles (melanosome stage I). The vesicles then enlarge and elongate to form an oval organelle (melanosome stage II, previously called premelanosome) in which develops a characteristic patterned membranous structure, the three-dimensional morphology of which is difficult to interpret. The internal structure has been regarded as a folded membrane, a concentric sheet, or a helical tubular structure with a space of about 100 Å between each turn of the coil.* Deposition of melanin on the membranous structure heralds the next stage (melanosome stage III, or partially melanized melanosome), and the completion of this process produces a uniformly electron-dense granule without discernible internal structure (melanosome stage IV, mature melanosome or melanin granule).

Variations in the size and shape of the melanosomes, depending on site and species, are known to occur. Breathnach (1969) reported that mature melanosomes of dark human skin measure 0·37 by 1·15 μ, that of the hair bulbs 0·3 by 0·7 μ, while melanosomes from the pigmented epithelium in the eye can measure up to 1·4 μ in breadth and 1·9 μ in length. (Recent scanning electron microscope studies show that the last-named can be as much as 2·5 μ long.) In red hair and in

---

* In sectioned material various appearances are seen in stages II and III melanosomes. A common appearance is that of a series of parallel or concentric zig-zag or dotted lines (*Plate 165*). Another appearance seen is that of striated or banded material lying in the melanosome (*Plates 168 and 169*).

Plate 165

From the pigment epithelium of the eye of a 10-week-old human fetus. (*Ghadially and Ailsby, unpublished electron micrographs*)

Fig. 1. Numerous stage III (A) and IV (B) melanosomes are seen in these cells. ×6,500

Fig. 2. A stage II melanosome, showing membranous formations in its interior. ×39,000

Figs. 3–6. Stage III melanosomes. The difference in appearances seen can be related to (1) the size and shape of the melanosome, (2) the plane of sectioning and (3) the amount of melanin present. ×39,000; ×40,000; ×45,000; ×40,000

Fig. 7. Stage IV melanosomes or melanin granules are seen here. ×26,000

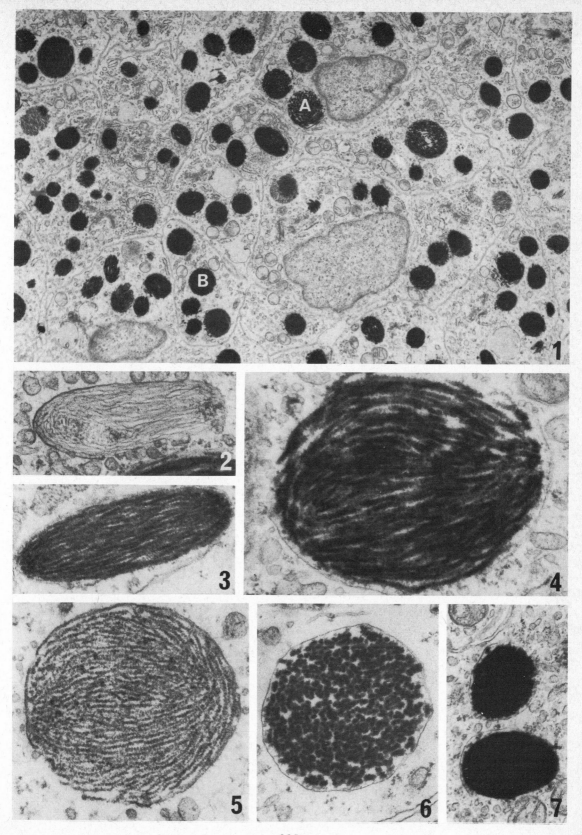

the relatively unpigmented skin between freckles in very pale caucasoids the melanosomes are more rounded (Birbeck and Barnicot, 1959; Breathnach, 1964). Differences in size, shape and internal structure, thought to be determined by genes, have been described in experimental animals such as mice (Moyer, 1961, 1963, 1966). Except in rare instances, melanosomes occur as discrete bodies in the melanocyte, but in the keratinocytes* and melanophages they also occur grouped together within single-membrane-bound bodies, which have at times been referred to as 'melanosome complexes' or 'compound melanosomes' (Drochmans, 1966). Because acid phosphatase activity has been demonstrated in these structures, they are regarded as lysosomes (Hori *et al.*, 1968). Fine granular material is also seen in these lysosomal bodies and this is regarded as material derived from the degradation of melanosomes and also perhaps other material incorporated within these lysosomes.

In caucasoids and mongoloids, groups of melanosomes occur within the lysosomes of the keratinocyte, but in the former they are not closely packed and fine granular material between them is more abundant (Szabo *et al.*, 1969). In negroids and Australian aborigines (Mitchell, 1968) the much larger melanosomes are dispersed individually within the keratinocyte, and characteristic 'complexes' with numerous melanosomes are not seen. Thus, a factor responsible for the more marked pigmentation of the negroid skin seems to be the persistence of pigment which, in the caucasoid, is destroyed by lysosomal activity.

Racial differences in pigmentation do not appear to be due to variations of population density of the melanocytes. The number of melanocytes varies with regions of the body, there being 2,000 or more melanocytes per square millimetre on exposed skin such as that of the forearm and face but only about 100 per square millimetre on the rest of the body in caucasoids, mongoloids and negroids (Szabo *et al.*, 1969). However, quantitative and qualitative differences between the melanosomes in the melanocyte occur among the races. Melanosomes are larger and more numerous in negroids and virtually all are stage III and IV melanosomes; stage II melanosomes are rarely seen. In very pale caucasoids with blue eyes and red hair, very few melanosomes are seen in the melanocytes and few, if any, stage III or IV melanosomes are found. In darker caucasoids the stage IV melanosome is rarely seen, but melanosomes stage I, II and III are present (Fitzpatrick *et al.*, 1971).

Ultraviolet radiation leads to a general increase in the number of melanosomes in all races. Qualitative changes are also noted; stage IV melanosomes develop in the skin of pale caucasoids and many more stage II and III melanosomes are found in negroids.

* Epidermal cells producing keratin are collectively referred to as keratinocytes. This includes basal cells and prickle cells.

Plate 166

Electron micrograph from normal human skin (caucasoid) showing a melanocyte (M) and a keratinocyte (K) separated from the dermis (D) by basement membrane (arrows). The melanocyte has a paler appearance and contains numerous discrete melanosomes (S). The keratinocyte has a darker appearance and contains numerous bundles of tonofilaments (T) and hemidesmosomes (H) along its basal border. Numerous large compound melanosomes (*) (formed by the aggregation of solitary melanosomes transferred from the melanocyte to the keratinocyte) are present. In some (C), the melanosomes within the compound melanosome can just be discerned. (See also *Plate 181.*) ×26,000

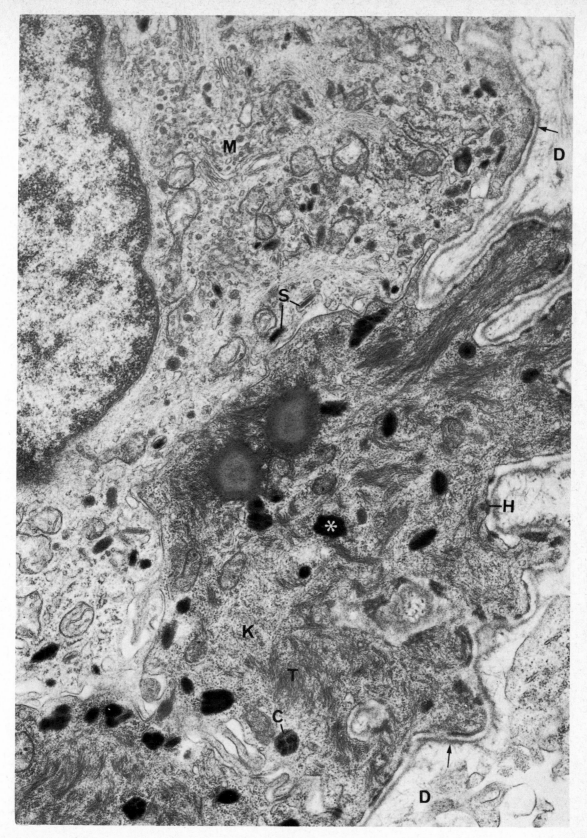

In addition to the normal variation in melanosome morphology, there also occur quantitative and qualitative variations associated with pigmentary disorders and melanomas. The largest single study on this point is by Mishima (1966), who described the melanosome morphology in various disorders such as Dubreuilh's melanosis, amelanotic and melanotic melanoma, junction naevus, intradermal naevus, juvenile melanoma, naevus of Ota, blue naevus, vitiligo and albinism. That considerable variation in melanosome morphology can occur in these conditions is evident from the illustrations in this paper, but how specific these alterations are has yet to be established.

It is well known that the amount of melanin in melanomas can vary markedly, and the naked-eye appearance of these tumours can range from black, through various shades of grey, to pink. This has been found to be so for melanomas of various animals including man and it is customary to refer to such tumours as melanotic, hypomelanotic or amelanotic melanomas. In the last instance melanin cannot be demonstrated unequivocally by histological examination of the tumour and the diagnosis of the lesion may become difficult or impossible. The amelanotic state indicates a loss of functional activity or dedifferentiation, and as such one may expect amelanotic melanomas to be more aggressive than melanotic melanomas (Illman and Ghadially, 1960; Ghadially and Illman, 1966). While this is, to some extent, correct, in man at least both well pigmented and non-pigmented malignant melanomas show a devastating capacity to metastasize.

It has already been noted (page 382) that the basic pigment cell of melanomas is the melanocyte. As well as the neoplastic melanocytes, however, there also occur numerous melanophages in the melanoma, and it is these cells which contain most of the pigment (*Plates 167 and 168*). Here, as in the normal state, the malignant melanocytes contain solitary or discrete melanosomes (many too small to be visualized by light microscopy) while the melanophages contain

---

Plate 167

Section from an equine melanoma showing a well differentiated melanocyte with melanosomes (M) in various stages of development and melanophages containing numerous compound melanosomes (C). × 13,500

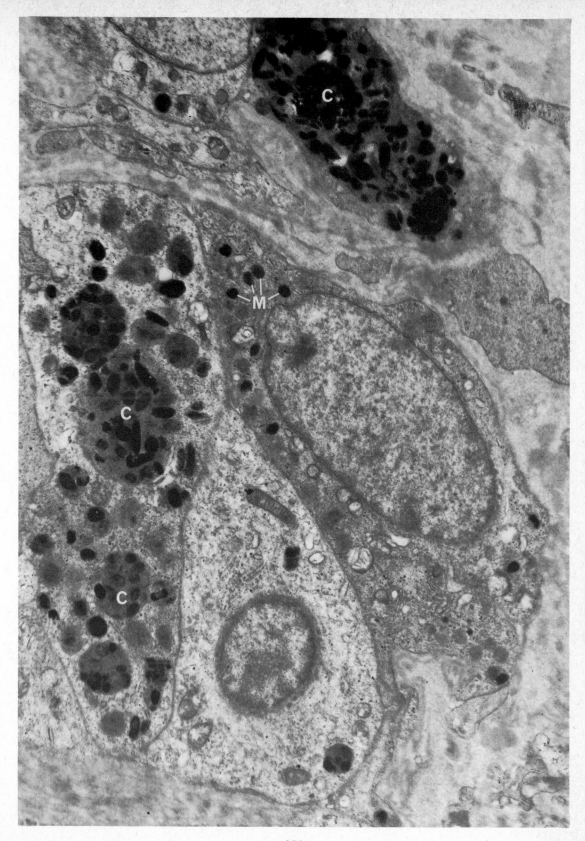

large compound melanosomes composed of numerous melanosomes derived from the malignant melanocytes. Such compound melanosomes contain recognizable melanosomes and also much granular material derived from their breakdown. Acid phosphatase activity has been demonstrated in such compound melanosomes, and they are thought to be a variety of phagolysosome. The melanosomes in the malignant melanocyte retain certain characteristic features of internal structure which permit their identification, but these organelles also show much variation in size, shape and internal organization (*Plate 169*).

Pigment-containing melanomas are easily diagnosed histologically, but when pigment production is sparse or absent this may be difficult (*Plate 169*). In such instances, electron microscopy may establish the diagnosis unequivocally by demonstrating small, poorly pigmented or unpigmented melanosomes in the tumour cells.

In hypomelanotic conditions such as human piebaldism and in recessively spotted guinea-pigs, melanocytes are absent from the 'white forelock' or the white skin areas (Breathnach *et al.*, 1965; Breathnach and Goodwin, 1965). In albino skin and hair follicles melanocytes and melanosomes are present, but they contain little or no melanin. In certain albino animals such as mice, there may be a total absence of melanin in the melanosomes (stage I and II melanosomes). This is not so in human oculocutaneous albinism, where stage III melanosomes with a minimal amount of melanin content also occur. The transfer of melanosomes from melanocytes to keratinocytes occurs as in the normal state. The basic defect in the human albino is subnormal melanogenesis, and this is determined genetically (inherited as a simple recessive trait). The subnormal melanogenesis is thought to be due to deficient tyrosinase synthesis but the unavailability of free tryosin or the presence of tyrosinase inhibitors may also be involved (Witkop *et al.*, 1963; Fitzpatrick and Quevedo, 1966; Chian and Wilgram, 1967).

In the low level of pigmentation seen in areas of chronic eczematous dermatitis (Pinkus *et al.*, 1959) the melanocytes become loaded with melanosomes, but few melanosomes are transferred to the keratinocytes. It is believed that the defect lies in the keratinocytes which are unable to accept the melanosomes. Such a mechanism also probably explains the hypomelanosis in

Plate 168

From a markedly melanotic malignant melanoma of human skin.

Fig. 1. Numerous pleomorphic melanosomes are seen in this malignant melanocyte. × 32,000

Fig. 2. Compound melanosomes found in a melanophage in this tumour. Besides recognizable melanin granules these single-membrane-bound bodies contain much granular material. Note that lipid droplets as found in lipofuscin granules are absent. Compare with *Plates 134, 135 and 152.* × 32,000

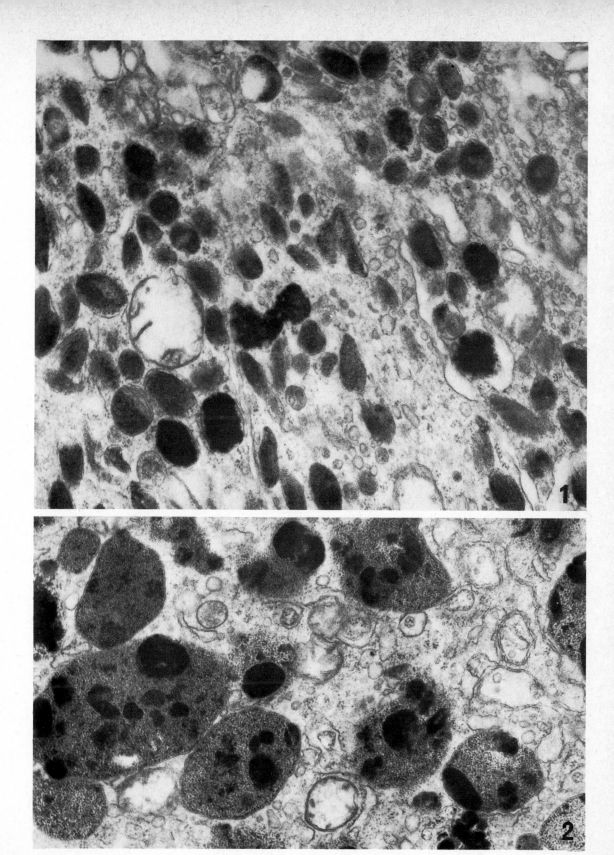

lupus erythematosus (Papa and Kligman, 1965). In psoriasis and verruca vulgaris there is also a low level of pigmentation which is believed to be due to an accelerated production of keratinocytes. This results in poor or brief contact with the dendrites of melanocytes, so that the normal complement of melanosomes is not transferred from melanocyte to keratinocyte (Fitzpatrick and Mihm, 1971).

However, failure of melanosome transfer may also be due to an abnormality of the dendritic processes of the melanocyte. Thus in certain mouse genotypes (Silvers, 1961; Quevedo and Smith 1963) and in chronically solar-irradiated human skin (Mitchell, 1963) poor pigmentation is associated with poorly developed or short and stumpy melanocytic dendrites, presumably incapable of transferring melanosomes to the keratinocytes.

White macules or 'depigmented naevi' occur in 90 per cent of patients with tuberous sclerosis. Since this may be the earliest sign of the disease (Gold and Freeman, 1965; Fitzpatrick et al., 1968; Fitzpatrick and Mihm, 1971), it is important to distinguish these lesions from the white macules seen in other conditions such as vitiligo. In vitiligo, there is a marked reduction or absence of melanocytes from the depigmented areas but this is not the case with the white macules of tuberous sclerosis. When melanocytes from normal surrounding skin are compared with those in the lesion, it is found that there is a marked reduction in the amount of melanin in the melanosome and there is also a marked decrease in the number and size of these organelles. The mechanism behind this defect is not understood, but Fitzpatrick and Mihm (1971) have suggested that 'the synthetic mechanisms for melanin are probably dampened'. It would appear that electron microscopy of these lesions in conjunction with clinical observations and histochemistry could play an important role in the early diagnosis of tuberous sclerosis.

Plate 169

Malignant melanoma of human skin. Histologically the primary tumour and numerous secondary deposits in grossly enlarged lymph nodes and elsewhere showed no pigment, but later at autopsy a small secondary deposit containing a little melanin was found in the brain. Light microscopy of the malignant effusion that developed in the patient showed numerous tumour cells but no melanin. At electron microscopy some of the tumour cells were found to contain melanosomes.

Fig. 1. A malignant melanocyte from peritoneal effusion, showing numerous small pleomorphic melanosomes (arrows). × 17,500

Fig. 2. High power view of atypical melanosomes. Some, however, show a characteristic internal pattern (arrows). × 112,000

Fig. 3. A rather large melanosome found in one of the tumour cells. A striated structure can just be discerned in its interior. × 70,000

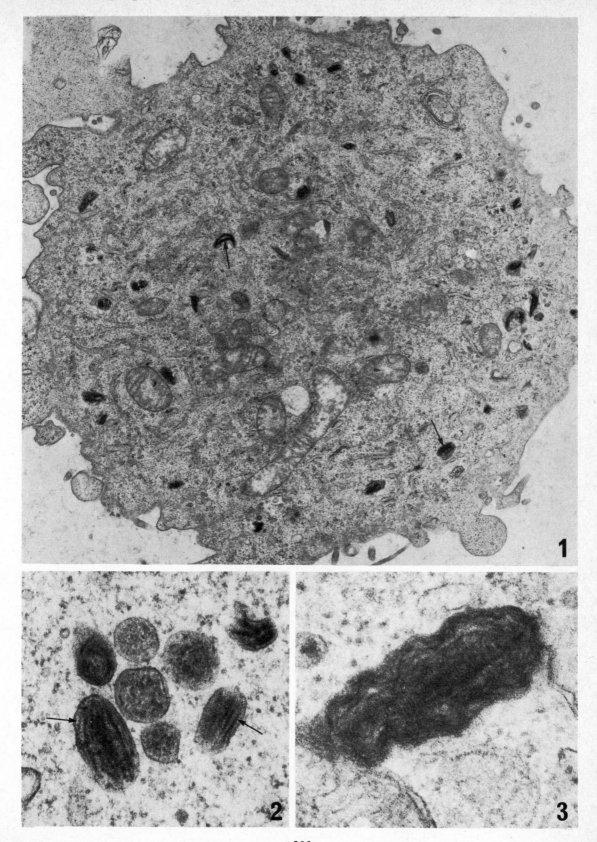

Birbeck, M. S. C. and Barnicot, N. A. (1959). 'Electron microscope studies on pigment formation in human hair follicles.' In *Pigment Cell Biology,* p. 549. Ed. by M. Gordon. New York: Academic Press

Bloch, B. (1927). 'Das Pigment.' *Jadassohn's Handb. Haut-Greschl. Krankh.* **1,** 434

Breathnach, A. S. (1964). 'Electron microscopy of melanocytes and melanosomes in freckled human epidermis.' *J. invest. Derm.* **42,** 388

— (1969). 'Normal and abnormal melanin pigmentation of the skin.' In *Pigments in Pathology,* p. 353. Ed. by M. Wolman. New York: Academic Press

— and Goodwin, D. (1965). 'Electron microscopy of non-keratinocytes in the basal layer of white epidermis of the recessively spotted guinea-pig.' *J. Anat., Lond.* **99,** 377

— Fitzpatrick, T. B. and Wyllie, L. M. A. (1965). 'Electron microscopy of melanocytes in human piebaldism.' *J. invest. Derm.* **45,** 28

Chian, L. T. Y. and Wilgram, G. F. (1967). 'Tyrosinase inhibition: its role in suntanning and in albinism.' *Science* **155,** 198

Drochmans, P. (1966). 'The fine structure of melanin granules (the early, mature and compound forms).' In *Structure and Control of the Melanocyte,* p. 90: Sixth Int. Pigment Cell Conf. sponsored by the International Union against Cancer. Ed. by G. Della Porta and O. Mühlbock. Berlin: Springer

Fitzpatrick, T. B. and Mihm, M. C., Jr. (1971). 'Abnormalities of the melanin pigmentary system.' In *Dermatology in General Medicine,* p. 1591. Ed. by T. B. Fitzpatrick, K. A. Arndt, W. H. Clark, A. Z. Eisen, E. J. Van Scott and J. H. Vaughan. New York and Maidenhead: McGraw-Hill

— and Quevedo, W. C., Jr. (1966). 'Albinism.' In *The Metabolic Basis of Inherited Disease,* 2nd ed, p. 324. Ed. by J. B. Stanbury, J. B. Wyngaarden and D. S. Fredrickson. New York and Maidenhead: McGraw-Hill

— Becker, S. W., Jr., Lerner, A. B. and Montgomery, H. (1950). 'Tyrosinase in human skin: demonstration of its presence and its role in human melanin formation.' *Science* **112,** 223

— Quevedo, W. C., Jr., Levene, A., McGovern, V. J., Michima, Y. and Oettle, A. G. (1966). 'Terminology of vertebrate melanin-containing cells: a report of the nomenclature committee of the Sixth International Pigment Cell Conference.' In *Structure and Control of the Melanocyte,* p. 1, Sixth Int. Pigment Cell Conf. sponsored by the International Union against Cancer. Ed. by G. Della Porta and O. Mühlbock. Berlin: Springer

— Szabo, G., Hori, Y., Simone, A. A. Reed, W. B. and Greenberg, M. H. (1968). 'White leaf-shaped macules: earliest visible sign of tuberous sclerosis.' *Archs Derm., Chicago* **98,** 1

— Quevedo, W. C., Jr., Szabo, G. and Seiji, M. (1971). 'Biology of the melanin pigmentary system.' In *Dermatology in General Medicine,* p. 117. Ed. by T. B. Fitzpatrick, K. A. Arndt, W. H. Clark, A. Z. Eisen, E. J. Van Scott and J. H. Vaughan. New York and Maidenhead: McGraw-Hill

Ghadially, F. N. (1969). *Advanced Aquarist Guide,* p. 202. New York and London: Pets Library

— and Barker, J. F. (1960). 'The histogenesis of experimentally-induced melanotic tumours in the Syrian hamster *(Cricetus auratus).'* *J. Path. Bact.* **79,** 263

— and Gordon, M. (1957). 'A localized melanoma in a hybrid fish *Lesbistes x mollienesia.'* *Cancer Res.* **17,** 597

— and Illman, O. (1964). 'The histogenesis of experimentally produced melanotic tumours in the Chinese hamster *(Cricetulus criseus).'* *Br. J. Cancer* **17,** 727

— — (1966). 'Small pigmented spots in hamsters.' In *Structure and Control of the Melanocyte,* p. 259, Sixth Int. Pigment Cell Conf. sponsored by the International Union against Cancer. Ed. by G. Della Porta and O. Mühlbock. Berlin: Springer

Gold, A. P. and Freeman, J. M. (1965). 'Depigmented nevi: the earliest sign of tuberous sclerosis.' *Pediatrics* **35** ,1003

Gordon, M. (1937). 'The production of spontaneous melanotic neoplasms in fishes by selective matings. II. Neoplasms with macromelanophores only. III. Neoplasms in day old fishes.' *Am. J. Cancer* **30,** 362

— (1948). 'Effects of five primary genes on the site of melanomas in fishes and the influence of two color genes on their pigmentation.' In *The Biology of Melanomas,* p. 216 (Special publications of the New York Academy of Sciences, Vol. IV). Ed by R. W. Miner and M. Gordon. New York: N.Y. Academy of Sciences

— (1953). 'Preface.' In *Pigment Cell Growth,* Proc. of the 3rd Conf. on the Biology of Normal and Atypical Pigment Cell Growth. Ed. by M. Gordon. New York: Academic Press

Grand, C. G., Gordon, M. and Cameron, G. (1941). 'Neoplasm studies. VIII. Cell types in tissue culture of fish melanotic tumors compared with mammalian melanomas.' *Cancer Res.* **1,** 660

Hori, Y., Toda, K., Pathak, M. A., Clark, W. H., Jr. and Fitzpatrick, T. B. (1968). 'A fine structure study of the human epidermal melanosome complex and its acid phosphatase activity.' *J. Ultrastruct. Res.* **25,** 109

Illman, O. and Ghadially, F. N. (1960). 'Coat colour and experimental melanotic tumour production in the hamster.' *Br. J. Cancer* **14,** 483

Masson, P. (1948). 'Pigment cells in man.' In *The Biology of Melanomas,* p. 15. (Special publications of the New York Academy of Sciences, Volume IV.) Ed. by R. W. Miner and M. Gordon. New York: N.Y. Academy of Sciences

Mishima, Y. (1966). 'Macromolecular characterizations in neoplastic and dysfunctional human melanocytes.' In *Structure and Control of the Melanocyte,* p. 133, Sixth Int. Pigment Cell Conf. sponsored by the international Union Against Cancer. Ed. by G. Della Porta and O. Mühlbock. New York: Springer

Mitchell, R. E. (1963). 'The effect of prolonged solar radiation on melanocytes of the human epidermis.' *J. invest. Derm.* **41,** 199

— (1968). 'The skin of the Australian aborigines; a light and electronmicroscopical study.' *Austral. J. Derm.* **9,** 314

Moyer, F. (1961). 'Electron microscopic observations on the origin, development and genetic control of melanin granules in the mouse eye.' In *The Structure of the Eye,* p. 469. Ed. by G. K. Smelser. New York: Academic Press

—(1963). 'Genetic effects on melanosome fine structure and ontogeny in normal and malignant cells.' *Ann. N.Y. Acad. Sci.* **100**, 584

—(1966). 'Genetic variations in the fine structure and ontogeny of mouse melanin granules.' *Am. Zool.* **6**, 43

Papa, C. M. and Kligman, A. M. (1965). 'The behaviour of melanocytes in inflammation.' *J. invest. Derm.* **45**, 465

Pinkus, H., Staricco, R. J. Kropp, P. J. and Fan, J. (1959). 'The symbiosis of melanocytes and human epidermis under normal and abnormal conditions.' In *Pigment Cell Biology*, p. 127. Ed. by M. Gordon. New York: Academic Press

Quevedo, W. C., Jr. and Smith, J. A. (1963). 'Studies on radiation-induced tanning of skin.' *Ann. N.Y. Acad. Sci.* **100**, 364

Rawles, M. E. (1947). 'Origin of pigment cells from the neural crest in the mouse embryo.' *Physiol. Zoöl.* **20**, 248

— (1948). 'Origin of melanophores and their role in development of color patterns in vertebrates.' *Physiol. Rev.* **28**, 383

Rosen, D. E. and Bailey, R. M. (1963). 'The Poeciliid fishes (cyprinodontiformes). Their structure, zoogeography and systematics.' *Bull. Am. Mus. nat. Hist.* **126**, 1

Seiji, M., Fitzpatrick, T. B. and Birbeck, M. S. C. (1961). 'The melanosome: a distinctive subcellular particle of mammalian melanocytes and the site of melanogenesis.' *J. invest. Derm.* **36**, 243

Silvers, W. K. (1961). 'Genes and the pigment cells of mammals.' *Science* **134**, 368

Szabo, G., Gerald, A. B., Pathak, M. A. and Fitzpatrick, T. B. (1969). 'Racial differences in the fate of melanosomes in human epidermis.' *Nature, Lond.* **222**, 1081

Toda, K., Hori, Y. and Fitzpatrick, T. B. (1968). 'Isolation of the intermediate "vesicles" during ontogeny of melanosomes in embryonic chick retinal pigment epithelium.' *Fedn Proc.* **27**, 722

Witkop, C. J., Jr., Van Scott, E. J. and Jacoby, G. A. (1963). 'Evidence for two forms of autosomal recessive albinism in man.' *Proc. 2nd Internat. Congr. on Human Genetics, Rome*, p. 1064. Rome: Istituto Gregorio Mendel

CHAPTER X

Rod-shaped Tubulated Bodies

INTRODUCTION

In 1964, Weibel and Palade described a new cytoplasmic component in the vascular endothelial cells of the rat, man and *Ambylostoma punctatum*. They called it a 'rod-shaped tubulated body', for ultrastructural studies showed this to be a long single-membrane-bound cylindrical body containing 6–26 microtubules set in an electron-dense matrix. Since then this organelle has been described by many other workers who have used various terms to describe it; these include 'Weibel–Palade bodies', 'rod-bodies', 'tubulated bodies' and 'specific organelle of endothelial cells'.

It is worth noting that prior to the study by Weibel and Palade (1964) such bodies had been observed in vascular endothelia by various workers on several occasions. Hibbs *et al.*, (1958) described dense cylindrical granules in the vasculature of human finger-tips, while micrographs published by Hatt *et al.* (1959) show similar bodies in arterioles and capillaries of human lung. Pease and Paule (1960) saw these bodies in the aortic endothelium of rats and described them as dense granules with a compartmentalized internal structure, while Bierring and Kobayasi (1963) described them in the same tissue as small, dense, osmiophilic bodies.

However, it was the classic study of Weibel and Palade (1964) which first clearly described and delineated this body from other cellular structures. Since then many publications dealing with the morphology and distribution of rod-shaped tubulated bodies in the vascular endothelia of various species have appeared, but the function of this organelle remains unclear although it has been suggested that it may be involved in intravascular clotting.

Variations that might occur in pathological states receive only passing mention in a few publications. Since this is a dense body it has at times been mistaken for a lysosome. Attempts to demonstrate acid phosphatase activity in these bodies have been unsuccessful (Lemeunier *et al.*, 1969).

Since their recognition by Weibel and Palade (1964), rod-shaped tubulated bodies have been described in the vascular endothelial cells of many vertebrates. These organelles usually appear scattered randomly in the cytoplasm of the endothelial cells of arteries, veins, capillaries and endocardium. Variations in structure and electron density occur, some of which are probably attributable to different techniques of fixation and the staining employed (*Plates 170 and 171*).

Basically this is a single-membrane-bound cylindrical rod-like body which contains a number of microtubules set in an electron-dense matrix. In ultrathin sections, this long organelle is rarely cut along its entire length, so that its true length is difficult to determine. The longest one seen by Weibel and Palade (1964) measured 3·2 μ, while that seen in the frog by Steinsiepe and Weibel (1970) measured 2 μ. The diameter of these bodies, as reported by various workers, ranges from 0·1 to 0·5 μ (human about 0·15 μ), and that of the microtubules in its substance from 150 to 270 Å (human, about 200 Å). The matrix varies from moderately to highly electron dense and appears granular in nature. The microtubules generally pursue a straight parallel course along the long axis of the organelle; sometimes, however, they show a twisted, spiral or whorled configuration. In some studies a central filament has been observed within the microtubules (e.g. Weibel and Palade, 1964; Ghadially and Roy, 1969).

These bodies appear to develop from the Golgi complex (Matsuda and Sugiura, 1970; Sengel and Stoebner, 1970). The first detectable stage of the process seems to be the formation of fine microtubular elements in enlarged sacs of the Golgi complex (*Plate 171, Figs. 2 and 3*). At this stage the matrix of the body is of low electron density. The body is then probably released into the cytoplasm by a process of pinching off from the Golgi stacks. The possibility that these bodies or their contents may be discharged into the blood stream has often been considered but contact between them and the cell membrane is not seen as a rule. Although vesicular structures have at times been shown attached to their surface (Steinsiepe and Weibel, 1970), from such static pictures it is difficult to say whether this represents material coming into or leaving these bodies.

Rod-shaped tubulated bodies have been seen in various species besides man. These include: (1) rat (Weibel and Palade, 1964; Fuchs and Weibel, 1966; Matthews and Gardner, 1966; Roy and Ghadially, 1967); (2) mouse (Clementi and Palade, 1969); (3) rabbit (Rhodin, 1968; Ghadially

---

Plate 170

Fig. 1. Blood vessel from a human lymph node, showing lumen containing an erythrocyte (E) and vascular endothelial cells containing markedly electron-dense rod-shaped tubulated bodies (R). × 32,000

Fig. 2. Vascular endothelial cell from subsynovial tissue of an osteoarthritic joint. The length of these organelles is difficult to appreciate in sectioned material, but here one of the rod-shaped tubulated bodies (R) has been sectioned quite a distance along its length. Another, cut transversely, shows tubules (arrow) in its interior. Note also the multivesicular body (M) which is frequently found in vascular endothelial cells × 84,000 (*From Ghadially and Roy, 1969*)

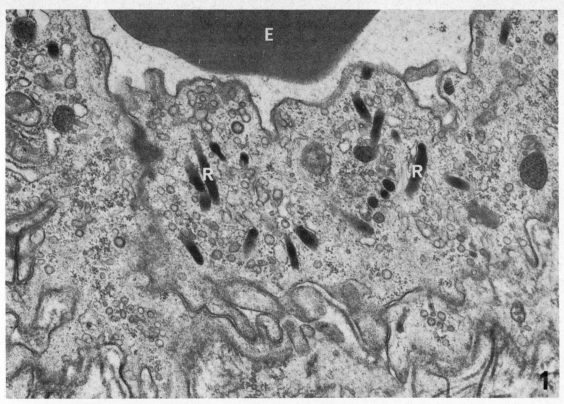

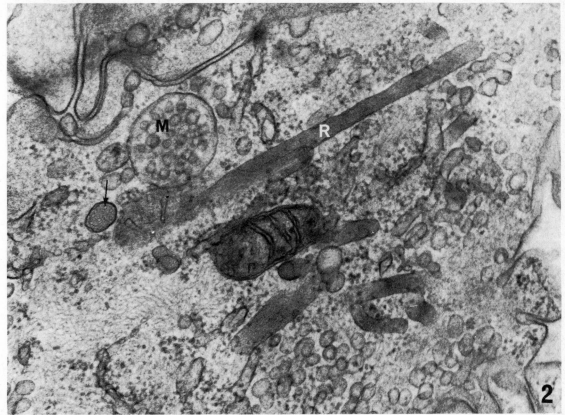

and Roy, 1969); (4) dog (Sun and Ghidoni, 1969); (5) pigeon (Raviola and Raviola, 1967); (6) frog (Stehbens, 1965; Steinsiepe and Weibel, 1970); and (7) *Amblystoma punctatum* larvae (Weibel and Palade, 1964).

In man these bodies have been described in blood vessels of: (1) umbilical cord (said to occur more frequently in the vein than the artery) (Dubois *et al.*, 1965; Parry and Abramovich, 1972); (2) carotid body and paraganglia (Grimley and Glenner, 1966, 1968); (3) kidney (Jacobsen *et al.*, 1966); (4) skin (White and Clawson, 1967); (5) lymph node (*Plate 170, Fig. 1*); (6) synovial membrane in normal subjects and in cases of traumatic arthritis, rheumatoid arthritis and osteoarthritis (Roy and Ghadially, 1967; Ghadially and Roy, 1969) (*Plate 170, Fig. 2*); (7) eye (Vegge and Ringvold, 1969; Matsuda and Sugiura, 1970) (*Plate 171*); (8) senile cutaneous angiomas (Stehbens and Ludatscher, 1968); (9) glomus tumours (Venkatachalam and Greally, 1969); and (10) parathyroid adenomas (Elliot and Arhelger, 1966).

Quantitative studies on the distribution of these bodies in various parts of the vascular system in the rat and frog (Fuchs and Weibel, 1966; Steinsiepe and Weibel, 1970) show that these are ubiquitous bodies found in vessels of all calibres and also in the endocardium. In the rat, the cytoplasmic volume occupied by these bodies in endothelial cells is said to be directly proportional to the size of the vessel, but in the frog this is said to depend more on the distance from the heart than on vessel size. In the frog the volume density of these organelles in endothelial cell cytoplasm is reported to be: thoracic aorta, 8 per cent; abdominal aorta, 6·6 per cent; capillaries, 0·3 per cent; vena abdominalis, 6·7 per cent; vena cava, 3·7 per cent; endocardium, 0·5 per cent.

Such a distribution correlates neither with hydrostatic pressure nor with oxygen or carbon dioxide tension of the blood. It has been suggested that these bodies are involved in blood coagulation because these granules are thought to resemble α-granules of thrombocytes (Weibel, 1964) and probably contain platelet factor 3 (Siegel and Lüscher, 1967). Some support for this idea may also be found in the work of Shimamoto and Ishioka (1963), who showed that after administration of adrenalin the aortic wall of the rabbit produces a coagulation-enhancing substance, and Burri and Weibel (1968), who found that in segments of rat aorta incubated *in vitro* for short periods with adrenalin there is a quantitative loss of up to 40 per cent of these bodies from the endothelium.

Plate 171

Rod-shaped tubulated bodies from vascular endothelial cells of the iris from a case of Behcet's disease. (*From Matsuda and Sugiura, 1970*)

Fig. 1. A number of rod-shaped tubulated bodies (R) are seen in a vascular endothelial cell. × 33,000

Figs. 2 and 3. A possible way in which these bodies are formed is depicted here. Near the Golgi complex are seen structures acceptable as enlarged Golgi sacs containing microtubules (T). One of these appears to be in the process of being pinched off from the Golgi stacks (arrow). × 42,000; × 60,000

Figs. 4 and 5. Longitudinal and transverse sections of rod-shaped tubulated bodies, showing the microtubules in their interior. × 147,000; × 168,000

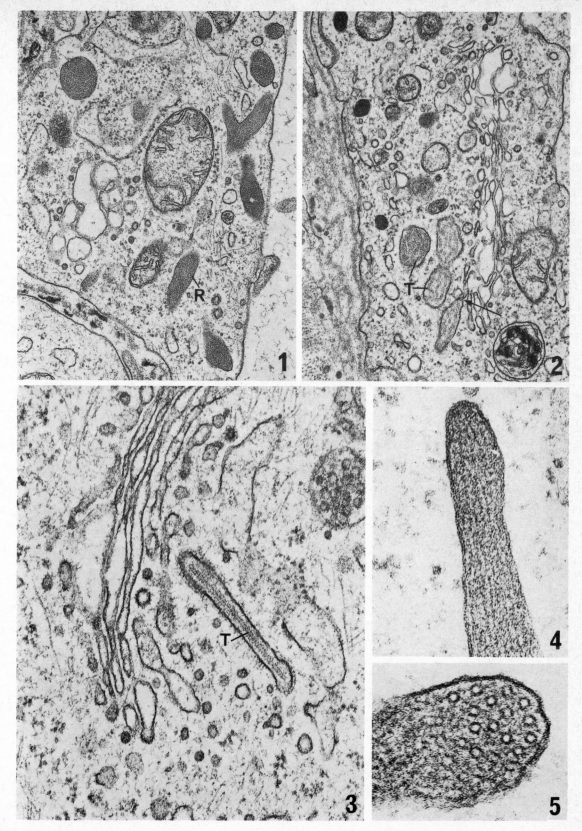

401

REFERENCES

Bierring, F. and Kobayasi, T. (1963). 'Electron microscopy of the normal rabbit aorta.' *Acta path. microbiol. scand* **57**, 154

Burri, P. H. and Weibel, E. R. (1968). 'Beeinflussung einer spezifischen Cytoplasmatischen Organelle von endothel-zellen durch Adrenalin.' *Z. Zellforsch. mikrosk. Anat.* **88**, 426

Clementi, F. and Palade, G. E. (1969). 'Intestinal capillaries. I. Permeability to peroxidase and ferritin.' *J. Cell Biol.* **41**, 33

Dubois, P., Dumont, L. and Lieux, J. M. (1965). 'Observation au microscope électronique des cellules endothéliales des vaisseaux ombilicaux à des strades précoces dévelopment embryonnaire chez l'homme.' *C.r. Soc. Biol., Paris* **159**, 2206

Elliot, R. L. and Arhelger, R. B. (1966). 'Fine structure of parathyroid adenomas, with special reference to annulate lamellae and septate desmosomes.' *Archs Path.* **81**, 200

Fuchs, A. and Weibel, E. R. (1966). 'Morphomestrische untersuchung der verteilung einer spezifishen cytoplasmatischen organelle in endothelzellen der ratte.' *Z. Zellforsch. mikrosk. Anat.* **73**, 1

Ghadially, F. N. and Roy, S. (1969). *Ultrastructure of Synovial Joints in Health and Disease.* London: Butterworths

Grimley, P. M. and Glenner, G. G. (1966). 'Histology and ultrastructure of carotid body paragangliomas. Comparison with normal gland.' *Cancer, Philad.* **20**, 1473

—— (1968). 'Ultrastructure of the human carotid body. A perspective on the mode of chemoreception.' *Circulation* **37**, 648

Hatt, P. Y., Rouiller, C. and Grosgogeat, Y. (1959). 'Les ultrastructures pulmonaires et le régime de la petite circulation.' *Path. Biol., Paris* **7**, 515

Hibbs, R. G., Burch, G. E. and Phillips, J. H. (1958). 'The fine structure of the small blood vessels of normal human dermis and subcutis.' *Am. Heart. J.* **56**, 662

Jacobsen, N. O., Jorgensen, F. and Thomsen, A. C. (1966). 'An electron microscopic study of small arteries and arterioles in the normal human kidney.' *Nephron* **3**, 17

Lemeunier, A., Burri, P. H. and Weibel, E. R. (1969). 'Absence of acid phosphatase activity in specific endothelial organelles.' *Histochemie* **20**, 143

Matsuda, H. and Sugiura, S. (1970). 'Ultrastructure of "tubular body" in the endothelial cells of the ocular blood vessels.' *Invest. Opthal.* **9**, 919

Matthews, M. A. and Gardner, D. L. (1966). 'The fine structure of the mesenteric arteries of the rat.' *Angiology* **17**, 902

Parry, E. W. and Abramovich, D. R. (1972). 'The ultrastructure of human umbilical vessel endothelium from early pregnancy to full term.' *J. Anat.* **111**, 29

Pease, D. C. and Paule, W. J. (1960). 'Electron microscopy of elastic arteries: the thoracic aorta of the rat.' *J. Ultrastruct. Res.* **3**, 469

Raviola, E. and Raviola, G. (1967). 'A light and electron microscopic study of pecten of pigeon eye.' *Am. J. Anat.* **120**, 427

Rhodin, J. A. G. (1968). 'Ultrastructure of mammalian venous capillaries, venules and small collecting veins.' *J. Ultra-struct. Res.* **25**, 452

Roy, S. and Ghadially, F. N. (1967). 'Aetiological significance of rod-shaped bodies in rheumatoid synovia.' *Nature, Lond.* **213**, 1139

Sengel, A. and Stoebner, P. (1970). 'The origin of tubular inclusions in endothelial cells.' *J. Cell Biol.* **44**, 223

Shimamoto, T. and Ishioka, T. (1963). 'Release of a thromboplastic substance from arterial walls by epinephrine.' *Circulation Res.*, **12**, 138

Siegel, A. and Lüscher, E. F. (1967). 'Non-identity of the α-granules of human blood platelets with typical lysosomes.' *Nature, Lond.* **215**, 745

Stehbens, W. E. (1965). 'Ultrastructure of the frog vascular endothelium.' *Q. Jl exp. Physiol.* **50**, 375

— and Ludatscher, R. M. (1968). 'Fine structure of senile angiomas of human skin.' *Angiology* **19**, 581

Steinsiepe, K. F. and Weibel, E. R. (1970). 'Electron microscopic studies on specific organelles of endothelial cells in the frog (*Rana temporaria*).' *Z. Zellforsch. mikrosk. Anat.* **108**, 105

Sun, C. N. and Ghidoni, J. J. (1969). 'Membrane-bound microtubular and crystalline structures in endothelial cells of normal canine aorta.' *Experientia* **25**, 301

Vegge, T. and Ringvold, A. (1969). 'Ultrastucture of the wall of human iris vessels.' *Z. Zellforsch. mikrosk. Anat.* **94**, 19

Venkatachalam, M. A. and Greally, J. G. (1969). 'Fine structure of glomus tumor: similarity of glomus cells to smooth muscle.' *Cancer, Philad.* **23**, 1176

Weibel, E. R. (1964). 'Neue cytoplasmatische komponenten von Endothelzellen.' *Acta anat.* **59**, 390

— and Palade, G. E. (1964). 'New cytoplasmic components in arterial endothelia.' *J. Cell Biol.* **23**, 101

White, J. G. and Clawson, G. G. (1967). 'Blood cells and blood vessels.' In *Ultrastructure of Normal and Abnormal Skin*, p. 261. Ed. by A. S. Zelickson. Philadelphia, Pa: Lea & Febiger

CHAPTER XI

Myofilaments and Other Intracytoplasmic Filaments

INTRODUCTION

Intracytoplasmic fine filaments approximately 40–120 Å thick and of indefinite length appear to be a common, or perhaps even a universal, component of the cytoplasmic matrix. However, most cell types contain only rare filaments or a few filaments scattered at random in the cytoplasm. These, as a rule, attract little attention; it is only when such filaments are abundant that curiosity as to their nature and significance is aroused.

An example of this are the tonofibrils seen with the light microscope in cells of squamous epithelia. The electron microscope shows that the tonofibrils are in fact bundles or sheaves of fine filaments, some of which terminate in desmosomes. The idea that these filaments represent keratin or its precursor is difficult to support on available evidence.* Intracytoplasmic filaments varying in orientation and abundance have been seen in a variety of cell types. They tend to be quite prominent in chondrocytes, astrocytes and neurons. Somewhat less abundant, but still quite characteristic, are the filaments in vascular endothelial cells, podocytes of the renal glomerulus, mesothelial cells and many others. There is also evidence that an increase in fine filaments occurs with age, at least in some cell types (e.g. chondrocytes of articular cartilage) and examples may also be found where such an increase is associated with pathological processes (page 426). Little is known about the chemical composition of these filaments, but they are thought to contain mainly protein. The question as to whether they represent a common structural protein in cells, or whether their composition varies from one cell type to another, is not resolved.

Myofilaments comprise a special class of intracytoplasmic filaments. Two types of filaments—thick (about 100 Å in diameter) and thin (about 60 Å)—are recognized in striated muscle cells. The former contain myosin, the latter actin and some tropomycin B (see also page 406). In striated muscle the two types of filaments are set side by side. They slide past one another during contraction. In the usual preparations of vertebrate smooth muscle, most of the filaments are very fine (40 Å) and only occasional thicker filaments (80 Å) are seen. However, there is now

---

* Keratohyalin first appears as an electron-dense substance between and around tonofilaments which probably serve as a scaffolding for its deposition. It is claimed that this substance can be removed selectively, leaving behind the filaments. For more details on this controversial subject, see Breathnach (1971).

a mounting body of evidence that the thicker myosin filaments are present in substantial numbers in smooth muscle also, but special methods are required to preserve and demonstrate them.

The term 'other intracytoplasmic filaments' is used to describe intracytoplasmic filaments other than myofilaments. The term 'fine filamentous fibres' (FFF) has been used frequently to describe the intracytoplasmic filaments in chondrocytes, but this term has not gained wide acceptance. Finally, it is worth noting that recent studies have clearly shown that some of the so-called 'other intracytoplasmic filaments' are, in fact, myofilaments.

Since intracytoplasmic filaments seen in cells other than muscle are also of a similar dimension and a limited ability to contract is a well known property of 'protoplasm', it is thought that all intracytoplasmic filaments may have a contractile rather than a cytoskeletal function.

It has already been noted that two types of myofilaments—thick and thin (myosin and actin)—occur in striated muscle (page 403). Such filaments are arranged in a highly ordered fashion to form contractile elements called myofibrils. Numerous myofibrils occur in the cytoplasmic matrix (sarcoplasm) of a skeletal muscle fibre, which in effect is a long cylindrical cell which, in addition to myofibrils, contains various organelles such as numerous nuclei, mitochondria and endoplasmic reticulum (page 218), and also inclusions such as glycogen and lipid. Under polarized light the myofibrils and myofibres display alternating bright anisotropic bands (A-bands) and dark isotropic bands (I-bands). In stained preparations viewed with ordinary light, the densities are reversed. Other features that can be shown in suitable preparations by light microscopy but are more clearly demonstrable by electron microscopy (*Plate 172*) include: (1) a dark line (Z-line or Zwischenscheibe) which traverses the middle of the I-band; (2) a pale zone (H-band or Hensen's stripe) which bisects the A-band; and (3) a narrow dark line (M-line or Mittelscheibe) which traverses the centre of the H-band. The portion of a myofibril between two consecutive Z-lines is called a sarcomere. This is the contractile unit of striated muscle. At the Z-line the thin actin filaments from two neighbouring sarcomeres are believed to be attached laterally to one another. In cross-section the Z-line shows a lattice pattern (for references and details, see page 412). The relative lengths of the I- and A-bands are dependent upon the state of contraction or relaxation of the myofibril. The A-band remains quite constant in length, but the I-band is longest when the muscle is stretched, medium sized when it is relaxed, and shortest when the muscle is contracted. The thin actin filaments in the I-band extend into the A-band which contains the thick myosin filaments. Cross-sections through the A-band of vertebrate skeletal and cardiac muscle show that the thick filaments form a hexagonal array.

The thin filaments are interposed between the thick filaments at the trigonal points in the hexagonal array so that each thick filament is seen surrounded by six thin filaments, the ratio of thin to thick filaments being 2 to 1. The longer, thicker myosin filaments of invertebrate striated muscle are capable of interacting with a greater number of thin filaments. In muscle from various species, thin to thick filament ratios varying from 3 to 1 to 6 to 1 have been found.

During contraction the thin filaments slide over the thick filaments and extend deeper into the A-band. This draws the two Z-lines closer together and reduces the length of the sarcomere with resultant shortening of the fibre. In relaxed muscle the thin filaments extending into the A-band from opposite ends do not meet at the M-line, but leave a gap which determines the width of the H-band. The H-band is thus the region of the A-band from which thin filaments are absent at any given moment. This explains why the H-band is wide in stretched muscle, of a medium size in relaxed muscle, and very narrow or entirely absent when the muscle is in the contracted state (*Plate 172*). (For references to the literature on myofibrils and structure of striated muscle, see Spiro and Hagopian, 1967; Mair and Tomé, 1972.)

Plate 172

Figs. 1 and 2. Stretched and contracted skeletal muscle, respectively, are shown. The principal features are identified in these electron micrographs as follows: sarcomere (S), A-band (A), I-band (I), H-band (H), M-line (M) and Z-line (Z). Note the wide H-band and I-band in the stretched myofibrils shown in *Fig. 1*, and the absence of an H-band and a narrow I-band in the contracted myofibrils shown in *Fig. 2*. Although the two muscle specimens illustrated here are similar in appearance, one is from a rabbit (*Fig. 1*) and other from a man (*Fig. 2*). ×30,000; ×30,000

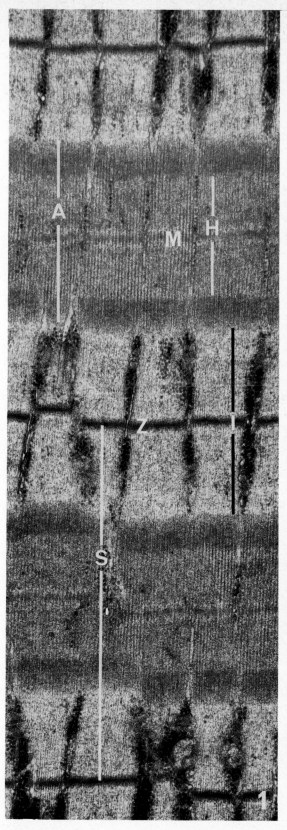

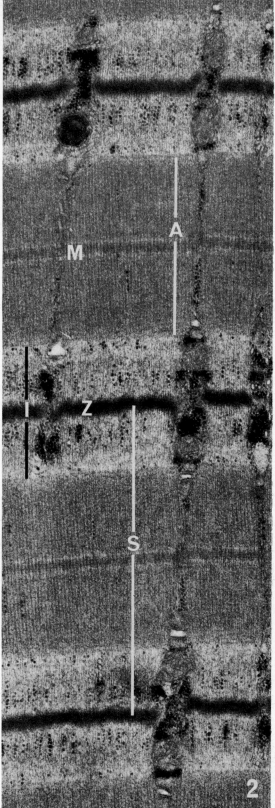

The term 'ring fibre' (striated annuli, ringbinden) designates a muscle fibre with an aberrant set of circumferentially placed myofibrils which follow a spiral or circular course, forming a collar around the usual central longitudinal core of myofibrils. Thus a cross-section through the ring fibre shows longitudinally arranged myofibrils encircling transversely cut myofibrils in the centre. In longitudinal sections through a ring fibre the collar of encircling myofibrils is seen in cross-section while the main central mass of myofilaments is cut longitudinally. No membrane separates the two sets of myofibrils. The long axes of the muscle nuclei are often parallel to the aberrant collar of myofibrils rather than to the central, longitudinally orientated myofibrils.

Ring fibres have been noted in: (1) amphibian muscle (Bataillon, 1891; Weiss and James, 1955; Jonecko, 1962); (2) muscle from amputation stumps (Apatenko, 1964); (3) apparently normal muscle, especially from the external ocular muscle of elderly subjects (Rubinstein, 1960; Bethlem and van Wijngaarden, 1963); (4) muscle from various conditions such as myasthenia gravis, dermatomyositis, periarteritis nodosa, scleroderma, sarcoidosis and disorders affecting the lower motor neuron (for references, see Schotland et al., 1966); and (5) muscular dystrophies, particularly myotonic dystrophy (Engel, 1962; Lapresle et al., 1964, 1966; Schotland et al., 1966; Lapresle and Fardeau, 1968: Schroeder and Adams, 1968; Hayward and Mair, 1970). Ring fibres have also been noted in the myocardium (Le Menn and Emeriau, 1970) in cases of obstructive cardiomyopathy, being particularly frequent in a case of aortic stenosis.

The function and significance of ring fibres are not well understood. The suggestion that they might be a fixation artefact (Adams et al., 1962) is not tenable and finds no support in recent papers on this subject. Ring fibres can be produced experimentally by interrupting the continuity of muscle between its origin and insertion by cutting either the muscle fibres or its tendon (Rumyantseva, 1957; Morris, 1959; Bethlem and Wijngaarden, 1963). In such instances the number of ring fibres increases with the passage of time. There is evidence that in man their number increases with advancing age. These findings taken in conjunction with their frequent occurrence in diseased human muscle have led Schotland et al. (1966) to suggest that 'ring fibers are reactive structures developing in response to pathologic alterations within the muscle fiber'.

Plate 173

Transverse section through a ring fibre, showing a band of myofibrils encircling a core of normally orientated myofibrils. From a case of Duchenne muscular dystrophy. ×2,100 (*From Oteruelo, 1972*)

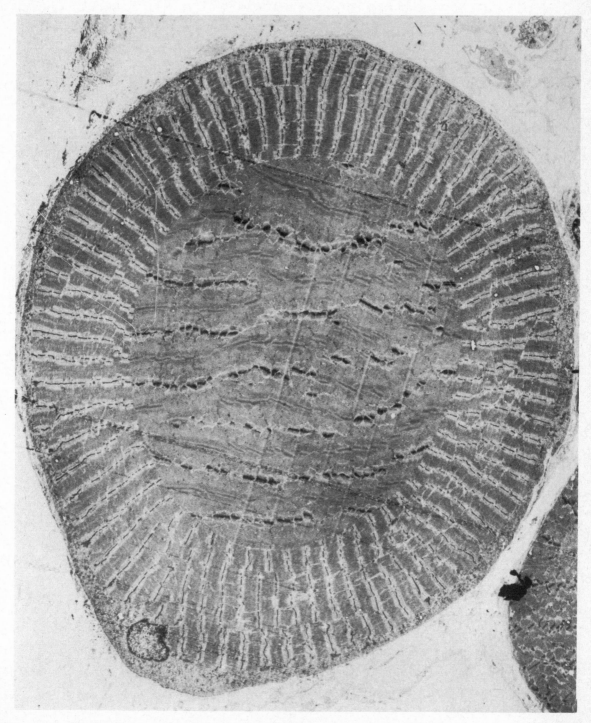

The term 'myofibrillary degeneration' is used to describe changes affecting myofilaments and Z-lines in myofibres undergoing degeneration and atrophy from various causes. Degeneration and atrophy of myofibres has been observed in a variety of pathological states affecting muscle. These include denervation, deprivation of blood supply, metabolic insufficiency, cachexia, mechanical compression, drug action and many other diseases, including muscular dystrophy and myositis (Stenger *et al.*, 1962; Pellegrino and Franzini, 1963; Gonatas *et al.*, 1965; Zacks, 1970; Mair and Tomé, 1972).

The degenerating myofibres and myofibrils show a variety of untrastructural alterations but none of these is specific or pathognomonic for any particular muscular disease or disorder. Depending upon the severity and stage reached by the degenerative process, various morphological changes are seen. Thus, in early or mild lesions there is a decrease in the width of the myofibrils due to a loss of peripheral myofilaments but the normal sarcomere structure is preserved. More marked changes include the destruction and loss of myofibrils over one or more sarcomere lengths (*Plate 174*), and various changes in the Z-line (which are discussed on page 412). As a consequence of such loss of myofibrils, there is a relative abundance of intervening sarcoplasm, and various structures such as mitochondria, triads and glycogen particles, which persist for a time, appear more prominent. The loss of myofibrils leads to a shrinkage of the myofibre so that its surface becomes scalloped or markedly irregular. Dissociation of the folded cell membrane from the basal lamina is also sometimes seen. The undulating configuration of the surface of the fibre produces sarcoplasmic projections or masses called sarcoplasmic pads. These contain occasional nuclei, many mitochondria, glycogen, lipid and disorientated disintegrating filaments. When a substantial loss of myofilaments has occurred the size and shape of the myofibre are grossly altered. Progressive changes along this line lead ultimately to necrosis of the muscle fibre.

Plate 174

The loss of myofilaments from the periphery of myofibrils and the disappearance of entire sarcomeres are evident in this degenerating myofibre from an atrophic deltoid muscle of man. Monoparticulate glycogen (arrows), lipid (L), triads (T) and transversely orientated mitochondria (M) (instead of the normal vertically disposed ones) are seen in the sarcoplasm (S) from which the myofilaments have disappeared. × 20,000 (*Ghadially and Ailsby, unpublished electron micrograph*)

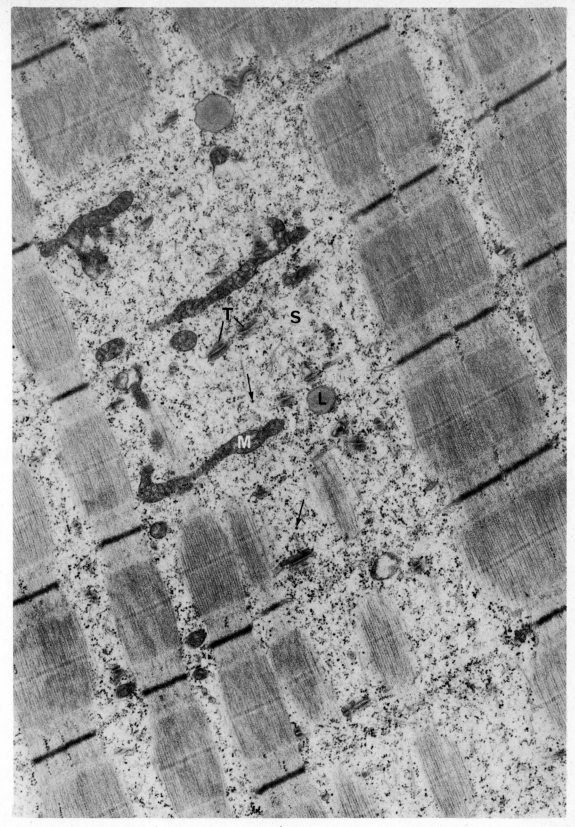

The Z-line in normal skeletal muscle varies between 500 and 1,000 Å in thickness. It is wider in red than white fibres (Shafiq *et al.*, 1966; Tice and Engel, 1967) and in glutaraldehyde-fixed material as compared to osmium-fixed material (Engel and MacDonald, 1970).

The structure of the Z-line has been studied by many workers (for references, see Landon, 1970), most of whom have found that in osmium-fixed material transverse sections through this structure present the appearance of a square lattice composed of 50 Å filaments with a spacing of 220 Å. The similarity between the crystalline lattice of the Z-line and tropomyosin B crystals has often been pointed out (Fawcett, 1968) but there is controversy as to whether tropomyosin occurs in this region or in the I-band region as suggested by immunofluorescence studies.

Alterations in Z-line morphology have been seen in various diseases of muscle and also at times in normal or apparently normal muscle. One such change is streaming of the Z-line (*Plate 175*). In such instances the Z-line develops a zig-zag appearance and the Z-band material extends into the I- and A-bands. Such a change may affect one or more sarcomeres in a single myofibril or affect many adjacent myofibrils. A more advanced stage of streaming leads to a disintegration of the Z-lines which then present as dispersed dense masses of Z-line material.

Light microscopists are familiar with the appearances called 'target' and 'targetoid' fibres, seen in diseased muscle (see below). Here, sarcomeres of several adjacent myofibrils are replaced by patchy electron-dense material, presumably derived from disintegrating Z-lines and myofibrils. It is thought that this change is also probably related to Z-line streaming and disintegration (Mair and Tomé, 1972). The target fibre derives its name from the light microscopic appearance of such fibres seen in transverse section. Three concentric zones are seen: (1) a central pale-staining zone lacking striations, but showing fine wavy filaments; (2) an intermediate zone which stains faintly but in which cross-striations can be detected by polarized light; and (3) a peripheral zone which is more or less normal looking but may show histochemical abnormalities. In targetoid fibres the intermediate zone is lacking. Engel (1961) reported the occurrence of target fibres in denervated muscle and thought that this was a sign of denervation. However, since then, such fibres have been found in a variety of other pathological states by numerous workers (Shafiq *et al.*, 1967; Schotland, 1969; Tomonaga and Sluga, 1969, 1970; Mair and Tomé, 1972).

Plate 175

From the same specimen as *Plate 174*. (*Ghadially and Ailsby, unpublished electron micrographs*)

Fig. 1. Streaming of three Z-lines (arrows) of adjacent sarcomeres is seen here. × 25,000

Fig. 2. Several adjacent myofibrils, showing a more advanced streaming leading to a disintegration of the Z-lines and of the sarcomeres. × 18,500

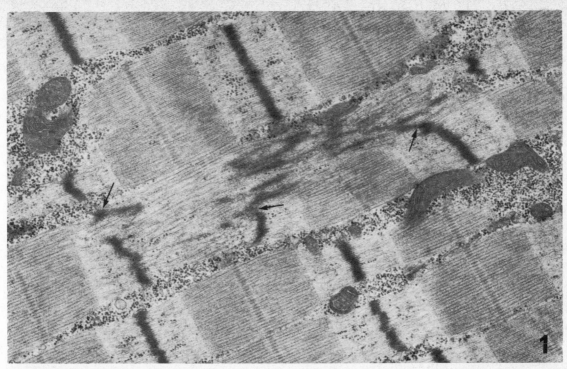

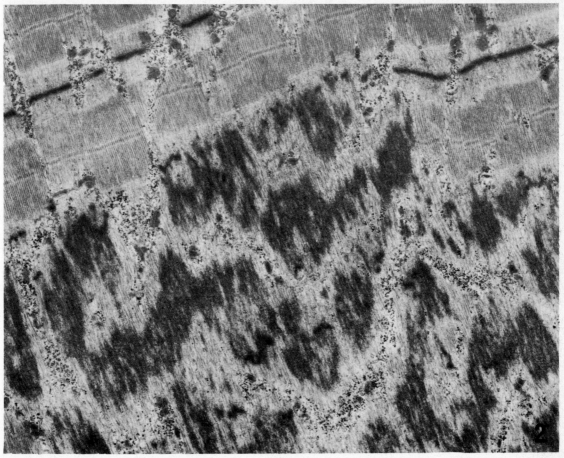

413

However, the most interesting change affecting the Z-line is the formation of dense rods (*Plate 176, Fig. 1*). Such rods may be solitary or multiple and small or large (up to 5 μ long and 1 μ in diameter). These structures were first described by Shy *et al.* (1963) in a familial myopathy characterized by non-progressive weakness. In histological preparations, rod-like or thread-like structures were found; hence they named the condition 'nemaline myopathy' (Gr. *nema* = thread). The origin of these rods from the Z-line was noted by Price *et al.* (1965) and it was suggested that they might contain tropomyosin B. Since then, however, rod formation has been reported in a variety of other myopathies and muscle diseases, including denervation and polymyositis (for references, see Mair and Tomé, 1972), and in the apparently normal heart of aged cats and dogs (Fawcett, 1968; Munnell and Getty, 1968).

According to Engel and MacDonald (1970), the rods are characterized by their origin from Z-lines and their continuity with the I-filaments. They also display a periodic pattern of lines parallel and perpendicular to the long axis of the rod. In fact, the ultrastructure of the rods and their lattice pattern are identical to that of Z-lines with which they are sometimes continuous (Mair and Tomé, 1972).

Yet another anomaly of the Z-lines seen in diseased muscle is a structure called the cytoplasmic body (MacDonald and Engel, 1969). It has a density and granularity similar to the Z-line and is hence believed to be derived from it. However, unlike the rods, it does not show a periodic structure, for it is composed of randomly orientated filaments; those in the centre are compacted and appear electron dense, while those at the periphery form a lighter halo.

Various other anomalies of the Z-lines have also been described. These include fragmentation and disappearance, widening and doubling of the Z-lines (*Plate 176, Fig. 2*). Doubling of Z-lines has been reported in diseased muscle but is also seen in normal muscle fibres at the myotendinous junction and in extraocular muscles (Grabow and Chou, 1968: Engel and MacDonald, 1970; Mair and Tomé, 1972).

Of the numerous alterations of Z-line morphology, three have received more study than others. These include Z-line streaming, rod formation and cytoplasmic bodies. It is clear that these are related anomalies of structure which, in their earlier stages of formation, resemble each other so closely as to be indistinguishable (Engel and MacDonald, 1970). Furthermore, it is clear that while there might be a tendency for one or other variety of Z-line anomaly to be prominent in a given muscular disorder, it is also evident that on the whole such changes are common to a variety of different pathological states affecting muscle.

Plate 176

Fig. 1. The rod (R) in this illustration is clearly seen to be derived from a Z-line. Continuity between the thin filaments of the I-band and the filaments in the rod is evident, as is the periodic parallel arrangement of the filaments in the rod. Below and to the left of the rod is another, less compact, rod-like formation. From atrophic deltoid muscle of man; same case as *Plate 184.* × 70,000 (*Ghadially and Ailsby, unpublished electron micrograph*)

Fig. 2. Doubling of Z-lines in a dystrophic human muscle. × 35,000 (*Ghadially and Ailsby, unpublished electron micrograph*)

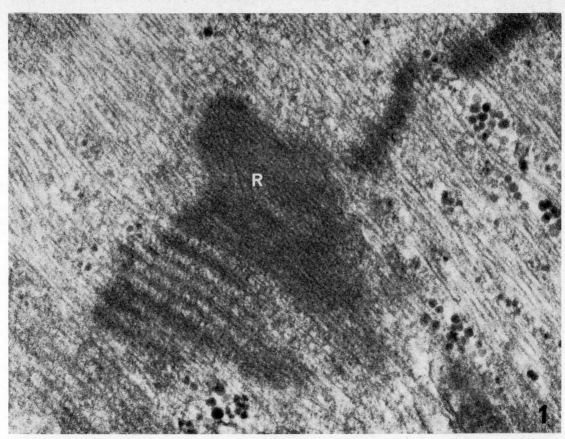

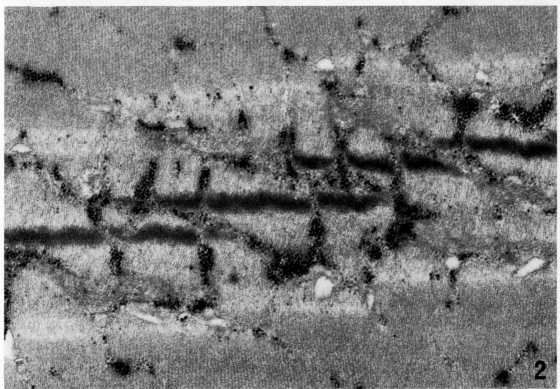

In routinely prepared tissues fixed in osmium or glutaraldehyde the cytoplasm of smooth muscle cells has a somewhat dense homogeneous appearance because the very fine filaments present here are difficult to resolve except at quite high magnifications. Nevertheless, these myofilaments are morphologically distinguishable from many other intracytoplasmic filaments (e.g. tonofilaments in keratinocytes and intracytoplasmic filaments in chondrocytes) because they show an orderly parallel arrangement and focal densities along their course (*Plate 177*). In addition to the presence of such filaments, the typical smooth muscle cell as found in the wall of the gut or uterus is characterized by its spindle shape, a nucleus which is folded when the muscle is contracted, a relative scarcity of endoplasmic reticulum and Golgi complex and an abundance of micropinocytotic vesicles which are frequently referred to in this instance as plasmalemmal vesicles.

Until recently it was thought that smooth muscle contained only thin actin filaments, or at the most only a few thick myosin filaments. During the last few years the arrangement of filaments in vertebrate smooth muscle has been the subject of intense study and the existence or non-existence of organized myosin filaments has been debated extensively.

Early studies revealed two sizes of filaments in some invertebrate smooth muscle but not in vertebrate smooth muscle (Hanson and Lowy, 1960, 1964a, b). Similarly early x-ray diffraction studies also failed to detect myosin filaments (Elliot, 1964, 1967). Recent studies, however, have shown reflections attributable to myosin filaments in the taenia coli of the guinea-pig (Lowy et al., 1970), and various authors have now also demonstrated the presence of thick filaments in preparations containing isolated filaments and in ultrathin sections of vertebrate smooth muscle (for references, see Newstead, 1971; Garamvolgyi et al., 1971). In some instances quite an impressive number of such thick filaments surrounded by thin filaments have been demonstrated. The difficulty of demonstrating thick filaments in smooth muscle led Kelly and Rice (1968) to suggest that thick filaments were formed when the muscle contracted, but others contended that this might be due to poor preservation of smooth muscle by conventional methods of tissue fixation. Recent studies tend to support the latter concept.

Plate 177

Fig. 1. Smooth muscle cells from the wall of human small intestine, showing myofilaments with focal densities (F) along their course, micropinocytotic vesicles (V), folded nucleus (N) and numerous mitochondria (M), but the Golgi complex and endoplasmic reticulum are not clearly evident. × 21,000

Fig. 2. Muscularis mucosae from the same specimen as *Fig. 1*. Note the abundance of micropinocytotic vesicles (arrows). × 28,000

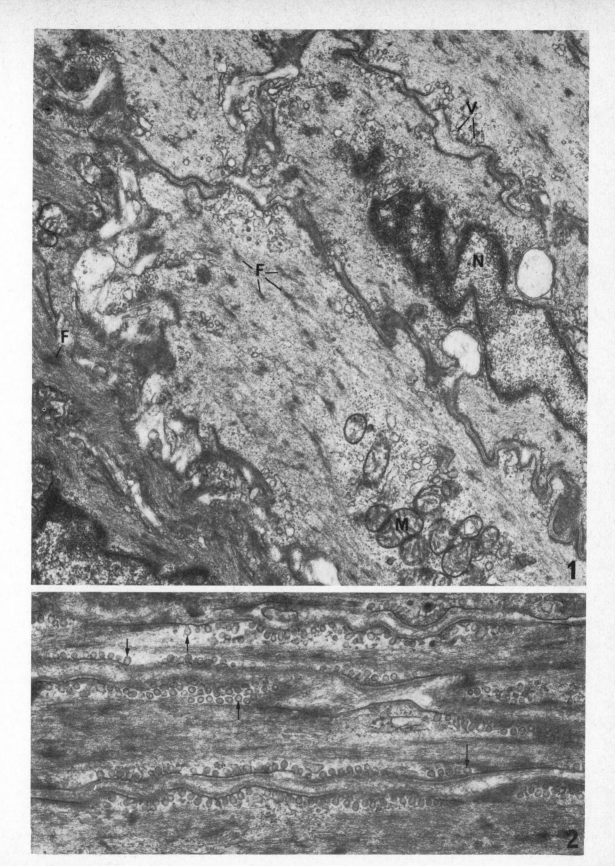

MYOFILAMENTS IN CELLS OTHER THAN MUSCLE

As noted in the previous section, the presence of filaments with focal densities along their course is a characteristic feature of typical smooth muscle cells found in sites such as the uterus or gut. However, the presence of such filaments is by no means the hallmark of a smooth muscle cell, for some other cells of substantially different morphology and function also contain filaments which show focal densities along their course. Furthermore, there are cells which are suspected of pronounced contractile activity where an orderly arrangement of filaments ranging in size from 30 to 170 Å (depending to some extent on preparative procedures) have been found. At least in some instances, correlated histochemical studies show that myosin is associated with such filaments (for more details and references, see Newstead, 1971).

An example of this is seen in the epithelial cells of renal tubules where tracts of filaments occur orientated circumferentially around the tubules (*Plate 178, Fig. 1*). The presence of myosin has been demonstrated here by histochemical methods, and the contractile nature of these filaments is also evidenced by the folding of the basal lamina seen in electron micrographs of this region (Newstead, 1971). Furthermore, recent studies on glycerol-extracted rat kidney tubule cells show that both actin and myosin are present and it is suggested (Rostgaard *et al.*, 1972) that this provides strong evidence that a two-filament contractile system, based on the interaction of actin and myosin, exists here.

Similarly, filamentous elements have been described in the endothelial cells of many small vessels (Hama, 1961; Dubois *et al.*, 1966; Florey, 1966; Majno *et al.*, 1970; Chen and Weiss, 1972) and in some examples (particularly in arterial endothelia) a band of filaments (called a 'myoid zone') is seen on the basal aspect of the endothelial cells (Parry and Abramovich, 1972). It has been shown that some endothelia have the power of independent contraction (Majno *et al.*, 1970) and evidence has also been presented that actomyosin occurs in endothelial cells (Becker and Murphy, 1969).

An example of a myofilament-containing cell well known to the light microscopist is the myoepithelial cell. These cells have been observed in the prostate gland, Harderian gland, apocrine glands, exocrine sweat glands and mammary glands (Richardson, 1949; Hurley and Shelly, 1954; Silver 1954; Hibbs, 1958, 1962; Hollman, 1959; Munger and Brusilow, 1961; Munger *et al.*, 1961; Rowlatt and Franks, 1964; Murad and von Haam, 1968). Such cells and their numerous branching processes form a basket-like structure around the gland acinus, a shape quite different from the spindle-shaped classical smooth muscle cell. These cells lie on the epithelial side of the basement membrane. They are of ectodermal origin, in contrast to muscle cells which derive from the mesenchyme. On rare occasions a desmosomal junction may be noted between the myoepithelial cells and the overlying secretory cell as well as occasional tight junctions between adjacent myoepithelial cells.

Plate 178

Fig. 1. Basal portion of a proximal tubule epithelial cell from a rat kidney, showing a circumferentially orientated tract of filaments (F). It would appear that in this specimen (fixed by perfusion with glutaraldehyde) an agonal contraction of the filamentous band occurred, producing a fold in the basal lamina (arrows). Within the pocket so created lies some extruded cellular material. × 19,000 (*Newstead, unpubllished electron micrograph*)

Fig. 2. A cell from Wharton's jelly, packed with fine filaments which are difficult to resolve. Some of the focal densities are randomly distributed (arrows) while others are aligned to form irregular dense bands (B). From a collapsed human umbilical cord. × 24,000 (*From Parry, 1970*)

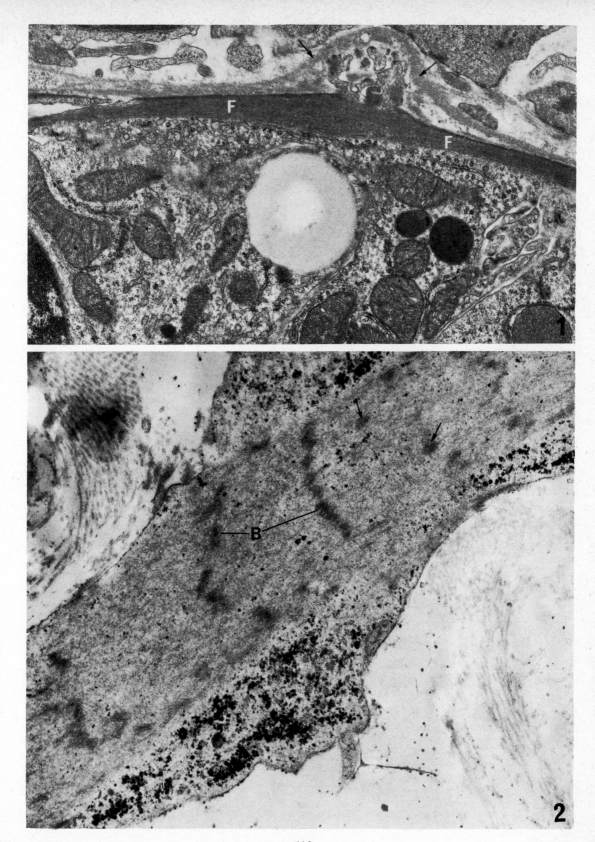

419

Like the smooth muscle cell, the myoepithelial cell is contractile, and electron microscopy has revealed typical myofilaments with focal densities along their course, both in the cell processes and in the cell body. In sclerosing adenosis of the human breast, nodules of myoepithelial cells are seen surrounded by a dense collagenous stroma. It has therefore been suggested that these cells can also produce tropocollagen from which the matrical collagen fibres are formed (Murad and von Haam, 1968).

Ultrastructural studies (Parry, 1970) have shown that Wharton's jelly contains long ribbon-like cells well endowed with myofilaments. The classical 'stellate fibroblast' appearance presented by the cells of Wharton's jelly at light microscopy is produced when the cord collapses after cutting and release of intravascular pressure. Differences between these myofilament-containing cells and typical smooth muscle cells include the occurrence of oriented focal densities which produce irregular bands (*Plate 178, Fig. 2*), the infrequency of plasmalemmal vesicles (micropinocytotic vesicles) and a relative abundance of elements of the rough endoplasmic reticulum and Golgi complex. Furthermore, the branched or stellate appearance assumed by these cells when tissue tension is released is characteristic of this cell but not of typical smooth muscle cells. The presence of rough endoplasmic reticulum and Golgi complex in these cells and the fact that typical fibroblasts are not found here indicate that the mucoid jelly and collagen fibres seen in this region are produced by these cells.

Perhaps the most important example of myofilament-containing cells capable of performing multiple functions is that found in the arterial wall, as reported to occur in ageing and atherosclerosis in man and various experimental animals (Flora *et al.*, 1967; Knieriem, 1967; Peterson *et al.*, 1971). During the formation of fatty streaks and atheromatous plaques, lipid accumulates within a cell called the foam cell. According to some authors, all such foam cells contain a few or many typical or not so typical myofilaments, while others have contended that not only smooth muscle cells or smooth muscle-like cells but also macrophages laden with lipid occur. In a singularly interesting and provocative editorial, Wissler (1967) has pointed out that no fibroblasts occur in this region and that the cells of the arterial wall should be regarded as multifunctional mesenchymal cells capable not only of producing myofilaments and trapping lipoproteins but also of synthesizing material, leading to the formation of other structures such as collagen fibres, elastic fibres, the mucopolysaccharide matrix and basement membrane. The term 'multifunctional mesenchymal cell resembling smooth muscle' seems singularly suitable

---

Plate 179

Portion of ganglion wall. The surface facing the ganglion cavity is not included, but it lay just beyond the top left corner of the picture. Numerous strap-like cells are seen lying in the collagen-fibre-rich intercellular matrix (M). The cytoplasmic matrix appears dense because it is packed with fine myofilaments which are difficult to resolve. However, focal densities can be detected quite frequently (arrows). Dilated cisternae of the rough endoplasmic reticulum (R) are seen in one cell, and another placed closer to the surface than the rest shows numerous vacuoles and a disorganized internal structure. Note the absence of cells acceptable as fibroblasts. × 7,000 (*From Ghadially and Mehta, 1971*)

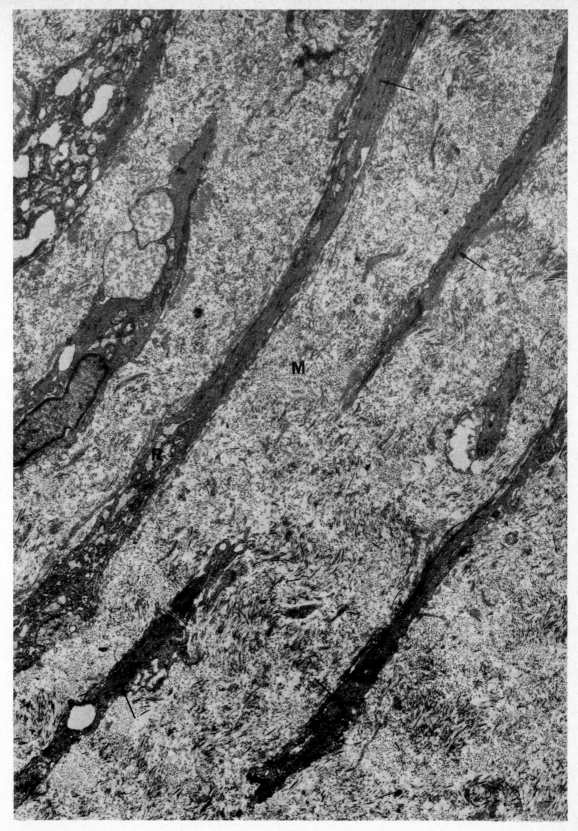

for describing these cells, for clearly the 'smooth muscle cell' here has a very different functional potential from typical smooth muscle cells found elsewhere.

In a recent study on ganglia in the region of the wrist joints of five patients, we (Ghadially and Mehta, 1971) found that in all instances the wall of this cystic structure contained multifunctional mesenchymal cells resembling smooth muscle and not fibroblasts and cells showing a synovial type of differentiation as had been thought in the past. Cells acceptable as fibroblasts were consistently absent or seen only in rare instances in only a few of the many samples of ganglion wall examined. Low power views of the ganglion wall show (*Plate 179*) that it is composed of elongated strap-like cells set in a fibrous and mucopolysaccharide matrix. These cells showed many morphological variations but a common feature was the presence of intracytoplasmic filaments which, in favourable sections, showed indubitable focal densities or attachment sites such as are known to occur among myofilaments. In some instances a small or large segment of the cell cytoplasm was occupied by rough endoplasmic reticulum often with markedly dilated cisternae, while in others a prominent Golgi complex and many smooth-walled vesicles containing secretory material were present (*Plate 180*).

Thus our study indicates that, except for a rare fibroblast and an occasional macrophage, the wall of the ganglion contains variants of only one cell type and that it resembles the smooth muscle cell rather than any other variety of mesenchymal cell. We can further argue that, since this is virtually the only cell type seen, it must be responsible for the production of the various components of the matrix; namely, collagen fibres, elastic fibres, and the mucopolysaccharide-containing ground substance or the interfibrillary matrix. That these cells are capable of achieving this end is attested to also by their ultrastructural appearance, for these cells are often well endowed with rough endoplasmic reticulum and Golgi complex. Interesting though these finding are, they do not help to resolve the long-standing dilemma as to the aetiology, pathogenesis and nature of these common lesions. Where these particular cells come from and why they proliferate and degenerate to form the ganglion and its fluid content remain a mystery.

Plate 180

A cell from ganglion wall. (*From Ghadially and Mehta, 1971*)
Fig. 1. High power view, showing cytoplasm packed with filaments that are difficult to resolve and numerous focal densities (arrows). × 36,000
Fig. 2. Dilated cisternae (C) of the rough endoplasmic reticulum and a dense myofilament-rich (M) cytoplasm. × 16,000
Fig. 3. The cytoplasmic matrix is packed with myofilaments (M), Golgi complex (G) and numerous smooth-walled vacuoles (V), some apparently about to open or opening into the matrix (arrows). × 20,000

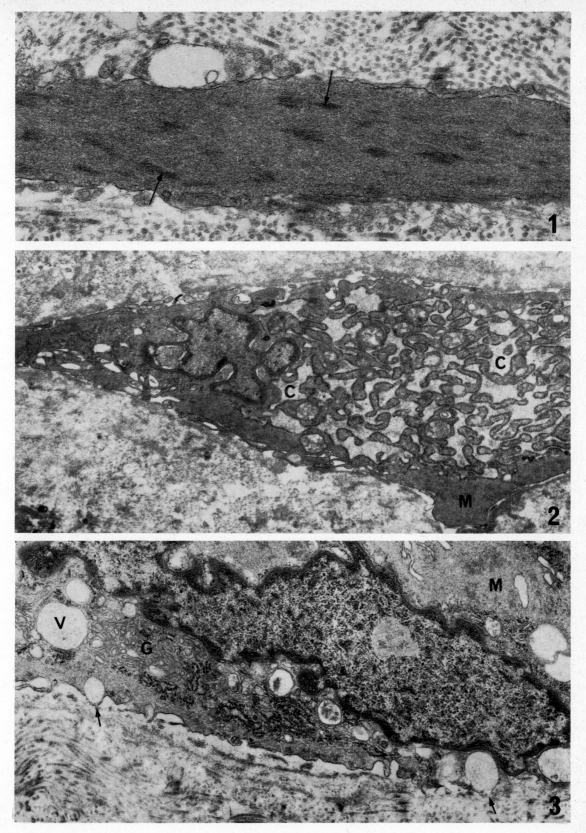

OTHER INTRACYTOPLASMIC FILAMENTS

Intracytoplasmic filaments similar in thickness to myofilaments but of unknown chemical composition are of common occurrence in a variety of cells. A convenient term covering all such intracytoplasmic filaments has not yet been coined. Terms such as 'other intracytoplasmic filaments', 'cytoplasmic fine filaments', 'fine filamentous fibres (or fibrils)', and 'FFF' have been used for this purpose. In the text that follows the term 'cytoplasmic filaments' is used in a restricted sense to mean all intracytoplasmic filaments except myofilaments.

It must, however, be realized that lack of knowledge about the chemical composition of these filaments and the suspicion that quite a few of them may be myofilaments after all precludes even a rough classification of the type suggested above. The text that follows must be read with this limitation in mind.

The myofilaments of striated muscle are easily recognized by their highly ordered arrangement (this is what produces the striated appearance). The myofilaments of smooth muscle are characterized by their orderly arrangement and the occurrence of focal densities along their course. But cytoplasmic filaments possess no such constant or characteristic distinguishing feature. Some differences in orientation are, however, seen. For example, the filaments comprising the tonofibrils of squamous epithelia are usually arranged in bundles or sheaves which at times terminate or loop through the plaques of desmosomes (Kelly, 1966) (*Plate 181*); those in chondrocytes show a whorled fascicular arrangement (*Plate 182*) while those in peritoneal macrophages are often straight, rigid-looking and short (*Plate 183*). Yet exceptions to such generalizations are seen at times.

The position of cytoplasmic filaments in the cell is also quite variable. They may be scattered diffusely in the cell or they may show a perinuclear or juxtanuclear distribution. At times such filaments may appear to arise as bushy outgrowths from the nuclear envelope, a mitochondrion or a lipid droplet. Such images are explicable on the basis of sectioning geometry and superimposition but the possibility that true continuity between the filaments and such structures may exist cannot be ruled out.

An increase in the cytoplasmic filament content of the cells has been noted in various experimental and pathological situations. Such an increase has been detected in cells that are often fairly well endowed with filaments (e.g. chondrocytes) and also in others where no filaments are said to occur (e.g. lymphocytes from peripheral blood) or only a few filaments are seen (e.g. vascular endothelial cells and synovial intimal cells).

An increase in the cytoplasmic filament content of cells has been noted in the following cell types and conditions: (1) chondrocytes of rabbit articular cartilage as a result of ageing (Barnett *et al.*, 1963), experimentally produced chronic haemarthrosis (Roy, 1968), experimentally produced lipoarthrosis (Ghadially *et al.*, 1970) and after the production of superficial defects in articular cartilage (Fuller and Ghadially, 1972); (2) synovial intimal cells in rheumatoid arthritis (for references, see Ghadially and Roy, 1969); (3) vascular endothelial cells of synovial blood

---

Plate 181

From normal human skin.

Fig. 1. This electron micrograph shows a basal cell containing loosely arranged tonofilaments (T) and a prickle cell containing tonofibrils (F) where the individual filaments are difficult to discern. Desmosomes (D) with attached tonofilaments are also evident. Note the transversely cut melanocyte dendrites containing melanosomes (M) and the much larger, compound melanosomes (C) in the keratinocytes. (See also *Plate 166*.) × 18,500

Fig. 2. High power view of tonofilaments (T) and desmosomes (D) with attached filaments. × 47,000

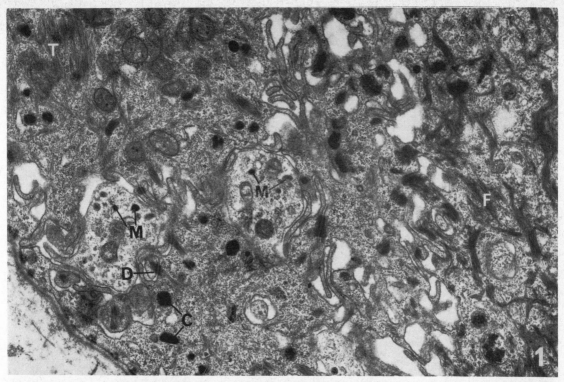

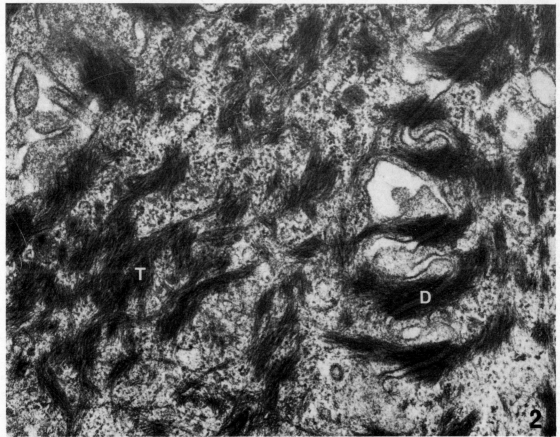

vessels in rheumatoid arthritis (Ghadially and Roy, 1967); (4) peritoneal macrophages in cases of malignant ascites (an example of this is shown in *Plate 183*); (5) human neurons in cases of sporadic motor neuron disease, infantile neuroaxonal dystrophy, vincristine neuropathy, Pick's disease and neurons of experimental animals in aluminium encephalopathy, spindle inhibitor encephalopathy, lathyrogenic encephalopathy, vitamin E deficiency, copper deficiency, and retrograde and Wallerian degeneration (Terry and Pena, 1965; Wisniewski *et al.*, 1970; Terry, 1971); (6) human lymphocytes from thoracic duct (Zucker-Franklin, 1963); (7) activated lymphocytes from mixed lymphocyte cultures but not those activated by phytohaemagglutinin (Parker *et al.*, 1967); (8) lymphomas and leukaemias (including plasma cell and myeloid leukaemia) (for references, see Rangan *et al.*, 1971; Beltran and Stuckey, 1972).

Cytoplasmic filaments have been noted in a wide variety of experimentally produced and human tumours. Prominent juxtanuclear filamentous aggregates and psammoma bodies were found in a papillary adenocarcinoma of the endometrium by Hameed and Morgan (1972). These authors suggest that such aggregates of cytoplasmic filaments provide the scaffolding for calcification and psammoma body formation, not only in the tumour studied by them but also in other tumours such as meningiomas. Furthermore, they and others who have studied fine filaments in lymphomas and leukaemias have proposed that such an increase indicates a state of heightened metabolic activity associated with an active or neoplastic state.

However, many workers have taken a contrary view and suggested that the accumulation of cytoplasmic filaments even in tumours is a sign of degeneration and impending necrosis. Such a view has been expressed about: (1) pituitary adenomas where focal whorls of cytoplasmic filaments occur (Cardell and Knighton, 1966; Peillon *et al.*, 1970; Schochet *et al.*, 1972); (2) Chang cells cultured with activated lymphocytes (Biberfeld, 1971); and (3) human breast carcinoma cells in culture where massive accumulation of 110 Å thick filaments occurs in declining cells in no longer dividing cultures (Tumilowicz and Sarkar, 1972).

Perhaps the most compelling evidence that accumulation of filaments represents a regressive or degenerative change comes from the study of such filaments in neurons (for references, see above), and here quite aptly the term 'neurofibrillary degeneration' has been coined to describe this phenomenon. My studies on articular tissues also support this idea, for the change is seen where degenerative changes may be expected or are known to occur. This is also in keeping with the observation (both in articular tissues and in neurons) that, as cytoplasmic filaments accumulate, cell organelles are first displaced and then destroyed so that ultimately the cytoplasm contains little besides filaments.

Plate 182

Fig. 1. Chondrocyte from articular cartilage of a rabbit that had received repeated injections of blood and autologous fat into the knee joint. The cytoplasm is packed with filaments (F), some of which appear to radiate from a lipid droplet (L). Also seen are many glycogen particles (G) and part of the nucleus (N). The usual cell organelles are not evident in this plane of sectioning. × 15,000

Fig. 2. High power view of intracytoplasmic filaments in a chondrocyte. From rabbit articular cartilage where a partial thickness defect had been made 3 months prior to collection of the specimen. × 85,000

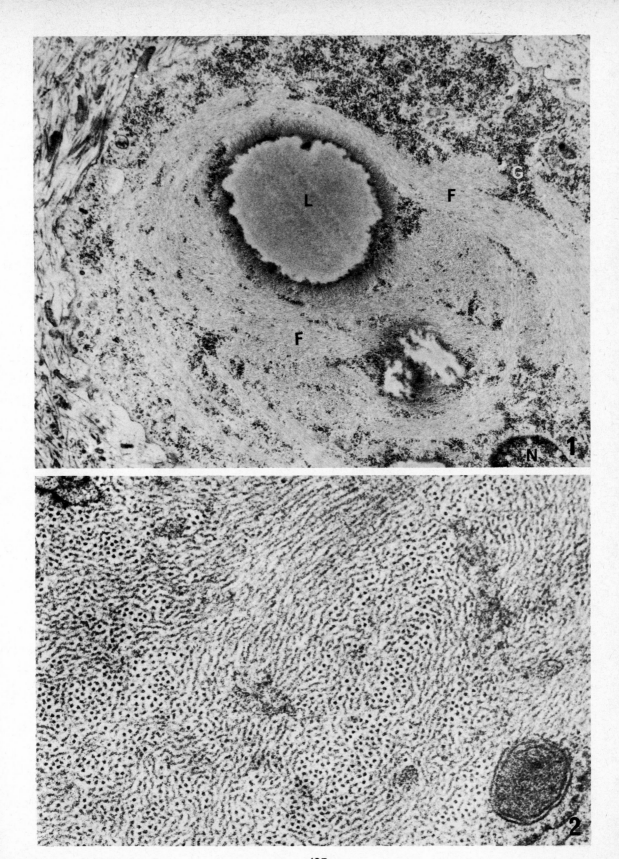

As noted earlier, the only serious dissenting vote comes from students of haemopoietic cells and their neoplasms, who consider the accumulation of intracytoplasmic filaments as a sign of heightened activity rather than degeneration. Therefore it behoves us to re-examine the situation and see if alternative explanations can be proposed. It seems to me that in the case of lymphomas and leukaemias one can argue that, in this, as in other neoplasms, there are both populations of actively growing cells and senescent and dying cells, and it is possible that it is the latter group which accumulate filaments. The observation that 'stimulated' lymphocytes in mixed lymphocyte cultures contain increased amounts of filaments but not those stimulated by phytohaemagglutinin is particularly intriguing, for one can contend that this shows that stimulation *per se* is not the common operative factor which leads to filament accumulation in lymphocytes. One can also point out that the mixed lymphocyte culture is not a market garden where lymphocytes thrive and multiply but a battle ground where strains of lymphocytes are injured and killed and that it is such cells that probably accumulate filaments in their cytoplasm. Such contentions are also supported by the observations that in cultures of Chang cells and lymphocytes stimulated with phytohaemagglutinin it is the injured and dying tumour cells which develop masses of cytoplasmic filaments and not the attacking lymphocytes.

Thus, it would appear that there is now a massive body of evidence which indicates that a gross increase in intracytoplasmic filaments is a sign of regressive and degenerative changes in a variety of cell types.

An interesting observation, whose significance is not entirely clear, is that in encephalopathy induced by treatment with spindle inhibitors (e.g. colchicine) or in cultures of neurons treated *in vitro* with such drugs there is a prompt disappearance of normal microtubules (240 Å diameter) and a massive replacement by cytoplasmic filaments.* This change, however, is reversible, for subsequently the filaments disappear and an increased population of microtubules (called neurotubules in this site) is seen (Wisniewski *et al.*, 1968; Terry, 1971).

It would appear that HeLa cells in culture respond similarly to neurons when treated with colchicine (Robbins and Gonatas, 1964; Bensch and Malavista, 1969). Here, too, filamentous proliferation is seen and it has been shown that the antimitotic effect of this drug is due to binding with spindle microtubular protein which suffers depolymerization. The capacity of this drug to bind to other cytoplasmic microtubules, including neurotubules, has also been demonstrated (Borisy and Taylor, 1967).

The tentative conclusion drawn from such studies (Wisniewski *et al.*, 1970) is that the subunits of intracytoplasmic filaments and microtubules are probably identical and interchangeable.

* For further examples of this phenomenon, see Chapter XII.

Plate 183

Fig. 1. Macrophage from ascitic fluid, showing sheaves of intracytoplasmic filaments (F). (From the same specimen as *Plate 169*). × 16,500

Fig. 2. High power view of the filaments shown in *Fig. 1.* × 50,000

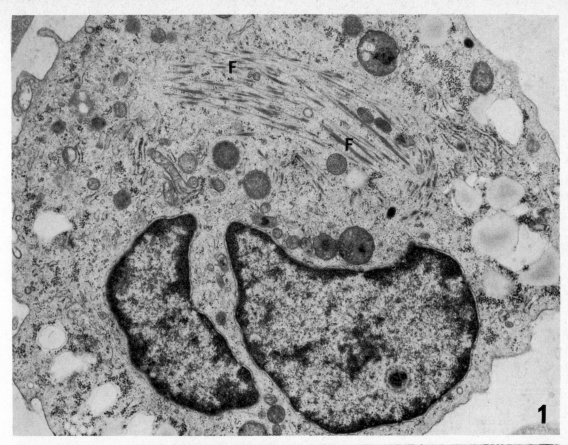

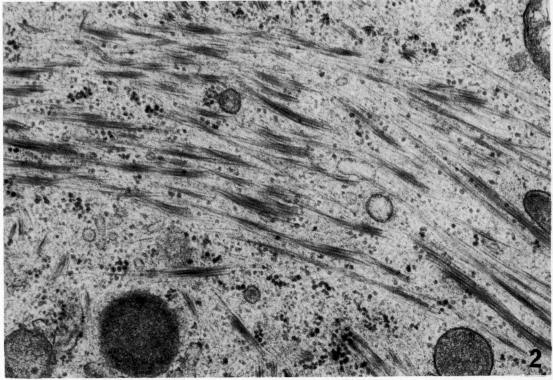

429

REFERENCES

Adams, R. D., Denny-Brown, D. and Pearson, C. M. (1962). *Diseases of Muscle,* 2nd edn., p. 585. New York: Hoeber Med.

Apatenko, A. K. (1964). 'Formation of annular fibrils in muscles of amputated stumps.' *Fedn Proc.* **23,** T71

Barnett, C. H., Cochrane, W. and Palfrey, A. J. (1963). 'Age changes in articular cartilage of rabbits.' *Ann. rheum. Dis.* **22,** 389

Bataillon, E. (1891). 'Recherches anatomiques et experimentales sur la metamorphose des amphibiens anoures.' *Annls Univ. Lyon* **2,** 1

Becker, C. G. and Murphy, G. E. (1969). 'Demonstration of contractile protein in endothelium and cells of heart valves, endocardium, intima, arterosclerotic plaques and Aschoff bodies of rheumatic heart disease.' *Am. J. Path.* **55,** 1

Beltran, G. and Stuckey, W. J. (1972). 'Nuclear lobulation and cytoplasmic fibrils in leukemic plasma cells.' *Am. J. clin. Path.* **58,** 159

Bensch, K. G. and Malawista, S. E. (1969). 'Microtubular crystals in mammalian cells.' *J. Cell Biol.* **40,** 95

Bethlem, J. and van Wijngaarden, G. K. (1963). 'The incidence of ringed fibres and sarcoplasmic masses in normal and diseased muscles.' *J. Neurol. Neurosurg. Psychiat.* **26,** 326

Biberfeld, P. (1971). 'Cytotoxic interaction of phytohemagglutin-stimulated blood lymphocytes with monolayer cells. A study by light and electron microscopy.' *Cellular Immunol.* **2,** 54

Borisy, G. G. and Taylor, E. W. (1967). 'The mechanism of action of colchicine. Binding of colchicine-^{3}H to cellular protein.' *J. Cell Biol.* **34,** 525

Breathnach, A. S. (1971). *The Ultrastructure of Human Skin.* Edinburgh and London: Churchill Livingstone

Cardell, R. R., Jr. and Knighton, R. S. (1966). 'The cytology of a human pituitary tumor: an electron microscopic study.' *Trans. Am. microsc. Soc.* **85,** 58

Chen, L. and Weiss, L. (1972). 'Electron microscopy of the red pulp of human spleen.' *Am. J. Anat.* **134,** 425

Dubois, P., Dumont, L. and Lieux, J. (1966). 'Histogenese de l'artere ombilicale humaine aux 3 et 4 mois du developpement embryonnaire etudie en microscopie electronique.' *Bull. Ass. Anat., Paris* **51,** 344

Elliot, G. F. (1964). 'X-ray diffraction studies on striated and smooth muscle.' *Proc. R. Soc. B* **160,** 467

— (1967). 'Variations of the contractile apparatus in smooth and striated muscle.' *J. gen. Physiol.* **50,** Supp. 171

Engel, W. K. (1961). 'Muscle target fibres, a newly recognized sign of denervation.' *Nature, Lond.* **191,** 389

— (1962). 'Chemocytology of striated annulets and sarcoplasmic masses in myotonic dystrophy.' *J. Histochem. Cytochem.* **10,** 229

Engel, A. G. and MacDonald, R. D. (1970). 'Ultrastructural reactions in muscle disease and the light-microscopic correlates.' In *Proceedings of the International Congress on Muscle Diseases, Milan, 1969,* p. 71. Int. Congr. Ser. No. 199. Ed. by J. N. Walton, N. Canal and G. Scarlato. Amsterdam: Excerpta Medica

Fawcett, D. W. (1968). 'The sporadic occurrence in cardiac muscle of anomalous Z-bands exhibiting a periodic structure suggestive of tropomyosin.' *J. Cell. Biol.* **36,** 266

Flora, G., Dahl, E. and Nelson, E. (1967). 'Electron microscopic observations on human intracranial arteries.' *Archs Neurol., Chicago* **17,** 162

Florey, H. W. (1966). 'The endothelial cell.' *Br. med. J.* **2,** 487

Fuller, J. A. and Ghadially, F. N. (1972). 'Ultrastructural observations on surgically produced partial-thickness defects in articular cartilage.' *Clin. Orthop. Rel. Res.* **86,** 193

Garamvolgyi, N., Vizi, E. S. and Knoll, J. (1971). 'The regular occurrence of thick filaments in stretched mammalian smooth muscle.' *J. Ultrastruct. Res.* **34,** 135

Ghadially, F. N. and Mehta, P. N. (1971). 'Multifunctional mesenchymal cells resembling smooth muscle cells in ganglia of the wrist.' *Ann. rheum. Dis.* **30,** 31

— and Roy, S. (1967). 'Ultrastructure of synovial membrane in rheumatoid arthritis.' *Ann. rheum. Dis.* **26,** 426

— — (1969). *Ultrastructure of Synovial Joints in Health and Disease.* London: Butterworths

— Mehta, P. N. and Kirkaldy-Willis, W. H. (1970). 'Ultrastructure of articular cartilage in experimentally produced lipoarthrosis.' *J. Bone Jt Surg.* **52A,** 1147

Gonatas, N. K., Perez, M. C., Shy, G. M. and Evangelista, I. (1965). 'Central "core" disease of skeletal muscle. Ultrastructural and cytochemical observations in two cases.' *Am. J. Path.* **47,** 503

Grabow, J. D. and Chou, S. M. (1968). 'Thyrotrophin hormone deficiency with a peripheral neuropathy.' *Archs Neurol., Chicago* **19,** 284

Hama, K. (1961). 'On the existence of filamentous structures in endothelial cells of the amphibian capillary.' *Anat. Rec.* **139,** 437

Hameed, K. and Morgan, D. A. (1972). 'Papillary adenocarcinoma of endometrium with psammoma bodies. Histology and fine structure.' *Cancer* **29,** 1326

Hanson, J. and Lowy, J. (1960). 'Structure and function of the contractile apparatus in the muscles of invertebrate animals.' In *Structure and Function of Muscle,* Vol. 1, p. 265. Ed. by G. H. Bourne. New York and London: Academic Press

— — (1964a). 'Comparative studies on the structure of contractile systems.' *Circulation Res.* **15,** Supp. 1–2, 11–4

— — (1964b). Discussion following paper by D. M. Needham and C. F. Shoenberg. 'Proteins of the contractile mechanism of mammalian smooth muscle and the possible location in the cell.' *Proc. R. Soc. B* **160,** 523

Hayward, M. and Mair, W. G. P. (1970). 'The ultrastructure of ring fibres in dystrophic muscle.' *Acta neuropath.* **16,** 161

Hibbs, R. G. (1958). 'The fine structure of human eccrine sweat glands.' *Am. J. Anat.* **103,** 201

— (1962). 'Electron microscopy of human apocrine sweat gland.' *J. invest. Derm.* **38,** 77

Hollmann, K. H. (1959). 'L'ultrastructure de la glande mammaire normale de la souris en lactation.' *J. Ultrastruct. Res.* **2,** 423

Hurley, H. J., Jr. and Shelley, W. B. (1954). 'The role of the myoepithelium of the human apocrine sweat gland.' *J. invest. Derm.* **22,** 143

Jonecko, A. (1962). 'Die Ringbinden als eine allgemeine unspezifische Reaktion der quergestreiften Muskulatur.' *Experientia* **18,** 166

Kelly, D. E. (1966). 'Fine structure of desmosomes, Hemidesmosomes, and an adepidermal globular layer in developing newt epidermis.' *J. Cell Biol.* **28,** 51

Kelly, R. E. and Rice, R. V. (1968). 'Localization of myosin filaments in smooth muscle.' *J. Cell Biol.* **37,** 105

Knieriem, H. J. (1967). 'Electron microscopic study of bovine arteriosclerotic lesions.' *Am. J. Path.* **50,** 1035

Landon, D. N. (1970). 'The influence of fixation upon the fine structure of the Z-disc of rat striated muscle.' *J. Cell Sci.* **6,** 257

Lapresle, J. and Fardeau, M. (1968). 'Les desorganisations spatiales des myofibrilles, des sarcomeres et des myofilaments dans les zones peripheriques de fibres musculaires pathologiques étudiés en microscope électronique.' *Acta neuropath.* **10,** 105

— — and Milhaud, M. (1964). 'Sur un type particulier d'alterations de la structure myofibrillaire rencontrées dans cinq cas de dystrophie musculaire progressive.' *C.r. Seanc. Soc. Biol.* **158,** 1807

— — — (1966). 'Etude des ultrastructures dans les dystrophies musculaires progressives.' *Proc. 5th Int. Congr. Neuropath.*, p. 602. Amsterdam: Excerpta Medica

Le Menn, R. and Emeriau, J. P. (1970). 'Etude en microscopie electronique de fibres annulaires dans le myocarde humain.' *C.r. Soc. Biol.* **8–9,** 1684

Lowy, J., Poulsen, F. R. and Vibert, D. J. (1970). 'Myosin filaments in vertebrate smooth muscle.' *Nature, Lond.* **225,** 1053

MacDonald, R. D. and Engel, A. G. (1969). 'The cytoplasmic body: another structural anomaly of the Z disc.' *Acta neuropath.* **14,** 99

Mair, W. G. P. and Tomé, F. M. S. (1972). *Atlas of the Ultrastructure of Diseased Human Muscle.* Edinburgh and London: Churchill Livingstone

Majno, G., Gabbiani, G., Joris, I. and Ryan, G. B. (1970). 'Contraction of non-muscular cells: endothelium and fibroblasts.' *J. Cell Biol.* **47** (Abst. 334), 127a

Morris, W. R. (1959). 'Striated annulets (ringbenden).' *Archs Path.* **68,** 438

Munger, B. L. and Brusilow, S. W. (1961). 'An electron microscopic study of eccrine sweat glands of the cat foot and toe pads—evidence for ductal reabsorption in the human.' *J. biophys. biochem. Cytol.* **11,** 403

— — and Cooke, R. E. (1961). 'An electron microscopic study of eccrine sweat glands in patients with cystic fibrosis of the pancreas.' *J. Pediat.* **59,** 497

Munnell, J. F. and Getty, R. (1968). 'Rate of accumulation of cardiac lipofuscin in the aging canine.' *J. Gerent.* **23,** 154

Murad, T. M. and von Haam, E. (1968). 'Ultrastructure of myoepithelial cells in human mammary gland tumors.' *Cancer* **21,** 1137

Newstead, J. D. (1971). 'Filaments in renal parenchymal and interstitial cells.' *J. Ultrastruct. Res.* **34,** 316

Oternelo, F. T. (1972). 'Ultrastructure of muscle in typical and atypical Duchenne muscular dystrophy.' Thesis: University of Western Ontario, London, Canada

Parker, J. W., Wakasa, H. and Lukes, R. J. (1967). 'Cytoplasmic fibrils in mixed lymphocyte cultures.' *Blood* **29,** 608

Parry, E. W. (1970). 'Some electron microscope observations on the mesenchymal structures of full-term umbilical cord.' *J. Anat.* **107,** 505

— and Abramovich, D. R. (1972). 'The ultrastructure of human umbilical vessel endothelium from early pregnancy to full term.' *J. Anat.* **111,** 29

Peillon, F., Vila-Porcile, E. and Olivier, L. (1970). 'L'action des oestrogenes sur les adenomas hypophysaires chez l'homme.' *Annls Endocr.* **31,** 259

Pellegrino, C. and Franzini, C. (1963). 'An electron microscope study of denervation atrophy in red and white skeletal muscle fibres.' *J. Cell Biol.* **17,** 327

Peterson, M., Day, A. J., Tume, R. K. and Eisenberg, E. (1971). 'Ultrastructure, fatty acid content, and metabolic activity of foam cells and other fractions separated from rabbit atherosclerotic lesions.' *Expl Molec. Path.* **15,** 157

Price, H. M., Gordon, G. B., Pearson, C. M. Munsat, T. L. and Blumberg, J. M. (1965). 'New evidence for excessive accumulation of Z-band material in nemaline myopathy.' *Proc. natn. Acad. Sci. U.S.A.* **54,** 1398

Rangan, S. R. S., Calvert, R. C. and Vitols, K. (1971). 'Fibrillar bundles in canine lymphomas: an ultrastructural study.' *J. Ultrastruct. Res.* **36,** 425

Richardson, K. C. (1949). 'Contractile tissues in the mammary gland, with special reference to myoepithelium in the goat.' *Proc. R. Soc. B* **136,** 30

Robbins, E. and Gonatas, N. K. (1964). 'Histochemical and ultrastructural studies on HeLa cell cultures exposed to spindle inhibitors with special reference to the interphase cell.' *J. Histochem. Cytochem.* **12,** 704

Rostgaard, J., Kristensen, B. I. and Nielsen, L. E. (1972). 'Electron microscopy of filaments in the basal part of rat kidney. Tubule cells and their in situ interaction with heavy Meromyosin.' *Z. Zellforsch. mikrosk. Anat.* **132,** 497

Rowlatt, C. and Franks, L. M. (1964). 'Myoepithelium in mouse prostate.' *Nature, Lond.* **202,** 707

Roy, S. (1968). 'Ultrastructure of articular cartilage in experimental haemarthrosis.' *Archs Path.* **86,** 69

Rubinstein, L. J. (1960). *The Structure and Function of Muscle,* Vol. 3, p. 213. Ed. by G. H. Bourne. New York: Academic Press

Rumyantseva, O. N. (1957). *Izv. Akad. Nauk, SSSR., Ser. Biol.* **3,** 331

Schochet, S. S., McCormick, W. F. and Halmi, N. S. (1972). 'Acidophil adenomas with intracytoplasmic filamentous aggregates. A light and electron microscope study.' *Archs Path.* **94,** 16

Schotland, D. L. (1969). 'An electron microscopic study of target fibers, target-like fibers and related abnormalities in human muscle.' *J. Neuropath. exp. Neurol.* **28**, 214

— Spiro, D. and Carmel, P. (1966). 'Ultrastructural studies of ring fibers in human muscle disease.' *J. Neuropath. exp. Neurol.* **25**, 431

Schroeder, J. M. and Adams, R. D. (1968). 'The ultrastructural morphology of the muscle fiber in myotonic dystrophy.' *Acta neuropath.* **10**, 218

Shafiq, S. A., Gorycki, M., Goldstone, L. and Milhorat, A. T. (1966). 'Fine structure of fiber types in normal human muscle.' *Anat. Rec.* **156**, 283

— Milhorat, A. T. and Gorycki, M. A. (1967). 'Fine structure of human muscle in neurogenic atrophy.' *Neurology, Minneap.* **17**, 934

Shy, G. M., Engel, W. K., Somers, J. E. and Wanko, T. (1963). 'Nemaline myopathy. A new congenital myopathy.' *Brain* **86**, 793

Silver, I. A. (1954). 'Myoepithelial cells in the mammary and parotid glands.' *J. Physiol.* **125**, 80

Spiro, D. and Hagopian, M. (1967). 'On the assemblage of myofibrils.' In *Formation and Fate of Cell Organelles*, p. 71. Ed. by K. B. Warren. New York and London: Academic Press

Stenger, R. J., Spiro, D., Scully, R. E. and Shannon, J. M. (1962). 'Ultrastructural and physiologic alterations in ischemic skeletal muscle.' *Am. J. Path.* **40**, 1

Terry, R. D. (1971). Presidential address: 'Neuronal fibrous protein in human pathology.' *J. Neuropath. exp. Neurol.* **30**, 8

— and Pena, C. (1965). 'Experimental production of neurofibrillary degeneration. 2. Electron microscopy, phosphatase histochemistry and electron probe analysis.' *J. Neuropath. exp. Neurol.* **24**, 200

Tice, L. W. and Engel, A. G. (1967). 'The effects of glucocorticoids on red and white muscles in the rat.' *Am. J. Path.* **50**, 311

Tomonaga, M. and Sluga, E. (1969). 'Zur ultrastruktur der "Target-Fasern".' *Virchows Arch. path. Anat. Physiol.* **348**, 89

— — (1970). 'The ultrastructure and pathogenesis of "target fibres".' In *Proceedings of the International Congress on Muscle Diseases*, p. 120. Ed. by J. N. Walton, N. Canal and G. Scarlato. Int. Congr. Ser. No. 199. Amsterdam: Excerpta Medica

Tumilowicz, J. J. and Sarkar, N. H. (1972). 'Accumulating filaments and other ultrastructural aspects of declining cell cultures derived from human breast tumors.' *Expl Molec. Path.* **16**, 210

Weiss, P. and James, R. (1955). 'Aberrant (circular) myofibrils in amphibian larvae: an example of orthogonal tissue structure.' *J. exp. Zool.* **129**, 607

Wisniewski, H., Shelanski, M. L. and Terry, R. D. (1968). 'Effects of mitotic spindle inhibitors on neurotubules and neurofilaments in anterior horn cells.' *J. Cell Biol.* **38**, 224

— Terry, R. D. and Hirano, A. (1970). 'Neurofibrillary pathology.' *J. Neuropath. exp. Neurol.* **29**, 163

Wissler, R. W. (1967). Editorial: 'The arterial medial cell, smooth muscle, or multifunctional mesenchyme.' *Circulation* **36**, 1

Zacks, S. I. (1970). 'Recent contributions to the diagnosis of muscle disease.' *Human Path.* **1**, 465

Zucker-Franklin, D. (1963). 'The ultrastructure of cells in human thoracic duct lymph.' *J. Ultrastruct. Res.* **9**, 325

CHAPTER XII

Microtubules

INTRODUCTION

Microtubules, like intracytoplasmic filaments, are of widespread occurrence and have now been reported in a variety of plant and animal cells. At times, microfilaments and microtubules occur in close association, and pathological and experimental situations are known where a diminution in the number of microtubules is accompanied by an increase in intracytoplasmic filaments (see below and page 428).

Microtubules measure about 250 Å in diameter. Examination of suitably prepared plant and animal material has revealed that their wall contains 10–13 longitudinally orientated filaments (Behnke and Zelander, 1966).

Various functions have been ascribed to microtubules found in different situations and cell types. In cells such as the neurons, where they are of frequent occurrence in the dendrites and axons, they are thought to represent 'roads' (Plasmastrassen) along which intracytoplasmic substances and organelles may move. The microtubules of the mitotic spindle are responsible for the movement of chromosomes within the cell, and those in cilia and flagella for the movement of these structures. In some other instances microtubules are thought to have a cytoskeletal function; that is to say, they may be involved in maintaining cell shape. An example of this is the marginal band of microtubules found in the nucleated erythrocytes of fish, amphibians and birds, and in human platelets.

A protein dimer composed of two monomeric subunits (molecular weight approximately 55,000), differing from each other only in a few amino acid residues, comprises the basic structural unit of microtubules. This is found to be so for microtubules from such disparate sources as human neuroblastoma cells and protozoan flagella (Olmsted et al., 1971). Microtubular protein resembles actin in its general properties and amino acid composition.

Colchicine combines with the protein dimer of microtubules stoichiometrically (one molecule per dimer) and it has been shown that this drug can cause a disruption of normal microtubules and an accumulation of intracytoplasmic filaments (see page 428). It has hence been suggested (Wisniewski et al., 1970) that the subunits of intracytoplasmic filaments and microtubules are probably identical and interchangeable.

P

Microtubules approximately 250 Å thick have now been found in a variety of cells. They are, as a rule, not evident in osmium-fixed material; glutaraldehyde fixation is usually necessary to demonstrate them. De-The (1964) observed that 'visualization of cytoplasmic microtubules after glutaraldehyde fixation seems to be one of the main differences between this fixation and fixation with osmium tetroxide alone'. While this is true of most microtubules, certain others such as those in cilia and centrioles and, to a lesser extent, those in the mitotic spindle are seen in osmium-fixed material. It is worth noting that microtubules tend to disappear when subjected to cold. Thus, when the object is to demonstrate microtubules, it is better to fix tissues at room temperature or at 37°C rather than at the conventional 0–4°C. Occasional microtubules have now been demonstrated in such a large variety of cells that it would be difficult to list all the situations in which they have been seen. More fruitful would be to review those studies which indicate the role of these structures in cell economy.

Perhaps the best known and most studied microtubules are those of the mitotic apparatus. The electron microscope has revealed that the spindle fibres of the light microscopist are not filaments but microtubules approximately 250 Å in diameter. It is also clear that in many mammalian cells the separation of the two sets of chromosomes during mitosis is not the result of a contraction of microtubules joining the pole to the chromosomes (chromosomal fibres) because no increase in the thickness of these microtubules is evident as the chromosomes move apart. (There is, however, some shortening of the microtubules; see below). The main factor involved in the separation of chromosomes in many, but not all, cells is an abrupt elongation of the spindle (pole to pole fibres) at anaphase, so that the two poles move apart (Mazia, 1961; Inoue and Sato, 1967; Forer, 1969; Nicklas, 1970; Brinkley and Cartwright, 1971).

Since microtubules are sometimes seen in groups of two or more lying closely apposed and fine cross-bridges have been demonstrated between them, it has been speculated that a sliding action akin to that of thick and thin filaments of muscle may be involved.* However, recent studies—including one by Brinkley and Cartwright (1971)—do not support this concept. They state, 'although sliding or shearing of microtubules may occur in the spindle, such appears not to be the mechanism by which the spindle elongates in anaphase. Instead our data support the hypothesis that spindle elongation occurs by growth of prepositioned microtubules which "push" the poles apart.' This process is accompanied by a shortening of chromosomal microtubules as the chromosomes move to the poles, and it is thought that subunits derived from the breakdown of chromosomal microtubules may be added to the cytoplasmic pool of microtubular protein from which the elongating pole to pole microtubules are supplied. The abruptness with which the spindle elongates also favours the idea that subunits are derived from a pool and are not synthesized as needed. (There is evidence that little or no protein synthesis occurs after the initiation of prophase: see page 232).

Thus, in this example, the role of microtubules in moving structures within the cell has been clearly demonstrated. It is not unreasonable to suppose that the microtubules of the axial microtubule complex of cilia are responsible for ciliary movement, but the mechanics of this are less clearly understood. A gliding movement of microtubules or an actual contraction of the microtubules has been suggested to explain this phenomenon.

* The occurrence of cross-bridges is so sparse as to belie this idea quite effectively.

Plate 184

A neoplastic cell in mitosis, showing chromosomes (C) and microtubules (T) of the mitotic spindle. From the same specimen as *Plate 169.* × 56,000

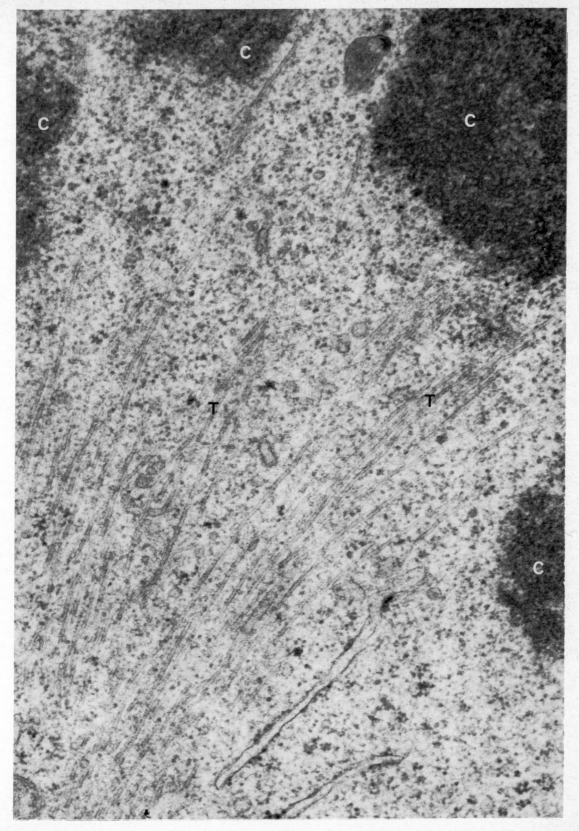

A number of observations suggest that in some instances microtubules are involved in the development and/or maintenance of cell form. The maintenance of cell form in metazoans depends upon many factors (for example, cell-to-cell attachment and mutual pressure), and microtubules play a minor, if any, role at all in most instances; but in some unicellular organisms such as the heliozoan, *Actinosphaerium nucleofilum* (Tilney, 1965), the numerous fine cell processes (axopodia) are supported by a complex array of microtubules. Such axopodia disappear and are not re-formed as long as the microtubules are kept in a dissociated state with hydrostatic pressure, low temperature or colchicine; but both microtubules and axopodia promptly reappear when such influences are removed (for references, see Tilney *et al.*, 1966; Tilney and Porter, 1967).

Similarly, it is thought that the flat discoid shape of the nucleated erythrocytes of birds, reptiles, amphibia and fish is maintained by a marginal bundle of microtubules (for references, see Grasso, 1966), and it has been shown that disruption of these by colchicine in developing erythroid cells of the chicken (Barrett and Dawson, 1972) leads to spherocytosis. In mature erythrocytes of man and laboratory animals such a band of microtubules has not been demonstrated. It has, however, been speculated that spherocytosis in man may be due to a defect in 'proteins of structure' because spherocytosis can be produced in normal erythrocytes by exposing them to antimitotic agents (Jacob *et al.*, 1972).

A marginal band of microtubules is found in human platelets, as well as numerous filaments in platelet pseudopodia (*Plate 185*). Furthermore, fibrillary material can be demonstrated in the platelet cytoplasm when its density is reduced by incubation in distilled water (Zucker-Franklin, 1969). Brief osmotic shock at low temperature leads to a disappearance of microtubules which are converted into filaments. The disappearance of microtubules was noted after colchicine treatment by Zucker-Franklin (1969) but this did not interfere with clot retraction. On the basis of the above-mentioned observations, she postulates that 'the contractile properties of the cells may be vested in the microfibrils, whereas the tubules may serve to maintain the highly asymmetric shape characteristic of circulating and irreversibly aggregated platelets'.

Although microtubules do not play a major role in the maintenance of cell shape in tissues of metazoans, they have been shown in some instances to be responsible for the development of cell shape. Evidence of this is found during the development of the primary mesenchyme in *Arabica punctulata* (Tilney and Gibbins, 1969), during the elongation of the primordial lens cells of the chick (Byers and Porter, 1964) and in the developing spermatid during the period of elongation to form the neck and midpiece when a cylindrical array of microtubules, called the caudal sheath or manchette, is formed (Burgos and Fawcett, 1956; Bloom and Fawcett, 1969).

A number of observations suggest that in some instances microtubules delineate pathways along which cytoplasmic organelles and inclusions move within the cell (see review by Porter, 1966). For example, such a system is thought to operate in the movement of: (1) melanin granules in the melanophores of *Fundulus heteroclitus* (Bikle *et al.*, 1966); (2) Golgi vesicles at the cell plate of plant cells (Whaley and Mollenhauer, 1963; Ledbetter and Porter, 1963); (3) cytoplasmic granules in the axopods of the heliozoan, *Actinosphaerium* (Tilney *et al*, 1966; Tilney and Porter, 1967); (4) endocytosed food particles along the tentacles of the suctorian, *Tokophrya* (Rudzinska,

---

Plate 185

Human platelets (*From Zucker-Franklin, 1969*).

Fig. 1. Human platelet, showing a marginal band of microtubules (arrow). × 42,000

Fig. 2. A platelet showing a cross-section through the marginal band of microtubules (arrow). × 39,000

Fig. 3. Fine filaments in a platelet psuedopod. × 75,000

Fig. 4. Microtubules (arrow) and fibrillar material which becomes apparent in the cytoplasm when platelets are incubated in distilled water at 37°C for 5 minutes. × 68,000

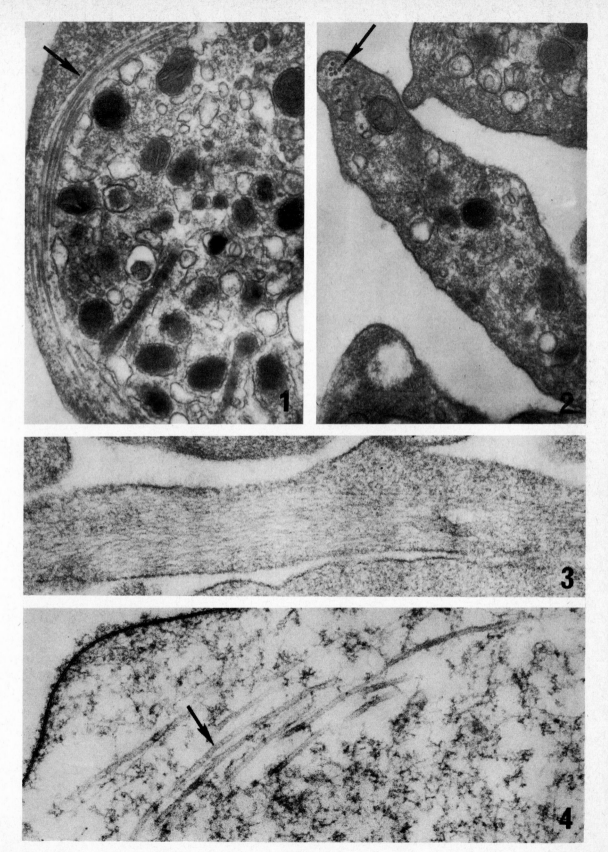

1965); and (5) nuclei of hamster kidney cells forming syncytia in culture after infection with parainfluenza virus SV5 (Holmes and Choppin, 1968). It has also been suggested that microtubules are involved in the movement and release of secretory products—such as insulin from β-cells, histamine from mast cells and catecholamines from the adrenal medulla (Thoa *et al.*, 1972).

In the above-mentioned examples there is no clear stable attachment between the moving 'particle' and microtubule akin to that seen in the case of chromosomes, although, in the case of virus-induced syncytia, rows of nuclei intimately associated with microtubules can be isolated from cell homogenates. In time-lapse movies of such cultures Holmes and Choppin (1968) found that migrating nuclei seemed to move as if there were channels through the cytoplasm, and they state that 'the nuclei within these channels move independently of each other and may revolve end-over-end as they migrate towards the center of the cell'. Electron microscopy showed that these channels are delineated by 250 Å diameter tubules and 80 Å thick filaments. Upon treatment of the cells with colchicine the microtubules were destroyed and there was an increase in the number of filaments. Such cells retain the power to fuse and form syncytia, but the nuclei do not migrate to form rows but remain randomly scattered in the syncytial cytoplasm.

The idea that microtubules in neurons (called neurotubules) also demarcate channels or 'roads' (Plasmastrassen) along which intracellular transport occurs has been frequently mooted (Andres, 1961; Bunge *et al.*, 1967; Billings, 1972). There is also evidence that, in pathological states or experimental situations (e.g. administration of colchicine, vinblastine or aluminium compounds) where microtubules are destroyed and an increase in intracytoplasmic filaments occurs, such movements are arrested (see page 428).

An interesting association between reovirus replication and microtubules has been demonstrated by many studies. Tournier and Plissier (1960) first demonstrated in tissue culture cells that cytoplasmic inclusions of reovirus formed along hollow tubular structures resembling tubules of the mitotic apparatus, and the studies of Dales and his associates (Dales, 1963; Dales *et al.*, 1965; Silverstein and Dales, 1968) have shown that, during virus development, the spindle microtubules become coated with a dense granular or fibrous material contiguous with aggregates of viral particles. A similar association of reovirus with neuronal microtubules and 50–65 Å kinky filaments has recently been noted in the brains of suckling mice infected with reovirus (Margolis *et al.*, 1971; Gonatas *et al.*, 1971). Here also, microtubules coated with 'fuzzy' material were seen in association with virus particles (*Plate 186*). A similar association of virus and microtubules or filaments has been noted by Hassan *et al.* (1965) in reovirus myocarditis and by Jenson *et al.* (1965) in reovirus encephalitis. The significance of this unique relationship of reovirus to microtubules is not clear, but Dales has pointed out that this association is not essential because destruction of the tubules by colchicine alters the site but not the rate of virus formation.

Plate 186

Mouse brain with experimentally produced reovirus type III encephalitis. (From *Gonatas, Margolis and Kilham, 1971*)

Fig. 1. Electron micrograph showing numerous neurotubules (T) and viral particles (V). Some of the tubules are coated with 'fuzzy' material (F). × 48,000

Fig. 2. Neurotubules with 'fuzzy' coat (F) and associated viral particles (V) are seen here, as are unaltered neurotubules (T). × 52,000

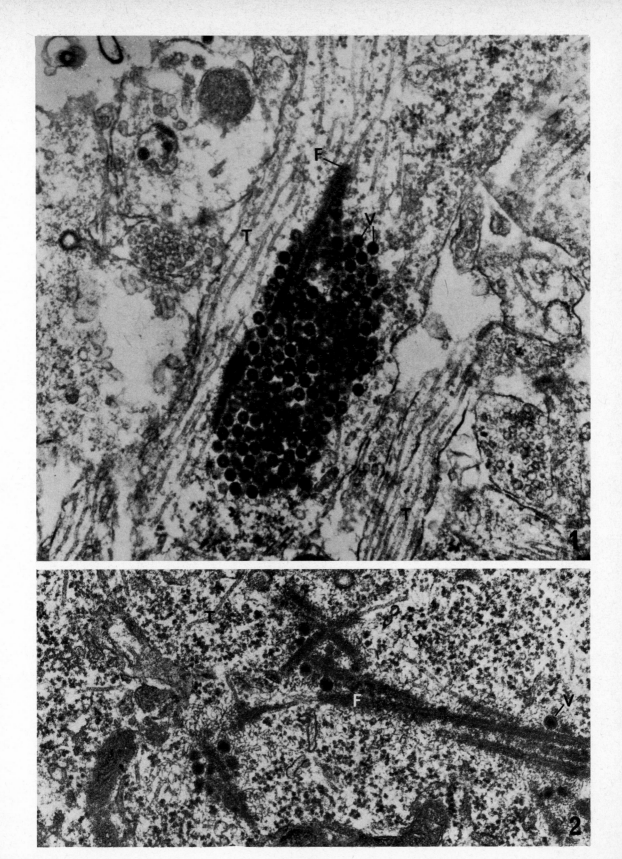

REFERENCES

Andres, K. H. (1961). 'Untersuchungen uber den Feinbau von spinalganglien.' *Z. Zellforsch. mikrosk. Anat.* **55**, 1

Barrett, L. A. and Dawson, R. B. (1972). 'Microtubules and erythroid cell shape.' *Fedn Proc.* **31**, 629

Behnke, O. and Zelander, T. (1966). 'Substructure in negatively stained microtubules of mammalian blood platelets.' *Expl Cell Res.* **43**, 236

Bikle, D., Tilney, L. G. and Porter, K. R. (1966). 'Microtubules and pigment migration in the melanophores of *Fundulus heteroclitus* L.' *Protoplasma* **61**, 322

Billings, S. M. (1972). 'Development of the mauthner cell in *Xenopus laevis*: a light and electron microscopic study of the perikaryon.' *Z. Anat. EntwGesch.* **136**, 168

Bloom, W. and Fawcett, D. W. (1969). *A Text Book of Histology,* 9th edn. Philadelphia and London: Saunders

Brinkley, B. R. and Cartwright, J., Jr. (1971). 'Ultrastructural analysis of mitotic spindle elongation in mammalian cells in vitro. Direct microtubule counts.' *J. Cell Biol.* **50**, 416

Bunge, M. B., Bunge, R. P. Peterson, E. R. and Murray, M. R. (1967). 'A light and electron microscope study of long-term organized cultures of rat dorsal root ganglia.' *J. Cell Biol.* **32**, 439

Burgos, M. H. and Fawcett, D. W. (1956). 'An electron microscope study of spermatid differentation in the toad *Bufo arenarum Hensel.*' *J. biophys. biochem. Cytol.* **2**, 223

Byers, B. and Porter, K. R. (1964). 'Oriented microtubules in elongating cells of the developing lens rudiment after induction.' *Proc. Natn. Acad. Sci., U.S.A.* **52**, 1091

Dales, S. (1963). 'Association between the spindle apparatus and reovirus.' *Proc. Natn. Acad. Sci., U.S.A.* **50**, 268

— Gomatos, P. J. and Hsu, K. C. (1965). 'The uptake and development of reovirus in strain L cells followed with labeled viral ribonucleic acid and ferritin–antibody conjugates.' *Virology* **25**, 193

De-The, G. (1964). 'Cytoplasmic microtubules in different animal cells.' *J. Cell Biol.* **23**, 265

Forer, A. (1969). 'Chromosome movement during cell division.' In *Handbook of Molecular Cytology,* p. 553. Ed. by A. Lima-de-Faria. Amsterdam: North Holland Publ.

Gonatas, N. K., Margolis, G. and Kilham, L. (1971). 'Reovirus type III encephalitis: observations of virus–cell interactions in neural tissues. II. Electron microscopic studies.' *Lab. Invest.* **24**, 101

Grasso, J. A. (1966). 'Cytoplasmic microtubules in mammalian erythropoietic cells.' *Anat. Rec.* **156**, 397

Hassan, S. A., Rabin, E. R. and Melnick, J. L. (1965). 'Reovirus myocarditis in mice: an electron microscopic immuno-fluorescent, and virus assay study.' *Expl Molec. Path.* **4**, 66

Holmes, K. V. and Choppin, P. W. (1968). 'On the role of microtubules in movement and alignment of nuclei in virus-induced syncytia.' *J. Cell Biol.* **39**, 526

Inoue, S. and Sato, H. (1967). 'Cell motility by labile association of molecules. The nature of mitotic spindle fibers and their role in chromosome movement.' *J. gen. Physiol.* **50**, 259

Jacob, H., Amsden, T. and White, J. (1972). 'Membrane microfilaments of erythrocytes: alteration in intact cells reproduces the hereditary spherocytosis syndrome.' *Proc. Natn. Acad. Sci., U.S.A.* **69**, 471

Jenson, A. B., Rabin, E. R., Phillips, C. A. and Melnick, J. L. (1965). 'Reovirus encephalitis in newborn mice. An electron microscopic and virus assay study.' *Am. J. Path.* **47**, 223

Ledbetter, M. C. and Porter, K. R. (1963). 'A microtubule in plant cell fine structure.' *J. Cell Biol.* **19**, 239

Margolis, G., Kilham, L. and Gonatas, N. K. (1971). 'Reovirus type III encephalitis: observations of virus–cell interactions in neural tissues. I. Light microscopy studies.' *Lab. Invest.* **24**, 91

Mazia, D. (1961). 'Mitosis and the physiology of cell division.' In *The Cell,* Vol. 3, p. 77. Ed. by J. Brachet and A. E. Mirsky. New York: Academic Press

Nicklas, R. B. (1970). 'Mitosis.' In *Advances in Cell Biology,* p. 225. Ed. by D. M. Prescott, L. Goldstein and E. H. McConkey. New York: Appleton-Century-Crofts

Olmstead, J. B., Witman, G. B. and Carlson, K. (1961). 'Comparison of the microtubule proteins of neuroblastoma cells, brain and Chlamydomonas flagella.' *Proc. Natn. Acad. Sci., U.S.A.* **68**, 2273

Porter, K. R. (1966). 'Cytoplasmic microtubules and their functions.' In *Principles of Biomolecular Organization,* p. 308. Ed. by G. E. W. Wolstenholme and M. O'Connor. Boston, Mass: Little, Brown and Co.

Rudzinska, M. A. (1965). 'The fine structure and function of the tentacle in *Tokophrya infusionum.*' *J. Cell Biol.* **25**, 459

Silverstein, S. C. and Dales, S. (1968). 'The penetration of reovirus RNA and initiation of its genetic function in L-strain fibroblasts.' *J. Cell Biol.* **36**, 197

Thoa, N. B., Wooten, G. F. and Axelrod, J. (1972). 'Inhibition of release of dopamine-β-hydroxylase and norepinephrine from sympathetic nerves by colchicine, vinblastine, or cytochalasin-B.' *Proc. Natn. Acad. Sci., U.S.A.* **69**, 520

Tilney, L. G. (1965). 'Microtubules in the heliozoan, *Actinosphaerium nucleofilum* and their relation to axopod formation and motion.' *J. Cell Biol.* **27**, 107A

— and Gibbins, J. R. (1969). 'Microtubules in the formation and development of the primary mesenchyme in *Arbacia punctulata*. II. An experimental analysis of their role in development and maintenance of cell shape.' *J. Cell Biol.* **41**, 227

— and Porter, K. R. (1967). 'Studies on the microtubules in heliozoa. II. The effect of low temperature on these structures in the formation and maintenance of the axopodia.' *J. Cell Biol.* **34**, 327

— Hiramoto, Y. and Marsland, D. (1966). 'Studies on the microtubules in heliozoa. III. A pressure analysis of the role of these structures in the formation and maintenance of the exopodia of *Actinosphaerium nucleofilum (Barrett).*' *J. Cell Biol.* **29**, 77

Tournier, P. and Plissier, M. (1960). 'Le developpement intracellulaire du reovirus observe au microscope electronique.' *Presse méd.* **68**, 683

440

Whaley, W. G. and Mollenhauer, H. H. (1963). 'The Golgi apparatus and cell plate formation—a postulate.' *J. Cell Biol.* **17,** 216

Wisniewski, H., Terry, R. D. and Hirano, A. (1970). 'Neurofibrillary pathology.' *J. Neuropath. exp. Neurol.* **29,** 163

Zucker-Franklin, D. (1969). 'Microfibrils of blood platelets: their relationship to microtubules and the contractile protein.' *J. clin. Invest.* **48,** 165

CHAPTER XIII

Cytoplasmic Inclusions

INTRODUCTION

The term 'cytoplasmic inclusions' has long been used by light microscopists to distinguish certain intracellular structures or bodies (consisting of accumulations of metabolites or cell products) from organelles which were looked upon as miniature organs or specialized units performing specific functions within the cell. Such inclusions include secretory granules, pigment granules and various accumulations of protein (crystalline inclusions), fat (lipid droplets) or carbohydrates (glycogen) in the cytoplasm. To this group of inclusions pathologists have added various other bodies found within the cell in diseased states, the best-known example being the 'inclusion bodies' found in virus-infected cells.

With the advent of electron microscopy and the acquisition of more precise knowledge about many cell structures and the discovery of others whose function is still obscure, it has become increasingly difficult to classify the various cellular structures into one or other category. An example of this is the rod-shaped tubulated body (Chapter X), a membrane-bound structure which is morphologically acceptable as an organelle, but which one feels reluctant to classify as such until its function is known. Another example is the melanosome (Chapter IX), a well-characterized enzyme-containing (tyrosinase) membrane-bound structure which performs a specific function, and hence deserves to be classified as an organelle, but which ultimately becomes an inclusion: the inert melanin granule. At what stage of development one should cease considering a melanosome as an organelle and call it an inclusion is debatable, for the intermediate stages of development contain both tyrosinase and melanin. Similar difficulties are also encountered with lysosomes, which at one stage are clearly organelles in every sense of the word, but which end up as lipofuscin granules or siderosomes.

There seems little point now in pursuing with vigour the exercise of classifying all structures as either organelles or inclusions, yet such classical terms and concepts can hardly be totally ignored. In this chapter only some of the classical cytoplasmic inclusions are discussed. Pigment granules are not mentioned here, for melanin granules are dealt with under melanosomes (Chapter IX) and deposits of lipofuscin and haemosiderin are now best studied with lysosomes (Chapter VII). Similarly, both convenience and logic dictate that secretory granules are best dealt with when considering the Golgi complex (Chapter IV).

Desmosomes are focal specializations of the cell surface which help to hold cells together, but sometimes they are found within the cytoplasm. Such intracytoplasmic desmosomes are best studied later (page 480) after various cell junctions have been described.

GLYCOGEN

Carbohydrate is stored in animal cells as a polysaccharide called glycogen. Light microscopy and enzyme histochemistry have long demonstrated its presence in the cytoplasm of various cell types and shown it to be abundant in hepatocytes and skeletal muscle. Electron microscopy has confirmed this and also demonstrated that lesser amounts of glycogen occur in many more cell types than had been suspected before. In routine preparations, cells of the erythropoietic series from normal humans do not show glycogen,* but substantial deposits of glycogen are found in certain pathological situations (Skinnider and Ghadially, 1973) (*Plate 187*).

Glycogen may be found not only in the cytoplasm but occasionally in other cell compartments also. Its occurrence in the nucleus (page 54), mitochondrion (page 162) and lysosome (page 356) has already been dealt with and will not be commented upon here. Suffice it to say that wherever it occurs, glycogen shows certain characteristic features which aid its identification.

In suitably stained ultrathin sections glycogen presents either as electron-dense granules approximately 150–300 Å in diameter (β particles or monoparticulate form) or as collections of such particles forming rosettes about 800–1,000 Å in diameter (α particles or rosette form). Atypical aggregations of monoparticulate glycogen generally larger than typical rosettes are sometimes seen. They are referred to as pseudorosettes. A faint but constant substructure is at times demonstrable in glycogen particles (β particles), and it is thought that monoparticulate glycogen may be composed of globular subunits about 30 Å in diameter. However, the possibility that this appearance might be due to a staining or focusing artefact is still debated.

It is now well established that solutions containing lead, such as lead citrate and lead hydroxide, stain glycogen intensely (Watson, 1958; Revel *et al.*, 1960; Vye and Fischman, 1970), while a staining of lesser intensity can be obtained with phosphotungstic and phosphomolybdic acid. Uranium stains glycogen very faintly or not at all.

The appearance presented by glycogen particles and deposits depends to some extent on the method of tissue fixation and preparation employed, for this determines the proportion of glycogen preserved in the tissue and that lost during processing. The appearance seen is also dependent on the method by which the sections are stained. A spectrum of appearances is seen, but the two extremes of the scale are represented by lead staining where the glycogen particles appear highly electron dense, and by uranium staining where solitary glycogen particles appear as 'holes' or very faintly stained particles, difficult to discern. In uranium-stained material collections of glycogen particles may present as lucent or faintly stained areas (glycogen lakes) within the cytoplasm (*Plate 188*).

Numerous other staining reactions for glycogen have been devised, some of which are said to stain glycogen in a more intense or selective manner than lead (see review by Vye and Fischman, 1971), yet unequivocal demonstration of glycogen still rests on evidence of diastase digestibility.

* It is worth noting, however, that a few particles of glycogen are demonstrable in normal erythroid cells by the periodic acid–thiosemicarbazide–silver proteinate reaction (Ackerman, 1973).

Plate 187

Glycogen-containing erythroid cells found in a case of erythroleukaemia.

Fig. 1. Mature erythrocyte with monoparticulate glycogen (arrows) in its cytoplasm × 25,000 (*Skinnider and Ghadially, unpublished electron micrograph*)

Fig. 2. This illustration demonstrates the occurrence of a dual population of erythroid cells in erythroleukaemia. A glycogen-laden normoblast (N) is adjacent to a glycogen-free late normoblast (L) and erythrocyte (E) of normal morphology. × 19,000 (*From Skinnider and Ghadially, 1973*)

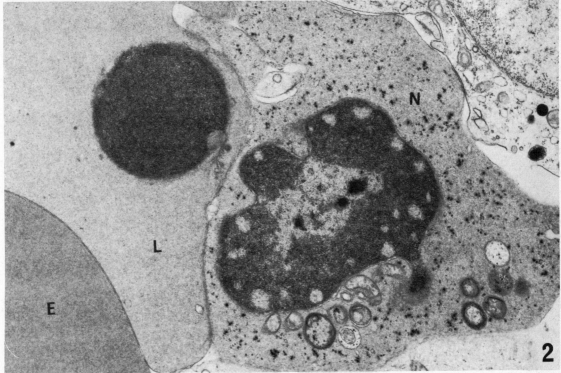

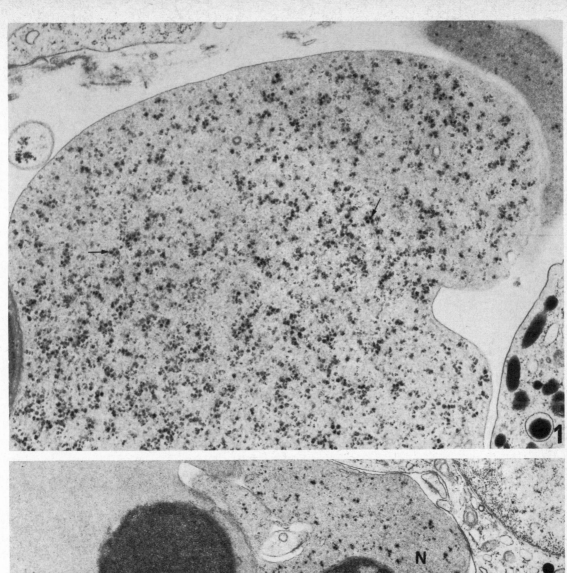

445

Unfortunately, this test cannot be executed on material routinely prepared for electron microscopy, since both osmium fixation and epoxy embedding render this impossible. The test for diastase digestibility has to be carried out on small blocks of aldehyde-fixed tissue, before post-fixation with osmium. However, such a method can only be operated with confidence when a fair amount of glycogen is present.

Glycogen particles of a small size (150–200 Å) are difficult to distinguish from ribosomes. Comparing adjacent sections—one stained with lead, the other with uranium—can help to resolve this difficulty, for ribosomes are visualized in preparations stained either with lead or with uranium but glycogen is evident only in the lead-stained sections.

A procedure which has gained much popularity in recent times is *en bloc* staining with un-buffered aqueous uranium acetate after fixation but prior to dehydration. This gives good visualization of general details and is particularly useful for the demonstration of the structure of cell membranes and cell junctions. The routine application of this technique is, however, hampered by the fact that much glycogen is extracted and what remains shows marked morphological alterations (Vye and Fischman, 1970).

It has been noted that two main forms of glycogen occur, namely the monoparticulate and the rosette form. Of these the monoparticulate form is by far the commoner and represents that usually encountered in most tissues. Rosettes are typical of glycogen deposits in the liver but examples of rosettes are found in other tissues also.

Biava *et al.* (1966) have found that while most of the kidney cells from normal human subjects contain monoparticulate glycogen, those in the collecting tubules contain glycogen rosettes also. However, in diabetic subjects, where there is a greater deposition of glycogen in the kidney, rosettes were found throughout the nephron, intermingled with larger deposits of monoparticulate glycogen. From observations made in various pathological states they conclude that 'in diseases associated with proteinuria, hypertrophic and hyperactive epithelial cells showed little or no glycogen. Conversely, glycogen tended to accumulate in atrophic cells and in cells, such as those of capsular epithelium in glomeruli, which are normally poorly differentiated and presumably less active.' My experience is in keeping with this, for it is in degenerating chondrocytes (articular cartilage) rather than in active ones that the larger deposits of glycogen occur. Glycogen also seems to be more abundant in the chondrocytes of old as compared to young animals. A similar situation prevails in the case of the polymorphonuclear neutrophil where glycogen accumulates as the cell gets older (*Plate 147*). Thus the collective evidence at hand suggests that there are instances where an increase in the amount of glycogen in the cell cytoplasm is an indicator of diminished usage and accumulation rather than a sign of increased metabolic activity.

Plate 188

Osmium-fixed (cacodylate buffer) zone III chondrocytes from the articular cartilage of a 2-year-old rabbit. Sections were cut from a single block of tissue. Some were stained with lead; others with uranium.

Fig. 1. In this lead-stained section large collections of intensely stained monoparticulate glycogen (G) are evident in the cytoplasm. Note also the poor visualization of the chromatin pattern in the nucleus (N) characteristic of lead staining and the abundance of cytoplasmic filaments (F). × 29,000

Fig. 2. In this uranium-stained chondrocyte, lakes of virtually unstained glycogen (G) are present. The boundary of one of these is indicated by arrowheads. Note also the good visualization of the chromatin pattern achieved in the nucleus (N) by uranium staining. × 29,000

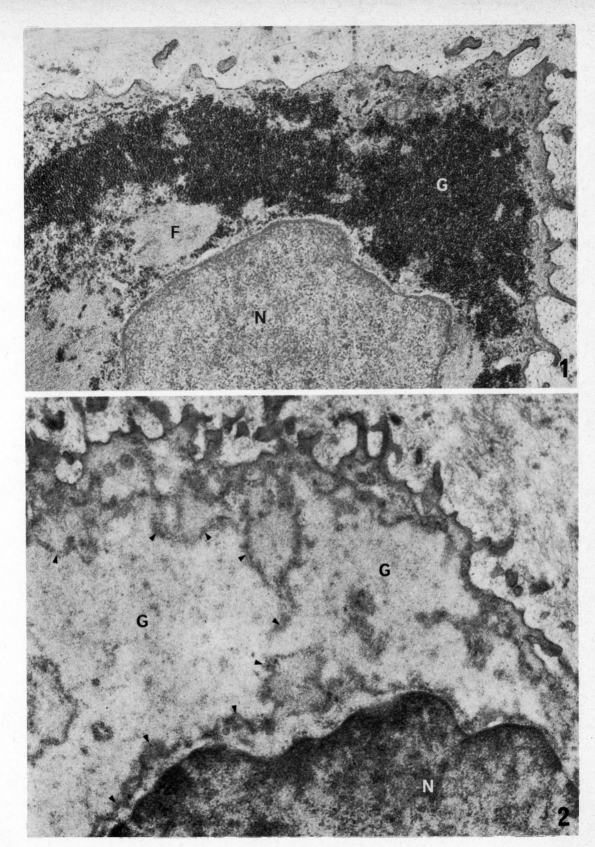

447

LIPID

Triglycerides of fatty acids represent the commonest form of lipid inclusion found in the cells of animals. In the mature adipocyte of white fat a large droplet of such lipid is found within the cell, but smaller lipid droplets are not uncommon in the cytoplasm of many other cell types. The size and number of such lipid droplets in cells of various tissues vary markedly in different physiological and pathological situations. A few lipid droplets are considered a normal inclusion of the cytoplasm and represent a potential source of energy and short carbon chains for the synthesis of cytomembranes and other lipid-containing material produced by cells. Gross deposits of lipid in parenchymatous cells (e.g. liver or myocardium) are pathological and constitute fatty degeneration.

Lipid droplets occur not only in the cytoplasm but at times also in other cell compartments, such as the nucleus (page 58), mitochondrion (page 166), Golgi complex (page 202), endoplasmic reticulum (page 248) and lysosome (page 306). It is worth noting that lipid droplets in these sites show the same variations of morphology as do lipid droplets in the cytoplasm.

The appearance of intracytoplasmic lipid in ultrathin sections is dependent upon various factors, such as size of the droplet, the method of fixation and tissue preparation, the saturated and unsaturated fatty acid content of the lipid and the degree of unsaturation of the fatty acids present. The basic form of the lipid droplet is spherical, and small droplets usually present in this manner; larger droplets tend to have a somewhat distorted or irregular outline. At times, lipid droplets can be markedly crenated. Large droplets are difficult to fix because they are poorly penetrated by fixatives, hence they tend to be extracted during processing. This is particularly so in the case of lipids with a high content of saturated fatty acids for such lipid does not bind osmium avidly.

The density of the lipid droplet as seen in electron micrographs varies from electron lucent to markedly electron dense. Roughly, this may be correlated with the saturated and unsaturated fatty acid content of the triglyceride and the degree of unsaturation of fatty acids present (*Plate 189*).

Plate 189

This plate demonstrates that one of the factors which determines the electron density of the lipid droplet is the saturated and unsaturated fatty acid content of the lipid. When lipid is injected into a joint (in this case, rabbit knee joint) some of it is taken up by the chondrocytes. If a lipid rich in saturated fatty acid is used (e.g. autologous depot fat) the chondrocytes come to contain electron-lucent lipid droplets. If corn oil (which is very rich in unsaturated fatty acid) is injected, the chondrocytes show numerous electron-dense lipid droplets.

Fig. 1. Chondrocytes from an autologous fat-injected joint, showing electron-lucent lipid droplets (L). × 8,000 (*From Mehta and Ghadially, 1973*)

Figs. 2 and 3. Chondrocytes from joints injected with corn oil, showing moderately to markedly electron-dense lipid droplets (L). × 23,000; × 15,500. (*Fig. 2, from Mehta and Ghadially, 1973; Fig. 3, Mehta and Ghadially, unpublished electron micrograph*)

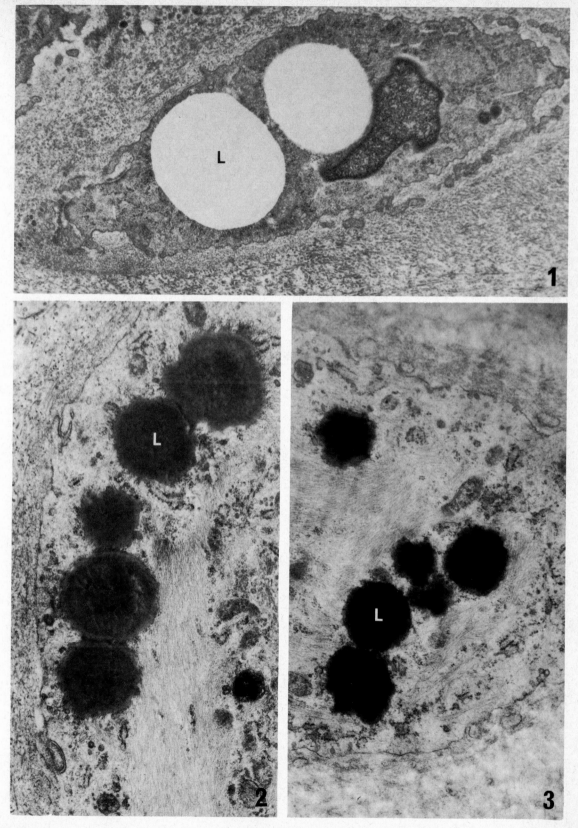

449

The greater the unsaturated fatty acid content and degree of unsaturation, the more electron-dense the lipid is likely to appear, for it will tend to bind more osmium.* The density of lipid droplets tends to be lower in glutaraldehyde-fixed material as compared to that fixed primarily with osmium.

Characteristically, intracytoplasmic lipid inclusions are not bounded by a true trilaminar membrane, but an osmiophilic 'ring' or a membrane-like structure is sometimes seen around a lipid droplet. This has at times been confused with a true limiting membrane. However, as already noted (page 248), membrane-bound lipid droplets called liposomes are known to occur in the cytoplasm, but these represent lipid lying in vesiculated endoplasmic reticulum and hence are not, strictly speaking, a true example of intracytoplasmic lipid.

Lipid droplets at times appear peppered with electron-dense particles, and occasionally accumulations of such particles are also seen on the periphery of the lipid droplet, forming granular irregular focal deposits (*Plate 190*). The nature of these particles and the significance of this phenomenon are not known.

Other interesting variations of lipid morphology occasionally encountered are droplets with a pale or clear centre (annular lipid inclusions) and droplets with a pale or clear halo (*Plate 190*). Such appearances are consistent with the idea that some material (presumably lipid) is removed from the centre or the periphery of the lipid droplet during tissue preparation, but why this should be so is not easy to understand. In the case of the annular lipid inclusion one may suggest that this is due to poor penetration of the fixative and a subsequent removal of the central unfixed lipid during tissue dehydration and clearing. Yet such a hypothesis obviously does not explain why lipid droplets sometimes have a clear halo.

A theory that could explain the occurrence of both types of partially extracted lipid droplets would be that such droplets are not homogeneous, and that there may be physical (e.g. state of hydration or emulsification) or chemical (e.g. saturated and unsaturated fatty acid content) differences within a lipid droplet that determine which part is fixed or not fixed and which part is retained or lost during tissue preparation (Parry and Ghadially, 1966). This, however, is pure speculation and, as mentioned earlier, the basis of this and some other variations of lipid morphology (e.g. the nature of the dense particles which pepper lipid droplets) has not as yet been satisfactorily explained.

* The primary site of reaction of osmium is with the $C=C$ double bonds of unsaturated fatty acids; 1 molecule of OsO_4 reacts with each double bond. Although at times the amount of osmium bound is less than that expected from the degree of unsaturation of the lipid, the general validity of the thesis that unsaturated lipids appear dense because of the osmium they bind cannot be doubted (Stockenius and Mahr, 1965).

Plate 190

Fig. 1. The medium-density lipid droplets (L) seen in this electron micrograph have a dense rim which in some places creates a false impression of a limiting membrane. The droplets are peppered with fine electron-dense particles (P) and there are also focal accumulations of such particles (arrows) in one area. From the liver of a rat bearing a carcinogen-induced sarcoma in its flank. × 26,000

Fig. 2. A lucent halo is seen around these lipid droplets found in a human hepatocyte. That this is no shrinkage artefact is evidenced by the well preserved mitochondria and other structures in the surrounding cytoplasm. × 18,000

Fig. 3. An annular lipid inclusion (i.e. a lipid droplet with a lucent centre) is seen in a chondrocyte. From the articular cartilage of a normal dog. × 42,000

Fig. 4. This cell, found in a cirrhotic human liver, shows lipid droplets of varying morphology. One of the droplets is lucent (L), some others of medium density (M) and there is one which has a clear centre (C). × 17,500

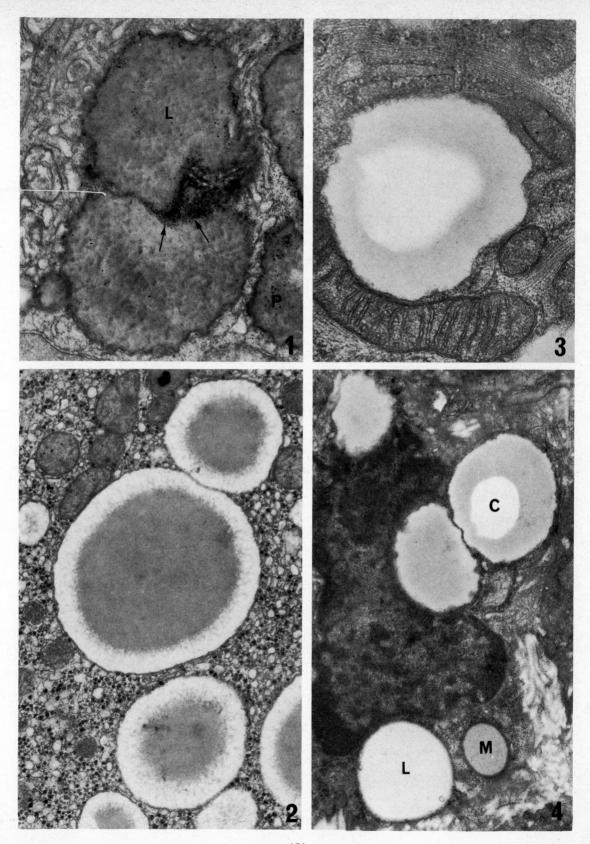

451

Crystalline inclusions thought to be protein or mainly protein in nature have been found in various cell compartments, such as the nucleus (page 62), mitochondrion (page 170), endoplasmic reticulum (page 244) and cytoplasmic matrix. However, translocation of a crystal from its site of genesis may occur so that at times it is difficult to label the crystal as belonging to one or other specific cell compartment.

An example of this is seen during yolk platelet formation in amphibian oöcytes, where crystals formed in the mitochondrion are extruded and come to lie in single-membrane-bound structures called yolk platelets (for references, see Karasaki, 1963; Massover, 1971). Similarly, in an alveolar soft part sarcoma Shipkey *et al.* (1964) have illustrated numerous small crystals in single-membrane-bound structures in the Golgi region and also larger crystals lying free in the cytoplasmic matrix. That the latter are derived from the former seems a reasonable assumption.

In contrast to this, the crystal of Reinke found in the interstitial cells of the human testis seems to evolve in the cytoplasmic matrix and is not membrane bound at any stage of development (*Plate 191*). Reinke's crystal has, however, also at times been found in the nucleus (page 62). Although at one time it was thought that these crystals were unique to interstitial cells of the human testis, similar crystals have now been found in: (1) the antebranchial organ of the ring-tailed lemur (*Lemur catta*) (Montagna, 1962; Sisson and Fahrenbach, 1967); (2) Leydig cells from an arrhenoblastoma (Berendsen *et al.*, 1969); (3) ovarian hilar cells (Sternberg, 1949; Gardner *et al.*, 1957); (4) numerous cases of hilar cell ovarian tumours (for references, see Merkow *et al.*, 1971); and (5) testicular interstitial cell tumours (Savard *et al.*, 1960; Silverberg *et al.*, 1966).

The ultrastructural morphology of Reinke's crystal in the interstitial cell of the human testis has been extensively investigated (Fawcett and Burgos, 1960; Yamada, 1962, 1965; Fawcett, 1967; De Kretser, 1967, 1968; Nagano and Ohtsuki, 1971). The structure of such crystals in some of the other sites mentioned above has also been described. Depending upon the plane of sectioning the crystal shows various patterns of dots, parallel lines or a prismatic or hexagonal lattice. From such images the structure of the crystal has been interpreted by various workers as composed of globular macromolecules 150 Å in diameter (Fawcett and Burgos, 1956, 1960), or 50 Å-thick filaments (Sisson and Fahrenbach, 1967; Nagano and Ohtsuki, 1971), or 200–300 Å hexagonal microtubules (Yamada, 1962, 1965; Merkow *et al.*, 1971). Despite the numerous studies the significance of Reinke's crystal remains obscure.

Besides the above-mentioned examples, intracytoplasmic crystals have been found in: (1) the lymphocytes from peripheral blood of patients with Down's syndrome (Smith *et al.*, 1967); (2) lymphocytes infiltrating the stroma of a basal cell carcinoma (Freidman *et al.*, 1971); and (3) L-strain fibroblasts and human leucocytes treated with vinca alkaloids (Bensch and Malawista, 1969; Krishan and Hsu, 1969). According to Bensch and Malawista (1969), the crystals formed after vinca alkaloid treatment consist mainly of microtubules, and this is accompanied by a disappearance of normal microtubules from the cell. The fact that such crystals form within polymorphonuclear neutrophils (a cell which in its adult form can synthesise little protein) and the speed (within 30 minutes) at which such crystals form in L-strain fibroblasts suggest that the crystals are formed from pre-existing microtubular protein and not from protein newly produced in the cell after exposure to vinca alkaloids.

Plate 191
Interstitial cell from human testis, showing several crystals of Reinke. These crystals have a polygonal shape. Note that each side of the crystal is parallel to the corresponding opposite side. × 23,000 (*From Nagano and Ohtsuki, 1971*)

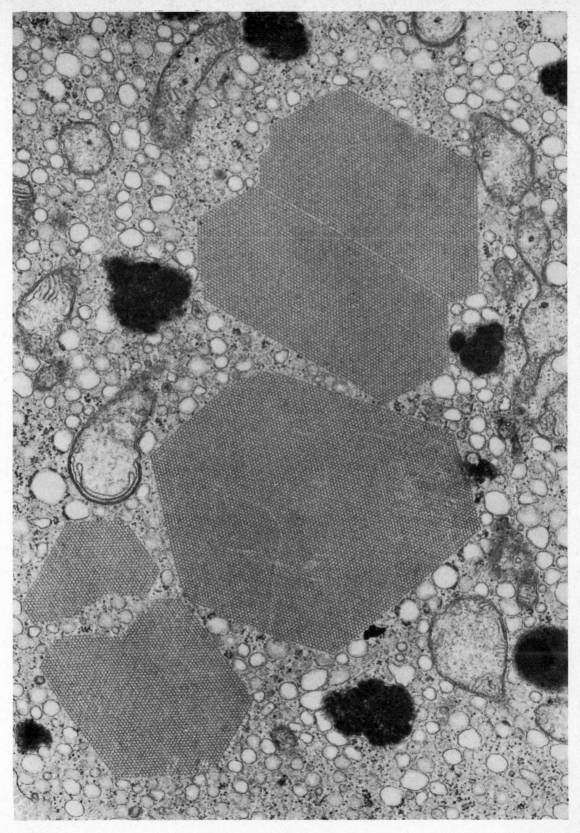

FIBRIN

Fibrin is not a normal intracytoplasmic inclusion but it has been seen in an intracellular location in certain experimental and pathological situations. Fibrin fibres are composed of numerous longitudinally orientated moderately dense fibrils. Unequivocal morphological identification of this fibrous protein is often possible because fibrin fibres show periodic striations 200–350 Å apart (Ruska and Wolpers, 1940; Hawn and Porter, 1947; Hall, 1949, 1963).

Although the spacings of the bands along a given fibre are remarkably constant, they may vary from fibre to fibre in the same specimen (Hall, 1949). Not all fibrin in a given sample appears banded, and at times known fibrin or fibrinoid deposits in pathological tissues or purified fibrin produced *in vitro* may fail to show striations (Haust *et al.*, 1965; Ghadially and Roy, 1969).

The reason for this is not clear but there is evidence that banding is better defined in clots formed at lower pH values (Hawn and Porter, 1947). The rate of clotting also seems to be important because clots formed very slowly in the presence of little or no thrombin show virtually no striations (Hall, 1949).

The occurrence of intracytoplasmic fibrin was noted by us (Parry and Ghadially, 1967) in the hepatocytes of regenerating post-hepatectomy liver in normal and tumour-bearing rats (*Plates 192 and 193*). Similar deposits lying free in the cytoplasm and also in membrane-bound vacuoles were seen by Reubner *et al.* (1970) in hepatitis produced by lasiocarpine in mice. In our material, in some cells, striated and non-striated fibrin (non-membrane-bound) was found in the cytoplasmic matrix lying intimately mingled with the cell organelles (*Plates 192*) while in other instances focal accumulations of fibrin were seen set in a light granular matrix (*Plate 193*). Some of these focal accumulations were at times partially delineated from the cell cytoplasm by a membrane, but completely sequestrated (membrane-bound) inclusions were not seen.

The situation here is reminiscent of that noted in studies on experimental malignant hypertension, where 'insudation' of plasma proteins into the vascular wall and fibrinoid or fibrin deposition is known to occur (Wiener *et al.*, 1965; Ooneda *et al.*, 1965; Hatt *et al.*, 1968; Still, 1968; Huttner *et al.*, 1968, 1969; Gardner and Matthews, 1969). In such instances, however, the

---

Plate 192
Partial hepatectomy was performed on a rat bearing a carcinogen-induced subcutaneous sarcoma. A specimen of liver was collected for electron microscopy 6 hours after operation. This electron micrograph shows fibrin lying in the cytoplasm of a hepatocyte; some of the fibrin shows characteristic banding (arrow). × 70,000 (*Parry and Ghadially, unpublished electron micrograph*)

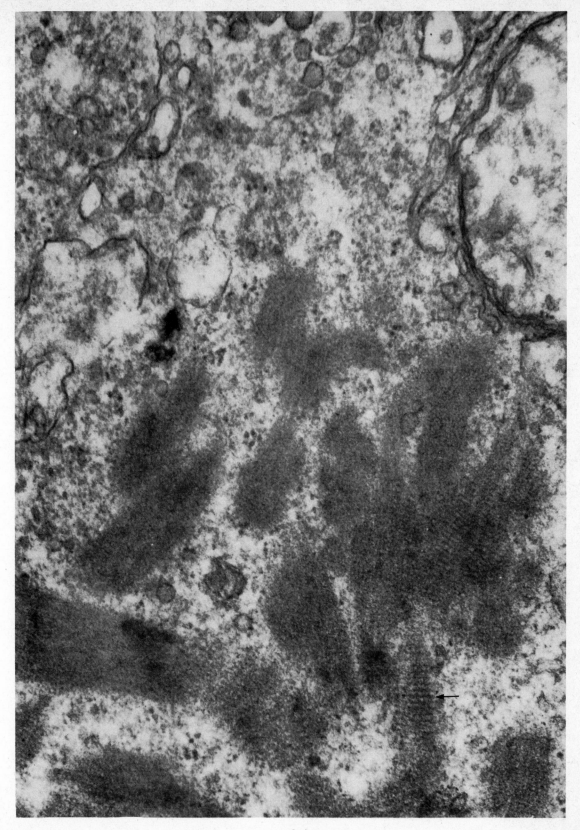

fibrin deposits are extracellular, although at times some fibrin is seen mingled with (or perhaps lying within) necrotic muscle fibres.

A phenomenon similar to the one reported by us (Parry and Ghadially, 1967) in hepatocytes has, however, been seen recently in cardiac muscle cells of the rat after experimentally produced malignant hypertension (Huttner *et al.*, 1971). The illustrations in this paper show most convincingly fibrin fibres intimately mingled with myofilaments in cells that do not appear severely damaged. These authors also found membrane-bound focal accumulations of fibrin and plasma in the cell cytoplasm (thought to be derived by invagination of cell membrane). Regarding the non-membrane-bound fibrin they state: 'the fine structural identification of fibrin in a true intracytoplasmic location can be considered as direct morphological evidence for plasma protein entrance into the injured cells, where fibrinogen polymerized intracellularly to fibrin'.

We (Parry and Ghadially, 1967) postulate that a similar mechanism probably operates in hepatocytes, after hepatectomy. The sequence of events seems to be: (1) an escape of plasma proteins from vessels; (2) entry of plasma proteins into cell cytoplasm (a phenomenon referred to as insudation); and (3) release of factors from injured cells which leads to the polymerization of fibrinogen to fibrin.

In our experience (Parry and Ghadially, 1967), the fibrin in most instances appears to lie in pools of finely granular material which probably represents a mixture of cytoplasmic matrix and plasma proteins (*Plate 193*). It is at the edge of such areas that the fibrin appears to lie in the cytoplasmic matrix in close association with cell organelles.

Plate 193

From the liver of a rat bearing a carcinogen-induced subcutaneous sarcoma. The specimen was collected 6 hours after partial hepatectomy. (*Parry and Ghadially, unpublished electron micrographs*)

Fig. 1. Collections of fibrin (arrows) and cell organelles are seen lying in a finely granular matrix (M) thought to represent a mixture of cytoplasm and insudated plasma proteins. × 18,500

Fig. 2. High power view of fibrin shown in *Fig. 1*. Note banding with a periodicity of approximately 245 Å. × 60,000

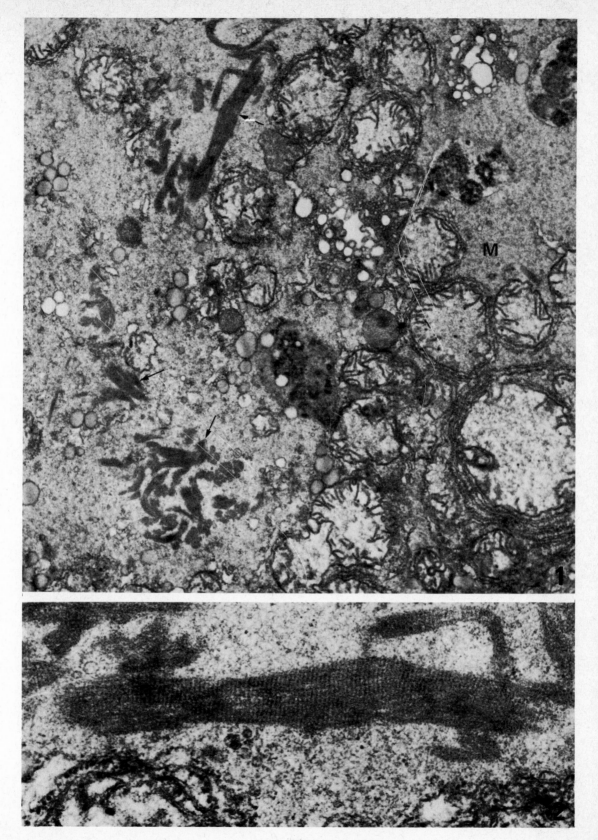

457

VIRAL INCLUSIONS

In previous chapters of this book have been described: (1) intranuclear viral inclusions (page 70) and other nuclear changes (page 24) produced by viruses; (2) viral inclusions in the endoplasmic reticulum and Golgi complex formed by budding of virus particles assembled on these membranes or in the adjacent cytoplasm (page 252); and (3) cytoplasmic inclusions of reovirus forming in association with microtubules (page 438). In order to avoid repetition only some remaining points of general interest will be mentioned here. Detailed references will not be quoted, since support for these statements may be found in many standard virology texts.

The term 'inclusion bodies' has long been employed by light microscopists to describe certain round, oval or irregular-shaped bodies found in the cytoplasm and/or nucleus of virus-infected cells. This morphological evidence of cell–virus interaction was first described by Findlay in 1938. Since then inclusion bodies have been examined extensively by light and electron microscopy as well as by fluorescent antibody staining methods. Although not all viral infections produce inclusion bodies and while structures resembling viral inclusions can at times be produced by other noxious agents, the value of such inclusion bodies in the diagnosis of many viral infections has been clearly demonstrated by light microscopy and improved and extended by electron microscopy.

Light microscopy studies have shown that inclusion bodies may be either basophilic or eosinophilic. Some show a clear halo around them but this is almost certainly a shrinkage artefact. Electron microscopy has clearly demonstrated that most but not all* inclusion bodies are sites of viral synthesis and/or maturation (referred to at times as 'factory areas' or 'viral factories'), as had indeed been suspected and in some instance fairly convincingly demonstrated long before the advent of electron microscopy.

Virtually all RNA viruses (except myxoviruses) are assembled in the cytoplasm and as such tend to produce inclusions in this region (*Plate 194*). However, inclusion bodies large enough to be seen with the light microscope are not formed in every case. Many of the small non-enveloped RNA viruses (e.g. poliovirus, Coxsackie virus and echovirus) and reovirus can, however, produce quite large inclusions which may progress to occupy most of the cytoplasm. Measles virus (an RNA virus) produces inclusions both in the nucleus and in the cytoplasm. At electron microscopy both the nuclear and cytoplasmic inclusions present as aggregates of tubules believed to be composed of viral nucleoprotein (*Plate 37*).

* For example, some of the prominent cytoplasmic eosinophilic inclusions of pox-virus infected cells (called 'A' bodies) are thought to reflect a late cellular response rather than a site of viral replication. (For details and references, see Fenner, 1968.)

Plate 194
Intracytoplasmic viral inclusions. (*Grodums, unpublished electron micrographs*)
Fig. 1. Reovirus inclusions (V) in LLCMK cell (a continuous cell line derived from monkey kidney). × 22,000
Fig. 2. Picornavirus (echo II) replicating in the cytoplasm of LLCMK cell. Granular (G), crystalline (C) and vermicellar (V) inclusions are seen in the cytoplasm of the infected cell. × 50,000
Fig. 3. Rhabdovirus inclusions (V) in an ependymal cell from the brain of a 3-week-old mouse. × 50,000

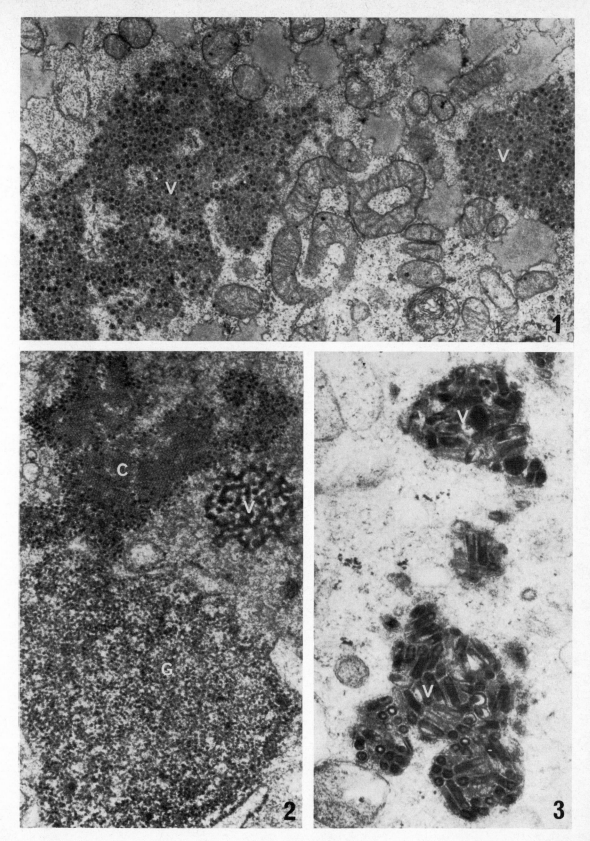

REFERENCES

Ackerman, G. A. (1973). 'Ultrastructural localization of glycogen in erythrocytes and developing erythrocytic cells in normal human bone marrow.' *Z. Zellforsch. mikrosk. Anat.* **140**, 433

Bensch, K. G. and Malawista, S. E. (1969). 'Microtubular crystals in mammalian cells.' *J. Cell Biol.* **40**, 95

Berendsen, P. B., Smith, E. B., Abell, M. R. and Jaffee, R. B. (1969), 'Fine structure of Leydig cells from an arrhenoblastoma of the ovary.' *Am. J. Obstet. Gynec.* **103**, 192

Biava, C., Grossman, A. and West, M. (1966). 'Ultrastructural observations on renal glycogen in normal and pathologic human kidneys.' *Lab. Invest.* **15**, 330

De Kretser, D. M. (1967). 'The fine structure of the testicular interstitial cells in men of normal androgenic status.' *Z. Zellforsch. mikrosk. Anat.* **80**, 594

— (1968). 'Crystals of Reinke in the nuclei of human testicular interstitial cells.' *Experientia* **24**, 587

Fawcett, D. W. (1967). *The Cell: Its Organelles and Inclusions,* p. 330. Philadelphia and London: Saunders

— and Burgos, M. H. (1956). 'Observations on the cytomorphosis of the germinal and interstitial cells of the human testis.' In Ciba Foundation Colloquia on *Aging,* Vol. 2, p. 86. Ed. by G. E. W. Wolstenholme and E. C. P. Millar. Boston, Mass: Little, Brown

——(1960). 'Studies on the fine structure of the mammalian testis. II. The human interstitial tissue.' *Am. J. Anat.* **107**, 245

Fenner, F. (1968). *The Biology of Animal Viruses. Molecular and Cellular Biology,* Vol. 1. New York and London: Academic Press

Findlay, G. M. (1938). In *Handbuch der Virusforschung,* p. 292. Ed. by R. Doerr and G. Hallauer. Erste Halfte. Wien: Julius Springer

Friedmann, I., Michaels, L. and Bird, E. S. (1971). 'Crystalline structures in lymphocytes.' *J. Path.* **105**, 289

Gardner, D. L. and Matthews, M. A. (1969). 'Ultrastructure of the wall of small arteries in early experimental rat hypertensions.' *J. Path.* **97**, 51

Gardner, G. H., Greene, R. R. and Peckham, B. (1957). 'Tumors of the broad ligament.' *Am. J. Obstet. Gynec.* **73**, 536

Ghadially, F. N. and Roy, S. (1969). *Ultrastructure of Synovial Joints in Health and Disease.* London: Butterworths

Hall, C. E. (1949). 'Electron microscopy of fibrinogen and fibrin.' *J. biol. Chem.* **179**, 857

— (1963). 'Electron microscopy of the fibrinogen molecule and the fibrin clot.' *Lab. Invest.* **12**, 998

Hatt, P. Y., Berjal, G. and Bonnet, M. (1968). 'L'artériopathie hypertensive expérimentale chez le rat (controverse sur le rôle de la thrombose murale dans les lésions (artérielles).' In Colloques Internationaux du C.N.R.S.: *Le rôle de la paroi artérielle dans l'athérogénèse,* p. 871. Paris: Centre National de la Recherche Scientique

Haust, M. D., Wyllie, J. C. and More, R. H. (1965). 'Electron microscopy of fibrin in human atherosclerotic lesions. Immunohistochemical and morphologic identification.' *Expl Molec. Path.* **4**, 205

Hawn, C. V. Z. and Porter, K. R. (1947). 'The fine structure of clots formed from purified bovine fibrinogen and thrombin: a study with the electron microscope.' *J. exp. Med.* **86**, 285

Hüttner, I., Jellinek, H. and Kerényi, T. (1968). 'Fibrin formations in vascular fibrinoid change in experimental hypertension: an electron microscopic study.' *Expl Molec. Path.* **9**, 309

— More, R. H., Rona, G. and Jellinek, H. (1969). 'Diversity of fibrin ultrastructure in experimental vascular fibrinoid.' *Lab. Invest.* (abstr.) **20**, 588

— Rona, G. and More, R. H. (1971). 'Fibrin deposition within cardiac muscle cells in malignant hypertension.' *Archs Path.* **91**, 19

Karasaki, S. (1963). 'Studies on amphibian yolk. I. The ultrastructure of the yolk platelets.' *J. Cell Biol.* **18**, 135

Krishan, A. and Hsu, D. (1969). 'Observations on the association of helical polyribosomes and filaments with vincristine-induced crystals in Earle's L-cell fibroblasts.' *J. Cell Biol.* **43**, 553

Massover, W. H. (1971). 'Intramitochondrial yolk-crystals of frog oöcytes. II. Expulsion of intramitochondrial yolk-crystals to form single-membrane bound hexagonal crystalloids.' *J. Ultrastruct. Res.* **36**, 603

Mehta, P. N. and Ghadially, F. N. (1973). 'Articular cartilage in corn oil-induced lipoarthrosis.' *Ann. rheum. Dis.* **32**, 75

Merkow, L. P., Slifkin, M., Acevedo, H. F., Pardo, M. and Greenberg, W. V. (1971). 'Ultrastructure of an interstitial (hilar) cell tumor of the ovary.' *Obstet. Gynec.* **37**, 845

Montagna, W. (1962). 'The skin of lemurs.' *Ann. N.Y. Acad. Sci.* **102**, 190

Nagano, T. and Ohtsuki, I. (1971). 'Reinvestigation on the fine structure of Reinke's crystal in the human testicular interstitial cell.' *J. Cell Biol.* **51**, 148

Ooneda, G. Ooyama, Y., Matsuyama, K., Takatama, M., Yoshida, Y., Sekiguchi, M. and Arai, I. (1965). 'Electron microscopic studies on the morphogenesis of fibrinoid degeneration in the mesenteric arteries of hypertensive rats.' *Angiology* **16**, 8

Parry, E. W. and Ghadially, F. N. (1966). 'The nature of some annular inclusions seen under the electron microscope.' *J. Path. Bact.* **91**, 93

—— (1967). 'Fibrin in hepatocytes.' *Naturwissenschaften* **20**, 541

Revel, J. P., Napolitano, L. and Fawcett, D. W. (1960). 'Identification of glycogen in electron micrographs of thin tissue sections.' *J. biophys. biochem. Cytol.* **8**, 575

Ruebner, B. H., Watanabe, K. and Wand, J. S. (1970). 'Lytic necrosis resembling peliosis hepatis produced by lasiocarpine in the mouse liver. A light and electron microscopic study.' *Am. J. Path.* **60**, 247

Ruska, H. and Wolpers, C. (1940). 'Zur struktur des liquor fibrins.' *Klin. Wschr.* **19**, 695

Savard, K., Dorfman, R. I., Baggett, B., Fielding, L. L., Engel, L. L., McPherson, H. T., Lister, L. M., Johnson, D. S., Hamblen, E. C. and Engel, F. L. (1960). 'Clinical, morphological and biochemical studies of a virilizing tumor in the testis.' *J. clin. Invest.* **39**, 534

460

Shipkey, F. H., Lieberman, P. H., Foote, F. W., Jr. and Stewart, F. W. (1964). 'Ultrastructure of alveolar soft part sarcoma.' *Cancer* **17**, 821

Silverberg, S. G., Thompson, J. W., Higashi, G. and Baskin, A. M. (1966). 'Malignant interstitial cell tumor of the testis: case report and review.' *J. Urol.* **96**, 356

Sisson, J. K. and Fahrenbach, W. H. (1967). 'Fine structure of steroidogenic cells of a primate cutaneous organ.' *Am. J. Anat.* **121**, 337

Skinnider, L. F. and Ghadially, F. N. (1973). 'Glycogen in erythroid cells.' *Archs Path.* **95**, 139

Smith, G. F., Penrose, L. S. and O'Hara, P. T. (1967). 'Crystalline bodies in lymphocytes of patients with Down's syndrome.' *Lancet* **2**, 452

Sternberg, W. H. (1949). 'The morphology, androgenic function, hyperplasia and tumors of the human ovarian hilus cells.' *Am. J. Path.* **25**, 493

Still, W. J. S. (1968). 'The pathogenesis of the intimal thickenings produced by hypertension in large arteries in the rat.' *Lab. Invest.* **19**, 84

Stoeckenius, W. and Mahr, S. C. (1965). 'Studies on the reaction of osmium tetroxide with lipids and related compounds.' *Lab. Invest.* **14**, 458

Vye, M. V. and Fischman, D. A. (1970). 'The morphologic alteration of particulate glycogen by en bloc staining with uranyl acetate.' *J. Ultrastruct. Res.* **33**, 278

—— (1971). 'A comparative study of three methods for the ultrastructural demonstration of glycogen in thin sections.' *J. Cell Sci.* **9**, 727

Watson, M. L. (1958). 'Staining of tissue sections for electron microscopy with heavy metals. II. Application of solutions containing lead and barium.' *J. biophys. biochem. Cytol.* **4**, 727

Wiener, J., Spiro, D. and Lattes, R. G. (1965). 'The cellular pathology of experimental hypertension. II. Arteriolar hyalinosis and fibrinoid change.' *Am. J. Path.* **47**, 457

Yamada, E. (1962). 'Some observations on the fine structure of the interstitial cell in the human testis.' In *Proceedings of the Fifth International Congress for Electron Microscopy*, Vol. 2. Ed. by S. S. Breese, Jr. New York: Academic Press

— (1965). 'Some observations on the fine structure of the interstitial cell in the human testis as revealed by electron microscopy.' *Gunma Symp. Endocr.* **2**, 1

CHAPTER XIV

Cell Membrane and Junctions

INTRODUCTION

At the cell surface or the limiting boundary which demarcates the cell from its surroundings, two structures are usually seen: a membrane composed of lipids and proteins called the 'cell membrane', 'plasmalemma' or 'plasmalemmal membrane' (which shows a characteristic trilaminar structure), and frequently but not invariably also a polysaccharide-rich layer adjacent to or attached to the external surface of the cell membrane called the 'cell coat' or 'glycocalyx'. In certain sites this polysaccharide-rich layer is firmly bound to the cell membrane (e.g. on intestinal microvilli) and it is hence thought by some to be an integral part of the cell membrane. On the other hand, the polysaccharide-rich layer which forms the basal lamina found at the base of various epithelia is often separated from the cell membrane by a lucent interval. A similar but thinner layer also invests many cells such as smooth and striated muscle cells, fibroblasts and Schwann cells. This is referred to as the external lamina (Fawcett, 1967). These structures at least are clearly a component of the matrix and not a part of the cell membrane itself. The cell coat therefore receives only passing mention in this book devoted to the cell.

In the pre-electron-microscope era, Danielli and Davson (1935) proposed a theory of membrane structure, based on the then available evidence about the chemical composition, surface tension, permeability and electrical properties of membranes. According to this theory the membrane was thought to consist of a central lipid layer covered by monolayers of protein. With the advent of electron microscopy the proposed trilaminar structure was visualized in sections through the cell membrane as two dense lines separated by a lucent interval. The over-all thickness of the cell membrane was found to be about 80–100 Å, each layer being about 30 Å in thickness. This characteristic trilaminar structure is now often referred to as the 'unit membrane' or 'Robertson's unit membrane'.

Based on extensive studies on the structure of cell membranes and other cytomembranes, Robertson (see his 1969 review for history and details) has proposed that the central lipid layer is a bimolecular lipid leaflet (with the polar groups pointing outwards) and that the boundary protein layers are chemically asymmetrical (i.e. they have a different chemical composition). In keeping with this is the fact that in quite a few membranes a morphological asymmetry is also demonstrable, the inner lamina (adjacent to cytoplasm) being thicker than the external lamina (Koss, 1969).

Various other concepts and models of membrane structure have been proposed (see the review by Stoeckenius and Engelman, 1969) but space permits the mention of only one other, called the 'fluid mosaic model of membrane structure' (Singer and Nicolson, 1972). This theory views various cytomembranes (i.e. cell membrane and various intracellular membranes) as a mosaic composed of globular molecules of proteins embedded in a phospholipid matrix, with the polar groups protruding from the membrane into the aqueous phase. The bulk of the phospholipid is thought to be organized as a discontinuous fluid bilayer. Thus the matrix of the mosaic is thought to be lipid in which float the proteins which constitute the pieces of the mosaic. A somewhat similar concept of membrane structure is also proposed for mitochondrial membranes by Packer (1972).

Specialized areas of cell surface serving to bind that surface to another cell surface or non-cellular structure are referred to as junctions. Many morphological and functional varieties of junctions have been described. While the sole function of some seems to be the provision of sites of firm attachment, others also act as watertight seals or as areas of low electrical resistance across which ions can flow. The structure of such junctions and their variations form the main topic of this chapter.

It has already been noted that the cell is demarcated from its environment by a trilaminar membrane and also quite often by a cell coat (*Plates 195 and 196*). However, this trilaminar structure of the cell membrane is not easily demonstrated in many routinely prepared tissues used for electron microscopy. Excellent visualization is obtained when fixed blocks of tissue are stained with uranium (*en bloc* staining) prior to dehydration.

Besides the method of tissue preparation, one must also consider the problems of sectioning geometry. It takes little imagination to see that unless the cell membrane is cut at right angles to its surface and the segment of membrane lying in the thickness of the section is straight and does not bend or fold, there will be little chance of demonstrating the characteristic trilaminar structure. It is therefore common experience that in many routine preparations, the trilaminar structure is difficult to demonstrate, and is at best visualized only in small segments of the cell membrane. More frequently, the cell membrane presents as a single dense line or as a blurred line or band, depending upon the plane of sectioning.

The chances of demonstrating the trilaminar structure of the membrane are enhanced when a relatively flat expanse of membrane is encountered, as when a cell is apposed to another cell or to some firm structure (*Plate 195, Fig. 2*). Favourable also is the situation in the case of microvilli covering the surface of intestinal mucosa. Here an accurately placed transverse section gives a beautiful demonstration of the trilaminar structure, even in routinely fixed and stained material (*Plate 196, Fig. 1*), for a straight tubular segment of the microvillus lies vertically within the section thickness.

Although the morphological features of cell membranes from various cells show a remarkable similarity, detectable differences in over-all thickness and in the symmetry, thickness and spacing of the laminae have been noted in different parts of the same cell and in cells from various tissues and organs (Yamamoto, 1963). For example, the membrane covering the free surface of a cell is usually slightly thicker than that covering its lateral surface. In keratinizing epithelia the more mature keratinizing cells have a thicker cell membrane, with a wider central lipid layer than the cell membrane of the basal cells from which they stem.

The varying physiological properties and functions of cell membranes from different sites clearly indicate that within the basic unit membrane lie different systems of lipids and enzymes, although these are not demonstrable in routine electron micrographs. That specialized areas exist in or on cell membranes is, however, shown when ultrastructural studies are combined with ferritin labelling (Lee and Feldman, 1964; Nicolson *et al.*, 1971) and cytochemical techniques (for references, see page 468). Such studies show, for example, that blood group antigens and some enzymes have a characteristic pattern of distribution on or in the cell membrane.

Singularly interesting are the studies with freeze-cleaving and freeze-etching techniques. With this method (freeze-cleaving) the specimen, frozen in liquid nitrogen, is cleaved and the fractured surface replicated by platinum–carbon shadowing. Such preparations show surfaces (fracture-faces) covered by 80–100 Å diameter particles.

Plate 195

Fig. 1. Longitudinal section of microvilli of intestinal brush border, showing the continuous mucopolysaccharide layer which constitutes the surface coat (∗). × 37,000 (*Ghadially and Ailsby, unpublished electron micrograph*)

Fig. 2. Two endothelial cells (E) from a fenestrated capillary, showing the characteristic trilaminar structure of the cell membrane and some 'fuzzy' material which represents the cell coat. The diaphragm (arrow) stretching across the pore does not have a trilaminar structure. Vascular lumen (L). From the kidney of a desert rat (*Perognathus boylei*). × 235,000 (*Newstead, unpublished electron micrograph*)

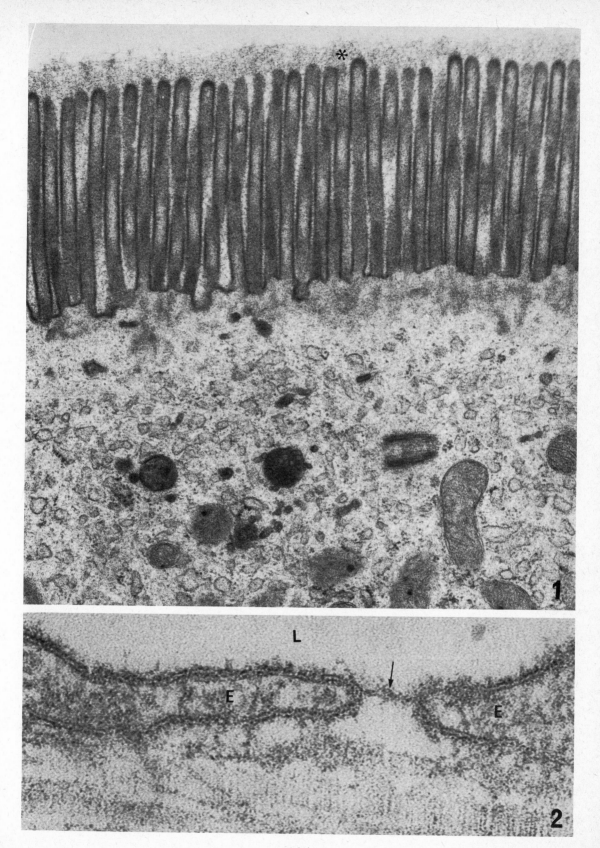

467

Although at first it was not at all clear exactly where these particles lay (a fundamental difference of opinion had developed as to the plane along which cleavage occurs) (Friederici, 1969), it is now reasonably well established that the fracture splits the membrane down its hydrophobic centre and that the particles seen are protein components protruding into the central regions of the membrane (Branton, 1966; Muhlethaler, 1971). Freeze-etching, a process whereby ice is allowed to sublime from the fractured specimen after cleaving, exposes the membrane surfaces (Tillack and Marchesi, 1970). Such surfaces are, relatively speaking, quite smooth (*Plate 196, Figs. 2 and 3*).

Active transport (i.e. against a concentration gradient) of ions across cell membranes requires expenditure of energy; so also does the transport of particulate material and fluid by mechanisms such as phagocytosis and micropinocytosis. In keeping with this is the demonstration of ATPase activity on the inner or outer surfaces of the cell membrane of various cell types by cytochemical methods (Ashworth *et al.*, 1963; Marchesi and Barrnett, 1963; Bartoszewicz and Barrnett, 1964; Marchesi *et al.*, 1964; Otero-Vilardebo *et al.*, 1964; Torack and Barrnett, 1964; Wachstein and Besen, 1964; Kaye and Pappas, 1965; Farquhar and Palade, 1966; Kaye and Tice, 1966; Kaye *et al.*, 1966; Santos-Buch, 1966; Campbell, 1968). The distribution of the reaction product is variously described by different authors but, generally, micropinocytotic vesicles show much activity, as also do membranes of cells known to be engaged in active transport. Furthermore, it would appear that in the case of some epithelia, only certain segments of the cell membrane exhibit overt ATPase activity and that this can be correlated with the known functional activity of the organ.

Thus in the normal liver (Wills and Epstein, 1966) ATPase activity is mainly localized at the luminal aspect of the bile canalicular membrane and microvilli (i.e. the part of the cell membrane actively involved in the transport of bile). In obstructive jaundice, both microvilli and enzyme activity tend to disappear from the distended bile canaliculi.

Few authors comment about the structure of the cell membrane (or alterations that might have occurred) when describing tissues of experimental animals or pathologically altered human tissues. To some extent this is due to the difficulty of demonstrating the trilaminar structure in routine preparations, and also because most biological work is done at quite low magnifications. Little information therefore is available on this point. The diminished power of adhesion of cancer cells, and the loss of contact inhibition shown by certain strains of cancer cells in tissue culture do not appear to be correlated with a detectable morphological alteration in the cell membrane itself. Such phenomena are probably explicable on the basis of alterations in the cell coat or cell junctions, but the evidence on these points is as yet scanty and no generalizations are possible.

Plate 196

Fig. 1. Cross-section of human intestinal microvilli, showing the characteristic trilaminar structure (i.e. two dense lines separated by a light intermediate zone) of the unit membrane. × 200,000

Fig. 2. Platinum–carbon replica of a freeze-cleaved human red blood cell ghost suspended in distilled water. The internal layer of the cell membrane bearing 85 Å particles (P) is revealed by this procedure. The junction of the particulate face and the surrounding ice is indicated by the arrow. × 60,000 (*From Tillack and Marchesi, 1970*)

Fig. 3. Platinum–carbon replica of a freeze-cleaved and deep-etched red blood cell ghost. The cloven convex face of the ghost is again seen to be covered with 85 Å particles (P). However, sublimation of the ice (I) during the etching process has revealed a smooth surface (S) which is the actual outer surface of the red blood cell membrane. × 60,000 (*From Tillack and Marchesi, 1970*)

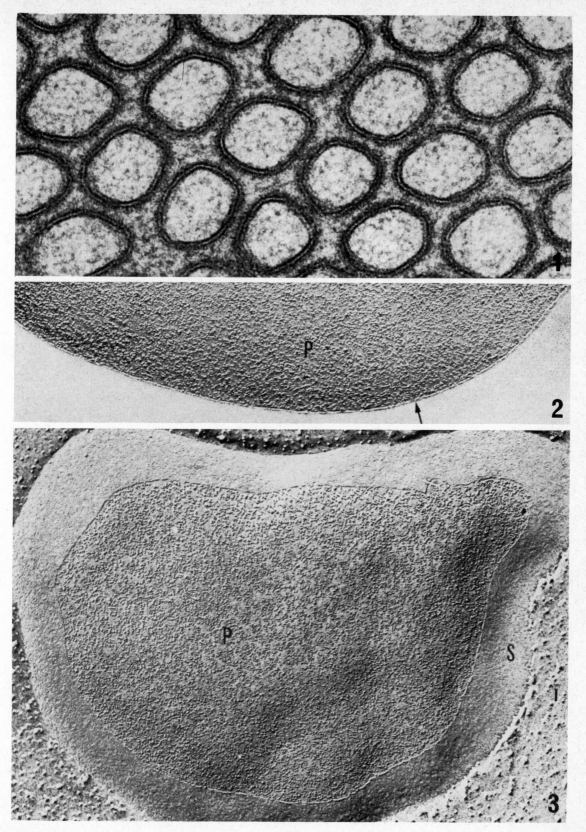

CELL JUNCTIONS

The narrow intercellular space which separates the apposed lateral surfaces of epithelial and endothelial cells contains a material which in the past was often referred to as the cement substance. It is now thought that this mucopolysaccharide-rich layer is a part of the cell coat, although it has properties somewhat different from other specialized parts of the cell coat such as the surface coat and the basal lamina.

The relatively constant interval (150–200 Å wide) and the parallel orientation of the apposed lateral surfaces of cells constituting epithelia and endothelia suggest the presence of a cohesive force operating over these surfaces. Often such apposed surfaces are amplified by the formation of a few or many complex interdigitating folds which probably play an additional role in cell-to-cell adhesion. Besides evidence of such a generalized mechanism, one also finds focal areas of specialization of the cell surface called junctions, which are thought to represent zones of firmer cell-to-cell attachment.

Perhaps the best-known examples of junctions seen at light microscopy are the so-called 'intercellular bridges' found between the prickle cells of the epidermis. Such bridges present as fine processes or fibrils traversing a clear space between adjacent cells, and it is this which gives the prickly appearance to prickle cells. The belief that such bridges represent tonofibrils crossing over from the cytoplasm of one cell into the next one, or that the cytoplasm of neighbouring cells is continuous at such sites is not borne out by electron microscopy. It would appear that this phenomenon is largely a shrinkage artefact, the bridges being no more than plaques or zones of firm attachment (in the past referred to as 'granules of Ranvier' or 'nodes of Bizzozero', now as desmosomes) which become drawn out as the cells shrink away from each other during fixation.

Although ultrastructural studies show that no true intracytoplasmic bridges establishing continuity between the cytoplasm of neighbouring cells are found in squamous epithelia, such bridges do occur between developing male germ cells (primary spermatocyte to late spermatid stage) and female germ cells and between certain cells in *Daphnia* and *Hydra* (Fawcett, 1961; Nagano, 1961; Zamboni and Gondos, 1968). More slender connections called 'plasmadesmata' are known to occur between adjacent cells of *Nitella* (Spanswick and Costerton, 1967).

Another example of junctions seen at light microscopy are the terminal bars demonstrable by classical histological methods near the surface of various epithelia, particularly the small intestine. In ultrathin sections the terminal bar is seen to be a junctional complex, comprising three morphologically distinct types of junctions. Starting from the lumen of the gut one finds a tight junction followed by an intermediate junction and some desmosomes (*Plate 197*). Similar

---

Plate 197

The terminal bar of the junction complex between adjacent intestinal epithelial cells of man is illustrated here. The tight junction (T) is seen near the lumen of the gut lined by microvilli (M). It presents as a dense line both in the low (*Fig. 1*) and in the high (*Fig. 2*) power views shown. The fusion of the outer leaflets of the plasma membrane characteristic of this type of junction is not revealed in these electron micrographs. Below the tight junction lie an intermediate junction (I) and some desmosomes (D). The desmosomes show dense plaques with attached filaments on their cytoplasmic surfaces. Less well oriented filamentous material is seen adjacent to the intermediate junction and some cytoplasmic 'fuzz' is also seen near the tight junction. In the desmosomes and intermediate junction the intercellular gap is widened. The parallel alignment of the cell membranes and the constancy of the intercellular gap (G) is clearly demonstrated in *Fig. 2*. The complex interdigitating folds (F) which are also thought to help to hold cells together are seen in *Fig. 1*. × 31,000; × 63,000 (*Ghadially and Ailsby, unpublished electron micrographs*)

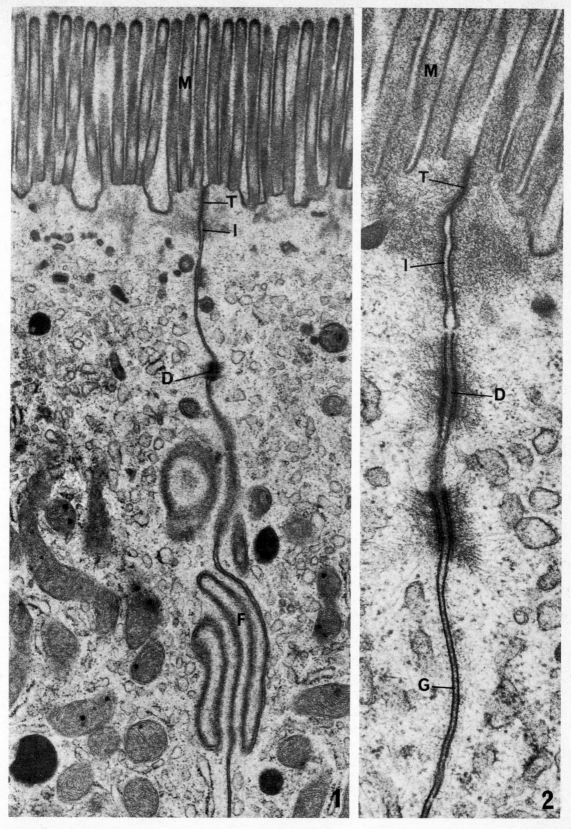

471

junction complexes have been described in various epithelia (Farquhar and Palade, 1963, 1965). However, the constant feature here is the tight junction which seals the intercellular space from the external environment (e.g. contents of gut, duct, acinus, etc.). The arrangement, number and type of the junctions which follow are quite variable.

The three types of junctions mentioned above and also other types have now been seen in a variety of tissues, and junctions have also been seen between cells in culture (Locke, 1965; Bullivant and Loewenstein, 1968; Brightman and Reese, 1969; Cobb and Bennett, 1969; Flaxman *et al.*, 1969; Schatzki, 1969; Goodenough and Revel, 1970; Martinez-Palomo, 1970; Sanel and Serpick, 1970; Nunez, 1971; Scalletta and MacCallum, 1972). It is important to note, however, that some of the literature that has accumulated is confusing and misleading. It is now known that examination of tissues prepared in the routine manner is not adequate to demonstrate and distinguish certain types of junctions. Studies using tissues stained *en bloc* with uranyl acetate (which gives better visualization of the structure of certain junctions), and studies using various tracers such as lanthanum hydroxide (which permeates the intercellular space and allows one to determine the degree and extent of obliteration of this space achieved in junctions), have helped to clarify the situation in recent years (*Plate 198*). In the light of such studies, one may briefly summarize what is currently thought about the structure and function of some junctions.

In ultrathin sections of tissues stained *en bloc* with uranium, the tight junctions of the junction complex of epithelia are characterized by punctate and linear fusion of the outer leaflets of the cell membrane of adjacent cells. (The fusion of the outer leaflets of the two apposing trilaminar membranes results in a pentalaminar structure, hence these junctions are at times referred to as pentalaminar junctions.) Lanthanum, which readily permeates the intercellular gap, may also invade part of the zone of punctate fusion, but it does not traverse the fusion line. Thus the collective evidence indicates that in this region the intercellular gap is obliterated. Since in epithelia such junctions occur as a continuous band around cells (but not in all endothelia, see below), it follows that tight junctions act as an effective seal which isolates the epithelial surfaces from the intercellular spaces. The term 'zonula occludens', used to describe these structures, is therefore quite appropriate.

In routine preparations, structures morphologically acceptable as tight junctions have been seen in a wide variety of tissues. In such preparations, however, and also in permanganate-fixed material it is difficult to distinguish a tight junction where the intercellular gap is obliterated from what is now known as a gap junction where the intercellular gap is reduced to a width of about 20–30 Å. Yet another problem is distinguishing what are known as 'labile or simple appositions of the cell membrane' from true tight junctions. Labile appositions are thought to be either transient associations of the cell membrane or an artefact producing a pentalaminar structure. Their incidence varies with preparative techniques and such structures, comprising apposed rather than fused membranes, do not impede the passage of tracers. They lack the zone of increased cytoplasmic density (cytoplasmic fuzz) seen adjacent to true tight junctions and their over-all width is not less than the combined width of the two membranes forming the junction, as is the case with true tight junctions.

Plate 198

Fig. 1. A tight junction between acinar cells of mouse mammary gland, showing the characteristic pentalaminar structure (see also *Plate 200*). The line of fusion of the outer leaflets of adjoining cell membranes is indicated by an arrow. Sections of microvilli (M), showing the characteristic trilaminar structure of the cell membrane, are seen within the lumen of the acinus. Tissue stained *en bloc* with uranium. × 120,000 (*Martinez-Palomo, unpublished electron micrograph*)

Fig. 2. Rat myocardium, showing a gap junction (between arrows) permeated by lanthanum. The intercellular gap (G) between the muscle fibres is abruptly narrowed in the junction which extends over quite a distance. × 84,000 (*Martinez-Palomo, unpublished electron micrograph*)

472

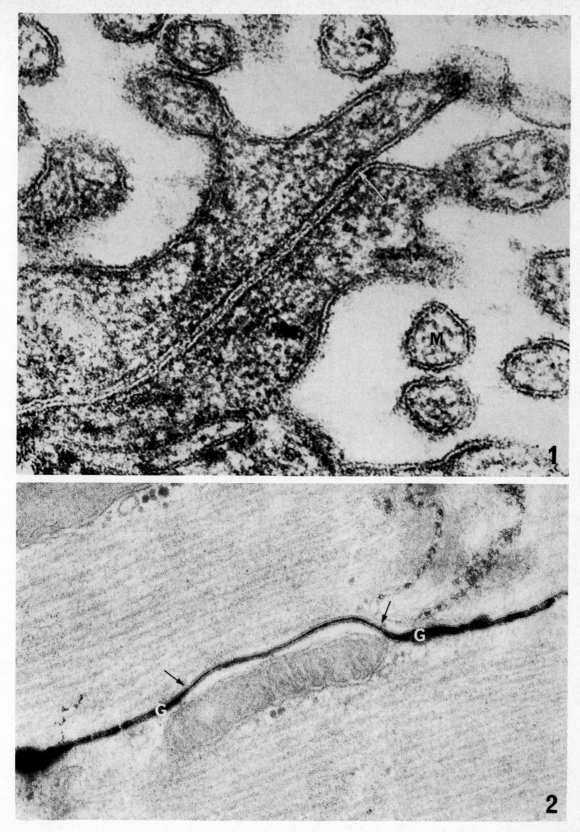

The points made above are clearly brought out by the meticulous studies of Brightman and Reese (1969) on junctions found in the vertebrate brain. They show that tight junctions which retain their pentalaminar appearance in tissues stained *en bloc* with uranium are restricted to the endothelium of capillaries and the epithelium of the choroid plexus. Such junctions are neither circumvented* nor penetrated by tracers such as lanthanum or horse-radish peroxidase, but various other junctions between astrocytes and between some neurons which, in the past, had been regarded as tight junctions are in fact gap junctions which are readily permeated by tracers. Gap junctions seem to be very widely distributed and have been seen in many tissues. In many studies a polygonal lattice has been demonstrated within the gap of the gap junction. There is much evidence that the gap junction represents a site of electrical coupling between cells. This is thought to be so for gap junctions found in mammalian heart, smooth muscle, Mauthner cell and liver (for details and references, see Goodenough and Revel, 1970).

Intermediate junctions and desmosomes are fundamentally different from tight junctions and gap junctions in that the width of the intercellular gap is either unaltered or widened but not narrowed. Even so, both these types of junctions are known to be sites of firm cell-to-cell attachment. Desmosomes are widely distributed and have been seen in many epithelia (*Plate 199*) and also between vascular endothelial cells of some species (Fawcett, 1967). However, they are singularly well developed and numerous in squamous epithelia, particularly the epithelium of the skin. The morphology and size of desmosomes are quite variable but they are readily identified by the presence of a dense plaque and filaments on their cytoplasmic faces. The widened intercellular space often contains a dense material and a dense line which suggests a modification of the cell coat at this site. Desmosomes are button-like structures which bind cells together; hence the desmosome is at times referred to as a 'macula adherens'. Their prominence in the epidermis and also in the intercalated disc of cardiac muscle indicates that this is the mechanically strongest type of junction. Not all desmosomes, however, bind adjacent cells together. On rare occasions a desmosome is seen binding an area of cell surface to another area on the surface of the same cell. This is referred to as an autodesmosome. The term 'hemidesmosome' is used for the 'half desmosomes' that bind an area of cell surface to some other non-cellular structure such as a basement membrane, an area of tooth surface, or a plastic membrane such as that used in tissue culture (Kelly, 1966; Flaxman *et al.*, 1968). Hemidesmosomes are of common occurrence along the dermo-epidermal junction.

A common type of cell junction seen in the epithelia of invertebrates is called the 'septate desmosome'. It bears little resemblance to the desmosomes described above. This is a cell junction with a gap about 150 Å wide, traversed by numerous septa or lamellae at right angles to the membrane surfaces. Tangential sections show that these septa are not straight sheets but a hexagonal network of septa demarcating symmetrical intercellular compartments. It is thought that septate desmosomes are involved in cell-to-cell electronic coupling (Locke, 1965; Bullivant and Loewenstein, 1968).

* Junctions in many capillaries outside the brain are known to be circumvented by tracers for they do not extend as a continuous band around the cells.

Plate 199

Fig. 1. Desmosomes from human skin. Note the dense plaque (P), filaments (F) and dense line (D) in the intercellular space. × 96,000

Fig. 2. Hemidesmosomes (arrows) are seen at the junction of the epidermis (E) and dermis (D). Also seen is the basal lamina (B), separated from the epithelium by a less dense or lucent zone. From the same specimen as *Fig. 1*. × 94,000

Fig. 3. Autodesmosome (arrow) from placental amnion of a 23-week-old human fetus. × 30,000. (*Parry, unpublished electron micrograph*)

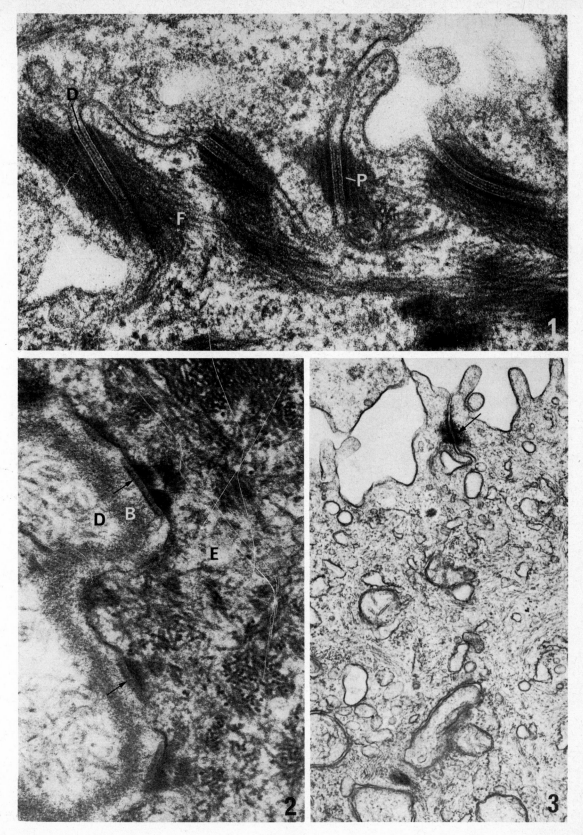

475

ALTERATION OF CELL JUNCTIONS IN NEOPLASIA

A fair-sized literature has now accumulated on this topic, and the prevailing impression is that there is a reduction in the number of various types of junctions and a widening of the inter-cellular spaces in malignant tumours and during carcinogenesis (Easty and Mercer, 1960; Bruni *et al.,* 1961; Friedmann, 1961; Vandrewalla and Sirsat, 1963; Hruban *et al.,* 1965; Ghadially and Parry, 1966; Ma and Webber, 1966; Mao *et al.,* 1966; Benedetti and Emmelot, 1967; Murad and Scarpelli, 1967; Usui, 1967; Shingleton *et al.,* 1968; Sugar, 1968; Sirsat and Shanbhag, 1969; Watanabe and Essner, 1969; Martinez-Palomo, 1970; Harris *et al.,* 1971).

It is said that, while there is a marked reduction in the number of desmosomes and a loss of structural cohesion in squamous carcinoma of the skin, in basal cell carcinomas a close mutual adhesion is maintained between adjacent cells (Vandrewalla and Sirsat, 1963). In human warts an increase in the number of desmosomes has been reported to occur (Chapman *et al.,* 1963). In keratoacanthomas desmosomes are plentiful (Fisher *et al.,* 1972) and, according to Takaki *et al.* (1971), increased in numbers. This seems to be a point worth pursuing for keratoacanthomas have frequently been mistaken for squamous carcinoma (Ghadially, 1971). The presence or absence of junctions, particularly desmosomes, is a useful factor in deciding whether an anaplastic tumour (or some rare tumour whose histogenesis is in doubt) is a carcinoma or a sarcoma. While the absence of desmosomes may not be too helpful (for this could be due to dedifferentiation), the presence of desmosomes of characteristic morphology would favour the diagnosis of a carcinoma, because desmosomes are characteristic of epithelial tissues and only on rare occasions have junctions resembling desmosomes been seen in connective tissues (see page 478). As a rule junctions are not seen in sarcomas, but intercellular junctions (some of which were thought to be atypical or poorly differentiated desmosomes) have been reported in 3-methylcholanthrene-induced mouse sarcomas (Clarke, 1970).

Earlier ultrastructural studies were concerned mainly with alterations in desmosomes but recently much interest has been directed to changes that might occur in tight junctions and gap junctions in tumours. Such junctions are thought to represent sites of electrical coupling, ion exchanges, and intercellular communication (Loewenstein, 1966; Furshpan and Potter, 1968). It is thought that alterations in such junctions might result in faulty co-ordination of cellular activity (Loewenstein and Kanno, 1966, 1967; Potter *et al.,* 1966). Electrophysiological studies have revealed that some cancer cells are electrically coupled but that others are not (Johnson and Sheridan, 1971). The recent elegant studies of Martinez-Palomo (1970) show that in many epithelial tumours tight junctions are absent between tumour cells, and gap junctions tend to be sparse (*Plate 200*).

How far one can implicate the changes seen in various types of cell junctions with tumour infiltration remains debatable. Clearly such changes relate only to carcinomas and not to sarcomas, for many connective tissue cells (from which sarcomas arise) do not have any cell junctions to begin with, and are yet quite capable of infiltrating and metastasizing.

Plate 200

Normal acinus from a mouse mammary gland (*Fig. 1*) and acinus from a mouse mammary carcinoma (*Fig. 2*) are compared here. Tissues were treated with lanthanum hydroxide, which presents here as a highly electron-dense linear deposit in the intercellular spaces. (*From Martinez-Palomo, 1970*)

Fig. 1. The lateral intercellular space is permeated with lanthanum except in the apical region, where the tight junctions (arrows) have occluded the intercellular space. × 13,500

Fig. 2. The absence of tight junctions in the tumoural acinus is evidenced by the fact that the lanthanum has permeated the four intercellular spaces up to the lumen of the acinus (arrows). × 23,000

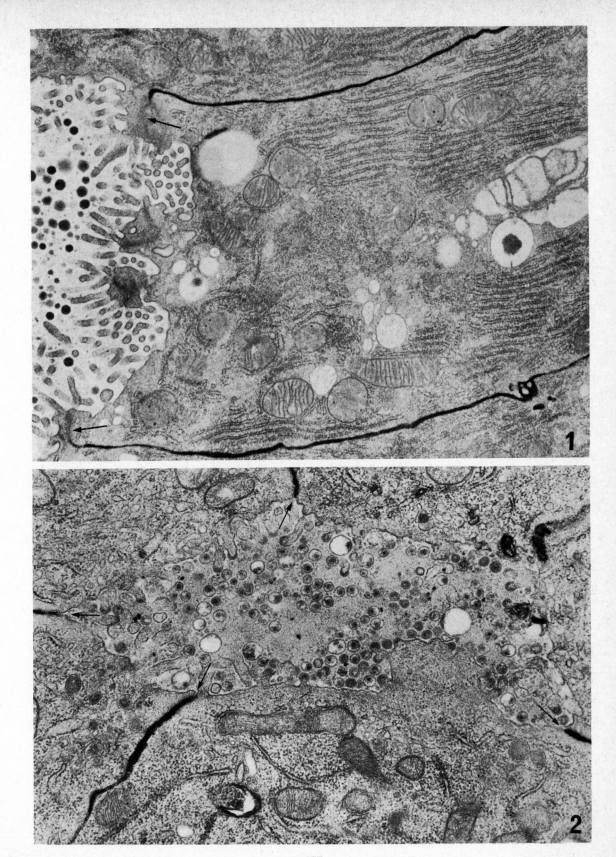

Although the factors leading to the production of intercellular junctions are by no means clear, an obvious minimum requirement would be a close apposition of neighbouring cell surfaces. In keeping with this is the observation that in fibrous tissue, synovial tissue, or cartilage where the cells are usually separated by a fair amount of matrix, junctions are, as a rule, not seen.

However, examples may be quoted where such junctions do develop in such tissues, and this is usually seen in situations where cellular proliferation has brought such cells close together. Thus tight junctions or close junctions (gap said to be 25–100 Å wide) have been noted between embryonic connective tissue cells (Trelstad *et al.*, 1966, 1967), and 'close association regions,' where the cell membranes of adjacent cells were in intimate contact, have been described in adult guinea-pig fibroblasts proliferating in cell culture (Devis and James, 1964). Sites of attachment resembling intermediate junctions have been demonstrated between a variety of embryonic connective tissue cells (Ross and Greenlee, 1966). That a neoplastic proliferation of connective tissue cells may lead to formation of cell junctions is evidenced by the report of Clarke *et al.* (1970), who found specialized attachments resembling intermediate junctions, and poorly formed or atypical desmosomes, in subcutaneous sarcomas of the mouse produced by the implantation of 3-methylcholanthrene.

The chondrocytes of articular cartilage usually lie apart, separated from one another by abundant matrix. Even between chondrocyte pairs there is a fair amount of intervening matrix. However, occasionally such cells may lie very close together and in one such instance the occurrence of a desmosome has been reported (Palfrey and Davis, 1966).

The synovial intima in most species is composed of one to four layers of cells set in a modest amount of matrix. In normal rabbit, guinea-pig and human synovial membrane the intimal cells are loosely arranged to form a fairly compact but not continuous lining layer like that found in various epithelia. The cell surfaces are rarely closely apposed and junctions have not been found in the normal synovial membrane of these species (Barland *et al.*, 1962; Wyllie *et al.*, 1964; Ghadially and Roy, 1966, 1969). The synovial intima of the rat is, however, much more richly endowed with cells and the matrix is scanty. The cells are closely packed and interdigitations between the cell membranes of adjacent cells are frequently seen. Here structures acceptable as desmosomes (and also perhaps tight junctions, but this was in routinely prepared material) have been found between the synovial cells (*Plate 201, Fig. 1*) (Roy and Ghadially, 1967). It is interesting to note that, although in normal human synovial membrane intercellular junctions are not found, in the hyperplastic synovial membrane of traumatic arthritis and rheumatoid arthritis the closely packed cells do develop desmosomes or desmosome-like attachment plaques (Grimley and Sokoloff, 1966; Ghadially and Roy, 1969). We have recently seen desmosome-like structures in the synovial intima of a case of villonodular synovitis (*Plate 201, Figs. 2 and 3*).

Plate 201

Desmosome or desmosome-like junctions (arrows) found in synovial tissue are depicted here.

Fig. 1. Normal rat synovial intima, showing junctions between closely apposed synovial cells. × 36,000 (*From Roy and Ghadially, 1967*)

Fig. 2. Junctions found in the synovial intima from a case of rheumatoid arthritis. × 48,000

Fig. 3. Junctions found in the synovial tissue from a case of villonodular synovitis. × 35,000

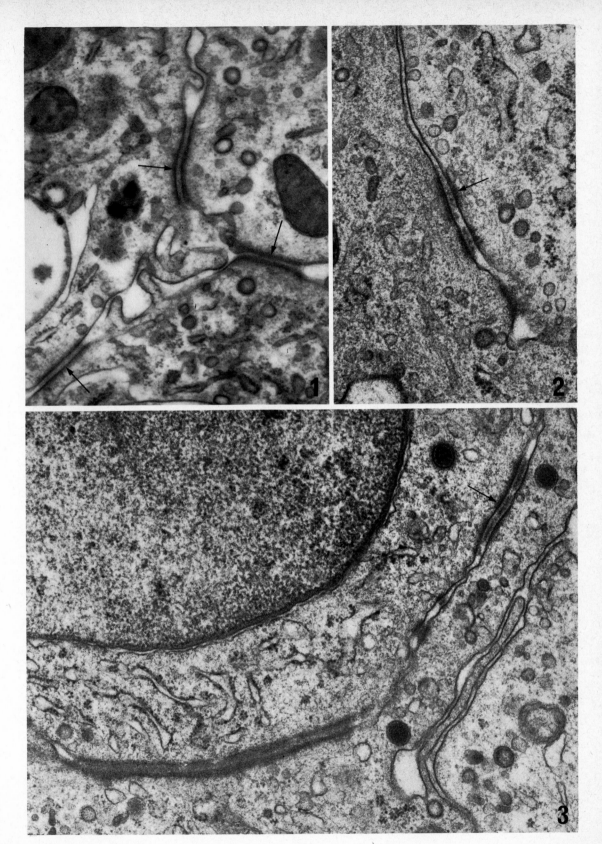

Intracytoplasmic desmosomes may occur when cells connected by desmosomes fuse to produce multinucleated giant cells or syncytial sheets. After fusion the intervening cell membranes suffer fragmentation and dissolution but the less vulnerable desmosomes tend to persist awhile and are hence seen lying free in the cytoplasm.*

Perhaps the best-known example of intracytoplasmic desmosomes is that known to occur in syncytiotrophoblasts which develop by fusion of cytotrophoblasts (Pierce et al., 1964; Enders, 1965; Boyd and Hamilton, 1966; Okudaira and Strauss, 1967; Garancis et al., 1970). After such fusion one may find: (1) fragments of cell membranes lying within the cytoplasm; (2) intrasyncytial clefts with desmosomes (i.e. paired membranes with accompanying desmosomes); (3) intracytoplasmic desmosomes; and (4) electron-dense rods (thought to be residual bodies derived by degradation of desmosomes).

In primary cultures of human amnion cells infected with varicella zoster virus (DNA virus of herpes type), giant cells (polykaryocytes) containing intracytoplasmic desmosomes were found by Cook and Stevens (1970). These authors postulate the same mechanism for the formation of intracytoplasmic desmosomes as mentioned earlier, but add the interesting observation that 'the formation of polykaryocytes and "cytoplasmic desmosomes" may be mediated by the exportation of hydrolytic enzymes since we have seen acid phosphatase positive deposits between the plasma membranes of adjacent cells in infected cultures'.

The occurrence of intracytoplasmic desmosomes does not always indicate cell fusion, for this phenomenon is not restricted to multinucleate cells. For example, intracytoplasmic desmosomes have been seen in the cells of human keratoacanthoma (Bülow and Klingmüller, 1971; Takaki et al., 1971; Fisher et al., 1972) and the cytoplasm of dyskeratotic cells undergoing mitosis in Bowen's disease (Seiji and Mizuno, 1969). The last-named authors suggest that such dyskeratotic cells may lose contact with neighbouring epidermal cells during mitosis and incorporate the desmosomes into their cytoplasm.

Multinucleate cells produced by repeated division of the nucleus without cell division can hardly be expected to contain intracytoplasmic desmosomes. Hence when intracytoplasmic desmosomes are found in a multinucleate cell this argues strongly in favour of the idea that such a giant cell has resulted from a fusion of cells. However, not all multinucleate cells produced by fusion can be expected to show intracytoplasmic desmosomes, for, clearly, desmosomes linking the cells have to be present in the first instance. An example of this is seen in developing muscle, at the stage when myotubes are formed by fusion of myoblasts. Attachment plaques (described as close junctions) develop between the adjacent cell membranes of the myoblasts, which are about to fuse (Mendell et al., 1972), but such junctions do not persist within the cytoplasm of the multinucleate myotube which develops. Cell junctions other than desmosomes have not been reported in an intracytoplasmic position. One would imagine that they are far more vulnerable than desmosomes.

* Although the term 'intracytoplasmic desmosome' is convenient and describes the situation adequately, it should be remembered that a major part of even the normal desmosome (i.e. dense plaques and filaments) is intracellular.

Plate 202

Fig. 1. Intracytoplasmic desmosomes (arrows) found in a varicella zoster virus-infected human amnion cell in culture. The cell appears to have at least two nuclei. Some of the intracytoplasmic desmosomes lie in the intervening cytoplasm. × 21,000 (*From Cook and Stevens, 1970*)

Figs. 2 and 3. High power view of intracytoplasmic desmosomes. The dense plaques and radiating filaments characteristic of this type of junction are clearly visualized. × 98,000; × 98,000 (*From Cook and Stevens, 1970*)

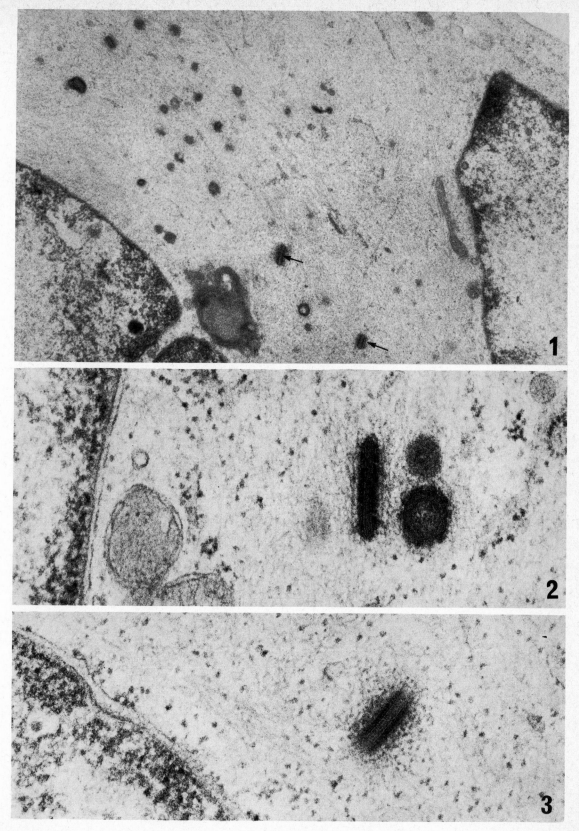

481

REFERENCES

Ashworth, C. T., Luibel, F. J. and Stewart, S. C. (1963). 'The fine structural localization of adenosine triphosphatase in the small intestine, kidney and liver of the rat.' *J. Cell Biol.* **17**, 1

Barland, P., Novikoff, A. B. and Hamerman, D. (1962). 'Electron microscopy of the human synovial membrane.' *J. Cell Biol.* **14**, 207

Bartoszewicz, W. and Barrnett, R. J. (1964). 'Fine structural localization of nucleoside phosphatase activity in the urinary bladder of the toad.' *J. Ultrastruct. Res.* **10**, 599

Benedetti, E. L. and Emmelot, P. (1967). 'Studies on plasma membranes, IV. The ultrastructural localization and content of sialic acid in plasma membranes isolated from rat liver and hepatoma.' *J. Cell Sci.* **2**, 499

Boyd, J. D. and Hamilton, W. J. (1966). 'Electron microscopic observations on the cytotrophoblast contribution to the syncytium in the human placenta.' *J. Anat.* **100**, 535

Branton, D. (1966). 'Fracture faces of frozen membranes.' *Proc. Natn. Acad. Sci., U.S.A.* **55**, 1048

Brightman, M. W. and Reese, T. S. (1969). 'Junctions between intimately apposed cell membranes in the vertebrate brain.' *J. Cell Biol.* **40**, 648

Bruni, C., Gey, M. K. and Svotelis, M. (1961). 'Changes in the fine structure of HeLa cells in relation to growth.' *Bull. John Hopkins Hosp.* **109**, 160

Bullivant, S. and Loewenstein, W. R. (1968). 'Structure of coupled and uncoupled cell junctions.' *J. Cell Biol.* **37**, 621

Bülow, M.v. and Klingmüller, G. (1971). 'Elektronenmikroskopische untersuchungen des Keratoakanthoms. Vorkommen intracytoplasmatischer Desmosomen.' *Arch. Derm. Forsch.* **241**, 292

Campbell, W. G., Jr. (1968). 'Localization of adenosine 5'-triphosphatase in vascular and cellular synovium of rabbits.' *Lab. Invest.* **18**, 304

Chapman, G. B., Drusin, L. M. and Todd, J. E. (1963). 'Fine structure of the human wart.' *Am. J. Path.* **42**, 619

Clarke, M. A. (1970). 'Specialized intercellular junctions in tumor cells—an electron microscope study of mouse sarcoma cells.' *Anat. Rec.* **166**, 199

Cobb, J. L. S. and Bennett, T. (1969). 'A study of nexuses in visceral smooth muscle.' *J. Cell Biol.* **41**, 287

Cook, M. L. and Stevens, J. G. (1970). 'Replication of varicella-zoster virus in cell culture: an ultrastructural study.' *J. Ultrastruct. Res.* **32**, 334

Danielli, J. R. and Davson, H. A. (1935). 'A contribution to the theory of permeability of thin films.' *J. Cell comp. Physiol.* **5**, 495

Devis, R. and James, D. W. (1964). 'Close association between adult guinea pig fibroblasts in tissue culture, studied with the electron microscope.' *J. Anat.* **98**, 63

Easty, G. C. and Mercer, E. H. (1960). 'An electron microscopic study of the surfaces of normal and malignant cells in culture.' *Cancer Res.* **20**, 1608

Enders, A. C. (1965). 'Formation of syncytium from cytotrophoblast in the human placenta.' *Obstet. Gynec.* **25**, 378

Farquhar, M. G. and Palade, G. E. (1963). 'Junctional complexes in various epithelia.' *J. Cell Biol.* **17**, 375

—— (1965). 'Cell junctions in amphibian skin.' *J. Cell Biol.* **26**, 263

—— (1966). 'Adenosine triphosphatase localization in amphibian epidermis.' *J. Cell Biol.* **30**, 359

Fawcett, D. W. (1961). 'Intercellular bridges.' *Expl Cell Res.* Suppl. 8, 174

— (1967). *The Cell: An Atlas of Fine Structure*. Philadelphia and London: Saunders

Fisher, E. R., McCoy, II, M. M. and Wechsler, H. L. (1972). 'Analysis of histopathologic and electron microscopic determinants of keratoacanthoma and squamous cell carcinoma.' *Cancer* **29**, 1387

Flaxman, B. A., Lutzner, M. A. and van Scott, E. J. (1968). 'Ultrastructure of cell attachment to substratum *in vitro*.' *J. Cell Biol.* **36**, 406

— Revel, J. P. and Hay, E. D. (1969). 'Tight junctions between contact-inhibited cells *in vitro*.' *Expl Cell Res.* **58**, 438

Friederici, H. H. R. (1969). 'The surface structure of some renal cell membranes.' *Lab. Invest.* **21**, 459

Friedmann, I. (1961). 'Electron microscopy of human biopsy material.' *Proc. R. Soc. Med.* **54**, 1064

Furshpan, E. J. and Potter, D. D. (1968). 'Low-resistance junctions between cells in embryos and tissue culture.' *Curr. Top. Devl Biol.* **3**, 95

Garancis, J. C., Pattillo, R. A., Hussa, R. O., Schultz, J. and Mattingly, R. F. (1970). 'Electron microscopic and biochemical patterns of the normal and malignant trophoblast.' *Am. J. Obstet. Gynec.* **108**, 1257

Ghadially, F. N. (1971). 'Keratoacanthoma.' In *Dermatology in General Medicine,* p. 425. Ed. by T. B. Fitzpatrick and D. P. Johnson. New York and Maidenhead: McGraw-Hill

Ghadially, F. N. and Parry, E. W. (1966). 'Ultrastructure of a human hepatocellular carcinoma and surrounding non-neoplastic liver.' *Cancer* **19**, 1989

— and Roy, S. (1966). 'Ultrastructure of rabbit synovial membrane.' *Ann. rheum. Dis.* **25**, 318

—— (1969). *Ultrastructure of Synovial Joints in Health and Disease*. London: Butterworths

Goodenough, D. A. and Revel, J. P. (1970). 'A fine structural analysis of intercellular junctions in the mouse liver.' *J. Cell Biol.* **45**, 272

Grimley, P. M. and Sokoloff, L. (1966). 'Synovial giant cells in rheumatoid arthritis.' *Am. J. Path.* **49**, 931

Harris, C. C., Sporn, M. B., Kaufman, D. G., Smith, J. M., Baker, M. S. and Saffiotti, U. (1971). 'Acute ultrastructural effects of benzo(a)pyrene and ferric oxide on the hamster tracheobronchial epithelium.' *Cancer Res.* **31**, 1977

Hruban, Z., Swift, H. and Rechcigl, M. (1965). 'Fine structure of transplantable hepatomas of the rat.' *J. Natn Cancer Inst.* **35**, 459

Johnson, R. G. and Sheridan, J. D. (1971). 'Junctions between cancer cells in culture: ultrastructure and permeability.' *Science* **174**, 717

Kaye, G. I. and Pappas, G. D. (1965). 'Studies on the ciliary epithelium and zonule. III. The fine structure of the rabbit ciliary epithelium in relation to the localization of ATPase activity.' *J. Microscopy* **4**, 497

— and Tice, L. W. (1966). 'Studies on the cornea. V. Electron microscopic localization of adenosine triphosphatase activity in the rabbit cornea in relation to transport.' *Invest. Ophthal.* **5**, 22

— Wheeler, H. O., Whitlock, R. T. and Lane, N. (1966). 'Fluid transport in the rabbit gallbladder. A combined physiological and electron microscopic study.' *J. Cell Biol.* **30**, 237

Kelly, D. E. (1966). 'Fine structure of desmosomes, hemidesmosomes and adepidermal globular layer in developing newt epidermis.' *J. Cell Biol.* **28**, 51

Koss, L. G. (1969). 'The asymmetric unit membranes of the epithelium of the urinary bladder of the rat. An electron microscopic study of a mechanism of epithelial maturation and function.' *Lab. Invest.* **21**, 154

Lee, R. E. and Feldman, J. D. (1964). 'Visualization of antigenic sites of human erythrocytes with ferritin-antibody conjugates.' *J. Cell Biol.* **23**, 396

Locke, M. (1965). 'The structure of septate desmosomes.' *J. Cell Biol.* **25**, 166

Loewenstein, W. R. (1966). 'Permeability of membrane junctions.' *Ann. N.Y. Acad. Sci.* **137**, 441

— and Kanno, Y. (1966). 'Intercellular communication and the control of tissue growth: lack of communication between cancer cells.' *Nature, Lond.* **209**, 1248

—— (1967). 'Intercellular communication and tissue growth. 1. Cancerous growth.' *J. Cell Biol.* **33**, 225

Ma, M. H. and Webber, A. J. (1966). 'Fine structure of liver tumours induced in the rat by 3'-methyl-4-dimethylamino-azobenzene.' *Cancer Res.* **26**, 935

Mao, P., Nakao, K. and Angrist, A. (1966). 'Human prostatic carcinoma. An electron microscopic study.' *Cancer Res.* **26**, 955

Marchesi, V. T. and Barrnett, R. J. (1963). 'The demonstration of enzymatic activity in pinocytic vesicles of blood capillaries with the electron microscope.' *J. Cell Biol.* **17**, 547

— Sears, M. L., and Barrnett, R. J. (1964). 'Electron microscopic studies of nucleoside phosphatase activity in blood vessels and glia of the retina.' *Invest. Ophthal.* **3**, 1

Martinez-Palomo, A. (1970). 'Ultrastructural modifications of intercellular junctions in some epithelial tumors.' *Lab. Invest.* **22**, 605

Mendell, J. R., Roelofs, R. I. and Engel, W. K. (1972). 'Ultrastructural development of explanted human skeletal muscle in tissue culture.' *J. Neuropath. exp. Neurol.* **31**, 433

Muhlethaler, K. (1971). 'Studies on freeze-etching of cell membranes.' *Int. Rev. Cytol.* **31**, 1

Murad, T. M. and Scarpelli, D. (1967). 'The ultrastructure of medullary and scirrhous mammary duct carcinoma.' *Am. J. Path.* **50**, 335

Nagano, T. (1961). 'The structure of cytoplasmic bridges in dividing spermatocytes of the rooster.' *Anat. Rec.* **141**, 73

Nicolson, G. L., Masouredis, S. P. and Singer, S. J. (1971). 'Quantitative two-dimensional ultrastructural distribution of $Rh_0(D)$ antigenic sites on human erythrocyte membranes.' *Proc. natn. Acad. Sci., U.S.A.* **68**, 1416

Nunez, E. A. (1971). 'Secretory processes in follicular cells of the bat thyroid.' *Am. J. Anat.* **131**, 227

Okudaira, T. and Strauss, L. (1967). 'Ultrastructure of molar trophoblast. Observations on hydatidiform mole and chorioadenoma destruens.' *Obstet. Gynec.* **30**, 172

Otero-Villardebo, L. R., Lane, N. and Godman, G. C. (1964). 'Localization of phosphatase activities in colonic goblet and absorptive cells.' *J. Cell Biol.* **21**, 486

Packer, L. (1972). 'Functional organization of intramembrane particles of mitochondrial inner membranes.' *Bioenergetics* **3**, 115

Palfrey, A. J. and Davis, D. V. (1966). 'The fine structure of chondrocytes.' *J. Anat.* **100**, 213

Pierce, G. B., Jr., Midgley, A. R., Jr. and Beals, T. F. (1964). 'An ultrastructural study of differentiation and maturation of trophoblast of the monkey.' *Lab. Invest.* **13**, 451

Potter, D. D., Furshpan, E. J. and Lennox, E. S. (1966). 'Connections between cells of the developing squid as revealed by electrophysiological methods.' *Proc. natn. Acad. Sci., U.S.A.* **55**, 328

Robertson, J. D. (1969). 'Molecular structure of biological membranes.' In *Handbook of Molecular Cytology,* p. 1404. Ed. by A. Lima-de-Faria. Amsterdam and London: North-Holland Publ.

Ross, R. and Greenlee, T. K., Jr. (1966). 'Electron microscopy: attachment sites between connective tissue cells.' *Science* **153**, 997

Roy, S. and Ghadially, F. N. (1967). 'Ultrastructure of normal rat synovial membrane.' *Ann. rheum. Dis.* **26**, 26

Sanel, F. T. and Serpick, A. A. (1970). 'Plasmalemmal and subsurface complexes in human leukemic cells: membrane bonding by zipperlike junctions.' *Science* **168**, 1458

Santos-Buch, C. A. (1966). 'Extrusion of ATPase activity from pinocytotic vesicles of abutting endothelium and smooth muscle to the internal elastic membrane of the major arterial circle of the iris of rabbits.' *Nature, Lond.* **211**, 600

Scaletta, L. J. and MacCallum, D. K. (1972). 'A fine structural study of divalent cation-mediated epithelial union with connective tissue in human oral mucosa.' *Am. J. Anat.* **133**, 431

Schatzki, P. F. (1969). 'Bile canaliculus and space of Disse. Electron microscopic relationships as delineated by lanthanum.' *Lab. Invest.* **20**, 87

Seiji, M. and Mizuno, F. (1969). 'Electron microscopic study of Bowen's disease.' *Archs Derm., Chicago* **99**, 3

Shingleton, H. M., Richart, R. M., Wiener, J. and Spiro, D. (1968). 'Human cervical intraepithelial neoplasia. Fine structure of dysplasia and carcinoma *in situ*.' *Cancer Res.* **28**, 695

Singer, S. J. and Nicolson, G. L. (1972). 'The fluid mosaic model of the structure of cell membranes.' *Science* **175**, 720

Sirsat, S. M. and Shanbhag, U. V. (1969). 'Histochemical and submicroscopic studies on sialic acid in induced epidermal cancer in relation to cell detachment and metastasis.' *Indian J. Cancer* **6**, 133

Spanswick, R. M. and Costerton, J. W. F. (1967). 'Plasmodesmata in *Nitella translucens*; structure and electrical resistance.' *J. Cell Sci.* **2**, 451

Stoeckenius, W. and Engelman, D. M. (1969). 'Current models for the structure of biological membranes.' *J. Cell Biol.* **42**, 613

Sugar, J. (1968). 'An electron microscope study of early invasive growth in human skin tumours and laryngeal carcinoma.' *Eur. J. Cancer* **4**, 33

Takaki, Y., Masutani, M. and Kawada, A. (1971). 'Electron microscopic study of keratoacanthoma.' *Acta derm.-vener.* **51**, 21

Tillack, T. W. and Marchesi, V. T. (1970). 'Demonstration of the outer surface of freeze-etched red blood cell membranes.' *J. Cell Biol.* **45**, 649

Torack, R. M. and Barrnett, R. J. (1964). 'The fine structural localization of nucleoside phosphatase activity in the blood–brain barrier.' *J. Neuropath. exp. Neurol.* **23**, 46

Trelstad, R. L., Revel, J. P. and Hay, E. D. (1966). 'Tight junctions between cells in the early chick embryo as visualized with the electron microscope.' *J. Cell Biol.* **31**, C6

— Hay, E. and Revel, J. P. (1967). 'Cell contact during early morphogenesis in the chick embryo.' *Devl Biol.* **16**, 78

Usui, T. (1967). 'Electron microscopic study of the ascites hepatoma. Comparative studies.' *Gann* **58**, 229

Vandrewalla, A. and Sirsat, S. M. (1963). 'Differential metastasis in epidermal neoplasms—a comparative electron microscopic and histochemical study.' *Indian J. Cancer* **1**, 1

Wachstein, M. and Besen, M. (1964). 'Electron microscopic study in several mammalian species of the reaction product enzymatically liberated from adenosine triphosphate in the kidney.' *Lab. Invest.* **13**, 476

Watanabe, H. and Essner, E. (1969). 'A comparative cytologic study of the cultivation of hepatomas of different growth rates.' *Cancer Res.* **29**, 631

Wills, E. J. and Epstein, M. A. (1966). 'Subcellular changes in surface adenosine triphosphatase activity of human liver in extrahepatic obstructive jaundice.' *Am. J. Path.* **49**, 605

Wyllie, J. C., More, R. H. and Haust, M. D. (1964). 'The fine structure of normal guinea pig synovium.' *Lab. Invest.* **13**, 1254

Yamamoto, T. (1963). 'On the thickness of the unit membrane.' *J. Cell Biol.* **17**, 413

Zamboni, L. and Gondos, B. (1968). 'Intercellular bridges and synchronization of germ cell differentiation during oogenesis in the rabbit.' *J. Cell Biol.* **36**, 276

CHAPTER XV

Endocytotic Structures and Cell Processes

INTRODUCTION

Extensions of the cell cytoplasm covered by cell membrane are collectively referred to as cell processes. Since some of these processes engage in endocytotic activity (e.g. pseudopodia in phagocytosis), it is convenient to consider together various cell processes and structures involved in endocytosis, and endocytotic phenomena such as: (1) micropinocytosis, whereby vesicles (called caveolae) springing from the cell membrane transport material into the cell; (2) micropinocytosis vermiformis, whereby material is transported via tubular channels; and (3) Langerhans cell granule, a structure of unique morphology which is also thought to be involved in the transport of material into the cell.

A variety of cell processes are known to occur on the cell surface and attempts have been made to classify them in various ways. Thus one may try to divide them into motile and non-motile processes, and into stable and ephemeral or transient processes. Such attempts are not too successful, for within a single morphological category different patterns of function and behaviour may be found (e.g. both motile and non-motile cilia are known to occur) and there is controversy regarding the nature and function of others. For example, it is not clear whether microvilli, which are considered a stable differentiation of the cell surface, represent merely a passive expansion of the cell surface providing an increased area for absorption, or whether they are contractile structures with a more complex mode of action.

However, the morphological distinctions between most cell processes are reasonably clear-cut. Cilia and flagella are distinguished by the presence of a basal body and an axial microtubule complex (page 508). In the striated or brush border of absorptive cells occur numerous uniform, slender processes called microvilli. A few microvilli occur also in a variety of other cells.

Pseudopodia are an example of blunt transient processes employed by cells such as amoeba or the neutrophil leucocyte for locomotion and the uptake of food particles and/or other extraneous matter. In ultrathin sections of tissues, long slender processes are at times encountered in some cells. Such an appearance often represents sections through folds or ruffles of the cell membrane. Cells in culture demonstrate that fusion of the margins of such folds leads to the formation of a vacuole in which impounded fluid is transported by a process called pinocytosis. No convenient acceptable term has been coined to describe those long slender 'cell processes' seen in sectioned material. Such processes abound in synovial intimal cells and students of this tissue have adopted the term 'filopodia' to describe them (*L. filium* = thread. Examples of true

485

filopodia are found in protozoa), yet such filopodia may or may not all be thread-like (three-dimensionally) and they certainly are not little feet or locomotor organs. However, the lack of a better term, and ignorance of the three-dimensional morphology of most of these processes, forces us to use the term 'filopodia' and even to extend its usage to other sites and situations where slender cell processes are seen in sectioned material.

In pathological and experimental situations processes may develop on cells that do not normally bear such processes, or have only a few processes. There is a tendency to call such processes microvilli, although often they bear little resemblance to these structures as they are neither uniform in size nor regularly arranged. Examples of such processes may be seen in cells in ascitic and other effusions and also in cells in oedematous tissues and in culture. These slender processes are more akin to filopodia than microvilli. Atypical cell processes may be found in tumour cells. The most florid example of this is the processes seen in a condition called 'hairy cell leukaemia (page 502).

ENDOCYTOTIC VESICLES AND VACUOLES

There are many ways by which substances can move in and out of the cell across the selective, semipermeable barrier imposed by the cell membrane. These include: (1) active transport, whereby substances are driven against a concentration gradient with energy originating from cell metabolism (e.g. from ATP; see page 468); (2) passive transport, whereby substances are driven across the cell membrane with energy supplied from external sources (e.g. osmotic forces or the application of an electrical potential); and (3) vesicular transport, whereby material is transported within single-membrane-bound vesicles or vacuoles derived from the cell membrane. Vesicular and vacuolar transport into the cell is now described by the term 'endocytosis', whereby the engulfed material ultimately comes to lie in a cytoplasmic vesicle or vacuole derived from the cell membrane. Similarly, vesicular transport out of the cell is spoken of as exocytosis, whereby a membrane-bound structure such as a secretory granule, a telolysosome or a vesicle derived by endocytosis fuses with the cell membrane and discharges its contents into the external environment.

In some instances the material leaving the cell takes with it a coat derived from the cell membrane. Examples of this are seen in the case of viruses, and particles of milk-secretion, which are liberated by a process of evagination and pinching off of the cell membrane (for references supporting the statements made above, see Bennett 1969a, b; Schoffeniels 1969a, b).

The first two methods of transport (active and passive) which are sometimes collectively referred to as transmembrane transport, or permeation, do not concern us here, for the ions and small molecules moved in this fashion are not directly demonstrable in electron micrographs.

Some 23 or more names have been coined by various workers to describe the process of endocytosis as seen in different sites and by different techniques. Fortunately, only three terms—namely, phagocytosis, pinocytosis and micropinocytosis—are in current use and seem adequate to describe most observed phenomena (*Plates 203–205*).

The terms 'phagocytosis' and 'pinocytosis' derive from the Greek roots for 'eating' and 'drinking' respectively.* Both phenomena are observable by light microscopy and have been recognized by students of the cell for a long time. The term 'phagocytosis' was coined by Metchinikoff (1883) to describe the process by which cells ingest food, and later he extended this to his well known concept of microphages (neutrophils) and macrophages and their role in defence mechanisms. Based on morphological differences of vacuole content, size of particles ingested and other small differences, a host of names were coined by other workers (e.g. colloidoplexy, chromopexy,

---

* The distinction between particulate uptake (eating) and fluid uptake (drinking) relate more to the resolving power of the microscope (light or electron) rather than the true state of affairs, for in the final analysis all matter is particulate. However, there is some value in retaining such distinctions from the morphological point of view.

Plate 203

Fig. 1. A human neutrophil leucocyte from peripheral blood, showing a pseudopod (P), which consists mainly of ectoplasm. The various organelles are confined to the endoplasm. The amoeboid movement of these leucocytes is accomplished by such pseudopodia. × 13,000

Fig. 2. The pseudopodia (P) on this leucocyte found in human bone marrow appear to be about to phagocytose a cell fragment. × 14,000

Fig. 3. Neutrophils phagocytosing staphylococci (S). From an *in vitro* preparation consisting of buffy coat of blood mixed with staphylococci. The cells were fixed 1 minute after the addition of the organisms. × 20,000 (*Skinnider and Ghadially, unpublished electron micrograph*)

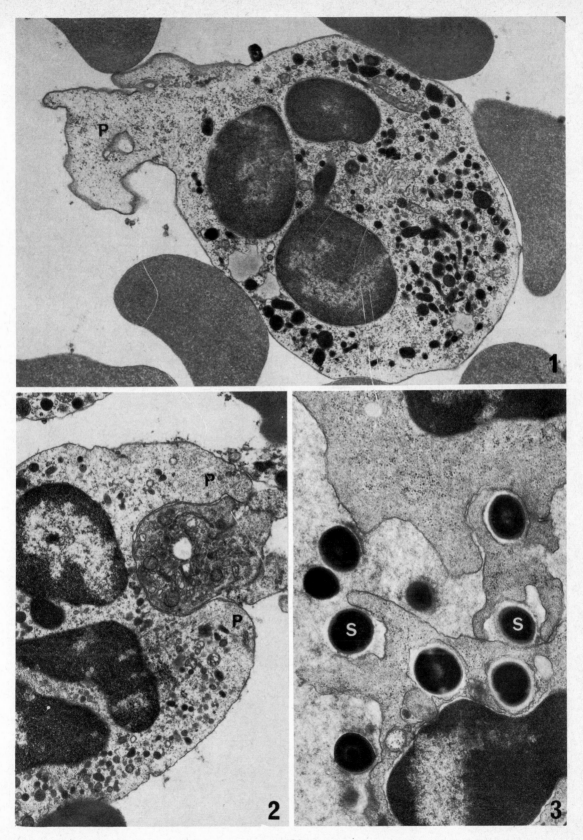

athrocytosis, phagotrophy and granulocytosis) to describe this phenomenon but these names are no longer used. The term 'phagocytosis' has, however, survived. Here it is envisaged that blunt pseudopodia arising from a cell such as a polymorphonuclear leucocyte (*Plate 203*) or an amoeba encircle some 'solid' particle or particles, and that fusion of such processes results in the trapping of the exogenous material in a membrane-bound vacuole which then moves into the cell. Usually, only the ectoplasmic zone of the cytoplasm is involved in the formation of pseudopodia. The major cytoplasmic organelles and inclusions as a rule do not flow into pseudopodia.

The term 'pinocytosis' was coined by Lewis (1931) to designate the vacuolar uptake of fluid by macrophages and sarcoma cells observed with phase-contrast microscopy. This phenomenon is commonly seen in tissue culture, where constantly moving and altering transient thin folds or ruffles are seen on the cell surface. Every now and again the margins of such folds fuse, or the margin of a fold fuses with the cell membrane to trap a droplet of fluid which then moves into the cytoplasm as a clear vacuole. It has long been debated whether such a phenomenon occurs *in vivo*. Certainly electron-microscopic images consistent with such a concept are seen, but, as is only to be expected, such folds and ruffles present as slender cell processes (filopodia) in sectioned material. Fawcett (1967) illustrates this in cells lining capillary endothelia, and the same is seen in the case of synovial cells which, with the aid of slender cell processes, can trap not only fluid but also fibrin and a variety of other materials (*Plate 204* and *Plate 154*) (Ghadially and Roy, 1969).

Electron microscopy reveals that, besides fluid, pinocytotic vacuoles may contain particulate matter, and in some instances quite large particulate material (e.g. entire erythrocytes) can be impounded by the filopodia of synovial cells. Thus the distinction between pinocytosis and phagocytosis is singularly tenuous. Except for the size and shape of the cell process, there is little that distinguishes the two in electron micrographs. Certainly cell 'eating' and cell 'drinking' are not such separate and distinct events, for both fluid and particulate matter are often impounded in a single gulp (see footnote on page 488).

Morphologically quite distinct from the above-mentioned processes is the process of micropinocytosis. Here small invaginations of the plasma membrane occur and later these detach by pinching off to form little vesicles which move into the cell. Both fluid and small particulate matter (e.g. ferritin, carbon or Thorotrast) is transported in this manner.

Plate 204

Synovial cells from an arthritic knee joint. (*Figs. 1 and 4 from Ghadially, Oryschak and Mitchell, 1974*)

Figs. 1 and 2. Filopodia wrapping around fibrin (F). Also seen are dense bodies (D) in the cell cytoplasm which represent phagosomes and phagolysosomes derived from the endocytosed fibrin. For a more detailed account of this phenomenon, see the legend to *Plate 154*. × 26,000; × 25,000

Fig. 3. Here again, filopodia are seen trapping fibrin. An unusual feature here is that part of the wall of an endocytotic vacuole is markedly thickened and electron dense (arrow). × 30,000

Fig. 4. At higher magnification, another forming or formed vacuole from the same specimen as *Fig. 3* shows that the thickening is due to the deposition of fuzzy electron-dense material on the cytoplasmic side of the cell membrane. Electron-dense material also coats the inner surface of the vacuole, but it is separated from the cell membrane by a less dense layer. × 65,000

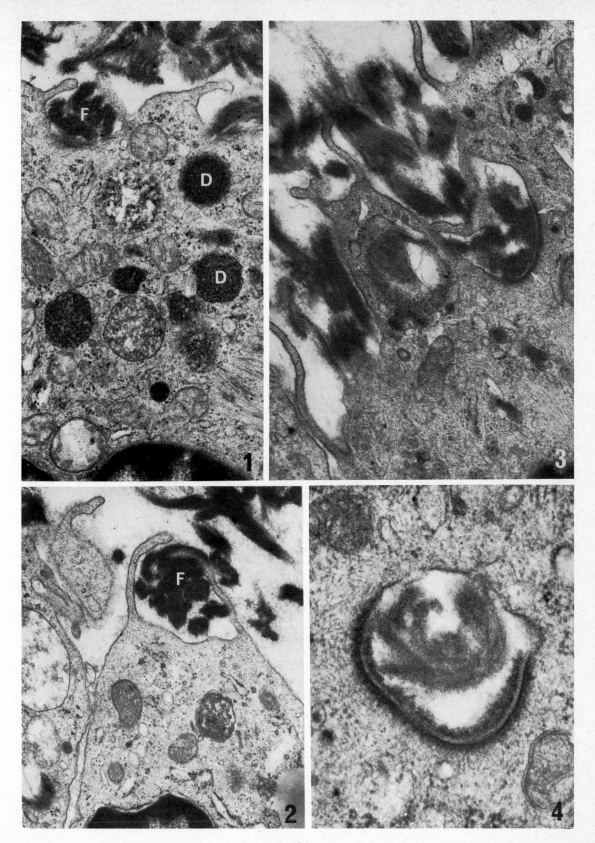

491

Micropinocytotic vesicles present in electron micrographs as alveolate or flask-shaped structures of uniform size (400–800 Å in diameter) attached to the cell membrane. Such an appearance could represent either a vesicle about to form and move into the cell (endocytosis) or a vesicle which has fused with the cell membrane and is discharging its contents into the cell environment (exocytosis). Since such distinctions cannot be made in a routine electron micrograph, it has been suggested that a morphologically descriptive but non-committal term such as 'caveolae' (first proposed by Yamada in 1955) would be more appropriate to describe these structures than 'micropinocytotic vesicles', which has functional connotations. Although this is a perfectly logical suggestion, the term 'caveolae' is used only occasionally.

A few micropinocytotic vesicles may be found in most cell types. but they are particularly common in capillary endothelia and in smooth and striated muscle (*Plate 205*; also *Plate 177*). Such vesicles are also at times quite numerous in synovial cells and chondrocytes. An abundance of micropinocytotic vesicles is an indication of heightened endocytotic activity, and it is said that this can be provoked by presenting the cell with material which is ingested by this mechanism (Stockem and Wohlfrath-Bottermann, 1969).

Various terms such as 'fuzzy vesicles', 'coated vesicles', 'alveolate vesicles', 'acanthosomes' and 'decorated vesicles' have been used to describe micropinocytic vesicles bearing filamentous and spiny adornments on their limiting membrane. Fuzzy micropinocytotic vesicles form when protein is being transported into the cell. An example of this is the fuzzy or spiny vesicle which is believed to transport ferritin destined for haemoglobin synthesis into the erythroblast (*Plate 205*). Fuzzy vesicles have been seen in many other situations, but the most conspicuous examples are found (Fawcett. 1967) in the oöcytes of insects at a stage when rapid uptake of protein is occurring.

We (Ghadially *et al.*, 1974) have recently noted that much larger endocytotic vacuoles may also develop a fuzzy or coated appearance when fibrin is being endocytosed by synovial cells. This was seen in a patient who had long-standing multiple sclerosis, psoriasis and arthritis. Here however the vacuoles were only partially coated, in the sense that only a portion of the circumference of the vacuole was coated and bore filamentous decorations on its cytoplasmic surface (*Plate 204*, *Figs. 3 and 4*).

Phagocytosis, pinocytosis and micropinocytosis all lead to the formation of a single-membrane-bound structure containing engulfed material. We have seen that distinction between these processes is at times subtle and difficult. Endocytosis may be followed by exocytosis so that the material is transported across the cell from one border to another (e.g. in capillary endothelium), but often the endocytotic vacuole is a phagosome which subsequently fuses with a primary lysosome or lysosomes to form a phagolysosome. The development and fate of these structures has been dealt with in Chapter VII.

Plate 205

Fig. 1. A vascular capillary from normal rabbit synovial membrane, showing unusually numerous caveolae (arrows). The nucleus of an endothelial cell (N), the lumen of a vessel (L) and the basal lamina (B) are easily identified. × 56,000 (*Ghadially and Roy, unpublished electron micrograph*)

Fig. 2. Erythroblast (normoblast) from human bone marrow, showing three fuzzy vesicles (arrowheads) in the process of formation from the cell membrane. × 17,500

Figs. 3, 4 and 5. Depict the manner in which fuzzy vesicles transporting ferritin develop. *Fig. 3* shows the cell membranes of two erythroblasts which were lying side by side. One of these shows a saucer-shaped depression where the cell membrane has acquired a fuzzy coat and some electron-dense particles (arrowhead) believed to be ferritin. *Fig. 4* shows two vesicles (arrowheads) which depict further stages of development, while *Fig. 5* shows a vesicle about to be detached or recently detached from the cell membrane. × 90,000; × 90,000; × 90,000

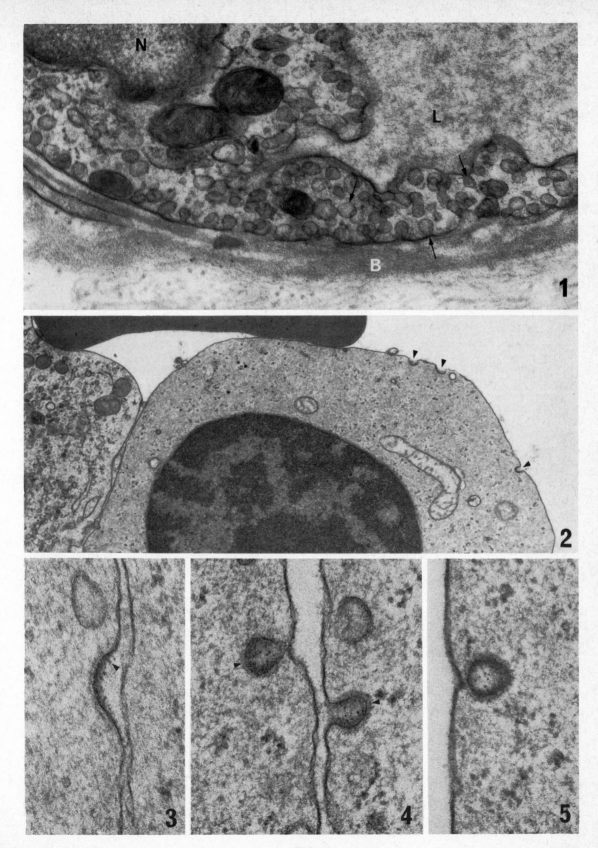

Micropinocytosis vermiformis, a term coined by Matter *et al.* (1968), is used to describe a unique type of endocytotic activity executed via certain worm-like structures first described by Toro *et al.* (1962) in the Kupffer cells of the rat liver. In favourable sections these formations are seen to be lamellar invaginations of the cell membrane of a fairly constant width (800–1,250 Å) which meander into the cell.

Also seen is a dotted or shaggy median line running along their length, produced by apposition of the free margins of the doubled-up cell coat as it extends into these invaginations. Fuzzy or coated vesicles, at times continuous with these lamellae, are also seen. This may represent fusion of pre-existing vesicles with the lamellae or the genesis of fuzzy vesicles from the wall of this structure.

Micropinocytosis vermiformis is not routinely seen in Kupffer cells; when present, it is thought to represent an exaggerated or intensified form of endocytosis. Since the discovery of this structure by Toro *et al.* (1962), various other workers have seen micropinocytosis vermicularis in Kupffer cells of the rat and rabbit under normal and experimental situations (Rohlich and Toro, 1964; Melis and Orci, 1967; Orci *et al.*, 1967; Matter *et al.*, 1968; Horn *et al.*, 1969; Wisse and Daems, 1970a, b; Pfeifer, 1970; Fahimi, 1970; Emeis and Wisse, 1971).

These studies have shown that micropinocytosis vermiformis (in Kupffer cells and occasionally also in splenic macrophages) can be induced by the injection of a variety of substances or by partial hepatectomy. Micropinocytosis vermiformis has also been demonstrated in macrophages harvested from the peritoneal cavity of the rat (Brederoo and Daems, 1972). These authors report that the omission of washing and centrifugation prior to fixation was important in preserving these structures and they point out that in previous studies where micropinocytosis vermiformis has been demonstrated in the Kupffer cells, *in situ* fixation by vascular perfusion has been employed.

It has long been suspected from observations on animals injected with colloidal substances that Kupffer cells can migrate to the lung (Simpson, 1922; Irwin, 1932; Nicol and Bilbey, 1958; Patek and Bernick, 1960; Collet and Policard, 1962; Frankel *et al.*, 1962), and it has been suggested that alveolar macrophages may derive from such cells trapped in pulmonary capillaries (Florey, 1958).

These ideas gain fresh support from the elegant experiments of Schneeberger-Keeley and Burger (1970). In these experiments Kupffer cells of cats were first labelled with a critical dose of colloidal carbon. When such animals were subjected a week later to one hour of open-chest ventilation the lungs came to contain numerous cells similar to Kupffer cells, showing both micropinocytosis vermiformis and vacuoles containing the carbon label. Hardly any cells showing micropinocytosis vermiformis were seen in the lungs of control animals. These authors conclude that 'the manipulations and drugs used in open-chest ventilation are powerful enough stimuli in the cat to induce migration of hepatic macrophages to the lung and cause micropinocytosis vermiformis in them'.

Plate 206

Fig. 1. An air space (A) and two pulmonary capillaries lined by endothelial cells (E) are seen here. Each capillary contains a phagocytic cell (P) showing micropinocytosis vermiformis (arrows). From the lung of a cat subjected to open-chest ventilation. (Kupffer cells were not labelled with carbon in this experiment.) × 15,000 (*From Schneeberger-Keleey and Burger, 1970*)

Fig. 2. Periphery of a phagocytic cell, showing micropinocytosis vermiformis. Numerous lamellae with a shaggy median line (M) are seen. Also present are coated vesicles (V), one of which (arrow) is continuous with a lamella. × 56,000 (*From Schneeberger-Keleey and Burger, 1970*)

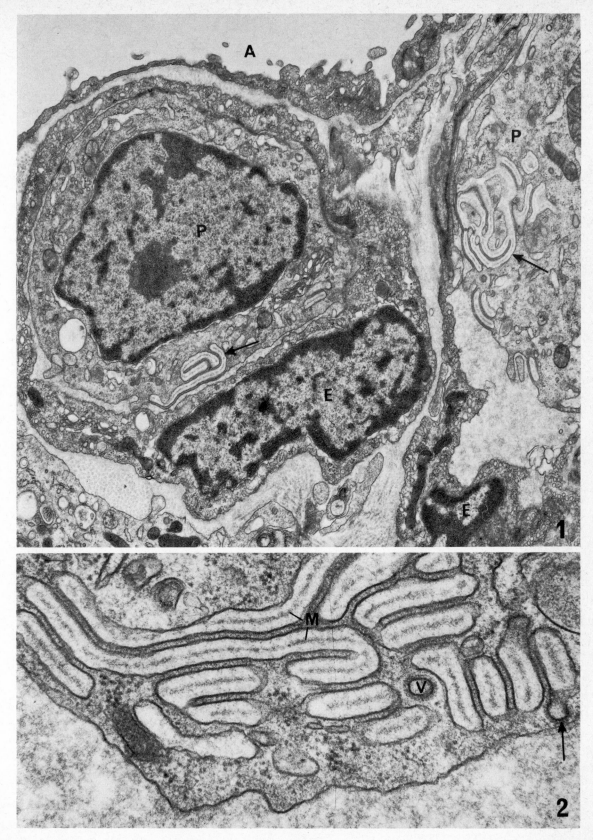

495

The intraepidermal gold-chloride-positive dendritic cells described by Langerhans (1868) were at one time regarded either as intraepidermal neural elements (see Niebauer, 1968) or as effete melanocytes (Masson, 1948, 1951; Billingham and Medawar, 1953; Billingham and Silvers, 1960). Ultrastructurally, this cell is characterized by the presence of cytoplasmic granules which present rod-shaped, flask-shaped or tennis-racket-shaped profiles in sectioned material. The rod-shaped structure or the handle of the racket shows a median striated line. Three-dimensional reconstruction of these granules by Wolff (1967) and Sagebiel and Reed (1968) show that they are basically discoid bodies (straight, curved or cup-shaped) with a focal vesicular expansion at the margin of the disc. The stippled line represents sections through paracrystalline nets or lattices with a periodicity of 90 Å.

Since Langerhans cell granules have at times been seen in continuity with the cell membrane, it is thought that they are produced here and represent a unique variety of endocytosis or that they are 'secretory' granules arising from the Golgi discharging their contents on to the cell surface. It is the former hypothesis which is now generally accepted (Hashimoto, 1970).

Langerhans cells characterized by the presence of these specific granules have now been found in various squamous epithelia such as cutaneous, ungual, gingival, buccal, glossal and cervical of man and experimental animals (Birbeck et al., 1961; Breathnach, 1964, 1965; Schroeder and Theilade, 1966; Hackemann et al., 1968; Hashimoto, 1970, 1971; Hutchens et al., 1971). Occasionally, melanin granules have been demonstrated in Langerhans cells (Breathnach and Wyllie, 1965) but they take the form of compound melanosomes as seen in keratinocytes and melanophages, so there is no reason to believe that melanosome formation and melanin synthesis occur here as in melanocytes. In achromic skin such as that found in vitiligo, pinta, the halo of halo naevus, the forelock area of human skin in piebaldism and the white areas of skin from recessively spotted black and white guinea-pigs, there is said to be an increase in the number of Langerhans cells and a diminution or absence of melanocytes (for references, see Rodriguez et al., 1971). This suggests a close relationship between melanocytes and Langerhans cells, but it is now difficult to accept that Langerhans cells are derived from melanocytes or that these two share a common lineage because cells containing these characteristic granules have been seen in: (1) the histiocytes of numerous cases of histiocytosis X (Hand–Schuller–Christian disease, Letterer–Siwe disease and eosinophil granuloma) (Basset et al., 1965; Turiaf and Basset, 1965; Basset and Nezelof, 1966; Hashimoto and Tarnowski, 1967; Cancilla et al., 1967; Tarnowski and Hashimoto, 1967; Cancilla, 1968; Gianotti and Caputo, 1969; De Man, 1968; Morales et al., 1969; Carrington and Winkelmann, 1972); (2) reticulum cell sarcoma and macrophages of pityriasis rosea (Hashimoto and Tarnowski, 1968); (3) human lymph nodes of dermatopathic lymphadenopathy (Jimbow et al., 1969); (4) normal lymph nodes of rabbit (Kondo, 1969); and (5) hyperplastic lymph nodes of man (Shamoto et al., 1971).

Thus it is now thought that the Langerhans cell is not related to melanocytes and that the characteristic granule is a feature of mesenchymal or certain histiocytic cells. Since such cells have now been seen crossing the basement membrane by more than one observer, and such cells have also been observed dividing, Hashimoto and Tarnowski (1968) have proposed that they 'may constitute a self-perpetuating "intraepidermal phagocytic system" to which histiocytes from the dermis are added from time to time'.

Plate 207

Langerhans cell from human epidermis, showing granules presenting rod-shaped (R) and tennis-racket-shaped (T) profiles. The discoid shape of the granule and the paracrystalline lattice (L) is better appreciated in tangential cuts through these structures. × 58,000

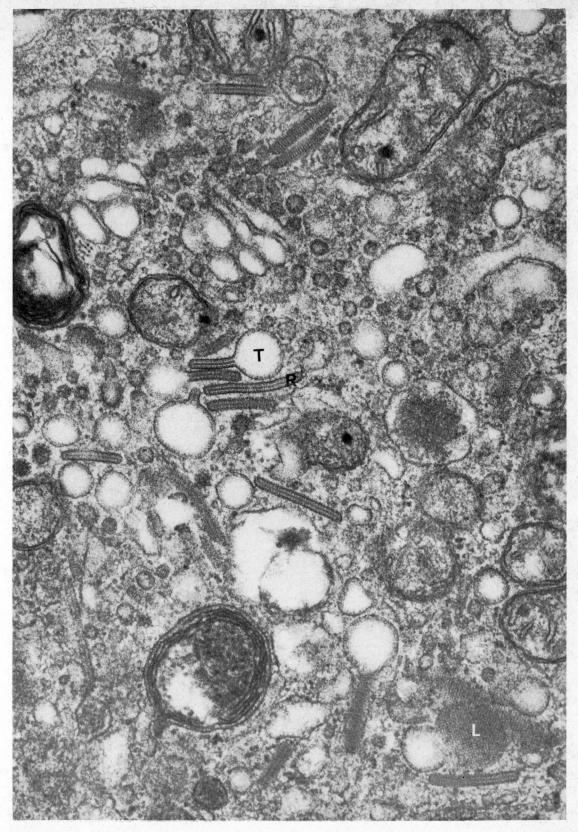

MICROVILLI

Numerous prominent, regularly arranged microvilli are usually found on the free surface of cells whose principal function is absorption. Fewer, less tidily arranged microvilli may, however, be seen on a variety of other cells. Microvilli are considered to be stable differentiations of the cell surface, in contrast to transient cell processes such as those formed during pinocytosis and phagocytosis. Microvilli are distinguished from cilia and flagella by the absence of a basal body and the characteristic 9 + 2 microtubule complex found in the latter two structures. It is thought that microvilli facilitate absorption by amplification of the cell surface.

Microvilli, remarkably uniform in size and shape, are found in the proximal convoluted tubule of the kidney and the intestinal mucosa (*Plates 195–197*), where they constitute the well known striated or brush border seen at light microscopy. Straight fine filaments run the length of such microvilli and extend downwards into the apical cell cytoplasm to mingle with the network of fine filaments in this region which forms the terminal web. Recent studies (Rostgaard and Thuneberg, 1972) on the isolated brush border of proximal tubule cells of mammalian kidneys have shown that the core of the microvillus contains filaments (50–70 Å in diameter) forming an axial bundle with a 6 + 1 configuration (i.e. one central filament surrounded by a ring of six filaments). These filaments are said to resemble actin filament and it is therefore thought that these microvilli have contractile properties which may play a part in absorptive processes.

Microvilli occur not only on absorptive surfaces but also at times on secretory and other surfaces. For example, in the liver, microvilli are found on both the absorptive (space of Disse) and secretory (bile canaliculus) poles of hepatocytes (*Plate 208, Fig. 1*). These microvilli are, however, not as regular in size or arrangement as those found in the gut.

Singularly long slender microvilli (three to four times longer than those seen in the brush border of the gut) are found on epididymal epithelium (*Plate 208, Fig. 2*). The term 'stereocilia' has long been used to describe these structures, but it is now evident that they are not cilia for they lack the characteristic basal body and axial microtubule complex (*Plate 213, Figs. 1 and 4*). Fine filaments are, however, readily demonstrated in these microvilli (*Plate 208, Figs. 3 and 4*). Another variation of microvillar form is the clavate microvillus found in the choroid plexus. These club-shaped microvilli show much irregularity of size, shape and arrangement.

Plate 208

Fig. 1. A bile canaliculus from cow liver, showing numerous microvilli. Note also the junction complexes between the adjacent hepatocyte cell membranes forming the canaliculus. × 27,000

Fig. 2. Stereocilia. From mouse epididymis. × 37,000

Figs. 3 and 4. Longitudinal and transverse sections through stereocilia, showing filaments (arrows) in their interior. From the same specimen as *Fig. 2*. × 68,000; × 98,000

498

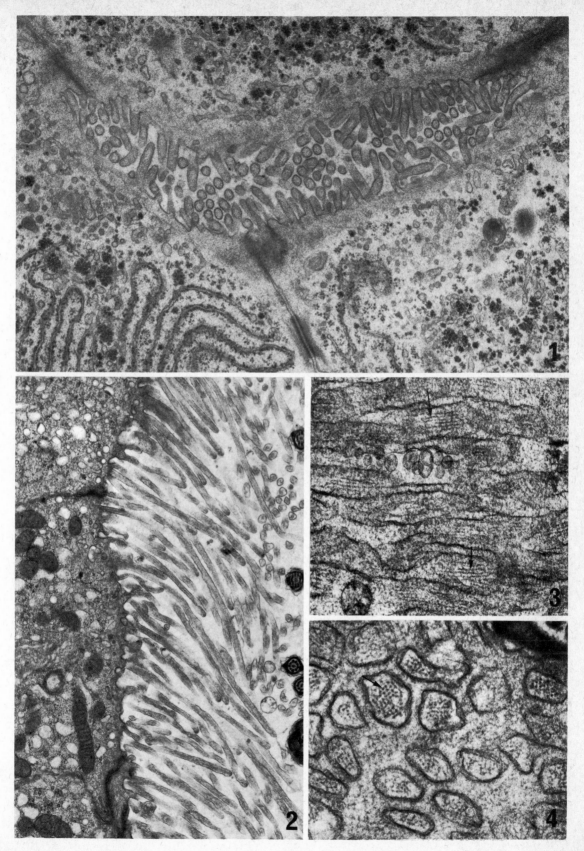

499

MORPHOLOGICAL ALTERATIONS IN MICROVILLI

Numerous alterations in microvilli have been noted in experimental situations and pathological states. Such changes include an increase or decrease in size and number of microvilli, ballooning of microvilli and fusion of microvilli. Such changes are quite common and only a few examples relating to microvilli in the liver and gut are presented here.

A reduction or absence of microvilli in bile canaliculi is seen after partial hepatectomy in the rat. This is part of the 'simplification' or dedifferentiation which occurs in hepatocytes preparing for mitosis. In hepatomas also, one of the ways in which the dedifferentiation of neoplasia may be expressed is by a loss of microvilli (Ghadially and Parry, 1966). We have seen a reduction of bile canalicular microvilli in the liver of rats bearing transplanted and carcinogen-induced tumours in their flanks (*Plate 209*). An increase in the number of microvilli in the space of Disse has been noted in: (1) rats after talcum-injury (Baum and Nishimura, 1964); (2) rabbits after injection of antigen–antibody complexes (Steiner, 1961); and (3) mice infected with hepatitis agent (Svoboda *et al.*, 1962). A ballooning of microvilli in the space of Disse 30 minutes after the administration of carbon tetrachloride was described by Reynolds (1963).

Alterations in the structure of intestinal villi and microvilli have received much attention. In coeliac sprue, electron microscopy of absorptive cells reveals an irregularity of arrangement, shortening, widening and fusion of microvilli (for references, see Trier and Rubin, 1965; Yardley *et al.*, 1962). Such changes are thought to reduce markedly the absorptive surface and impair the functional capacity of the gut. It is interesting to note, however, that in the majority of patients with clinically detectable malabsorption such morphological alterations are not evident. Such examples include postgastrectomy malabsorption, diabetic steatorrhea, pancreatic insufficiency and many others (Trier, 1967).

Dilatation and vesiculation of the microvilli have been observed in human jejunal biopsies after a single large dose of intravenous methotrexate (Trier and Rubin, 1965) and within 1 hour in mouse small intestine after a high dose of x-rays (Quastler and Hampton, 1962; Hugon *et al.*, 1963). At a later stage of the experiment the intestinal villi are populated by cuboidal cells with large nuclei and sparse short microvilli. Similar changes have also been described in the human small intestine after therapeutic field irradiation with 2,000–3,000 r (Trier and Browning, 1965).

In cholera a voluminous outpouring of fluid occurs from the surface of the intestinal mucosa and it is now well known that this loss occurs through a fairly intact mucosa and not through a necrotic mucosa denuded of cells. Ultrastructural studies (Chen *et al.*, 1971) have shown that fluid released from the vessels into the lamina propria is effectively prevented from reaching the lumen via an intercellular route by the tight junctions of the terminal bar. Instead, the fluid finds its way into the cells via the lateral cell borders and appears in vesicles and vacuoles formed from the endoplasmic reticulum. The final route of escape seems to be via the microvilli, for many bullous villi are seen containing either oedematous cytoplasmic material or numerous fluid-containing membrane-bound vacuoles.

Plate 209

Fig. 1. Bile canaliculus from the liver of a rat bearing a subcutaneous sarcoma. A portion of the canaliculus (between arrowheads) is well populated by microvilli and gives some idea as to what a normal canaliculus looks like (*see also Plate 208, Fig. 1*). The remainder of the canaliculus shows a paucity of microvilli. × 26,000 (*Ghadially and Parry, unpublished electron micrograph*)

Fig. 2. Bile canaliculus from another rat bearing a subcutaneous sarcoma, showing a more severe loss of microvilli. × 52,000 (*Ghadially and Parry, unpublished electron micrograph*)

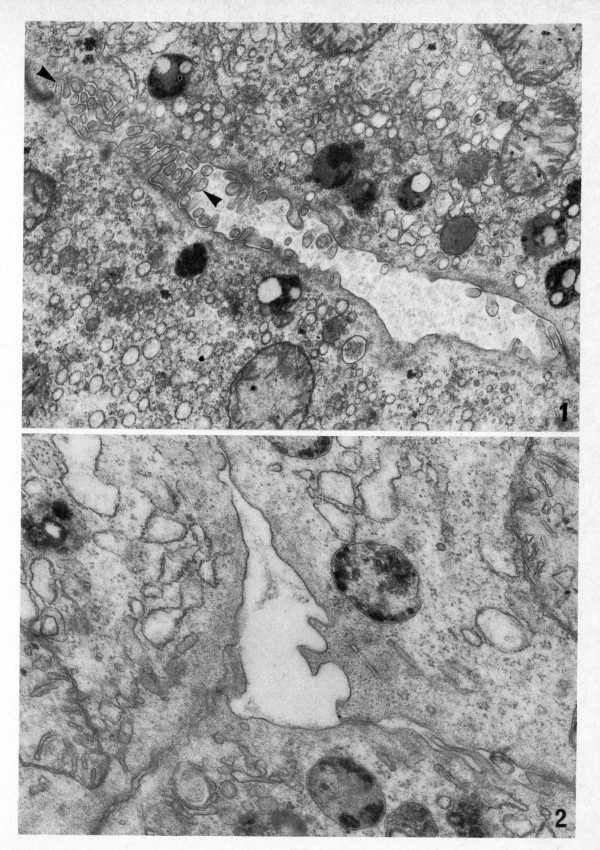

501

CELL PROCESSES IN HAIRY CELL LEUKAEMIA

Several cases of this unusual type of leukaemia, which is characterized by leukaemic cells with a ragged appearance and numerous cell processes, have been described (Mitus *et al.*, 1961; Schrek and Donnelly, 1966; Plenderleith, 1970; Mitus, 1971). It is now aptly called a 'hairy cell' leukaemia. It would appear that similar cases have also been reported by some authors (Ewald, 1923; Bouroncle *et al.*, 1958; Yam *et al.*, 1968, 1971) as leukaemic reticuloendotheliosis and reticulum cell leukaemia. The nature of the hairy cell and the classification of this leukaemia is uncertain.

At light microscopy the dense nucleus and scant cytoplasm lend support to the idea that this is a variety of lymphocyte, the only disconcerting feature being the cell processes which can be seen at light microscopy but are much more clearly demonstrated by electron microscopy. These cell processes are somewhat reminiscent of the filopodia seen on synovial cells, but they do not seem to be engaged in endocytotic activity, and in the case we studied (Ghadially and Skinnider, 1972), dense bodies acceptable as lysosomes were virtually absent.

Since reticulum cells and histiocytes are the only cells in the haemopoietic tissues well endowed with cell processes, attempts have been made to relate these hairy cells to reticulum cells or histiocytes. Katayama *et al.* (1972) did not succeed in demonstrating acid phosphatase activity in these cells with the Gomori method, but activity was demonstrated using an azo-dye method in some of the clear vacuoles in these cells. The cells illustrated in their paper are not particularly hairy, nor are the clinical and light microscopic findings presented. Neoplastic cells from three patients in the leukaemic phase of reticulum cell sarcoma have recently been described by Schnitzer and Kass (1973). Such cells have a few small processes but the authors quite rightly conclude that these cells are quite different from the hairy leukaemic cells.

Various other observations which suggest that hairy cell leukaemia is a variety of lymphocytic leukaemia and that these cells are not related to reticulum cells or monocytes are as follows: (1) reticulum cells and monocytic or histiocytic cells have a pale nucleus with a prominent nucleolus, but hairy cells have a dense nucleus and a small nucleolus; (2) the virtual absence of pinocytotic, micropinocytotic and lysosomal activity seen in our case (Ghadially and Skinnider, 1972), and the inability of hairy cells to phagocytose latex particles (Schrek and Donnelly, 1966), also argue against the idea that these cells are related to histiocytic cells; (3) it is now well documented that lymphocytes often cluster around and establish connections with macrophages, and we have shown that hairy cells behave in the same way (Ghadially and Skinnider, 1972); (4) a recent review of 100 cases of reticulum cell sarcoma has shown that in no instance did hairy cells appear in the blood, while cases of hairy cell leukaemia do not develop the characteristic lymph node masses and skin infiltrates of reticulum cell sarcoma; and (5) the average survival time for reticulum cell sarcoma is about 9 months, while for hairy cell leukaemia it is 4 years.

The reason for the hairiness of these cells remains obscure, but an interesting finding in our study (Ghadially and Skinnider, 1972) was that plasma cells and erythrocytic series of cells were also similarly affected. The latter phenomenon is discussed in the next section of this chapter.

Plate 210

Leukaemic cells from a case of hairy cell leukaemia. Note the dense nucleus, and the absence of dense bodies acceptable as lysosomes.

Fig. 1. Shaggy leukaemic cells with long cell processes. × 18,000

Fig. 2. A ragged leukaemic cell. × 7,500 (*From Ghadially and Skinnider, 1972*)

Fig. 3. A cell with relatively few short processes. × 13,500 (*From Ghadially and Skinnider, 1972*)

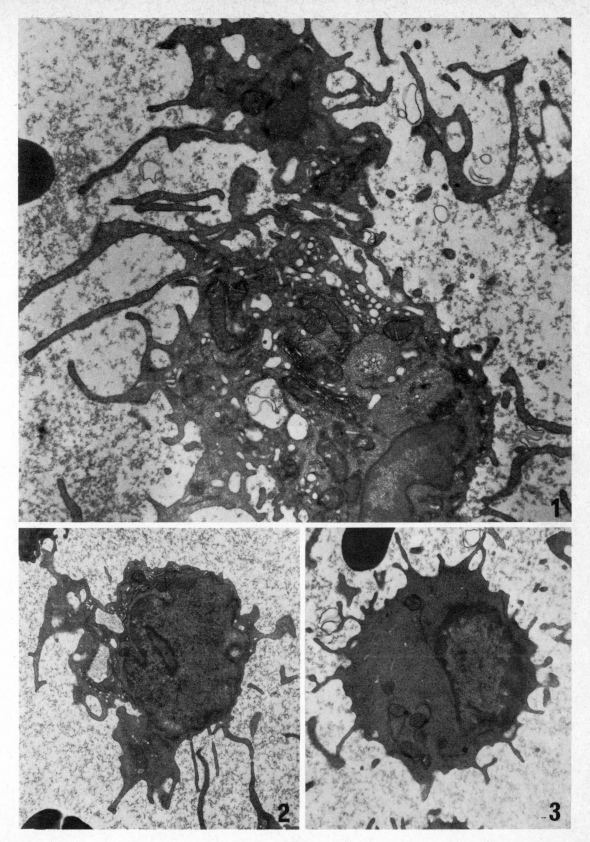

During the course of our studies (Ghadially and Skinnider, 1971, 1972) on a case of hairy cell leukaemia (page 502) we observed a remarkable abnormality in the form of the erythrocytes and their precursors. A normocytic, normochromic anaemia is commonly associated with this condition, but light microscopy of blood films and bone marrow shows no overt alterations of erythrocytic morphology, apart from the occurrence of an occasional burr cell.

However, ultrathin sections of marrow and peripheral blood from our case revealed complex alterations in the morphology of normoblasts (*Plate 211*), reticulocytes (*Plate 211*), and erythrocytes (*Plate 212*). The alterations in form are often quite complex, so that no two cells look exactly alike, but the basic feature here seems to be the occurrence of branched and unbranched cell processes which often appear club-shaped. It is worth noting that this is the appearance seen in ultrathin sections. It is more than likely that a three-dimensional view would reveal that many of these processes are complex folds or deep invaginations of the cell membrane.

Since the basic defect presents in ultrathin sections as club-shaped processes and the Greek for club is *ropalon*, we coined the term 'ropalocytosis' to describe this abnormality of erythrocytic form (Ghadially and Skinnider, 1971).

Since then a search for ropalocytes has also been made in the blood and bone marrow from patients with various haematological disorders (14 cases), and such cells have been seen in idiopathic thrombocytopenic purpura, pernicious anaemia and Hodgkin's disease involving the bone marrow (Skinnider and Ghadially, 1973).

It will be evident that ropalocytes are quite distinct and different from other well known forms of abnormal erythrocytes such as schistocytes, echinocytes and target cells. The abnormality of form that characterizes these latter cells is best recognized by light microscopy of entire erythrocytes. In ultrathin sections they present little evidence of their characteristic form and are thus difficult or impossible to recognize with any degree of confidence. In contrast to this, ropalocytosis is a fine structural manifestation and, as already noted, light microscopy gives no clear indication of its presence. A further distinguishing feature is that ropalocytosis affects the entire series of erythroid cells and not just mature erythrocytes.

Plate 211

Fig. 1. A normoblast showing a mild degree of focal ropalocytosis. × 16,000 (*From Skinnider and Ghadially, 1973*)

Fig. 2. Normoblasts showing marked ropalocytosis. The entire cell has a ragged appearance produced by the abundance of processes and vacuoles. Fine vesicles are seen in the main cytoplasmic mass and also in the cell processes. × 15,000 (*From Skinnider and Ghadially, 1973*)

Fig. 3. A reticulocyte showing short club-shaped, sessile and pedunculated processes. × 11,000 (*Ghadially and Skinnider, unpublished electron micrograph*)

Fig. 4. A reticulocyte from peripheral blood, showing a picturesque alteration of over-all shape and cell processes. × 10,500 (*From Ghadially and Skinnider, 1971*)

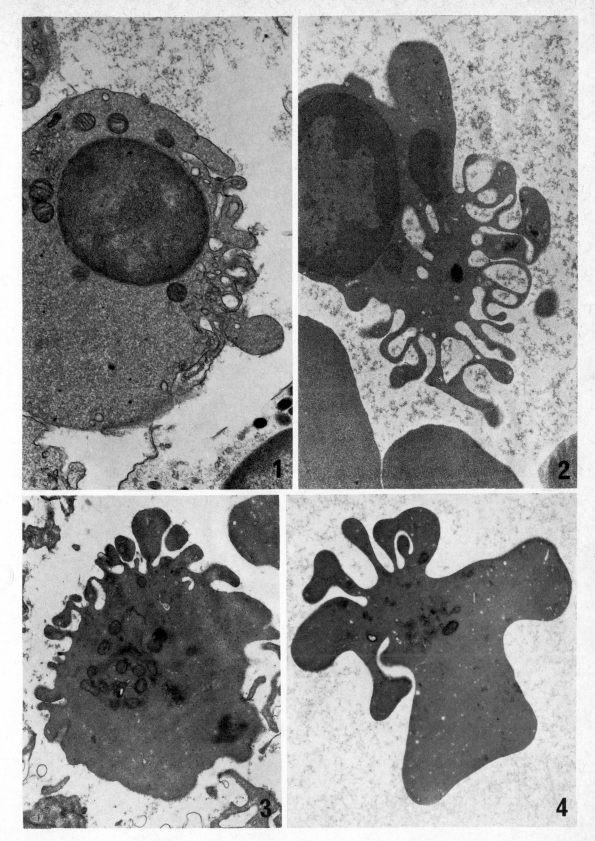

505

As noted earlier, this change is seen in erythrocytes (*Plate 212*), reticulocytes (*Plate 211*) and normoblasts (*Plate 211*), but in every case where this defect has been found the reticulocytes were most frequently involved, the defect being less frequent in normoblasts and quite rare in erythrocytes. Although at times the entire cell may be grossly deformed, with numerous processes springing from its entire surface, in most instances the defect is focal, with only a segment of the cell affected.

The significance of this change and the manner in which it is produced is obscure. In studies on the denucleation of normoblasts in dogs rendered anaemic by various means, Simpson and Kling (1967) noted the occurrence of numerous small vesicles on the 'underside' of the nucleus apposed to the cell membrane. They postulated that fusion of such vesicles leads to the detachment of the marginated nucleus and may leave behind a ragged area of cell wall. This in some instances bears a resemblance to the change we are describing (see their Fig. 10). However, our experience with denucleating normoblasts in human bone marrow is not in keeping with this and the fact that ropalocytosis is seen in normoblasts with intact nuclei argues against the idea that ropalocytosis is produced in this fashion (Skinnider and Ghadially, 1973).

It is noted in Chapter VII that cytolysosomes occur in erythrocytes (page 326) and that when their contents are discharged or when such bodies are removed by the spleen, clear tracts extending from within the cell to its surface are left behind. The possibility that ropalocytosis results from a heightened activity of this kind was not borne out by our investigations, for there was no positive correlation between the occurrence of cytolysosomes and ropalocytosis in the cases we studied.

The only positive correlation seemed to be between the occurrence of vesicles in these cells and ropalocytosis. It is likely that some but not all such vesicles represented sections through invaginations of the plasma membrane, for often such vesicles were too numerous, not near the cell surface, and quite small.

It seems to us that both pinocytotic and micropinocytotic activity are heightened in these cells (Skinnider and Ghadially, 1973), but the stimulus which provokes this change remains obscure. If this tentative supposition is correct, then one could speculate that it could be due to a deficiency of some factor needed by the cell, or to the presence of some stimulating agent in the cell environment.

Plate 212

Fig. 1. Two cells showing ropalocytosis are seen here. The one in the top right-hand corner may be regarded as an erythrocyte and the one in the bottom left-hand corner as a late reticulocyte, for it contains a few ribosomes (not clearly evident here but seen at higher magnification). Note also the numerous fine vesicles in its cytoplasm. Three normal-looking erythrocytes are seen in the bottom right-hand corner. × 10,000 (*From Skinnider and Ghadially, 1973*)

Fig. 2. An erythrocyte showing ropalocytosis. × 14,000 (*From Skinnider and Ghadially, 1973*)

Fig. 3. A singularly picturesque alteration of erythrocytic morphology is seen here. Islands and bands of erythroid substance are seen as a network or a maze from which spring many club-shaped processes. The general pattern here is continuous and the over-all maximum dimension is about 6 µ; hence it is conceivable that this is a single altered erythrocyte rather than two or more erythrocytes lying close to one another, but one cannot be certain. × 22,000 (*From Ghadially and Skinnider, 1972*)

506

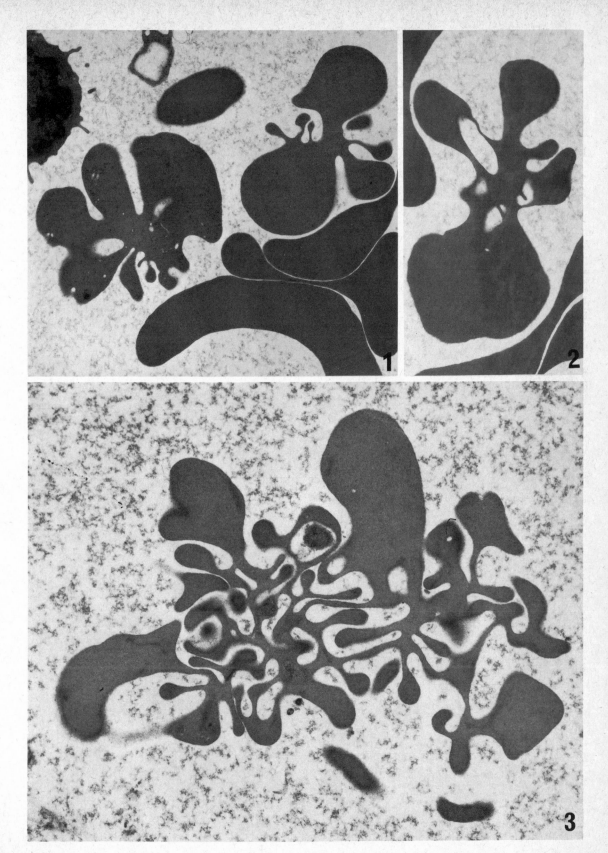

Certain cylindrical, hair-like motile processes first observed on some protozoa and later on certain epithelia of higher animals, have long been known to light microscopists as cilia and flagella. It has been customary to call relatively short numerous processes arising from a cell 'cilia' while the term 'flagella' has been reserved for longer, solitary or not too numerous processes arising from the cell. According to Fawcett (1967), 'The shaft of the cilium is 0·2 to 0·25 μ in diameter and 5 to 10 μ long. Flagella range from this length to 150 μ or more.' Ultrastructural studies have shown that the basic structure of cilia and flagella is identical. Many cell processes which in the past were classified as flagella are now called cilia and the term 'cilia' is often used in a collective sense when referring to both cilia proper and flagella.

In suitable preparations examined with the light microscope, a small granular body can be seen in the cell close to the base of the cilium, as can an axial filament (axoneme) which arises from this structure and runs along almost the entire length of the cilium. Ultrastructural studies show that the granular body referred to as a 'basal body', 'basal corpuscle', 'basal granule', 'kinetoplast' or 'blepharoplast' is in fact a hollow cylinder with the same structure as a centriole. The homology of these two structures, recognized long ago by cytologists (Henneguy, 1897; Lenhossek, 1898), has now been confirmed by electron microscopists (see page 93). On the basis of fine structural variations of morphology, about six types of basal bodies have been identified (Fawcett, 1961; Randall and Hopkins, 1962). Striated rootlets (usual periodicity about 700 Å), apparently serving to anchor the basal bodies, are often seen associated with most types of cilia, as are microtubules or filaments connected to the basal bodies and rootlets (*Plate 213, Fig. 1*). Whether these filaments or microtubules are anchoring devices or play a role in the co-ordination and propagation of the ciliary wave has been frequently debated (Parducz, 1967).

The electron microscope shows that the axial filament of the light microscopist is not a single filament but a bundle of microtubules (called filaments by some workers; for discussion on this point, see page 94). This structure, now referred to as the 'axial filament complex', 'axoneme' or 'axial microtubule complex', shows nine pairs of microtubules arranged in a circle around the periphery of the cilium, and two microtubules in the centre. This is referred to as the '9 + 2'

Plate 213

Fig. 1. The proximal portions of cilia from human bronchial mucosa are depicted here (for a low power view, see *Plate 59*). Besides the cilia with their axial microtubule complex (A), some microvilli (M) are seen, springing from the cell surface. Also seen are basal bodies (B), striated rootlets (R) and associated filaments (F). × 40,000

Fig. 2. Transversely cut cilia from the bronchial mucosa of a cow, showing the characteristic 9 + 2 pattern of microtubules. × 89,000

Fig. 3. Transverse section of cilia near their terminal part. The microtubules terminate at variable distances as the tip of the cilium is approached so that fewer microtubules are seen and doublets are replaced by singlets (arrow). × 83,000

Fig. 4. A 9 + 2 cilium from human bronchial mucosa. Note the trilaminar structure of the ciliary membrane, the central microtubules (C) and the peripheral doublets comprising microtubules A and B, and the short arms (arrowheads) arising from microtuble A. × 160,000

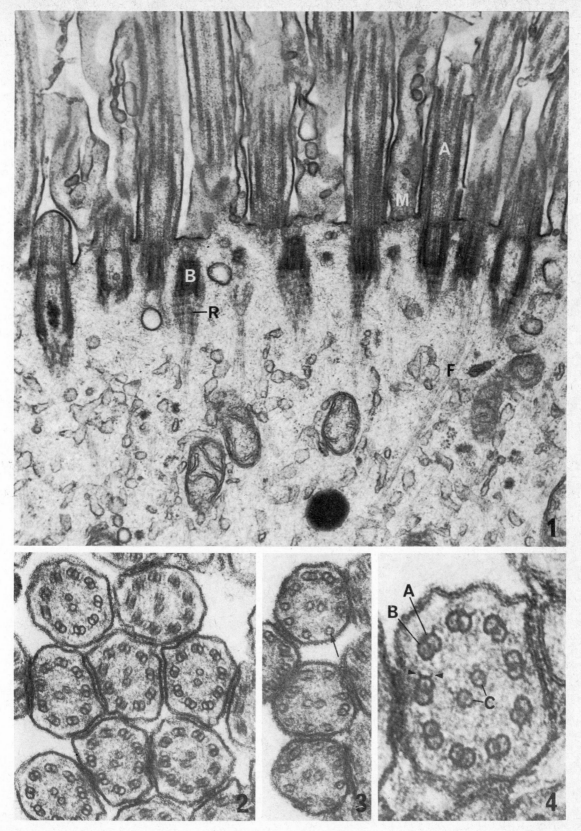

509

pattern of organization. The significance of this pattern, which is remarkably constant for many cilia and flagella throughout the plant and animal kingdoms has yet to be elucidated. Although numerous variations of the 9 + 2 pattern have been seen, most of these can be looked upon as variations of the same master plan. It is the universality and constancy, rather than the variations of the 9 + 2 pattern, which are intriguing. What advantage such a plan of organization has in evolutionary terms that it should have been adopted by such diverse forms of life remains unexplained.

In transverse sections of cilia (*Plate 213, Figs. 2–4*), the central microtubules present discrete circular profiles, but the peripheral doublets show a figure-of-eight configuration. One of these tubules, which at times appears solid or filament-like and also often carries short 'arms' is designated microtubule A or subfilament A. The other microtubule is designated microtubule B or subfilament B. It is said that the direction of the ciliary beat occurs in a plane perpendicular to the plane joining the two central microtubules.

The two central microtubules have often been considered essential for motility and such motile cilia (9 + 2) are at times referred to as kinocilia. This contrasts them to cilia which are not motile, such as the connecting cilium of the vertebrate retinal rod cell (De Robertis, 1956), which has a 9 + 0 pattern of organization. Ultrastructural studies have shown that a large variety of cells possess an occasional or a few cilia (page 512) and that many such cilia show the 9 + 0 pattern, but not much is known about their motility. However, the motile sperm tails of *Myzostommium cirriferum* have a 9 + 0 pattern of organization. Their motion, although sluggish compared to 9 + 2 sperm tails, is not restricted to one plane (Afzelius, 1961, 1962). One may therefore argue that the central microtubules determine the direction of the beat, rather than the motility or otherwise of the cilium.

The tails of many but not all non-mammalian vertebrate spermatozoa are remarkably similar to the cilia and flagella described above. The tail of the mammalian sperm is more complex, but it too bears an axial microtubule complex with the 9 + 2 pattern. The main difference here is the occurrence of a further set of dense rods or fibres around the axial microtubule complex (*Plate 214*).

The term 'stereocilia' has been used in classical histology to describe certain long slender cell processes such as those seen on the pseudo-stratified columnar epithelium of the epididymis and the hair cells of the vestibular labyrinth (Bloom and Fawcett, 1969; Lentz, 1971). These processes do not contain an axial microtubule complex, nor are they associated with basal bodies, and as such they are no longer considered to be cilia but a variety of microvilli (page 498).

Plate 214

Sections through mouse spermatozoa cut in various planes. (The sperm has a head and a tail; the tail is further subdivided into the neck, middle piece, principal piece and end piece (Bloom and Fawcett, 1969).)

Fig. 1. Longitudinal section showing the head (H), neck (N) and middle piece with its gyres of helically arranged mitochondria (M), axial microtubule complex (A) and the outer dense rods of fibres (D). × 28,000

Fig. 2. Longitudinal section through the principal piece, showing the ribbed fibrous sheath (F), outer dense fibres (D) and the central microtubules of the axial microtubule complex (A). × 81,000

Fig. 3. Transverse sections through sperm tails. The one on the left, passing through the middle piece, shows the mitochondrial sheath (M), nine peripheral dense fibres (D) and the 9 + 2 microtubule complex. The one on the right passing through the distal part of the principal piece, shows only four dense fibres (D), the others having terminated higher up the tail. × 76,000

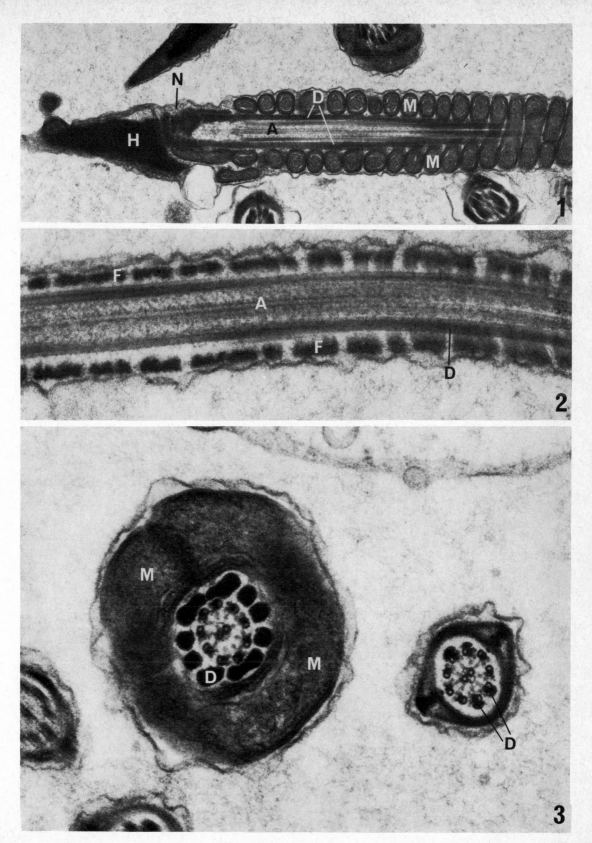

SINGLE, PRIMARY OR OLIGOCILIA

Electron microscopy has now revealed the presence of single cilia or a few cilia on a large variety of cells (*Plates 215–218*). However, these structures, whose function and significance still elude us, had been noted on a few cells with the light microscope, the first such report being by Zimmermann in 1898. In light microscopic studies and also in some early electron microscopic studies these structures were referred to as 'central flagella' or 'isolated flagella'. In more recent studies these structures have been called 'solitary cilia', 'single cilia' or 'primary cilia'. None of these terms is particularly suitable. It is clear now that in some examples of so-called 'single cilia', two or more cilia may be found on a single cell, while other cells in the same sample may show only a single cilium. Such variations reflect the difficulty of ascertaining the number of cilia per cell from a random ultrathin section, and also, no doubt, the biological variation in the number of cilia truly present.

The term 'primary cilia' was coined by Sorokin (1968) to describe cilia with a 9 + 0 structure which develop in fetal rat lung, long before the abundant 9 + 2 cilia form in the bronchial mucosa. Since then, some authors have tried to extend this term to cover various examples of single or few cilia seen in other tissues. This seems undesirable, for such a sequence of formation of primary (9 + 0) cilia followed by the formation of secondary (9 + 2) cilia has been demonstrated only in the lung. It should be noted that primary cilia as reported by Sorokin had a 9 + 0 structure. While this is true of many of the single or few cilia seen in other sites, one can also cite examples where 9 + 2 and other patterns of microtubular arrangement have been found (see below for further discussion on primary cilia).

Indeed, the only consistent difference between the classical cilia of ciliated epithelia and the ones considered here is that, while in the former instance there are hundreds of cilia per cell, in the latter their numbers are quite small. Hence it seems appropriate to coin a new term 'oligocilia' (meaning 'few cilia') to describe them. Under this term shall be described various examples of single or few cilia, wherever found and whatever their structure.

Oligocilia have now been observed in the cells of a wide variety of tissues and organs. These include: (1) adenohypophysis of mouse, rat, rabbit, dog and man (Barnes, 1961; Salazar, 1963; Ziegler, 1963; Kagayama, 1965; Wheatley, 1967; Dingemans, 1969); (2) adrenals of rat and hamster (De Robertis and Sabatini, 1970; Propst and Muller, 1966); (3) thyroid of man, chicken and dog (Kano, 1952; Fujita, 1963); (4) parathyroid of mouse, deer and man (also human parathyroid adenoma) (Munger and Roth, 1963; Stoeckel and Porte, 1966; Black *et al.*, 1970; Roth, 1970; Altenahr and Seifert, 1971) (*Plate 218, Fig. 3*); (5) follicular epithelium of rat and guinea-pig ovary (Bjorkman, 1962; Adams and Hertig, 1964); (6) stromal cells of rat uterus (Tachi *et al.*, 1969); (7) rete testis of rat (Leeson, 1962); (8) seminal vesicles of mouse (Deane and Wurzelmann, 1965); (9) pancreas of chicken, mouse and rat (exocrine, endocrine and ductular cells) (Munger, 1958; Zeigel, 1962; Baradi and Brandis, 1969); (10) intrahepatic bile duct of rat and man with biliary obstruction (Steiner *et al.*, 1962; Grisham, 1963; Grisham and Porta, 1963; Steiner and Carruthers, 1963); (11) kidney tubules of mammals, including man (Leeson, 1960; Latta *et al.*, 1961;

Plate 215

Fig. 1. A human synovial cell showing a cilium (C) arising from one member of a centriolar pair. The cilium is seen lying in an obliquely sectioned tunnel (T) or vacuole. × 55,000 (*From Ghadially and Roy, 1969*)

Fig. 2. A chondrocyte from rabbit articular cartilage, showing a cilium (C) similar to that in *Fig. 1.* × 71,000

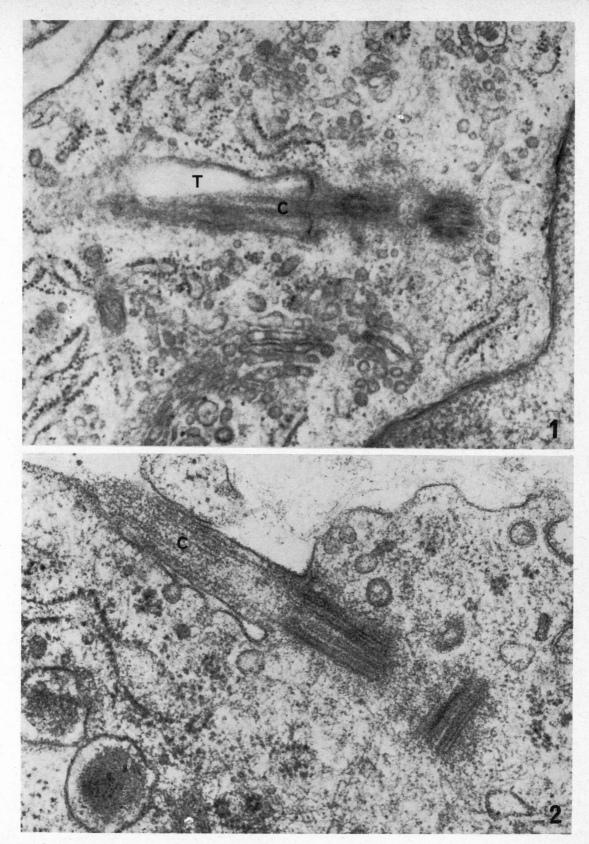

Myers *et al.*, 1966; Tisher *et al.*, 1966);* (12) fetal kidney of man (Zimmermann, 1971); (13) Wilm's tumour but not other human kidney tumours (Tannenbaum, 1971); (14) experimentally produced kidney tumours in hamsters (Mannweiler and Bernhard, 1957); (15) cultured monkey kidney cell infected with herpesvirus (*Plate 217*); (16) renal cells from cases of lupus nephritis (Latta *et al.*, 1967; Rossmann and Galle, 1968; Larsen and Ghadially, 1974) (*Plate 216, Fig. 2*); (17) basal cells of epidermis and basal cell carcinoma of man (Wilson and McWhorther, 1963); (18) gingiva of man and oral mucosa of rat (Nikai *et al.*, 1970); (19) sensory cells of inner ear of guinea-pig (Wersall, 1956; Engstrom and Wersall, 1958); (20) choroid plexus of rabbit (Millen and Rogers, 1956); (21) retina of rabbit, guinea-pig, cat and man (Sjostrand, 1953; De Robertis, 1956; De Robertis and Lasansky, 1958; Tokuyasu and Yamada, 1959; Allen 1965); (22) a variety of cells from the nervous system of goldfish, rat, rabbit, and man (Palay, 1961; Taxi, 1961; Dahl, 1963; Grillo and Palay, 1963) (*Plate 218, Fig. 5*); (23) fibroblasts (in culture and from various tissues) of chicken, mouse, rat, man and Chinese hamster (Sorokin, 1962; Schuster, 1964; Wilson and McWhorther, 1963; Stubblefield and Brinkley, 1966; Wheatley, 1969) (*Plate 216, Fig. 1; Plate 218, Figs. 1, 2 and 4*); (24) meningiomas (Cervos-Navarro and Vazquez, 1966); (25) smooth muscle (Sorokin, 1962); (26) reticular cells and unidentified cells from the spleen of rat, rabbit and chicken and haemopoietic cells from vitelline sac of embryos (De Harven and Bernhard, 1956; Bernhard and De Harven, 1960; Roberts and Latta, 1964; Abdel-Bari and Sorenson, 1965; Breton-Gorius and Stralin, 1967); (27) chondrocytes from epiphyseal and articular cartilage of mouse and rabbit (Scherft and Daems, 1967) (*Plate 215, Fig. 2*); (28) synovial cells of guinea-pig, man and rabbit (Wyllie *et al.*, 1964; Ghadially and Roy, 1969; Campbell and Callahan, 1971) (*Plate 215, Fig. 1*); (29) osteocytes in femoral cortical bone of mice (Tonna and Lampen, 1972); and (30) human ameloblastoma (Lee *et al.*, 1972).

Certain generalizations have frequently been made regarding oligocilia. It has been said that these cilia are solitary or few, that they have a diplosomal basal organization (i.e. they arise from one member of a pair of centrioles comprising the diplosome), a 9 + 0 axial microtubule complex and that they lie in a vacuole or a tunnel or invagination of the plasma membrane. It will be recalled that the usual variety of cilia is numerous, has a single centriole as a basal body, a 9 + 2 axial microtubule complex and arises near the cell surface.

---

* Kidney tubules of many lower vertebrates are endowed with numerous cilia. They cannot be accepted as examples of oligocilia. (For a review and references, see Larsen and Ghadially, 1974.)

Plate 216

Fig. 1. Evidence of more than one cilium per cell is seen here in a cultured mouse fibroblast. In a vacuole or transversely sectioned tunnel or invagination are seen the base of two cilia (C) cut obliquely. The transverse section of the cilium with the 9 + 0 structure (arrowhead) could be a resectioning of a cilium folded back on itself or a third example. × 60,000 (*Wheatley, unpublished electron micrograph*)

Fig. 2. Some 15 or more sections of cilia (9 + 2 structure) are seen within a transversely sectioned tunnel lying within a human kidney tubular epithelial cell. From a case of lupus nephritis. × 60,000 (*From Larsen and Ghadially, 1974*)

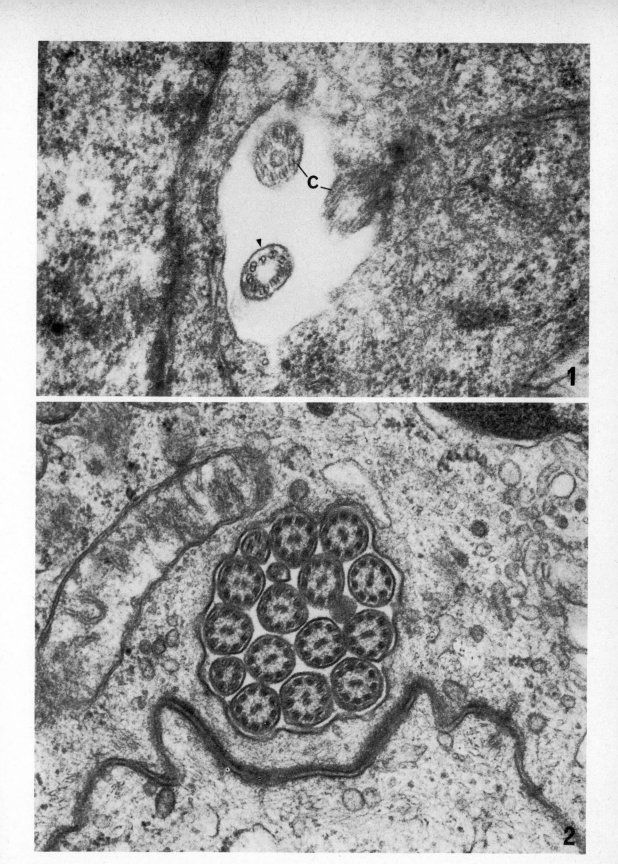

Exceptions and amplifications of the generalizations made above are as follows. Firstly, regarding the number of cilia per cell, one may observe that between the two extremes of single cilia and the hundreds of cilia per cell seen in typical ciliated epithelia lie examples where some cells with two (Stubblefield and Brinkley, 1966; Roth, 1970) or three or four (Millen and Rogers, 1956; Wheatley, 1969) cilia per cell have been seen, and in *Plate 216, Fig. 2*, is shown an example where it would appear that 15 or more cilia are arising from a human kidney tubular epithelial cell.

It is worth noting that, while many oligocilia have shown a 9 + 0 pattern, there are examples where the familiar 9 + 2 pattern has been observed (e.g. Wersall, 1956; Millen and Rogers 1956; Grisham and Porta, 1963). In the neurons of the rat, Dahl (1963) observed cilia which near the base showed the 9 + 0 pattern but higher up along the shaft one of the doublets was displaced to the centre so that an 8 + 1 configuration developed (*Plate 218, Fig. 5*). An 8 + 1 pattern was noted by Munger and Roth (1963) for the cilia in parathyroid gland, and Stoeckel and Porte (1966) reported that the peripheral microtubular pairs may vary from 6 to 9. In pathological renal tissue the commonest type of cilium encountered is the 9 + 2 cilium, but rare examples of 9 + 0, 9 + 1, 8 + 0, 8 + 1, 8 + 2 and 7 + 2 cilia have also been reported to occur (for references, see Larsen and Ghadially, 1974). In some studies microtubular complexes were found to be completely or almost completely lacking in the oligocilia (Sorokin, 1962; Adams and Hertig, 1964; Scherft and Daems, 1967). In many studies the microtubular pattern is not reported simply because the number of cilia seen was too few and transversely sectioned shafts were not encountered.

Reports of oligocilia arising from a single centriole or basal body rather than one member of a pair of centrioles may also be found in the literature. In some instances, particularly when but a single cilium has been seen, it seems highly probably that this was due to one member of the pair of centrioles not being included in the section rather than being truly absent. Where two cilia have been seen it is at times evident that both members of the diplosome have formed cilia.

Oligocilia often, but not invariably, appear to lie in a vacuole or a tunnel. It is conceivable that in some instances the 'vacuole' is no more than an oblique section through an invagination of the plasma membrane communicating with the exterior. In other instances, however, it is likely to be a stage in the growth of the cilium, for a vesicle is known to be associated with early stages of ciliary development in many sites (Sotelo and Trujillo-Cenoz, 1958).

The function and significance of most oligocilia remain obscure.* Since often the two central microtubules of the complex are absent, it is thought that these cells are not motile. In fact, proof regarding the motility of virtually all oligocilia is lacking, for they have been visualized in

---

* The function of some of these cilia is well established. For example, the 9 + 0 cilium of the vertebrate retinal rod cell has a photoreceptor function. In certain lower animals, rare examples of 9 + 2 and 8 + 1 cilia with photoreceptor function are also known to occur. The solitary 9 + 2 cilium on the sensory cells of the inner ear is considered to have a mechanoreceptor function. (See Afzelius, 1969, for further examples and references.)

Plate 217

This electron micrograph shows a small, superficially placed cilium found in a monkey kidney cell from a culture infected with herpesvirus. Only one centriole forming the basal body of the cilium is clearly seen but the presence of the other member of the pair can be just discerned (∗). × 67,000

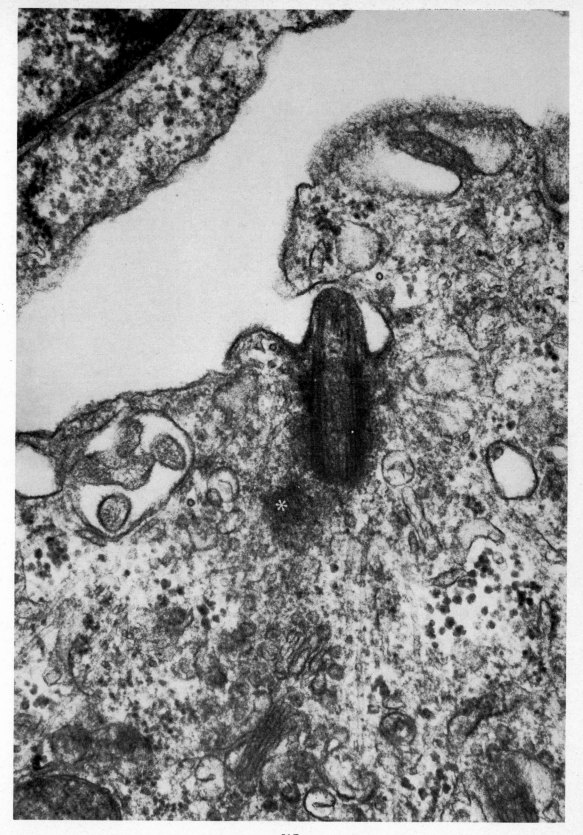

electron micrographs and not in living cells. An exception to this are the oligocilia produced in cultured fibroblasts exposed to Colcemid. Here Stubblefield and Brinkley (1966) found with the phase-contrast microscope that a few of the cilia were beating erratically.

Munger (1958) proposed a chemoreceptor function for cilia in endocrine organs, while the absence of the central microtubules led Barnes (1961) to conclude that oligocilia may have a sensory function. However, this view was not supported by Grillo and Palay (1963), who recalled that 'most of these examples do not involve known receptor cells', and by Sorokin (1962), who remarked that he could see 'no compelling reason for assigning a sensory function to these structures'.

From their study of cilia in the rat nephron, Latta et al. (1961) suggested that 'these structures may be viewed as an evolutionary remnant because cilia are found much more frequently in the excretory ducts of lower animals'. Similarly, Grisham and Porta (1963) and Grisham (1963) have pointed out that biliary epithelial cells of several non-mammalian vertebrates bear cilia and that their rare occurrence in rat and man 'may indicate a reversion to a more primitive condition'.

In some instances, such as thyroid follicular cells in the fowl and the oral epithelium of the rat (Fujita, 1963; Nikai et al., 1970), oligocilia have been noted to be more abundant in young or embryonic tissues as compared to the corresponding tissue in the adult, but in mouse osteocytes (Latta et al., 1961; Tonna and Lampen, 1972), the converse appears to be the case. Hence the often expressed idea that these cilia are primitive or embryonal structures deserving to be called primary cilia (in analogy with the situation in the lung) is not unequivocally supported by available evidence.

Ciliation has been induced in: (1) cultured fibroblasts treated with Colcemid or cytochalasin B (Stubblefield and Brinkley, 1966, 1967; Krishan, 1971); (2) neural and glial cells of cat brain brain by pargyline (Milhaud and Pappas, 1968); and (3) sea-urchin embryos by a variety of agents (Lallier, 1964). On the basis of such observations, Milhaud and Pappas (1968) have suggested that 'stimulation of centriolar reproduction without subsequent mitosis may lead to ciliary formation'. A negative correlation between mitosis and cilia production is also thought to occur in the adenohypophysis. Oligocilia are, relatively speaking, of fairly common occurrence in this region, but it is said that they are of less frequent occurrence in experimental situations where mitotic activity is enhanced, and Dingemans (1969) explains the situation by stating that 'centrioles cannot simultaneously be involved in mitosis and constitute a part of the basal structure of a cilium'.

As stated earlier, no unifying hypothesis regarding the significance of these cilia has been proposed and their function, if any, is unknown. The collective evidence, however, indicates that the ability of centrioles to form cilia exists and persists in virtually all cells, and that they can be provoked to produce cilia by a variety of natural and experimental stimuli.

Plate 218

Fig. 1. A fibroblast in culture, showing a cilium lying at the bottom of a deep invagination. × 16,000 (*From Wheatley, 1969*)

Fig. 2. A fibroblast in culture, showing a cilium arising from a centriole near the surface of the cell. × 38,000 (*Wheatley, unpublished electron micrograph*)

Fig. 3. A cell from a human parathyroid adenoma, showing a cilium lying in a characteristic vacuole or invagination. × 41,000 (*Larsen and Ghadially, unpublished electron micrograph*)

Fig. 4. Transverse section of a 9 + 0 cilium from a mouse fibroblast in culture. × 65,000 (*Wheatley, unpublished electron micrograph*)

Fig. 5. An 8 + 1 cilium from rat cerebral cortex. × 75,000 (*From Dahl, 1963*)

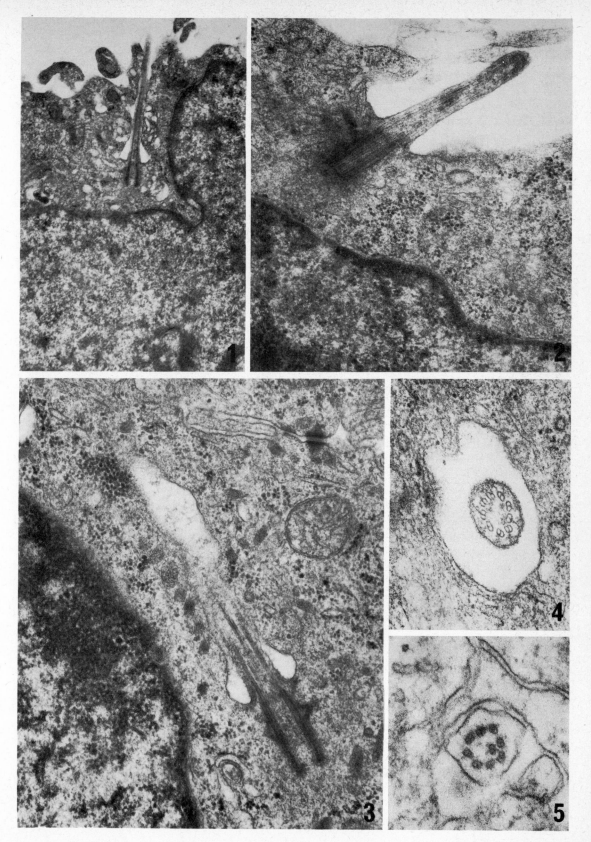

Atypical or pathologically altered cilia have been seen in the ciliated epithelium of the respiratory passages and also in a few other tissues. For descriptive purposes such altered cilia may be divided into five main groups: (1) compound cilia, that is to say, cilia containing multiple axial microtubule complexes set in a common matrix and enclosed in a single membrane (*Plate 219*; *Plate 220, Figs. 1 and 2*); (2) swollen cilia, where the prominent feature is an abundance of matrix as compared to the normal state (*Plate 220, Fig. 3*); (3) cilia showing various fine alterations of structure such as disorganization and/or loss of some of the microtubules from the complex (Ailsby and Ghadially, 1973), vesiculation of the ciliary membrane (Friedman and Bird, 1971); (4) intracytoplasmic cilia where the axial microtubule complex is deviated and follows an intracytoplasmic course rather than emerging as a free cilium from the surface (Wong and Buck, 1971; Larsen and Ghadially, 1974) (*Plate 220, Fig. 4*); and (5) cilia with an atypical basal body. An example of a cilium arising from a giant basal body, a little more than five times the length of a normal basal body, was found by us in a lupus kidney (Larsen and Ghadially, 1974). Needless to say, such categories are not clear-cut, and examples of cilia showing more than one of the above-mentioned morphological alterations may be found.

It is worth noting that the term 'compound cilia' has been used to describe the membranelle (composed of rows of cilia) and the cirrhus (a collection of cilia resembling a water-colour brush) of protozoa. In these instances the cilia are set in a common matrix (extracellular) to form what is called a 'compound motile organelle' (Fawcett, 1961). Such cilia beat in unison as if 'fused'. However, the individual cilia in these so-called 'compound cilia' can be separated by microdissection (Afzelius, 1969). It seems to me that these structures should be called compound motile organelles, as suggested by Fawcett, and not compound cilia so as to avoid confusion with cilia more deserving this appellation such as those shown in *Plate 219*. In order to avoid confusion some authors refer to such compound cilia as giant cilia. This term, however, is unsuitable for it does not indicate the main feature of this change, namely the presence of multiple axial microtubule complexes within a single ciliary sheath, but stresses the size, which can be quite variable. For example, many compound cilia contain only two or three axial microtubule complexes (*Plate 220, Fig. 1*) and are not particularly large. These can hardly be accepted as giant cilia.

Compound cilia (i.e. cilia containing multiple axial microtubule complexes within a single ensheathing ciliary membrane) have been found in: (1) epithelium lining of colloid cyst of the third ventricle (Coxe and Luse, 1964); (2) human malignant polycystic teratoma of the ovary (Luse and Vietti, 1968); (3) nasal papilloma in man (Gaito *et al.*, 1965); (4) human ovarian carcinoma (*Plate 220, Fig. 2*); (5) bronchial mucosa of a heavy smoker with bronchial carcinoma (Ailsby and Ghadially, 1973) (*Plate 219*); (6) antral mucosa of maxillary sinuses in allergic conditions and ventricular mucosa of the human larynx (Friedmann and Bird, 1971); (7) middle-ear mucosa of a deaf patient and an adult guinea-pig (Kawabata and Paparella, 1969); (8) embryonic chick otocyst in culture (Friedmann and Bird, 1971); and (9) tracheal epithelium of the fowl infected with infectious laryngotracheitis virus (Purcell, 1971).

Plate 219

From the bronchial mucosa of a man who had smoked 25 cigarettes per day over a period of 46 years and developed a bronchial carcinoma. The cilia shown here were found in a segment of apparently normal-looking mucosa collected well away from the tumour site. This electron micrograph shows two compound cilia (C) containing transversely and longitudinally sectioned axial microtubule complexes and numerous normal-looking cilia sectioned in various planes. × 22,000 (*From Ailsby and Ghadially, 1973*)

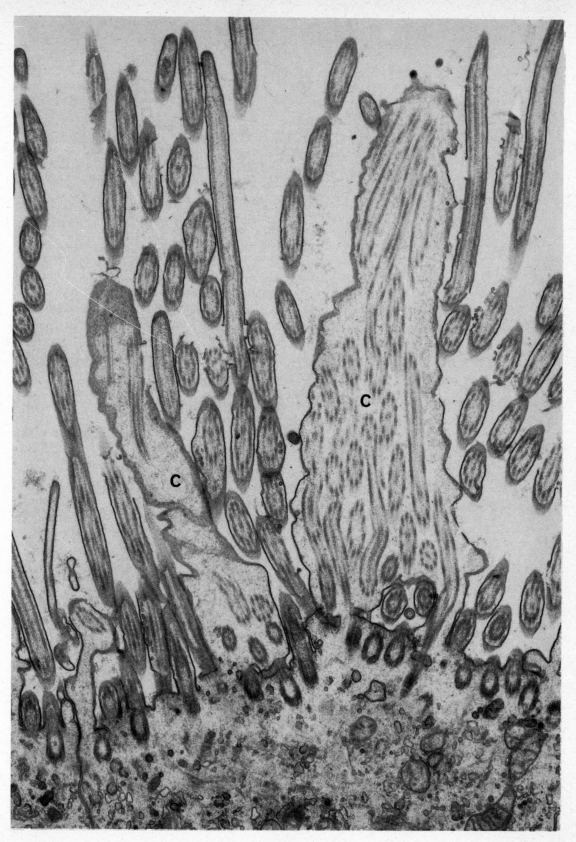

In many of the above-mentioned instances only one of a few compound cilia with two to four axial microtubule complexes were seen. The really large compound cilia have been seen mainly in the respiratory passages and in some tumours.

For example, in the bronchial mucosa of the patient reported by us (Ailsby and Ghadially, 1973) there were innumerable compound cilia containing two to four axial microtubule complexes. The largest compound cilium seen in transverse section probably contained about 27 axial microtubule complexes (see *Fig. 2* in Ailsby and Ghadially, 1973). Moreover, it was often observed that the microtubules within some of the complexes were disarranged. In other instances the central pair of filaments was absent (9 + 0 pattern). Absence of the central filaments was also quite frequently observed in otherwise normal-looking cilia. Failure to visualize these microtubules did not appear to be due to obliquity of sectioning or poor fixation, for peripheral microtubules were well resolved, and numerous cilia with the normal 9 + 2 pattern were also present, in close proximity to those showing a 9 + 0 organization.

Another somewhat rare abnormality was the occurrence of moderately to markedly swollen cilia containing only a single axial microtubule complex but more than the usual amount of matrix (*Plate 220, Fig. 3*). Swollen cilia of a somewhat different morphology have been reported by Duncan and Ramsey (1965) in the porcine nasal mucosa in *Bordetella-bronchiseptica*-induced rhinitis (*Plate 221*). In this example the swelling affected the distal part of the ciliary shaft so that an appearance akin to a balloon on a string, or a table tennis racket, was created. The magnitude of the swelling was also quite remarkable, the swollen portion of the cilium measuring approximately $1.5 \times 2.2 \mu$. The axial microtubule complex showed the characteristic 9 + 2 arrangement in the relatively unaltered stem of the cilium, but became disorientated and coiled in the distal swollen portion of the cilium.

The significance and mechanism of production of swollen cilia are not evident, but it would seem that such cilia may be functionally incompetent, for the axial microtubule complex may be inadequate to move the increased mass of the swollen cilium effectively.

Little is known about the manner in which compound cilia are produced, but one could propose that they are either produced by a fusion of pre-existing cilia, or arise as a result of multiple axial microtubule complexes entering a single large evagination of the plasma membrane. Whether such cilia are capable of beating is also not known. In the large compound cilia seen by

---

Plate 220

Fig. 1. Compound cilia (C) containing two or more axial microtubule complexes are seen here, as are numerous normal-looking cilia and some (arrows) where the central microtubules are missing. Note also the missing central microtubules (arrowhead) and disorganized complexes in the compound cilia. From the same case as *Plate 217*. × 25,000 (*Ailsby and Ghadially, unpublished electron micrograph*)

Fig. 2. A compound cilium seen in a tumour cell obtained from a malignant ascitic effusion. From a case of ovarian carcinoma. × 29,000

Fig. 3. A transversely cut swollen cilium. There is an excess of matrix but only a single axial microtubule complex is present. From the same case as *Plate 219*. × 34,000 (*From Ailsby and Ghadially, 1973*)

Fig. 4. A ciliated cell from the bronchial mucosa of a vitamin-A-deficient rat, showing intracytoplasmic cilia. A deviated axial microtubule complex (C) and attached basal body (B) are clearly seen in the cytoplasm. The presence of another such cilium is suggested by what appears to be a grazing cut along another microtubule complex (arrowhead). × 22,000 (*From Wong and Buck, 1971*)

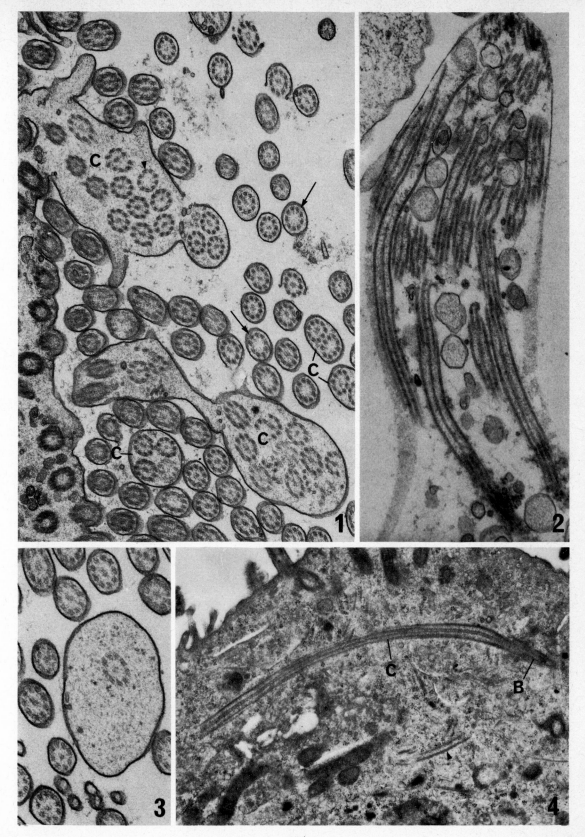

us, in the bronchial mucosa, the haphazardly distributed and poorly orientated axial microtuble complexes do not inspire confidence in the ability of such cilia to assist in the movement of the mucus blanket over the bronchial epithelium.

It has long been known that the ciliated epithelium of the respiratory tract may be damaged and undergo squamous metaplasia in a variety of chronic inflammatory states and in vitamin A deficiency (Straub and Mulder, 1948; Wilhelm, 1954; Wong and Buck, 1971). It has also been established that various noxious agents such as cigarette smoke, sulphur dioxide, formaldehyde and ammonia impair the movement of the mucus blanket (mucus-escalator) over the respiratory epithelium, by altering the viscosity of the mucus and causing a disturbance or paralysis of the ciliary beat (Hilding, 1956; Falk *et al.*, 1959; Kensler and Battista, 1963, 1966; Dalhamn, 1964). Light microscopic studies failed to show any overt morphological changes in the cilia themselves, but the electron microscope shows that many and varied are the morphological changes that can occur in the cilia of the respiratory passages. It would therefore appear that pathologically altered cilia may constitute yet another factor responsible for the sluggish movement of mucus and the pulmonary pathology which results from an impairment of this vital cleansing mechanism which helps to rid the respiratory tract of irritants, carcinogens and pathogenic organisms.

In the foregoing discussion attention has been concentrated on morphologically altered cilia. It is, however, worth noting that the various noxious agents which damage the respiratory epithelium also produce a widespread destruction and loss of cilia. One of the questions that has been asked is whether such damage can be repaired by the production of new cilia by the surviving deciliated cell?

According to Burian and Stockinger (1963) and Burian (1966), regeneration of cilia does occur after deciliation by various chemical agents, but Hilding (1965) reported that, in the calf trachea, deciliated cells produced by mild mechanical trauma were exfoliated within about 1 hour after injury, and were later replaced by immature cells from the deeper layers which then proceeded to form cilia. A similar experiment was performed on rabbits by Hilding and Hilding (1966) and they stated that, 'Removing cilia from rabbit cells by our methods results in so much disruption that it seems unlikely that the remaining fragments would survive'.

It would appear that there is as yet no compelling reason to believe that cilia destroyed by pathological agents can regenerate. Indeed, in view of the known rapid turnover of cells in most epithelia, one would imagine that a deciliated cell would be discarded and replaced by another cell.

Plate 221

Swollen cilia from the nasal mucosa of a pig with experimentally produced *Bordetella bronchiseptica* rhinitis. (*From Duncan and Ramsey, 1965*)

Fig. 1. Section through swollen cilia, showing the swollen distal portion and the normal-looking proximal portion of the ciliary shaft. × 18,000

Figs. 2 and 3. Coiling of the axial microtubule complex within the swollen portion of the cilia. × 44,000; 49,000

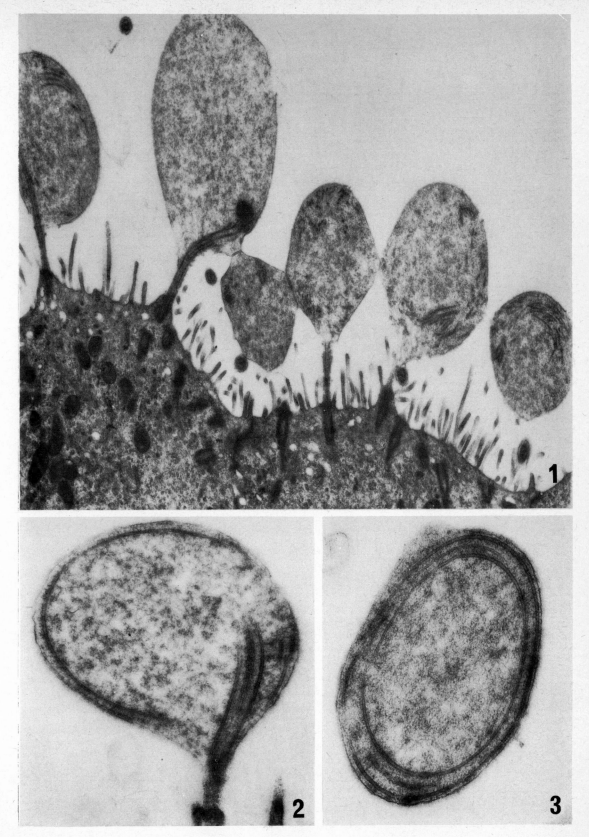

1

2

3

REFERENCES

Abdel-Bari, W. and Sorenson, G. D. (1965). 'Ciliated cells in the spleen of adult rats.' *Anat. Rec.* **152**, 481

Adams, E. C. and Hertig, A. T. (1964). 'Studies on guinea pig oocytes. I. Electron microscopic observations on the development of cytoplasmic organelles in oocytes of primordial and primary follicles.' *J. Cell Biol.* **21**, 397

Afzelius, B. (1961). 'Some problems of ciliary structure and ciliary function. Biological structure and function.' In *Proceedings of the first IUB/IUBS international symposium, Stockholm*, Vol. II, p. 557. Ed. by T. W. Goodwin and O. Lindberg. London and New York: Academic Press

— (1962). 'The contractile apparatus in some invertebrate muscles and spermatozoa M-1.' In *Proceedings of the Fifth International Congress for Electron Microscopy*, Vol. II. Ed. by S. S. Breese, Jr. New York and London: Academic Press

— (1969). 'Ultrastructure of cilia and flagella.' In *Handbook of Molecular Cytology*, p. 1220. Ed. by A. Lima-de-Faria. Amsterdam and London: North Holland Publ.

Ailsby, R. L. and Ghadially, F. N. (1973). 'Atypical cilia in human bronchial mucosa.' *J. Path.* **109**, 75

Allen, R. A. (1965). 'Isolated cilia in inner retinal neurons and in retinal pigment epithelium.' *J. Ultrastruct. Res.* **12**, 730

Altenahr, E. and Seifert, G. (1971). 'Ultrastruktureller Vergleich menschlicher Epithelkorperchen bei sekundaren Hyperparathyreoidismus und primarem Adenom.' *Virchows Arch. path. Anat. Physiol.* **353**, 60

Baradi, A. F. and Brandis, D. J. (1969). 'Observations on the morphology of pancreatic secretory capillaries.' *Z. Zellforsch. mikrosk. Anat.* **102**, 568

Barnes, B. G. (1961). 'Ciliated secretory cells in the pars distalis of the mouse hypophysis.' *J. Ultrastruct. Res.* **5**, 453

Basset, F. and Nezelof, C. (1966). 'Présence en microscopie électronique de structures filamenteuses originales dans les lésions pulmonaires et osseuses de l'histiocytose "X": etat actuel de la question.' *Bull. Soc. méd. Hôp. Paris* **117**, 413

— — Mallet, R. and Turiaf, J. (1965). 'Nouvelle mise en évidence, par la microscopie électronique, de particules d'allure virale dans une seconde forme clinique de l'histiocytose X, le granulome éosinophile de l'os.' *C.r. hebd. Séanc. Acad. Sci., Paris* **261**, 5719

Baum, J. H. and Nishimura, E. T. (1964). 'Alterations in the fine structure of liver cells during depressed catalase synthesis in the mouse.' *Cancer Res.* **24**, 2001

Bernhard, W. and De Harven, E. (1960). 'L'ultrastructure du centriole et d'autres elements de l'appareil achromatique.' *Proc. 4th Int. Conf. Electron Microscopy, Berlin*, Vol. II, p. 217. Berlin: Springer

Bennett, H. S. (1969a). 'The cell surface: components and configurations.' In *Handbook of Molecular Cytology*, p. 1261. Ed. by A. Lima-de-Faria. Amsterdam and London: North Holland Publ.

— (1969b). 'The cell surface: movements and recombinations.' In *Handbook of Molecular Cytology*, p. 1294. Ed. by A. Lima-de-Faria. Amsterdam and London: North Holland Publ.

Billingham, R. E. and Medawar, P. B. (1953). 'A study of the branched cells of the mammalian epidermis with special reference to the fate of their division products.' *Phil. Trans. R. Soc.* **237**, 151

— and Silvers, W. K. (1960). 'The melanocytes of mammals.' *Q. Rev. Biol.* **35**, 1

Birbeck, M. S., Breathnach, A. S. and Everall, J. D. (1961). 'An electron microscope study of basal melanocytes and high-level clear cells (Langerhans cells) in vitiligo.' *J. invest. Derm.* **37**, 51

Bjorkman, N. (1962). 'A study of the ultrastructure of the granulosa cells of the rat ovary.' *Acta anat.* **51**, 125

Black, W. C., Slatopolsky, E., Elkan, I. and Hoffsten, P. (1970). 'Parathyroid morphology in suppressible and nonsuppressible renal hyperparathyroidism.' *Lab. Invest.* **23**, 497

Bloom, W. and Fawcett, D. W. (1969). *A Text Book of Histology*, 9th edn. Philadelphia and London: Saunders

Bouroncle, B. A., Wiseman, B. K. and Doan, C. A. (1958). 'Leukemic reticuloendotheliosis.' *Blood* **13**, 609

Breathnach, A. S. (1964). 'Observations on cytoplasmic organelles in Langerhans cells of human epidermis.' *J. Anat.* **98**, 265

— (1965). 'The cell of Langerhans.' *Int. Rev. Cytol.* **18**, 1

— and Wyllie, L. M-A. (1965). 'Melanin in Langerhans cells.' *J. invest. Derm.* **45**, 401

Brederoo, P. and Daems, W. Th. (1972). 'Cell coat, worm-like structures, and labyrinths in guinea pig resident and exudate peritoneal macrophages, as demonstrated by an abbreviated fixation procedure for electron microscopy.' *Z. Zellforsch. mikrosk. Anat.* **126**, 135

Breton-Gorius, J. and Stralin, H. (1967). 'Formation de cils rudimentaires dans les cellules sanguines primitives du sac vitellin d'embryons de rat et de poulet.' *Nouv. Revue Franc. Hematol.* **7**, 79

Burian, K. (1966). 'Regeneration in respiratory epithelium.' *Proc. 8th Int. Congr. Oto-Rhinolaryngol.*, Tokyo, 1965. Amsterdam and New York: Excerpta Medica

— and Stockinger, L. (1963). 'Elektronenmikroskopische Untersuchungen an der Nasenchleimhaut. 1. Das Flimmerepithel Nach Lokalen Schadigungen.' *Acta oto-lar.* **56**, 376

Campbell, W. G. and Callahan, B. C. (1971). 'Regeneration of synovium of rabbit knees after total chemical synovectomy by ingrowth of connective tissue-forming elements from adjacent bone. A light and electron microscopic study.' *Lab. Invest.* **24**, 404

Cancilla, P. A. (1968). 'Demonstration of the Langerhans granule by lanthanum.' *J. Cell Biol.* **38**, 248

— Lahey, M. E. and Carnes, W. H. (1967). 'Cutaneous lesions of Letterer–Siwe disease: electron microscopic study.' *Cancer* **20**, 1986

Carrington, S. G. and Winkelmann, R. K. (1972). 'Electron microscopy of histiocytic diseases of the skin.' *Acta derm.-vener.* **52**, 161

Cervos-Navarro, J. and Vazquez, J. (1966). 'Elektronenmikroskopische Untersuchungen uber das Vorkommen von Cilien in Meningeomen.' *Virchows Arch. path. Anat. Physiol.* **341**, 280

Chen, Hai-Chin, Reyes, V. and Fresh, J. W. (1971). 'An electron microscopic study of the small intestine in human cholera.' *Virchows Arch. Abt. B. Zellpath.* **7**, 236

Collet, A. and Policard, A. (1962). 'Essai de localisation infrastructurale dans des poumons des elements du système reticuloendothelial.' *C.r. Acad. Sci., Paris* **156**, 991

Coxe, W. and Luse, S. A. (1964). 'Colloid cyst of third ventricle. An electron microscopic study.' *J. Neuropath. exp. Neurol.* **23**, 431

Dahl, H. A. (1963). 'Fine structure of cilia in rat cerebral cortex.' *Z. Zellforsch. mikrosk. Anat.* **60**, 369

Dalhamn, T. (1964). 'Studies on tracheal ciliary activity. Special reference to the effect of cigarette smoke in living animals.' *Am. Rev. resp. Dis.* **89**, 870

De Harven and Bernhard, W. (1956). 'Etude au microscope electronique de l'ultrastructure du centriole chez les vertebres.' *Z. Zellforsch. mikrosk. Anat.* **45**, 378

De Man, J. C. (1968). 'Rod-like tubular structures in the cytoplasm of histiocytes in "histiocytosis X".' *J. Path. Bact.* **95**, 123

De Robertis, E. (1956). 'Electron microscope observations on the submicroscopic organization of the retinal rods.' *J. biophys. biochem. Cytol.* **2**, 319

— and Lasansky, A. (1958). 'Submicroscopic organization of retinal cones of the rabbit.' *J. biophys. biochem. Cytol.* **4**, 743

— and Sabatini, D. D. (1970). In *Cell Biology*, 5th Edn. p. 1527. Ed. by E. De Robertis, W. W. Nowinsky and F. A. Saez, Philadelphia, Pa: Saunders

Deane, H. and Wurzelmann, S. (1965). 'Electron microscopic observations on the postnatal differentiation of the seminal vesicle epithelium of the laboratory mouse.' *Am. J. Anat.* **117**, 91

Dingemans, K. P. (1969). 'The relation between cilia and mitoses in the mouse adenohypophysis.' *J. Cell Biol.* **43**, 361

Duncan, J. R. and Ramsey, F. K. (1965). 'Fine structural changes in the porcine nasal ciliated epithelial cell produced by *Bordetella bronchiseptica* rhinitis.' *Am. J. Path.* **47**, 601

Emeis, J. J. and Wisse, E. (1971). 'Electron microscopic cytochemistry of the cell coat of Kupffer cells in rat liver.' In *The Reticuloendothelial System and Immune Phenomena*. Ed. by N. R. Di Luzio and K. Flemming. Proc. 6th Int. Meet. Reticuloend. Soc., Freiburg, 1970. *Adv. exp. Med. Biol.* **15**, 1–12. New York: Plenum Press

Engstrom, H. and Wersall, J. (1958). 'Structure and innervation of the inner ear sensory epithelia.' *Int. Rev. Cytol.* **7**, 535

Ewald, O. (1923). 'Die Leukemische Reticuloendotheliose.' *Deutsch. Arch. klin. Med.* **142**, 222

Fahimi, H. D. (1970). 'The fine structural localization of endogenous and exogenous peroxidase activity in Kupffer cells of rat liver.' *J. Cell Biol.* **47**, 247

Falk, H. L., Tremer, H. M. and Kotin, P. (1959). 'Effect of cigarette smoke and its constituents on ciliated mucus-secreting epithelium.' *J. natn. Cancer Inst.* **23**, 999

Fawcett, D. (1961). 'Cilia and flagella.' In *The Cell*, p. 217. Ed. by J. Brachet and A. E. Mirsky. New York and London: Academic Press

— (1967). *An Atlas of Fine Structure. The Cell, Its Organelles and Inclusions.* Philadelphia and London: Saunders

Florey, H. (1958). *General Pathology*, 2nd edn. Philadelphia, Pa: Saunders

Frankel, H. H., Patek, P. R. and Bernick, S. (1962). 'Long term studies of the rat reticuloendothelial system and endocrine gland responses to foreign particles.' *Anat. Rec.* **142**, 359

Friedmann, I. and Bird, E. S. (1971). 'Ciliary structure, ciliogenesis, microvilli.' *Laryngoscope* **81**, 1852

Fujita, H. (1963). 'Electron microscopic studies on the thyroid gland of domestic fowl with special reference to the mode of secretion and the occurrence of a central flagellum in the follicular cell.' *Z. Zellforsch. mikrosk. Anat.* **60**, 615

Gaito, R. A., Gaylord, W. H. and Hilding, D. A. (1965). 'Ultrastructure of a human nasal papilloma.' *Laryngoscope* **75**, 144

Ghadially, F. N. and Parry, E. W. (1966). 'Ultrastructure of a human hepatocellular carcinoma and surrounding non-neoplastic liver.' *Cancer* **19**, 1989

— and Roy, S. (1969). *Ultrastructure of Synovial Joints in Health and Disease*. London: Butterworths

— and Skinnider, L. F. (1971). 'Ropalocytosis—a new abnormality of erythrocytes and their precursors.' *Experientia* **27**, 1217

— — (1972) 'Ultrastructure of hairy cell leukemia.' *Cancer* **29**, 444

— Oryschak, A. F. and Mitchell, D. M. (1974). 'Partially coated vacuoles—a new type of endocytotic structure.' *Experientia* **30**, 649

Gianotti, F. and Caputo, R. (1969). 'Skin ultrastructure in Hand–Schuller–Christian disease. Report on abnormal Langerhans' cells.' *Archs Derm.* **100**, 342

Grillo, M. A. and Palay, S. L. (1963). 'Ciliated Schwann cells in the autonomic nervous system of the adult rat.' *J. Cell Biol.* **16**, 430

Grisham, J. W. (1963). 'Ciliated epithelial cells in normal murine intrahepatic bile ducts.' *Proc. Soc. exp. Biol. Med.* **114**, 318

— and Porta, E. A. (1963). 'Ciliated cells in altered murine and human intrahepatic bile ducts.' *Expl Cell Res.* **31**, 190

Hackemann, M., Grubb, C. and Hill, K. R. (1968). 'The ultrastructure of normal squamous epithelium of the human cervix uteri.' *J. Ultrastruct. Res.* **22**, 443

Hashimoto, K. (1970). 'Lanthanum staining of Langerhans' cell. Communication of Langerhans' cell granules with extracellular space.' *Archs Derm.* **102**, 280

— (1971). 'Ultrastructure of the human toenail. I. Proximal nail matrix. *J. invest. Derm.* **56**, 235

— and Tarnowski, W. M. (1967). 'Ultrastructural studies of racket-bodies in epidermal Langerhans cells and in histiocytosis X (abstract).' *Fedn Proc.* **26**, 370

— — (1968). 'Some new aspects of the Langerhans cell.' *Archs Derm.* **97**, 450

Henneguy, L. F. (1898). 'Les rapports des cils vibratiles avec les centrosomes.' *Archs Anat. Microscop.* **1**, 481

Hilding, A. C. (1956). 'On cigarette smoking, bronchial carcinoma and ciliary action. II. Experimental study on filtering action of cow's lungs, deposition of tar in bronchial tree and removal by ciliary action.' *New Engl. J. Med.* **254**, 1155

— (1965). 'Regeneration of respiratory epithelium after minimal surface trauma.' *Ann. Otol. Rhinol. Lar.* **74**, 903

527

Hilding, D. A. and Hilding, A. C. (1966). 'Ultrastructure of tracheal cilia and cells during regeneration.' *Ann. Otol. Rhinol. Lar.* **75**, 281

Horn, R. G., Koenig, M. G., Goodman, J. S. and Collins, R. D. (1969). 'Phagocytosis of *Staphylococcus aureus* by hepatic reticuloendothelial cells. An ultrastructural study.' *Lab. Invest.* **21**, 406

Hugon, J., Maisin, J. R. and Borgers, M. (1963). 'Modifications ultrastructurales précoces des cellules des cryptes duodénales de la Souris apres irradiation par rayons X.' *C.r. Soc. Biol., Paris* **157**, 2109

Hutchens, L. H., Sagebiel, R. W. and Clarke, M. A. (1971). 'Oral epithelial dendritic cells of the rhesus monkey—histologic demonstration, fine structure and quantitative distribution.' *J. invest. Derm.* **56**, 325

Irwin, D. A. (1932). 'Kupffer cell migration.' *Can. med. Ass. J.* **27**, 353

Jimbow, K., Sato, S. and Kukita, A. (1969). 'Langerhans' cells of the normal human pilosebaceous system' *J. jnvest. Derm.* **52**, 177

Kagayama, M. (1965). 'The follicular cells in the pars distalis of the dog pituitary gland: an electron microscopic study.' *Endocrinology* **77**, 1053

Kano, K. (1952). 'Zytologische Untersuchungen *k*ber die menschliche Schelddruse mit besonderel Berucksichtigung der Ausschwemmung des infrafollicularen Kolloides durch die interzellularen Kanalchen.' *Arch. histol. jap.* **4**, 245

Katayama, I., Li, C. Y. and Yam, L. T. (1972). 'Ultrastructural cytochemical demonstration of tartrate-resistant acid phosphatase isoenzyme activity in "hairy cells" of leukemic reticuloendotheiosis.' *Am. J. Path.* **69**, 471

Kawabata, I. and Paparella, M. (1969). 'Atypical cilia in normal human and guinea pig middle ear mucosa.' *Acta oto-lar* **67**, 511

Kensler, C. J. and Battista, S. P. (1963). 'Components of cigarette smoke with ciliary depressant activity. Their selective removal by filters containing activated charcoal granules.' *New Engl. J. Med.* **269**, 1161

—— (1966). 'Chemical and physical factors affecting mammalian ciliary activity.' *Am. Rev. resp. Dis.* **93**, 93

Kondo, Y. (1969). 'Macrophages containing Langerhans cell granules in normal lymph nodes of the rabbit.' *Z. Zellforsch mikrosk. Anat.* **98**, 506

Krishan, A. (1971). 'Fine structure of cytochalasin-induced multinucleated cells.' *J. Ultrastruct. Res.* **36**, 191

Lallier, R. (1964). 'Biochemical aspects of animalization and vegetalization in the sea urchin embryo.' *Adv. Morphogen.* **3**, 147

Langerhans, P. (1868). 'Uber die nerven der menschlichen haut.' *Virchows Arch.* **44**, 325

Larsen, T. E. and Ghadially, F. N. (1974). 'Cilia in lupus nephritis.' *J. Path.* **114**, 69

Latta, H., Maunsbach, A. B. and Madden, S. C. (1961). 'Cilia in different segments of the rat nephron.' *J. biophys. biochem. Cytol.* **11**, 248

—— and Osvaldo, L. (1967). In Ultrastructure of the Kidney, p. 14. Ed. by A. J. Dalton and F. Haguenau. New York and London: Academic Press

Lee, K. W., El-Labban, N. G. and Kramer, I. R. H. (1972). 'Ultrastructure of a simple ameloblastoma.' *J. Path.* **108**, 173

Leeson, T. S. (1960). 'Electron microscope studies of newborn hamster kidney.' *Norelco Reporter* **7**, 45

—— (1962). 'Electron microscopy of the rete testis of the rat.' *Anat. Rec.* **144**, 57

Lenhossek, M. von (1898). *Verh. deutsch. anat. Ges. Jena* **12**, 106

Lentz, T. L. (1971). *Cell Fine Structure.* Philadelphia and London: Saunders

Lewis, W. H. (1931). 'Pinocytosis.' *Bull. Johns Hopkins Hosp.* **49**, 17

Luse, S. A. and Vietti, T. (1968). 'Ovarian teratoma. Ultrastructure and neural component.' *Cancer, Philad.* **21**, 38

Mannweiler, K. L. and Bernhard, W. (1957). 'Recherches ultrastructurales sur une tumeur rénale experimentale du hamster.' *J. Ultrastruct. Res.* **1**, 158

Masson, P. (1948). 'Pigment cells in man.' In *The Biology of Melanomas*, p. 15 (Special publications of the New York Academy of Sciences, Volume IV.) Ed. by R. W. Miner and M. Gordon. New York: N.Y. Academy of Sciences

—— (1951). 'My conception of cellular nevi.' *Cancer* **4**, 9

Matter, A., Orci, L., Forssmann, W. G. and Rouiller, C. (1968). 'The stereological analysis of the fine structure of the "micropinocytosis vermiformis" in Kupffer cells of the rat.' *J. Ultrastruct. Res.* **23**, 272

Melis, M. and Orci, L. (1967). 'Sugli aspetti ultrastrutturali delle cellule di Kupffer nel ratto dopo epatectomia parziale.' *Fegato* **13**, 356

Metchnikoff, E. (1883). 'Untersuchungen uber die Mesodermalen Phagocyten einiger Wirbeltiere.' *Biol. Zbl.* **3**, 360

Milhaud, M. and Pappas, G. D. (1968). 'Cilia formation in the adult cat brain after pargyline treatment.' *J. Cell. Biol.* **37**, 599

Millen, J. W. and Rogers, G. E. (1956). 'An electron microscopic study of the choroid plexus in the rabbit.' *J. biophys. biochem. Cytol.* **2**, 407

Mitus, W. J. (1971). 'Hairy cells and isoenzymes.' *New Engl. J. Med.* **284**, 389

—— Mednicoff, I. B., Wittels, B. and Dameshek, W. (1961). 'Neoplastic lymphoid reticulum cells in the peripheral blood: a histochemical study.' *Blood* **17**, 206

Morales, A. R., Fine, G., Horn, R. C. and Watson, J. H. L. (1969). 'Langerhans cells in a localized lesion of the eosinophilic granuloma type.' *Lab. Invest.* **20**, 412

Munger, B. L. (1958). 'A light and electron microscopic study of cellular differentiation in the pancreatic islets of the mouse.' *Am. J. Anat.* **103**, 275

—— and Roth, S. I. (1963). 'The cytology of the normal parathyroid glands of man and Virginia deer.' *J. Cell. Biol.* **16**, 379

Myers, C. E., Bulger, R. E., Tisher, C. C. and Trump, B. F. (1966). 'Human renal ultrastructure. IV. Collecting duct of healthy individuals.' *Lab. Invest.* **15**, 1921

Nicol, T. and Bilbey, D. L. J. (1958). 'Elimination of macrophage cells of the reticuloendothelial system by way of the bronchial tree.' *Nature, Lond.* **182**, 192

Niebauer, G. (1968). *Dendritic Cells of Human Skin.* Basel: Karger

Nikai, H., Rose, G. G. and Cattoni, M. (1970). 'Electron microscopy of solitary cilia in human gingiva and rat oral mucosa.' *J. dent. Res.* **49**, 1141

Orci, L., Pictet, R. and Rouiller, C. (1967). 'Image ultrastructurale de pinocytose dans la cellule de Kupffer du foie de rat.' *J. Microscopie* **6**, 413

Palay, S. L. (1961). 'Structural peculiarities of the neurosecretory cells in the preoptic nucleus of the goldfish *Carassius auratus*.' *Anat. Rec.* **139**, 262

Parducz, B. (1967). 'Ciliary movement and co-ordination in ciliates.' *Int. Rev. Cytol.* **21**, 91

Patek, P. R. and Bernick, S. (1960). 'Time sequence studies of reticuloendothelial cell responses to foreign particles.' *Anat. Rec.* **138**, 27

Pfeifer, U. (1970). 'Uber endocytose in Kupfferschen sternzellen nach parenchymschadigung durch ¾ teilhepatektomie.' *Virchows Arch. Abt. B. Zellpath.* **6**, 263

Plenderleith, I. H. (1970). 'Hairy cell leukemia.' *Can. med. Assoc. J.* **102**, 1056

Propst, A. and Muller, O. (1966). 'Die Zonen der Nebennierenrinde der Ratte. Elektronenmikroskopische Untersuchung.' *Z. Zellforsch. mikrosk. Anat.* **75**, 404

Purcell, D. A. (1971). 'The ultrastructural changes produced by infectious laryngotracheitis virus in tracheal epithelium of the fowl.' *Res. Vet. Sci.* **2**, 455

Quastler, H. and Hampton, J. C. (1962). 'Effects of ionizing radiation on the fine structure and function of the intestinal epithelium of the mouse. I. Villus epithelium.' *Radiat. Res.* **17**, 914

Randall, J. T. and Hopkins, J. M. (1962). 'On the stalks of certain peritrichs.' *Phil. Trans. R. Soc., B* **245**, 59

Reynolds, E. S. (1963). 'Liver parenchymal cell injury. I. Initial alterations of the cell, following poisoning with carbon tetrachloride.' *J. Cell. Biol.* **19**, 139

Roberts, D. K. and Latta, J. S. (1964). 'Electron microscopic studies on the red pulp of the rabbit spleen.' *Anat. Rec.* **148**, 81

Rodriguez, H. A., Albores-Saavedra, J., Lozano, M. M., Smith, M. and Feder, W. (1971). 'Langerhans' cells in late pinta. Ultrastructural observations in one case.' *Archs Path.* **91**, 302

Rohlich, P. and Toro, I. (1964). 'Uptake of chylomicron particles by reticular cells of mesenterial lymph nodes of the rat.' In *Electron Microscopy*, Vol. B, p. 225, Proc. 3rd Europ. Reg. Conf. Prague 1964. Ed. by M. Titlbach. Prague: Publ. House Czechoslovak. Acad. Sci.

Rossmann, P. and Galle, P. (1968). 'Mise en evidence de cellules renales ciliees chez l'homme.' *Nephron* **5**, 426

Rostgaard, J. and Thuneberg, L. (1972). 'Electron microscopical observations on the brush border of proximal tubule cells of mammalian kidney.' *Z. Zellforsch. mikrosk. Anat.* **132**, 473

Roth, S. I. (1970). 'The ultrastructure of primary water-clear cell hyperplasia of the parathyroid glands.' *Am. J. Path.* **61**, 233

Sagebiel, R. W. and Reed, T. H. (1968). 'Serial reconstruction of the characteristic granule of the Langerhans cell.' *J. Cell Biol.* **36**, 595

Salazar, H. (1963). 'The pars distalis of the female rabbit hypophysis. An electron microscope study.' *Anat. Rec.* **147**, 469

Scherft, J. P. and Daems, W. Th. (1967). 'Single cilia in chondrocytes.' *J. Ultrastruct. Res.* **19**, 546

Schneeberger-Keeley, E. E. and Burger, E. J. (1970). 'Intravascular macrophages in cat lungs after open chest ventilation.' *Lab. Invest.* **22**, 361

Schnitzer, B. and Kass, L. (1973). 'Leukemic phase of reticulum cell sarcoma (histiocytic lymphoma).' *Cancer* **31**, 547

Schoffeniels, E. (1969a). 'Uptake mechanism of the cell, active transport.' In *Handbook of Molecular Cytology*, p. 1320. Ed. by A. Lima-de-Faria. Amsterdam and London: North Holland Publ.

— (1969b). 'Cellular aspects of membrane permeability.' In *Handbook of Molecular Cytology*, p. 1346. Ed. by A. Lima-de-Faria. Amsterdam and London: North-Holland Publ.

Schrek, R. and Donnelly, W. J. (1966). '"Hairy" cells in blood in lymphoreticular neoplastic disease and "flagellated" cells of normal lymph nodes.' *Blood* **27**, 199

Schroeder, H. E. and Theilade, J. (1966). 'Electron microscopy of normal human gingival epithelium.' *J. periodont. Res.* **1**, 95

Schuster, F. L. (1964). 'Ciliated fibroblasts from a human brain tumor.' *Anat. Rec.* **150**, 417

Shamoto, M., Kaplan, C. and Katoh, A. K. (1971). 'Langerhans cell granules in human hyperplastic lymph nodes.' *Archs Path.* **92**, 46

Simpson, M. E. (1922). 'The experimental production of macrophages in the circulating blood.' *J. med. Res.* **43**, 77

Simpson, C. F. and Kling, J. M. (1967). 'The mechanism of denucleation in circulating erythroblasts.' *J. Cell Biol.* **35**, 237

Sjostrand, F. S. (1953). 'The ultrastructure of the inner segments of the retinal rods of the guinea pig eye as revealed by electron microscopy.' *J. cell. comp. Physiol.* **42**, 45

Skinnider, L. F. and Ghadially, F. N. (1973). 'An ultrastructural study of ropalocytosis in human blood and bone marrow.' *J. Path.* **109**, 1

Sorokin, S. (1962). 'Centrioles and the formation of rudimentary cilia by fibroblasts and smooth muscle cells.' *J. Cell Biol.* **15**, 363

— (1968). 'Reconstructions of centriole formation and ciliogenesis in mammalian lungs.' *J. Cell Sci.* **3**, 207

Sotelo, J. R. and Trujillo-Cenozo (1958). 'Electron microscope study on the development of ciliary components of the neural epithelium of the chick embryo.' *Z. Zellforsch. mikrosk. Anat.* **49**, 1

Steiner, J. W. (1961). 'Investigations of allergic liver injury. I. Light, fluorescent and electron microscopic study of the effects of soluble immune aggregates.' *Am. J. Path.* **38**, 411

— and Carruthers, J. S. (1963). 'Electron microscopy of hyperplastic ductular cells in α-naphthyl isothiocyanate-induced cirrhosis.' *Lab. Invest.* **12**, 471

— — and Kalifat, S. R. (1962). 'The ductular cell reaction of rat liver in extrahepatic cholestasis. I. Proliferated biliary epithelial cells.' *Expl Molec. Path.* **1**, 162

Stockem, W. and Wohlfarth-Bottermann, K. E. (1969). 'Pinocytosis (endocytosis).' In *Handbook of Molecular Cytology*, p. 1373. Ed. by A. Lima-de-Faria. Amsterdam and London: North Holland Publ.

Stoeckel, M. E. and Porte, A. (1966). 'Observations ultrastructurales sur la parathyroide de souris. I. Etude chez la souris normale.' *Z. Zellforsch. mikrosk. Anat.* **73**, 488

Straub, M. and Mulder, J. (1948). 'Epithelial lesions and respiratory tract in human influenzal pneumonia.' *J. Path. Bact.* **60**, 429

Stubblefield, E. and Brinkley, B. R. (1966). 'Cilia formation in Chinese hamster fibroblasts *in vitro* as a response to colcemid treatment.' *J. Cell. Biol.* **30**, 645

—— (1967). 'Architecture and function of the mammalian centriole.' In *Formation and Fate of Cell Organelles,* Vol. 6, p. 175. Ed. by K. B. Warren. New York and London: Academic Press

Svoboda, D., Nielson, A., Werder, A. and Higginson, J. (1962). 'An electron microscopic study of viral hepatitis in mice.' *Am. J. Path.* **41**, 205

Tachi, S., Tachi, C. and Linder, H. R. (1969). 'Cilia-bearing stromal cells in the rat uterus.' *J. Anat.* **104**, 295

Tannenbaum, M. (1971). 'Ultrastructural pathology of human renal cell tumors'. *Path. A.* **6**, 249

Tarnowski, W. M. and Hashimoto, K. (1967). 'Langerhans' cell granules in histiocytosis X: the epidermal Langerhans' cell as a macrophage.' *Arch. Derm.* **96**, 298

Taxi, J. (1961). 'Sur l'existence de neurons cilies dans les ganglions sympathiques de certains vertèbres.' *C.r. Soc. Biol.* **155**, 1860

Tisher, C. C., Bulger, R. E. and Trump, B. F. (1966). 'Human renal ultrastructure. 1. Proximal tubule of the healthy individuals.' *Lab. Invest.* **15**, 1357

Tokuyasu, K. and Yamada, E. (1959). 'The fine structure of the retina studied with the electron microscope. IV. Morphogenesis of outer segments of retinal rods.' *J. biophys. biochem. Cytol.* **6**, 225

Tonna, E. A. and Lampen, N. M. (1972). 'Electron microscopy of aging skeletal cells. I. Centrioles and solitary cilia.' *J. Geront.* **27**, 316

Toro, I., Ruzsa, P. and Rohlich, P. (1962). 'Ultrastructure of early phagocytic stages in sinus endothelial and Kupffer cells of the liver.' *Expl Cell Res.* **26**, 601

Trier, J. S. (1967). 'Structure of the mucosa of the small intestine as it relates to intestinal function.' *Fedn Proc.* **26**, 1391

—— and Browning, T. H. (1965). 'Morphologic response of human small intestine to x-ray exposure.' *Clin. Res.* **13**, 263

—— and Rubin, C. E. (1965). 'Electron microscopy of the small intestine: a review.' *Gastroenterology* **49**, 574

Turiaf, J. and Basset, F. (1965). 'Histiocytose "X" pulmonaire: identification de particules de nature probablement virale dans un fragment pulmonaire preleve pour biopsie.' *Bull. Acad. natn. Méd.* **149**, 674

Wersall, J. (1956). 'Studies on the structure and innervation of the sensory epithelium of the cristae ampullares in the guinea pig. A light and electron microscopic investigation.' *Acta oto-lar.* Suppl. 126, 1.

Wheatley, D. N. (1967). 'Cells with two cilia in the rat adenohypophysis.' *J. Anat.* **101**, 479

—— (1969). 'Cilia in cell-cultured fibroblasts. I. On their occurrence and relative frequencies in primary cultures and established cell lines.' *J. Anat.* **105**, 351

Wilhelm, D. L. (1954). 'Regeneration of the tracheal epithelium in the vitamin A deficient rat.' *J. Path. Bact.* **67**, 361

Wilson, R. B. and McWhorther, C. A. (1963). 'Isolated flagella in human skin electron microscopic observations.' *Lab. Invest.* **12**, 242

Wisse, E. and Daems, W. Th. (1970a). 'Differences between endothelial and Kupffer cells in rat liver.' In *Microscopie Electronique,* Res. 7e Congr. Intern. Grenoble 1970. Vol. III, p. 57. Ed. by O. Favard. Paris: Societe Francaise de Microscopie Electronique

—— (1970b). 'Fine structural study on the sinusoidal lining cells of rat liver.' In *Mononuclear Phagocytes*, p. 200. Ed. by R. van Furth. Oxford: Blackwell Scientific

Wolff, K. (1967). 'The fine structure of the Langerhans cell granule.' *J. Cell. Biol.* **35**, 468

Wong, Y. C. and Buck, R. C. (1971). 'An electronmicroscopic study of metaplasia of the rat tracheal epithelium in vitamin A deficiency.' *Lab. Invest.* **24**, 55

Wyllie, J. C., More, R. H. and Haust, M. D. (1964). 'The fine structure of normal guinea pig synovium.' *Lab. Invest.* **13**, 1254

Yam, L. T., Castoldi, G. L., Garvey, M. B. and Mitus, W. J. (1968). 'Functional cytogenetic and cytochemical study of the leukemic reticulum cells.' *Blood* **32**, 90

—— Li, C. Y. and Lam, K. W. (1971). 'Tartrate-resistant acid phosphatase isoenzyme in the reticulum cells of leukemic reticuloendotheliosis.' *New Engl. J. Med.* **284**, 357

Yamada, E. (1955). 'The fine structure of the gall bladder epithelium of the mouse.' *J. biophys. biochem. Cytol.* **1**, 445

Yardley, J. H., Bayless, T. M., Norton, J. H. and Hendrix, T. (1962). Celiac disease: a study of the jejunal epithelium before and after a gluten-free diet.' *New Engl. J. Med.* **267**, 1173

Zeigel, R. F. (1962). 'On the occurrence of cilia in several cell types of the chick pancreas.' *J. Ultrastruct. Res.* **7**, 286

Ziegler, B. (1963). 'Licht- und Elektronenmikroskopische Untersuchungen an pars Intermedia und Neurohypophyse der Ratte. Zur Frage der Beziehungen Zwischen Pars Intermedia und Hinterlappen der Hypophys.' *Z. Zellforsch. mikrosk. Anat.* **59**, 486

Zimmermann, K. W. (1898). 'Beitrage zur kenntniss einiger Drusen und Epithelien.' *Arch mikrosk. Anat. EntwMech.* **52**, 552

Zimmermann, H. D. (1971). 'Cilien in der fetalen Nlere des Menschen.' *Beitr. path. Anat.* **143**, 227

Index*

* References to illustrations are italicized. For convenience the page number on which the plate appears is given rather than the plate number itself.

INDEX

540